Kostoris Library Christie
R02967L4988

KV-211-911

ANTICANCER DRUG TOXICITY

ANTICANCER DRUG TOXICITY

Prevention, Management, and Clinical Pharmacokinetics

edited by

Hans-Peter Lipp

Eberhard-Karls University
Tübingen, Germany

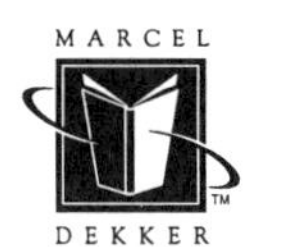

MARCEL DEKKER, INC.   NEW YORK • BASEL

ISBN: 0-8247-1930-1

This book is printed on acid-free paper.

Headquarters
Marcel Dekker, Inc.
270 Madison Avenue, New York, NY 10016
tel: 212-696-9000; fax: 212-685-4540

Eastern Hemisphere Distribution
Marcel Dekker AG
Hutgasse 4, Postfach 812, CH-4001 Basel, Switzerland
tel: 41-61-261-8482; fax: 41-61-261-8896

World Wide Web
http://www.dekker.com

The publisher offers discounts on this book when ordered in bulk quantities. For more information, write to Special Sales/Professional Marketing at the headquarters address above.

Current printing (last digit):
10 9 8 7 6 5 4 3 2 1

PRINTED IN THE UNITED STATES OF AMERICA

Preface

Within the past few years many significant developments have taken place in clinical oncology, such as the introduction of new drugs (e.g., the topoisomerase-I inhibitors and the taxanes) and new therapeutic strategies for supportive care.

Undoubtedly, our limited knowledge about the optimal dosing of anticancer drugs is still a great cause for debate. Because of the narrow therapeutic index of cytostatics, one has to be very careful to avoid producing severe toxicity by overdosing or impaired efficacy by underdosing. However, up to now the dosage of almost all anticancer drugs has been related to the patients' body surface area, and this method has been associated with unacceptably high variability in pharmacokinetics. As a consequence, it is important to establish more thorough and extensive therapeutic drug monitoring in clinical oncology practice.

In my first book, *Prevention and Management of Anticancer Drugs—The Significance of Clinical Pharmacokinetics*, published by the Universitaetsverlag Jena in 1995, I pointed out several interesting pharmacokinetic–toxicodynamic relationships in cytostatics and illustrated them with many tables and figures. When Marcel Dekker, Inc., prompted me to edit a more comprehensive, multiauthored work, I selected several renowned experts who deal with the clinical pharmacology of anticancer drugs as well as with supportive therapy.

This book summarizes the most important facts concerning clinical pharmacokinetics and toxicity of anticancer drugs and describes correlations between specific metabolic pathways and the development of toxic symptoms. Some aspects are much more extensively reviewed such as the hepatotoxicity of asparaginase preparations, the pharmacogenetics of 6-mercaptopurine, and the problems associated with extravasation or late side effects induced by cytostatics. Within the different chapters many management tips regarding dose calculation or supportive therapy are presented to simplify everyday clinical practice.

I am deeply grateful to the authors of this volume for their contributions in the various areas of anticancer drug toxicity. My special appreciation goes to Graham Garratt, Elyce Misher, and the staff at Marcel Dekker, Inc., for their roles in coordinating production of the book and their helpful discussions and stimulation.

I hope that many clinicians, pharmacists, and scientists working in clinical oncology can use the illustrated information presented in this book as an effective tool in their everyday clinical practice.

Hans-Peter Lipp

Contents

Preface *iii*
Contributors *vii*

PART I INTRODUCTION AND CLINICAL PHARMACOKINETICS

1 Introduction 3
Hans-Peter Lipp

2 Clinical Pharmacokinetics of Cytostatic Drugs: Efficacy and Toxicity 11
Hans-Peter Lipp and Carsten Bokemeyer

PART II TOXICITY OF CYTOSTATICS IN RAPIDLY PROLIFERATING NORMAL CELLS

3 Prophylaxis and Treatment of Neutropenia with Hematopoietic Growth Factors 205
Hartmut Link

4 Oral and Gastrointestinal Toxicity 235
Carsten Bokemeyer and J.T. Hartmann

5 Dermatological Toxicity and Hypersensitivity Reactions Associated with the Use of Cytostatics 263
Hans-Peter Lipp

PART III EXTRAVASATION AND PARAVASATION

6 Managing Extravasations of Vesicant Chemotherapy Drugs 279
Robert T. Dorr

PART IV ORGAN TOXICITY INDUCED BY CYTOSTATIC AGENTS

7 Nephrotoxicity and Urotoxicity of Chemotherapeutic Agents 321
Roderick Skinner

8 Hepatotoxicity Induced by Cytostatic Drugs 347
Hans-Peter Lipp, Joachim Boos, Eugen J. Verspohl, Eugene Y. Krynetski, and William E. Evans

9 Neurotoxicity (Including Sensory Toxicity) Induced by Cytostatics 431
Hans-Peter Lipp

10 Pulmonary Toxicity of Chemotherapeutic Agents 455
Jost Niedermeyer, H. Fabel, Carsten Bokemeyer, and Hans-Peter Lipp

11 Cardiotoxicity of Cytotoxic Drugs 471
Hans-Peter Lipp

PART V LATE SIDE EFFECTS OF CANCER CHEMOTHERAPY

12 Gonadal Toxicity and Teratogenicity After Cytotoxic Chemotherapy 491
Elizabeth B. Lamont and Robert L. Schilsky

13 Secondary Malignancies 525
Carsten Bokemeyer and Christian Kollmannsberger

Index *549*

Contributors

Carsten Bokemeyer, M.D. Department of Internal Medicine II (Hematology-Oncology), University of Tübingen Medical Center, Tübingen, Germany

Joachim Boos, M.D. Department of Pediatric Hematology and Oncology, University of Münster, Münster, Germany

Robert T. Dorr, M.D. Department of Pharmacology, College of Medicine, Pharmacology Research Program, Arizona Cancer Center, The University of Arizona, Tucson, Arizona

William E. Evans, Pharm.D. St. Jude Children's Research Hospital, Memphis, Tennessee

H. Fabel, M.D. Department of Respiratory Medicine, Medizinische Hochschule Hannover, Hannover, Germany

J.T. Hartmann, M.D. Department of Hematology/Oncology/Immunology/Rheumatology, Eberhard-Karls University, Tübingen, Germany

Christian Kollmannsberger, M.D. Department of Internal Medicine II (Hematology-Oncology), University of Tübingen Medical Center, Tübingen, Germany

Eugene Y. Krynetski, M.D. St. Jude Children's Research Hospital, Memphis, Tennessee

Elizabeth B. Lamont, M.D. Department of Hematology/Oncology, University of Chicago Pritzker School of Medicine, Chicago, Illinois

Hartmut Link, M.D., Ph.D. Department of Internal Medicine I, Westpfalz-Klinikum Kaiserslautern, Kaiserslautern, Germany

Hans-Peter Lipp, M.D. Department of Clinical Pharmacy, University of Tübingen, Tübingen, Germany

Jost Niedermeyer, M.D. Department of Respiratory Medicine, Medizinische Hochschule Hannover, Hannover, Germany

Robert L. Schilsky, M.D. Cancer Research Center, University of Chicago Pritzker School of Medicine, Chicago, Illinois

Roderick Skinner, Ph.D., M.R.C.P., B.Sc., M.B.Ch.B., DLH, FRCPCH Sir James Spence Institute of Child Health, University of Newcastle upon Tyne, Newcastle upon Tyne, England

Eugen J. Verspohl, Ph.D. Department of Pharmacology, Institute of Pharmaceutical Chemistry, University of Münster, Münster, Germany

I

INTRODUCTION AND CLINICAL PHARMACOKINETICS

1

Introduction

HANS-PETER LIPP
University of Tübingen, Germany

With the exception of methotrexate, most anticancer drugs were not until recently measured routinely in plasma regarding therapeutic drug monitoring (TDM) in clinical oncology [1–3].

However, particularly within the last 10 years, data have accumulated indicating that the measurement of drug concentrations in plasma or tissues seems to be very important for many reasons in clinical oncology [1]. Undoubtedly the routine procedure of dosing anticancer drugs according to patient's body surface area results in a 10- to 100-fold range of individual pharmacokinetics [4–14]. The underlying reasons are complex. Differences in elimination capacity particularly in regard to the glomerular filtration rate (GFR), the hepatic expression of cytochrome P450 isozymes, or biliary function, are important determinants for high pharmacokinetic variability among cancer patients [15–21].

Often the serum creatinine level is estimated to be a good predictor of renal function. However, despite normal serum creatinine values [0.6–1.2 mg/dl] the underlying GFR values may range from 30 to 180 mL/min and, thus, the pharmacokinetics of drugs such as methotrexate, bleomycin, or carboplatin may be interindividually highly variable [15]. As a consequence, without TDM management, patients with extraordinarily high or low anticancer drug plasma levels cannot be identified.

Particularly in the case of conventional carboplatin therapy it has been impressively demonstrated within the last few years that individualization of anticancer drug therapy is obviously warranted. Only patients within a defined therapeutic AUC (*area under the time vs. concentration curve*) range have a higher probability for partial or complete remission as well as for tolerable side effects. The establishment of simple formulas with which the absolute dose can be calculated to achieve a defined target AUC value based on the underlying creatinine clearance made progress with the individualization of carboplatin therapy. Though this example represents a very encouraging start of pharmacokinetically guided anticancer drug therapy, most other antineoplastic agents lag far behind for several reasons [22].

Whereas unchanged carboplatin elimination is closely correlated with the underlying creatinine clearance, many other drugs are excreted changed and unchanged via urine and feces [23]. Thus, for an accurate estimation of their pharmacokinetics, one has to consider GFR, constitutive cytochrome P450 activity, serum bilirubin, and sometimes (if the drug is extensively protein bound), the amount of serum albumin. As a consequence, formulas of AUC calculation are far more complex, as in the case of etoposide or docetaxel. However, efforts in this area seem to be well on the way to optimize anticancer drug therapy.

Additionally, the use of TDM can help to identify and understand important pharmacokinetic drug interactions between cytostatics and other drugs [24]. Enzyme inducers of cytochrome P450 3A4, such as phenytoin, carbamazepine, or rifampicin, may increase the clearance of cytostatics (e.g., that of vinca alkaloids, podophyllotoxin derivatives, or taxoids), whereas cytochrome P450 3A4 inhibitors, particularly itraconazole, may impair the metabolic clearance of these drugs. Definitive knowledge about these interactions seems to be very important to establish dosage recommendations. For example, since it has been demonstrated that phenytoin accelerates the metabolic clearance of busulfan, diazepam rather than phenytoin has been recommended as the anticonvulsant of first choice during high-dose therapy [25]. TDM may also be helpful to identify patients with pharmacogenetic deficiencies, particularly in regard to the metabolism of oxazaphosphorines, 6-mercaptopurine, and azathioprine as well as 5-fluorouracil [20].

Several studies indicate that TDM may help to predict the clinical efficacy of anticancer drug therapy [10,22]. One must be careful with extrapolation of results, however, because plasma levels do not reflect the extent of transmembrane drug uptake, intracellular anticancer drug pharmacokinetics, and overall blood perfusion of the tumor tissue [26]. In conclusion, TDM primarily helps to define the minimal therapeutic plasma concentrations that should be achieved to ensure clinical efficacy.

Some exciting data presented very recently indicate that the measurement of intracellular drug concentrations in the tumor cells of cancer patients is manageable. In the case of 5-fluorouracil (5-FU) noninvasive ^{19}F nuclear magnetic resonance spectroscopy allows the detection of 5-FU and its metabolites in tumor tissue. As a consequence, patients who will not respond to repeated 5-FU therapy because they cannot trap the drug within their tumor may be identified in time to try alternative therapies [27].

In the case of cytarabine (Ara-C), it has been demonstrated that the active intracellular metabolite, cytarabine triphosphate (Ara-CTP), can be subjected to quantitative analysis when leukemic cells are isolated after Ara-C infusion. Interestingly, these pharmacokinetic studies indicate that in some patients no correlation between Ara-C dose and intracellular Ara-CTP concentration can be detected, perhaps as a result of a transmembranaceous saturation mechanism. As a consequence, these patients may develop the same Ara-CTP levels in their malignant cells irrespective of whether they receive conventional or high-dose therapy. The possibility that these patients may gain higher probability of remission by high-dose Ara-C cannot be excluded, but they may suffer from increased overall systemic toxicity [28].

The criticism that the management of TDM is associated with high costs for the establishment of specialized techniques and staff is undoubtedly warranted. To enforce TDM in clinical oncology, however, the costs related to TDM management are to be compared with the therapeutic benefits. Recently it has been postulated that at the time of reinfusion of bone marrow or peripheral blood stem cells the persisting concentrations of cyctostatics (e.g., etoposide, TEPA) may be still high enough to impair a successful graft [29,30]. If these preliminary results are confirmed by further studies, individual TDM during high-dose chemotherapy will be an unquestionably far-sighted and cost-effective measure.

Much progress has been made in regard to the simplification of TDM in clinical practice. In several cases, such as the administration of etoposide, carboplatin, and busulfan, only one to three blood samples suffice for total AUC extrapolation [31–33]. Additionally, analytical methods of processing and sensitivity have been improved [34–36].

However, some problems remain unresolved: in the case of the nitrosoureas or oxazaphosphorines, the active metabolites rather than the parent compounds are responsible for efficacy as well as toxicity [23]. For these drugs, the quantification of the parent compound may not be very helpful. For example, it has to be questioned whether the carmustine AUC is really useful for the prediction of pulmonary toxicity, since the isocyanates rather than the parent compound have been shown to play an important role in the development of nitrosourea-induced lung toxicity [23,37].

In conclusion, if several reactive metabolic intermediates are formed which may be important for the prediction of efficacy as well as toxicity, further interpretation will be enhanced if the total metabolic profile is measured, rather than the parent compound. Indeed, the blood level of the very reactive intermediate 4-hydroxycyclophosphamide, rather than cyclophosphamide, appears to be a predictor for the risk of cardiotoxicity [38]. These intermediates cannot be easily quantified, however, because of their high reactivity and short half-lives. Often difficult derivatization techniques have to be developed to overcome rapid degradation processes. The extension of knowledge about the qualitative and quantitative roles of different metabolites in clinical efficacy and toxicity as well as the underlying stability of the parent compounds and the corresponding intermediates is a great challenge for scientists dealing with TDM [39,40]. The following important reasons prove the importance of extended TDM in clinical oncology.

1. Based on several studies, extended TDM can avoid extraordinarily high peak and trough levels or AUC values and thus improve the tolerability of conventional anticancer drug therapy. As a consequence, the probability of severe myelosuppression can be decreased by TDM management, which may result in hospital stays of shorter duration and less expensive supportive care (e.g., use of cytokines or blood products). Very probably prospective randomized trials confirming the advantage of individualized carboplatin therapy will be available in the near future [5,10,22].

2. If a correlation between plasma concentrations or AUC values and therapeutic efficacy of a certain drug exists, it seems very reasonable to avoid rapid progression of disease by achieving a defined therapeutic range. In the case of carboplatin or methotrexate, minimum AUC values or steady-state concentrations, respectively, have been defined. A patient who does not achieve these defined levels must be considered underdosed [5,10,22].

3. Concerning the transplantation of bone marrow (BMT) or peripheral blood stem cells, cytotoxic drug concentrations may persist in some patients for a longer period of time after high-dose chemotherapy. If this happens, these higher drug levels at the time of reinfusion of stem cells, may severely impair engraftment and hematopoietic recovery. If preliminary results are confirmed by further trials, TDM will help in the timely identification of such individuals [29,30].

4. Finally, the use of TDM not only helps to clarify special pharmacokinetic questions (e.g., distribution into intraperitoneal or intrapleural fluids), but also helps to identify pharmacogenetically based deficiencies and important pharmacokinetic drug interactions between cytostatics and other drugs [41,42]. Additionally, more knowledge about the pharmacokinetic characteristics of antineoplastic agents increases the reliability of the concrete dosing guidelines that are established for patients with impaired renal or hepatic function or with concomitant drug therapy [21,43].

REFERENCES

1. Obrecht JP, Obrist R. 50 years of cytostatic chemotherapy. Onkologie 1993: 16:142–146.

2. El-Yazigi A, Ezzat A. Pharmacokinetic monitoring of anticancer drugs at King Faisal Specialist Hospital, Riyadh, Saudi Arabia. Ther Drug Monit 1997:19: 390–393.
3. Stoller RG, Hande KR, Jacobs SA, et al. Use of plasma pharmacokinetics to predict and prevent methotrexate toxicity. N Engl J Med 1977:297:630–634.
4. Desoize B, Robert J. Individual dose adaptation of anticancer drugs. Eur J Cancer 1994:30A:844–851.
5. Freyer G, Ligneau B, Tranchard B, et al. Pharmacokinetic studies in cancer chemotherapy: Usefulness in clinical practice. Cancer Treatment Rev 1997:23: 153–169.
6. Sasaki Y. Pharmacological considerations in high-dose chemotherapy. Cancer Chemother Pharmacol 1997:40(suppl):S115–S118.
7. Kobayashi K, Ratain MJ. Individualizing dosing of cancer chemotherapy. Semin Oncol 1993:20:30–42.
8. Grochow LB, Baraldi C, Noe D. Is dose normalisation to weight or body surface area useful in adults? J Natl Cancer Inst 1990:82:323–324.
9. Workman P, Graham MA. Pharmacokinetics and cancer chemotherapy. Eur J Cancer 1994:30A:706–710.
10. Evans WE, Relling MV. Clinical pharmacokinetics-pharmacodynamics of anticancer drugs. Clin Pharmacokinet 1989:16:327–336.
11. Knoester PD, Underberg WJM, Beijnen JH. Clinical pharmacokinetics and pharmocodynamics of anticancer agents in pediatric patients. Anticancer Res 1993:13:1795–1808.
12. Workman P, Graham MA. Pharmacokinetics and cancer chemotherapy. Eur J Cancer 1994:30A:706–710.
13. Perry MC. Chemotherapy, toxicity and the clinician. Semin Oncol 1982:9: 1–4.
14. Reilly JJ, Workman P. Normalisation of anticancer drug dosage using body surface area: Is it worthwhile? A review of theoretical and practical considerations. Cancer Chemother Pharmacol 1993:32:411–418.
15. Reyno LM, Egorin J, Canetta RM, Jodree DJ, et al. Impact of cyclophosphamide on relationships between carboplatin exposure and response or toxicity when used in the treatment of advanced ovarian cancer. J Clin Oncol 1993:11: 1156–1164.
16. Kintzel PE, Dorr RT. Anticancer drug renal toxicity and elimination: Dosing guidelines for altered renal function. Cancer Treatment Rev 1995:21:33–64.
17. Kivistö KT, Kroemer HK, Eichelbaum M. The role of human cytochrome P450 enzymes in the metabolism of anticancer agents: Implications for drug interactions. Br J Clin Pharmacol 1995:40:523–530.
18. Spatzenegger M, Jaeger W. Clinical importance of hepatic cytochrome P450 in drug metabolism. Drug Metab Rev 1995:27(3):397–417.
19. Transon C, Lecoeur S, Leemann T, et al. Interindividual variability in catalytic activity and immunoreactivity of three major human liver cytochrome P450 isoenzymes. Eur J Clin Pharmacol 1996:51:79–85.
20. Chabot GG. Factors involved in clinical pharmacology variability in oncology. Anticancer Res 1994:14:2269–2272.

21. Koren G, Beatty K, Seto A, Einarson TR, Lishner M. The effects of impaired liver function on the elimination of antineoplastic agents. Ann Pharmacother 1992:26:363–371.
22. Bokemeyer C, Lipp H-P. Is there a need for pharmacokinetically guided carboplatin dose schedule? Onkologie 1997:20:343–345.
23. Lipp H-P. Prevention and management of anticancer drug toxicity—The significance of clinical pharmacokinetics. University of Jena, 1995.
24. Le Blanc GA, Waxman DJ. Interaction of anticancer drugs with hepatic monooxygenase enzymes. Drug Metab Rev 1989:20(2–4):395–439.
25. Fitzsimmons WE, Ghalie R, Kaizer H. The effect of hepatic enzyme inducers on busulfan neurotoxicity and myelotoxicity. Cancer Chemother Pharmacol 1990:37:226–228.
26. Ratain MJ, Schilsky RL, Conley BA, Egorin MJ. Pharmacodynamics in cancer therapy. J Clin Oncol 1990:8:1739–1753.
27. Presant CA, Wolf W, Albright MJ, et al. Human tumor fluorouracil trapping: Clinical correlations of in vivo ^{19}F-nuclear magnetic resonance spectroscopy pharmacokinetics. J Clin Oncol 1990:8:1868–1873.
28. Rustum YM, Riva C, Preisler HD. Pharmacokinetic parameters of 1-β-D-arabinofuranosylcytosine (Ara-C) and their relationship to intracellular metabolism of Ara-C, toxicity and response of patients with acute nonlymphocytic leukemia treated with conventional and high-dose Ara-C. Semin Oncol 1987: 14(suppl 1):141–148.
29. Rodman JH, Murry DJ, Madden T, Santana VM. Altered etoposide pharmacokinetics and time to engraftment in pediatric patients undergoing autologous bone marrow transplantation. J Clin Oncol 1994:12:2390–2397.
30. Przepiorka D, Madden T, Ippoliti C, et al. Dosing of ThioTEPA for myeloablative therapy. Cancer Chemother Pharmacol 1995:37:155–160.
31. Strömgren AS, Sorensen BT, Jakobsen P, Jakobsen A. A limited sampling method for estimation of the etoposide area under the curve. Cancer Chemother Pharmacol 1993:32:226–230.
32. Ghazal-Aswad S, Calvert AH, Newell DR. A single-sample assay for the estimation of the area under the free carboplatin plasma concentration versus time curve. Cancer Chemother Pharmacol 1996:37:429–434.
33. Hassan M, Fasth A, Gerritsen B, et al. Busulphan kinetics and limited sampling model in children with leukemia and inherited disorders. Bone Marrow Transplant 1996:18:843–850.
34. El-Yazigi A, Martin CR. Improved assay for etoposide in plasma by radial compression liquid chromatography with electrochemical detection. Clin Chem 1987:33:803–805.
35. El-Yazigi A, Martin CR. Rapid determination of methotrexate and 7-OH methotrexate in serum and cerebrospinal fluid by radical compression liquid chromatography. J Liq Chromatogr 1984:7:1579–1591.
36. Rifai N, Sakamoto M, Lafi M, Guinan E. Measurement of plasma busulfan concentration by high-performance liquid chromatography with ultraviolet detection. Ther Drug Monit 1997:19:169–174.

37. Jones RB, Matthes S, Shpall EJ, et al. Acute lung injury following treatment with high-dose cyclophosphamide, cisplatin and carmustine: Pharmacodynamic evaluation of carmustine. J Natl Cancer Inst 1993:85:640–647.
38. Slattery JT, Kalhorn TF, McDonald GB, et al. Conditioning regimen-dependent disposition of cyclophosphamide and hydroxycylophosphamide in human marrow transplantation patients. J Clin Oncol 1996:14:1484–1494.
39. Williams DA, Lokich J. A review of the stability and compatibility of antineoplastic drugs for multiple-drug infusions. Cancer Chemother Pharmacol 1992:31:171–181.
40. Trissel LA. Handbook on injectable drugs, 8th ed. American Society of Hospital Pharmacists, Bethesda, Maryland, 1994, pp 149–269.
41. Sauer HJ, Füger K, Blumenstein M. Modulation of cytotoxicity of cytostatic drugs by hemodialysis in vitro and in vivo. Cancer Treatment Rev 1990:17: 293–300.
42. Lee C, Marbury TC. Drug therapy in patients undergoing hemodialysis. Clinical pharmacokinetic considerations. Clin Pharmacokinet 1984:9:42–61.
43. van der Wall E, Beijnen JH, Rodenhuis S. High-dose chemotherapy regimens for solid tumors. Cancer Treatment Rev 1995:21:105–132.

2

Clinical Pharmacokinetics of Cytostatic Drugs: Efficacy and Toxicity

HANS-PETER LIPP
University of Tübingen, Tübingen, Germany
CARSTEN BOKEMEYER
University of Tübingen Medical Center, Tübingen, Germany

2.1 ALKYLATING AGENTS

2.1.1 N-Lost-Derivatives, Alkane Sulfonates, and Aziridines

The alkylating agents (Table 1) belong to the first type of clinically used anticancer drugs. Because of their steep dose–response curve, they have recently been the basis for many high dose chemotherapies [1–3].

Related to the chemical warfare agent sulfur mustard gas, the corresponding lead compound, nitrogen mustard (Fig. 1) exerts considerable antineoplastic efficacy but also possesses many severe side effects, particularly hematological toxicity as well as gonadal dysfunction [4,5].

Other alkylating agents, like melphalan, chlorambucil, and bendamustine (Fig. 1), were developed to increase antitumor selectivity [1–3]. Because of their very reactive nature, however, more comprehensive studies regarding their exact metabolism and pharmacokinetics are still warranted [6]. Because of their high reactivity toward DNA and the corresponding mutagenicity that is observed, alkylating agents have been classified as substantial carcinogens for human beings [7,8].

Table 1 Clinically Used Alkylating Agents: An Overview

N-Lost derivatives
Mechlorethamine
Chlorambucil
Melphalan
Bendamustine (Cytostasane)
Alkane sulfonates and related compounds
Busulfan
Treosulfan
Aziridines
Thiotepa
Oxazaphosphorines
Cyclophosphamide
Ifosfamide
Trofosfamide
Other types of alkylating agent
Procarbazine
Dacarbazine
Mitomycin C
Hexamethylmelamine
Nitrosoureas
Carmustine (BCNU)
Lomustine (CCNU)
Nimustine (ACNU)
Streptozocin
Fotemustine

Busulfan and treosulfan (= dihydroxybusulfan) represent alkane sulfonates (Fig. 1). Whereas the former exerts direct alkylating activity, treosulfan is a prodrug which is converted nonenzymatically under physiological conditions into the corresponding mono- and diepoxide (diepoxybutane) [2].

Thiotepa (Fig. 1) belongs to the aziridines. It is of clinical importance that its metabolites, particularly TEPA, (N,N′N″-triethylenephosphoramide) exert considerable antineoplastic activity [2]. Because of its ability to produce cerebrospinal fluid levels nearly identical to those achievable in plasma, this agent has been suggested as an interesting tool for the treatment of malignant brain tumors. However, its low therapeutic index even at conventional doses is disadvantageous [9].

2.1.1.1 N-Lost Derivatives

Mechlorethamine

Mechlorethamine (nitrogen mustard, N-lost) was one of the very first alkylating agents used in clinical oncology. Within the MOPP protocol developed for Hodgkin's disease it is still used in the USA in combination with vincristine, procarbazine, and prednisone in the protocol called MOPP [2,4,5].

In aqueous solutions mechlorethamine is rapidly converted to the ethylene immonium ion, which is considered to be able to alkylate nucleophilic molecule sites. The cytotoxic effect is particularly based on the covalent binding to the N-7 position of guanine, which results in inter- and intrastrand cross-links [2]. The bifunctional alkylating agent undergoes rapid chemical transformation. Thus, unchanged mechlorethamine is undetectable in the blood within minutes after intravenous administration. Less than 0.01% of an IV dose is excreted unchanged in the urine [10].

Chlorambucil

Chlorambucil is used in the treatment of chronic lymphatic leukemia, in low grade non-Hodgkin's lymphoma, in Waldenströms macroglobulinemia, and less frequently in advanced ovarian or breast cancer [1–3].

The toxicity pattern of chlorambucil includes myelosuppression, mild nausea and emesis (incidence <10%), a transient increase of liver enzymes, alopecia, infertility, cumulative pulmonary toxicity, and neurotoxic side-effects.

Chlorambucil is usually given orally (e.g., 0.1–0.2 mg/kg/d on days 1–14, or 0.4 mg/kg every 2 weeks). The parent compound seems to be rapidly and completely absorbed from the gastrointestinal tract. After a single oral dose of 0.6 mg/kg, a plasma concentration ranging from 2 to 6 μM was reached within 1 hour. There is some evidence that concomitant food intake may lead to an overall reduction in the maximum clearance and the area under the curve (AUC) values, and to a lengthening of the time to the c_{max} [11–13].

In plasma the bifunctional alkylating agent is highly bound (nearly 99%) to serum proteins, mainly albumin. The major metabolite, phenylacetic acid mustard, which still exerts considerable antiproliferative activity, is primarily formed by β-oxidation of the butyric acid side chain (Fig. 2). The half-life of chlorambucil and its major metabolite have been estimated to average 92 minutes and 2.5 hours, respectively.

Chlorambucil and its major metabolite hydrolyze spontaneously in plasma, resulting in the formation of inactive monohydroxy and dihydroxy derivatives. About 60% of the dose is excreted in urine within 24 hours,

$Cl-CH_2-CH_2$
$Cl-CH_2-CH_2$ N– (benzene ring) $-CH_2-CH_2-CH_2-COOH$

Chlorambucil (A)

$Cl-CH_2-CH_2$
$Cl-CH_2-CH_2$ N– (benzene ring) $-CH_2-CH(NH_2)-COOH$

Melphalan (A)

$Cl-CH_2-CH_2$
$Cl-CH_2-CH_2$ N– (benzimidazole, N–CH_3) $-(CH_2)_3-COOH$

Bendamustine (A)

$CH_3-SO_2-O-CH_2CH_2CH_2CH_2-O-SO_2-CH_3$

Busulfan (A)

$H_3C-SO_2-O-CH_2-C(HO)(H)-C(H)(OH)-CH_2-O-SO_2-CH_3$

Treosulfan (B)

S = P (N aziridine: H_2C–CH_2)$_3$

Thiotepa (A)

$Cl-CH_2-CH_2$
$Cl-CH_2-CH_2$ N–P=O (H–N–CH_2, CH_2, O–CH_2)

Cyclophosphamide (B)

$Cl-CH_2-CH_2-NH$–P(=O) (CH_2-CH_2-Cl –N–CH_2, CH_2, O–CH_2)

Ifosfamide (B)

$Cl-CH_2-CH_2$
$Cl-CH_2-CH_2$ N–P=O (CH_2-CH_2-Cl –N–CH_2, CH_2, O–CH_2)

Trofosfamide (B)

$CH_3-NH-NH-CH_2$– (benzene ring) $-CONH-CH(CH_3)_2$

Procarbazine (B)

(imidazole) $-C(=O)-NH_2$; $-N=N-N(CH_3)_2$

Dacarbazine (DTIC) (B)

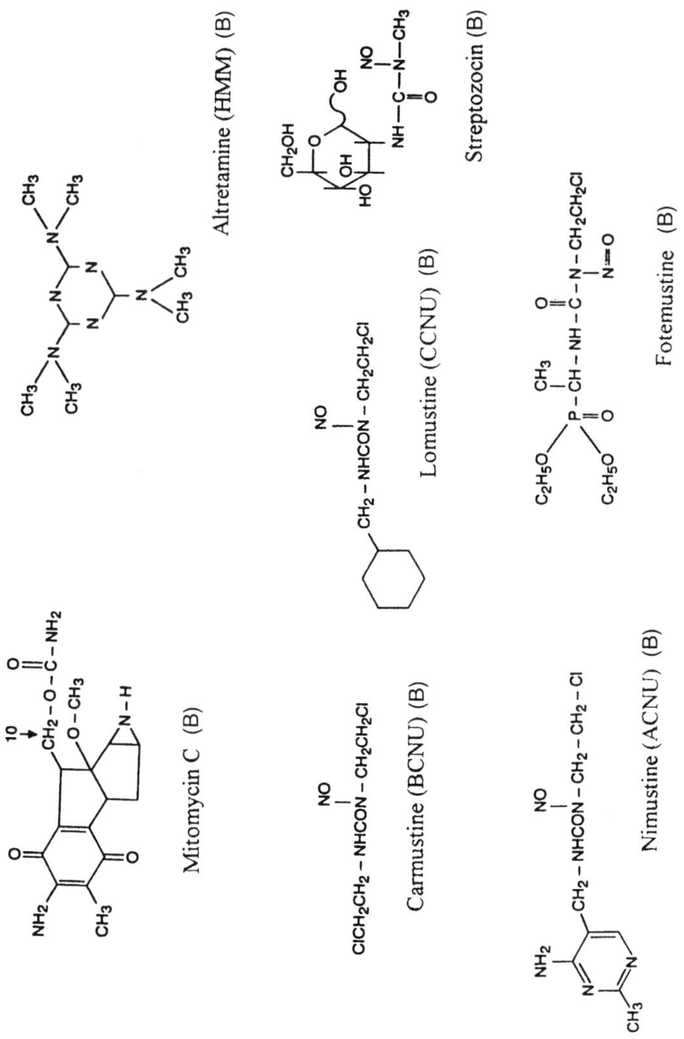

Mitomycin C (B)

Altretamine (HMM) (B)

Carmustine (BCNU) (B)

Lomustine (CCNU) (B)

Streptozocin (B)

Nimustine (ACNU) (B)

Fotemustine (B)

Fig. 1 Chemical structures of alkylating agents: (A) directly alkylating agents and (B) prodrugs.

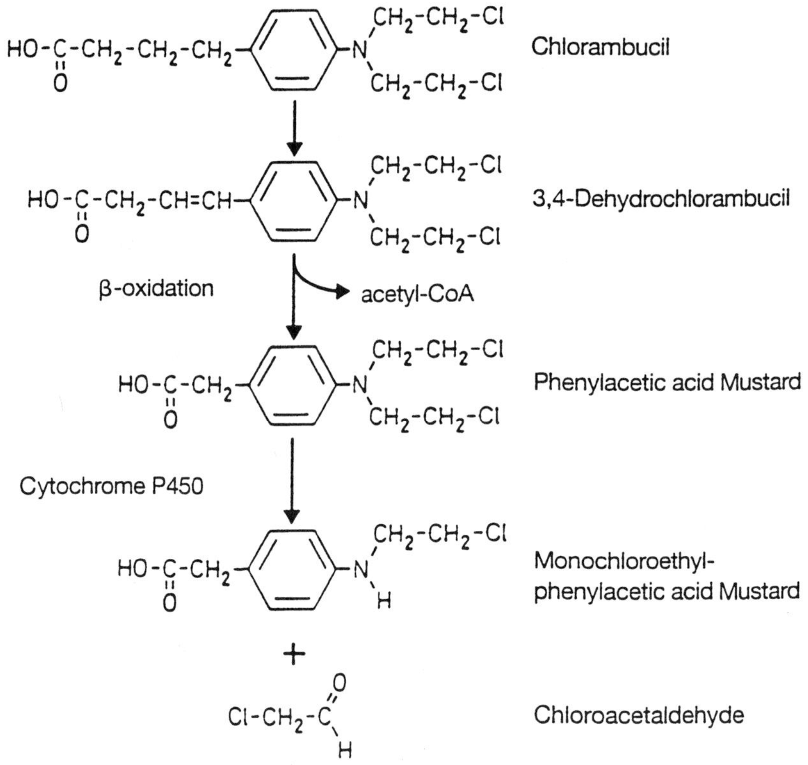

Chlorambucil

3,4-Dehydrochlorambucil

β-oxidation

acetyl-CoA

Phenylacetic acid Mustard

Cytochrome P450

Monochloroethyl-
phenylacetic acid Mustard

Chloroacetaldehyde

Fig. 2 Metabolism of chlorambucil: the major metabolite phenylacetic acid, which is formed by β-oxidation of the butyric acid side chain, is still cytotoxic. The release of the metabolite chloroacetaldehyde is mediated by cytochrome P450.

with 99% resembling hydrolyzed degradation products. Dosage adjustment is not indicated in the presence of decreased renal function [1–3,11–13].

Melphalan (Phenylalanine Mustard)

Conventional doses of melphalan (8–30 mg/m^2 IV every 2–6 weeks or 0.15–0.2 mg/kg/d on days 1–5 every 4 weeks) have proven to be active against multiple myeloma (plasmocytoma) and ovarian or breast cancer. High-dose melphalan (100–200 mg/m^2 IV) can be employed followed by the transplantation of bone marrow cells or peripheral blood progenitor cells (PBPC) [1–3,14].

The toxicity pattern of melphalan includes delayed myelosuppression, mild to moderate nausea and emesis (incidence: 10–30%), and gastrointestinal side effects.

The drug is administered via the oral or the parenteral route. However, oral administration is accompanied by high variability of absorption rate: 20–50% of an oral dose may be found in feces within 24 hours. Concomitant food intake results in a significant decrease in absolute bioavailability [12,15,16].

Comparing oral with intravenous administration of 0.6 mg/kg melphalan, the AUC value of the latter is found to be three times higher (150 vs. 53 $\mu g \times min/mL$). As a consequence, the parenteral route is often preferred in clinical practice [1–3].

In plasma the drug is highly bound to proteins. High doses of melphalan (e.g., 140 mg/m^2) as a slow bolus injection (e.g., over 5 min) are suggested rather than a 30-minute short-time infusion, to increase the free and bioavailable unbound fraction by oversaturating plasma protein binding [17,18].

The apparent volume of distribution after high-dose melphalan (e.g., 140 mg/m^2) has been estimated to range from 0.5 to 0.6 L/kg, approximately equivalent to 14.6 ± 5.1 L/m^2. The β-elimination half-life averages 45 minutes; the AUC approximates 423 $mg \times min/L$. There is some evidence that melphalan pharmacokinetics is not dose dependent [19–24].

Melphalan is rather rapidly hydrolyzed in aqueous solutions, particularly at acidic pH values (e.g., in 5% dextrose), which results in the formation of the corresponding mono- and dihydroxy derivatives, which can no longer cross-link DNA strands (Fig. 3). If freshly prepared melphalan concentrates have to be diluted for infusion, it appears most reasonable to use sodium chloride 3% because it has the highest documented physicochemical stability [25].

Another nonenzymatic deactivation pathway is the reaction of melphalan with glutathione (GSH) leading to 4-(glutathionyl)phenylalanine and other adducts (Fig. 3) [26,27]. This reaction is of particular importance in the development of melphalan-induced allergic reactions as well as in the increased intracellular resistance that occurs in tumor cells expressing high constitutive GSH levels [28–30].

There is evidence that individual glomerular filtration rate significantly correlates with melphalan clearance. Keeping in mind that renal excretion of melphalan is highly variable in cancer patients, ranging from 2 to 93%, it seems reasonable to recommend dosage adjustment in the presence of renal dysfunction [11]. Thus, especially in high-dose therapy, it has been recommended to use 85, 75, and 70% of the planned dose if the patient's creatinine clearance is reduced to 60, 45, and less than 30 mL/min, respec-

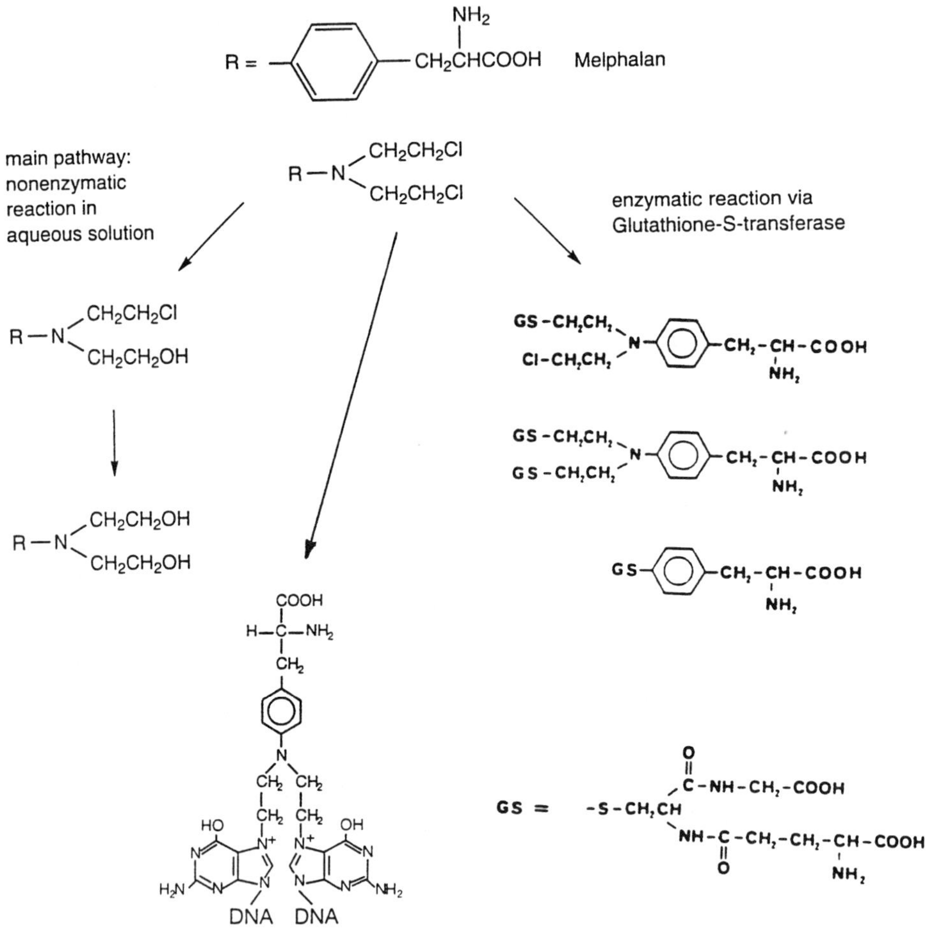

Fig. 3 The bifunctional alkylating agent melphalan, which is able to induce DNA cross-links, can hydrolyze rather rapidly in aqueous solutions or bind covalently with glutathione, leading to inactive products.

tively. However, the necessity of reducing the dose in patients with renal dysfunction is still a matter of controversy: several authors could not find any close correlation between GFR and the pharmacokinetic parameters of melphalan [11,19–24].

Clinical Pharmacokinetics Regarding Efficacy and Toxicity. Melphalan is used for high-dose chemotherapy with transplantation of bone marrow cells or blood progenitor cells for two reasons: (a) its toxicity is largely confined to myelosuppression, and (b) based on its short half-life, the PBSC can be reinfused shortly after high-dose chemotherapy.

Wide interindividual variations of AUC values as well as half-lives are common after intravenous high-dose therapy with melphalan (140 mg/m^2 as slow 5 min injection), ranging from 175 to 682 mg × min/L and 18 to 71 minutes, respectively. This may partially explain the large differences in the observed toxicity of melphalan [19–24].

An interesting method with which an optimization of high-dose therapy (HD melphalan) may be achievable is the characterization of the individual pharmacokinetic parameters by using a test dose of melphalan (e.g., 14 mg/m^2 melphalan). Because of the well-documented linearity of melphalan pharmacokinetics, it seems reasonable to calculate the optimal dose for achieving a target AUC by the formula:

$$\text{High-dose melphalan} = \text{test dose} \times \frac{\text{AUC target}}{\text{AUC test dose}}$$

However, the validity of this procedure must be established by further studies, particularly in regard to the optimal target AUC [31].

Bendamustine (Cytostasane)

Bendamustine is a bifunctional alkylating agent that is conventionally (e.g., 50–60 mg/m^2 IV, on days 1–3, every 3–4 weeks) used for the treatment of relapsed or refractory Hodgkin's and non-Hodgkin's lymphoma, plasmocytoma, chronic lymphocytic leukemia (CLL), or breast cancer.

Based on physico-chemical stability data bendamustine should only be diluted with sodium chloride 0.9%.

After IV administration, about 90% of the dose is bound to plasma proteins, with initial and terminal elimination half-life of about 10 and 36 minutes, respectively. The distribution volume in steady-state conditions approximates 20.5 L.

Bendamustine is metabolized by liver enzymes. The major metabolite is a hydroxy derivative in the butyric acid side chain, which exerts significant antiproliferative activity, too. The parent compound as well as its metabolites are primarily excreted in urine and only to a minor extent in bile. Thus, it has been recommended that the dose should be reduced in patients with impaired renal function [32].

2.1.1.2 Alkane Sulfonates and Related Compounds

Busulfan

The bifunctional alkylating agent busulfan is used for remission induction (e.g., 0.06 mg/kg/d PO) and remission maintenance (e.g., 0.5–2 mg/d PO) in CLL or essential thrombocytosis. High doses of oral busulfan (e.g., 1 mg/kg four times a day, days 1–4) have been administered in combination chemotherapy followed by autologous bone marrow reinfusion [33].

The toxicity pattern of busulfan includes dose-limiting myelosuppression, cumulative pulmonary toxicity, liver dysfunction, skin disorders, infertility, cataracts, and, rarely, hemorrhagic cystitis. Its emetogenic potency is generally low.

After oral administration the drug is rapidly and almost completely absorbed from the GI tract and widely distributed into body tissues [34]. Busulfan is able to cross the blood–brain barrier. The corresponding concentration in cerebrospinal fluid may be similar to that in plasma. Plasma protein binding is highly variable, ranging from 3 to 55% [33].

Peak plasma levels are obtained within 0.5–2 hours after oral application. Based on a half-life of about 2.5–3.4 hours, the steady-state concentrations are usually reached after 10–12 hours. Peak plasma concentrations average 65 and 1080 ng/mL after 4 mg (conventional dose) and 1 mg/kg (high dose), respectively. Less than 2% of the administered dose is recovered in urine as unchanged drug [35–38].

The only apparent metabolic catabolism of busulfan seems to be mediated by the enzyme glutathione-*S*-transferase (GST). Among the different human GST isozymes, GST-1 appears to play the most important role in busulfan metabolism. More than 10 metabolites have been identified so far, but many others have not yet been isolated. The major metabolites seem to be methanesulfonic acid and 3-hydroxytetrahydrothiophene-1,1-dioxide. Other known metabolites include sulfolane, 3-hydroxysulfolane, and tetrahydrothiopene [39,40] (Fig. 4). The possibility that the clearance of the drug will increase on repeated administration, perhaps by the induction of GST-1, cannot be excluded. This might be of clinical importance as a potential explanation of the increase of busulfan clearance during a treatment course [33].

The antiepileptic drug phenytoin is also able to increase busulfan clearance, very probably by GST induction. Thus, it is most reasonable to use diazepam rather than phenytoin to prevent seizures during high-dose busulfan therapy [41].

Clinical Pharmacokinetics Regarding Efficacy and Toxicity. Busulfan concentrations at steady-state conditions are believed to correlate well with regimen-related toxicity, particularly in regard to the risk of hepatic veno-occlusive disease (HVOD). Additionally, there may be an inverse relationship between busulfan AUC or busulfan steady-state concentrations and the probability of graft failure [42–50].

However, wide interindividual variations in AUC values as well as half-lives are common after oral high-dose therapy with busulfan in pediatric

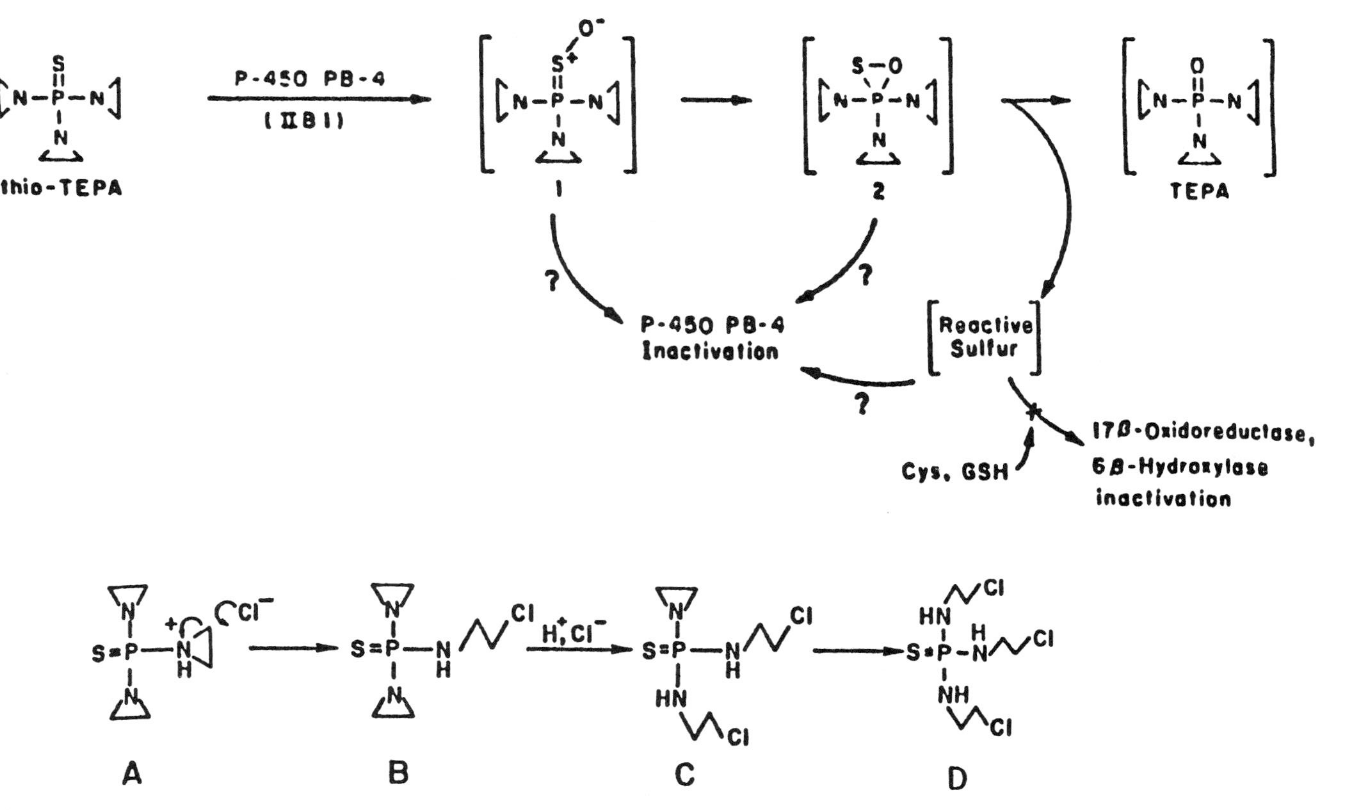

Fig. 5 Thiotepa is transformed enzymatically (to TEPA) or nonenzymatically to a variety of alkyating intermediates. (From Refs. 57 and 58.)

in the urine; the remainder is excreted as unidentified metabolites. This observation may be partially based on tendency of the low urinary pH as well as the physiological temperature to accelerate the nonenzymatic degradation of thiotepa and TEPA in substances that retain alkylating activity (Fig. 5) [58].

Regarding conventional and high-dose therapy, thiotepa has an initial and a β-elimination half-life averaging 10 minutes and 2 hours, respectively. However, there is some evidence that the metabolic clearance of thiotepa may be oversaturable at high-dose levels (e.g., 250 mg/m^2 IV on days 1–3), which may result in a prolonged initial and terminal half-life of 20 minutes and 4 hours, respectively [54–57,59].

Because less than 1.5% of unchanged drug is recovered in urine within 12 hours, it has been suggested that dosage adjustments are not warranted in the presence of decreased renal function. Since, however, remarkable alkylating activity is recovered in urine during thiotepa therapy, further studies are needed to establish definite dosage recommendations in patients with decreased creatinine clearance [58].

Clinical Pharmacokinetics Regarding Efficacy and Toxicity. Pharmacokinetic studies considering thiotepa and TEPA concentrations after high-dose therapy brought two very interesting aspects into discussion.

First, there seems to be a close correlation between thiotepa pharmacokinetics and grade 2–4 maximum related toxicity (MRT). Przepiorka et al. suggested that in patients given Thiotepa, peak concentrations exceeding 1.75 μg/mL and with AUC values (TEPA + thiotepa) exceeding 30 mg × h/L will be at a significantly higher risk of mucosal, liver, and central nervous system toxicity [60].

Second, the plasma decline of thiotepa and particularly TEPA varies considerably among patients. As a consequence, the possibility cannot be excluded that in some patients 18–20 hours after infusion, plasma TEPA concentrations may exceed levels that inhibit the growth of the reinfused hematopoietic stem cells [60]. Thus it has been suggested that if limited blood sampling is used on the first day of thiotepa administration, the doses on day 2 and 3 might be prospectively modified to achieve an ideal AUC level for thiotepa [60]. Generally, plasma probes containing thiotepa and TEPA should be handled rather quickly to avoid ex vivo degradation [61].

2.1.2 Oxazaphosphorines

In contrast to the above-mentioned agents, the oxazaphosphorines represent prodrugs that must be converted enzymatically into active compound (e.g., phosphoramide mustard). As a rule, they are far more stable physicochemically in aqueous solutions than directly alkylating agents. Additionally, their metabolic pathways are well defined [62,63].

2.1.2.1 Cyclophosphamide

Cyclophosphamide (Fig. 1) is an important component in combination chemotherapy of chronic lymphocytic and myelogenous leukemia (CLL), malignant lymphomas, or paraproteinemia (e.g., plasmocytoma, Waldenström macroglobulinemia) as well as ovary and small-cell lung cancer (SCLC), neuroblastoma. It is also frequently used in the treatment of autoimmune diseases. Conventional dosage recommendations range from 600 to 1200 mg/m^2 IV every 3–4 weeks or from 50 to 200 mg, PO, on days 1–14. High-dose cyclophosphamide (e.g., 60 mg/kg IV, day 1 + 2) is used in combination with other drugs followed by the transplantation of bone marrow or blood progenitor cells [64].

The toxicity pattern of cyclophosphamide includes dose-limiting myelosuppression, gastrointestinal side effects, a transient increase of liver enzymes, hemorrhagic cystitis, alopecia, and infertility. Particularly during high-dose therapy the risk for severe cardiotoxic side effects and pulmonary fibrosis is increased [62].

The drug can be administered orally or intravenously. However, the oral application route results in a considerably higher variability of absolute bioavailability, ranging from 74 to 97% [65]. Cyclophosphamide and its metabolites are widely distributed into body tissues. Cyclophosphamide has been reported to have an apparent distribution volume of about 0.7 L/kg after i.v. administration [65,66].

The oxazaphosphorine cyclophosphamide is a prodrug that must be bioactivated to its most active metabolite phosphoramide mustard via cytochrome P450 2C6/2C11 and Cyp 2B. After hydroxylation of the C-4 position, the formed metabolite, 4-hydroxycyclophosphamide, is in equilibrium with the ring-opened derivative aldophosphamide. If the latter is catabolized via a nonenzymatic β-elimination process, the bifunctional alkylating agent phosphoramide mustard and the highly urotoxic metabolite acrolein are released in equimolar amounts (Fig. 6) [67–69]. The incidence of any form of acute hemorrhagic cystitis induced by acrolein or 4-hydroxycyclophosphamide can be successfully prevented by the use of the thiol-containing agent mesna. This uroprotectant is usually administered if cyclophosphamide doses exceed 10 mg/kg or more than 750 mg [70–75]. Particularly during high-dose cyclophosphamide (e.g., 60 mg/kg as 2-hour infusion) the individual course of urinary alkylating activity may be highly variable.

Therefore, Fleming et al. recently suggested that it seems reasonable to combine intermittent bolus administrations (e.g., 25 mg/kg mesna at 0, 3,

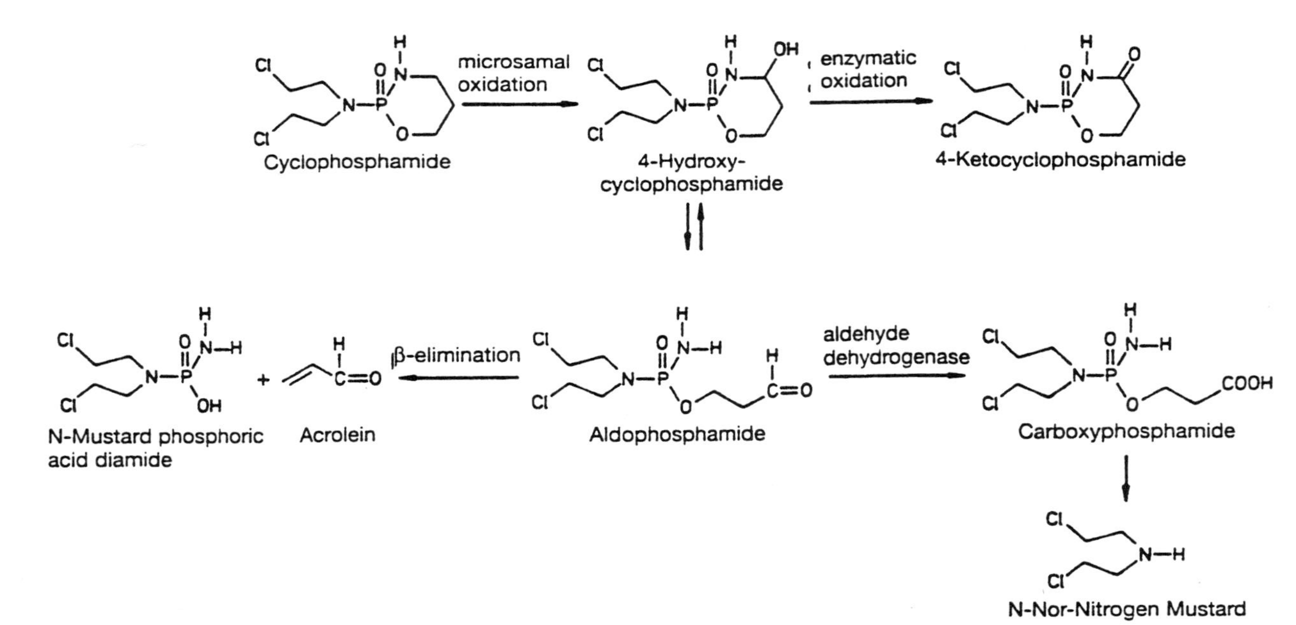

Fig. 6 Metabolic pathway of the prodrug cyclophosphamide. Its bioactivation is mediated via cytochromes P450 2C6/2C11 and 2B, which result in the formation of the corresponding 4-hydroxy-cyclophosphamide. A nonenzymatic β-elimination step regarding the ring-opened aldophosphamide leads to the bifunctional alkylating agent phosphoramide mustard and the urotoxic acrolein, which is released in equimolar amounts.

6, and 9 h) with a continuous mesna infusion (e.g., 60 mg/kg) over at least 24 hours, because this strategy may provide the highest degree of uroprotection [76]. However, this intensified treatment regimen is not yet widely used in clinical practice.

The bifunctional alkylating agent phosphoramide mustard can be hydrolyzed to a minor extent into nornitrogen mustard [bis(2-chlorethyl)amine] in vitro and in vivo [65,66].

Other metabolic pathways include the formation of 4-ketocyclophosphamide (via aldehyde oxidase) or carboxyphosphamide [via aldehyde dehydrogenase (ADH)]. Neither metabolite has any antiproliferative activity. N-Dechloroethylation pathways are of minor importance in cyclophosphamide metabolism [65,66].

Interestingly, there seems to exist a genetic polymorphism regarding ADH expression (Table 3). Thus, patients with a very low constitutive expression of this enzyme will develop very high concentrations of phosphoramide mustard and acrolein but only very low concentrations of carboxyphosphamide after conventional doses of cyclophosphamide [77].

The main elimination route of cyclophosphamide and its metabolites is renal excretion. About 36–99% of a conventional dose seems to be excreted in urine within 48 hours, carboxyphosphamide being the major metabolite and about 5–30% being unchanged drug. Less than 4% of the dose is recovered in feces. The terminal elimination half-life is estimated to be about 4 and 5–8 hours in pediatric and adult patients, respectively [65,66]. During high-dose therapy the β-elimination half-life decreases within a treatment cycle on days 2–4 (Table 4). The same is true for the cyclophosphamide clearance, which is increased from about 90 mL/min on day 1 to about

Table 3 Effect of "Low Carboxylator" (LC) and "High-Carboxylator" (HC) Phenotype on the Relative Percentage of Excretion (mean ± SD) of Each Cyclophosphamide Metabolite

	Phenotype		
Compound	LC	HC	*p*
Cyclophosphamide	19.4 ± 12.6	46.4 ± 15.5	0.006
4-Ketocyclophosphamide	3.1 ± 2.2	3.0 ± 1.9	0.962
Nornitrogen mustard	1.5 ± 1.1	2.2 ± 1.3	0.317
Carboxyphosphamide	0.34 ± 0.26	15.5 ± 11.5	<0.0001
Phosphoramide mustard	75.6 ± 13.9	33.0 ± 12.2	<0.0001

Source: Adapted from Ref. 77.

Table 4 Plasma Elimination Half Life $t_{1/2}$ and Volume of Distribution V_d of Cyclophosphamide in Patients Receiving 50 mg/kg/d on 4 Consecutive Days

Treatment day	Plasma $t_{1/2}$ (h)	V_d (L)
1	5.1	40.5
2	3.7	38.0
3	2.9	39.5
4	2.6	43.5

V_d: distribution volume (1 : liters).
Source: Adapted from Ref. 78.

180 mL/min on day 2. Probably the hepatic isozyme cytochrome P450 2B6 is autoinducible by cyclophosphamide itself within 24 hours, leading to higher phosphoramide mustard formation as well as increased antineoplastic activity on days 2 and 3 [78,79].

It has been recommended that dosage of cyclophosphamide be reduced if glomerular filtration rate is decreased. Between GFR values of 10–50 mL/min and values less than 10 mL/min, only 75 and 50% of the original dose should be given, respectively [11]. However, there is some controversy regarding the necessity of dosage reduction in patients with reduced creatinine clearance. Some pharmacokinetic data indicate that only about 15% of the parent compound and its alkylating metabolites is recovered in urine within 24 hours. Further data seem to be warranted for the establishment of definite dosage recommendations when kidney function is impaired. In patients with end-stage renal failure, cyclophosphamide and its metabolites are dialyzable [65,66].

It has been recorded that the dosage of cyclophosphamide should be reduced in patients with hyperbilirubinemia and elevated liver enzymes (e.g., a 75% or 25% dosage reduction has been recommended, if bilirubin and SGOT values range from 1.5–3.0 mg/dl and 60–180 IU/l or 3.1–5.0 mg/dl and more than 180 IU/l, respectively). However, one may speculate that constitutive bioactivation may be reduced in patients with liver dysfunction. As a consequence, the recommended dosage reduction might further diminish the percentage of phosphoramide mustard formed in the liver. Therefore, adequate dosing of cyclophosphamide appears to be difficult in patients with hepatic dysfunction [65].

Clinical Pharmacokinetics Regarding Efficacy and Toxicity

It has been reported that an infusion of high-dose cyclophosphamide (HD cyclophosphamide) over 2 hours rather than 1 hour may improve the acute tolerability regarding rhinitis, sneezing, or headache. One may speculate that these adverse affects may be correlated to high peak plasma levels of the unchanged drug [80,81].

Patients who died of acute HD-cyclophosphamide-induced cardiotoxicity revealed progressive hypotension associated with a marked decrease in systemic vascular resistance. However, cyclophosphamide is a prodrug. Thus, the quantification of the active metabolites, particularly hydroxycyclophosphamide and phosphoramide mustard, would appear to be a most reasonable route to the study of the role of pharmacokinetics in the cardiotoxic pathomechanism of HD cyclophosphamide. Possibly the cellular mechanisms of cardiotoxicity include the release of free oxygen radicals through intracellular phosphoramide mustard accumulation and glutathione depletion [81].

Recently, a clinically applicable method for the analysis of active metabolites, particularly 4-hydroxycyclophosphamide (HCY), has been presented based on derivatization to a stable *p*-nitrophenylhydrazone analogue. It must be kept in mind that HCY is a very unstable metabolite whose half-life averages 3 minutes in plasma. Based on preliminary results, it has been suggested that the AUC of HCY rather than the AUC of the parent compound may be an important determinant for cardiotoxic side effects [82].

There is marked intersubject variability concerning the AUC of cyclophosphamide and HCY after high-dose chemotherapy. In conclusion, more pharmacokinetic studies are needed to establish the correlation between HCY clearance and severe side effects as well as tumor response [83].

2.1.2.2 Ifosfamide

Ifosfamide (Fig. 1) is used in a variety of solid tumors (e.g., NSCLC, head and neck cancer and testicular cancer) as well as soft tissue sarcoma or relapsed NHL. Conventional dosage recommendations range from 1200 to 2400 mg/m^2 IV on days 1–3 (or 1–5) every 3–4 weeks. High-dose ifosfamide (e.g., 4000 mg/m^2 on days 1–4) can be used without stem cell rescue or in combination with carboplatin and etoposide (e.g., 5–12 g/m^2 ifosfamide) followed by transplantation of PBPC in the treatment of sarcoma or testicular cancer [84,85].

The toxicity pattern of ifosfamide includes dose-limiting myelosuppression, gastrointestinal side effects, a transient increase of liver enzymes, hemorrhagic cystitis, alopecia, and infertility. In contrast to cyclophosphamide high-dose regimens containing ifosfamide may result in acute and subacute neurotoxic symptoms as well as severe nephrotoxic side effects [84].

The oxazaphosphorine ifosfamide appears to exert greater cytotoxic activity than cyclophosphamide in several experimental tumor models and seems to produce less severe myelosuppressive side effects. The exocyclic chloroethyl group results in a drug that is more highly water soluble and has a different affinity to cytochrome P450 isozymes. Cytochrome 3A4, rather than cytochrome P450 2C or 2B (Cyp 2C, 2B) appears to be responsible for the bioactivation of ifosfamide in hepatic and extrahepatic tissues, in contrast to the behavior of the structurally related cyclophosphamide [67,68].

After i.v. administration, ifosfamide is widely distributed into body tissues. The parent compound has been recorded to have a volume of distribution which ranges from 32 to 40 L [87–92]. The drug is exclusively administered via the intravenous route, since oral administration results in inacceptably high neurotoxicity [93].

Like cyclophosphamide, ifosfamide is a prodrug that must be metabolized to the active metabolite isophosphoramide mustard via cytochrome P450. After hydroxylation of the C-4 position, the formed metabolite, 4-hydroxyifosfamide, is in equilibrium with the ring-opened derivative aldoifosfamide. If the latter is catabolized via a nonenzymatic β-elimination process, both the bifunctional alkylating agent isophosphoramide mustard and the highly urotoxic metabolite acrolein are released in equimolar amounts. Isophosphoramide mustard can be further hydrolyzed to chloroethylamine and phosphoric acid in vitro and in vivo (Fig. 7) [87–92].

To diminish the risk for oxazaphosphorine-induced urotoxicity and hemorrhagic cystitis, it is recommended to use the sulfhydryl compound mesna as well as appropriate hydration [94]. Other metabolic pathways include the formation of 4-ketoifosfamide (via aldehyde-oxidase) or carboxyifosfamide (via aldehyde dehydrogenase). A genetic ADH polymorphism, which may result in comparatively high levels of isophosphoramide mustard and acrolein in spite of conventional dosages, cannot be excluded [87–92].

The main elimination route of ifosfamide and its metabolites is renal excretion. About 70–86% of dose (e.g., after 3.8–5 g/m^2 IV) is excreted in urine within several days, 53% as unchanged drug. However, the percentage of drug excreted in urine within days varies highly among individuals. The terminal elimination half-life of the metabolites is estimated to be about 6 and 16 hours for conventional dosages (e.g., 1.5 g/m^2) and high dosages (e.g., 5 g/m^2), respectively. Thus it seems to be prudent to administer mesna at least up to 12 hours after the completion of ifosfamide when given as continuous infusion.

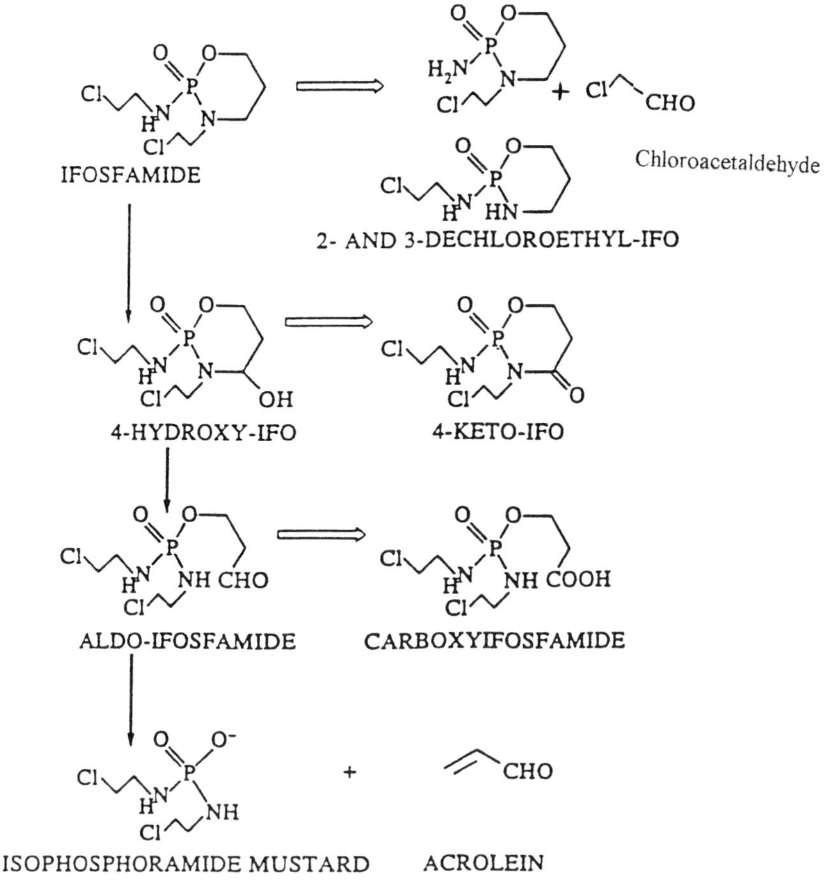

IFOSFAMIDE

Chloroacetaldehyde

2- AND 3-DECHLOROETHYL-IFO

4-HYDROXY-IFO

4-KETO-IFO

ALDO-IFOSFAMIDE

CARBOXYIFOSFAMIDE

ISOPHOSPHORAMIDE MUSTARD

ACROLEIN

Fig. 7 Metabolic pathways of ifosfamide, which are very similar to the structurally related cyclophosphamide. However, in contrast to the latter, dechloroethylation of the side chain, which results in the release of chloroacetaldehyde, is of quantitative importance, particularly regarding therapy with high-dose ifosfamide. (From Ref. 115.)

Similarly to cyclophosphamide, an increase of ifosfamide plasma clearance has been observed within a treatment cycle. This increase, evident as early as day 2, is probably based on an autoinduction of cytochrome P450 3A4 by ifosfamide itself [95,96]. It has not yet been fully understood why ifosfamide elimination seems to be prolonged in obese cancer patients [97].

Because renal excretion of unchanged drug is an important elimination pathway of ifosfamide, the avoidance of dose reduction in patients with renal dysfunction might lead to an increased risk of systemic toxicity, particularly nephrotoxicity, as well as CNS toxicity and severe myelosuppression [98–102]. As a consequence, it has been recommended to use 80, 75, and 70% of the usual dose if creatinine clearance approximates 60, 45, and 30 mL/min, respectively [11].

It has been recorded that overall pharmacokinetics is not significantly altered in the presence of hepatic insufficiency. Thus, a dosage modification does not seem to be warranted in patients with increased liver enzymes [87–92].

In contrast to cyclophosphamide, the structurally related ifosfamide can be significantly dechloroethylated at its side chain, resulting in 2-DCEI (dechloroethylifosfamide), 3-DCEI, and chloroacetaldehyde (Fig. 7). This biotransformation pathway catalyzed by Cyp 3A4 seems to be of major clinical concern regarding the onset of neurotoxic side effects (e.g., altered mental status, hallucinations) during or shortly after ifosfamide infusion. However, recent data indicate that chloroacetaldehyde may also contribute to the cytotoxic effect of ifosfamide on tumor cells [107].

The incidence of neurotoxicity has been estimated to average 13% during high-dose therapy [103–107]. Very probably chloroacetaldehyde and chloroethylamine can be further metabolized to corresponding ketimine structures, which seem to be very potent neurotoxins [108–114]. If ifosfamide is given orally there is—in contrast to the parenteral route—already a high first-pass effect via Cyp 3A4 when the drug passes the gut wall, resulting in abnormally high chloroacetaldehyde concentrations and corresponding neurotoxicity [93].

Boddy et al. reported no consistent difference between continuous infusion of 9 g/m^2 over 72 hours and repeated bolus administration (3 g/m^2 every 24 h on days 1–3) with respect to the quantitative metabolic pattern in plasma, the degree of enzymatic autoinduction, or the cumulative recovery of the parent compound and its metabolites in urine [115]. A somewhat smaller degree of dechloroethylation has been observed following bolus administrations, which may indicate that this metabolic pathway can be oversaturated by this mode of administration. These results must be classified as preliminary and do not allow a strict recommendation to avoid continuous ifosfamide infusion in conventional or high-dose therapy [115–118].

Clinical Pharmacokinetics Regarding Efficacy and Toxicity

Ifosfamide-induced nephrotoxicity is a well established side effect of this oxazaphosphorine and is mainly characterized by hypophosphatemic rickets and renal tubular acidosis (Fanconi-like syndrome). Important risk factors for the development of this severe side effect, particularly in pediatric patients, include pretreatment with cisplatin, nephrectomy, or pclvic disease and the cumulative dose of ifosfamide [98,99,119–122].

Any obvious correlation between chronic ifosfamide-induced nephrotoxicity and the pharmacokinetics and metabolism of the drug has not been exactly evaluated. It has been suggested by Boddy et al. that patients in whom the dechloroethylation is decreased between late and early courses may be at a higher risk of developing nephrotoxic side effects. This observation is rather surprising because it has been hypothesized that chloroacetaldehyde, which is released during dechloroethylation, may be responsible not only for neurotoxicity but also for nephrotoxicity [119–122].

There is some evidence that a special cytochrome P450 isozyme, Cyp 3A5, is constitutively expressed in the kidney, which catalyzes the formation of carboxyphosphamide. This metabolite is often undetectable in plasma, whereas it seems to be a major metabolite of ifosfamide recovered in urine (up to 25% of the administered dose). If the constitutive Cyp 3A5 level is very low, renal inactivation of ifosfamide will be diminished and the risk of nephrotoxicity may be increased. However, further studies are needed to confirm this hypothesis [119–122].

Recently, Wright et al. recorded that persistent high levels of the parent drug during continuous infusion may be a very critical parameter for the development of significant renal dysfunction. If 16–22 hours after the start of the continuous infusion of 4 g/m^2 ifosfamide (days 1–4) the corresponding plasma levels still exceed 150 μM, the risk of irreversible renal failure will be significantly increased. If this observation is confirmed by others, routine monitoring of ifosfamide during high-dose therapy might be prudent, to permit the timely interruption of the continuous infusion [120].

However, since the definite role of ifosfamide pharmacokinetics in the pathogenesis of nephrotoxicity is not yet fully understood, frequent monitoring of renal and tubular function as well as plasma bicarbonate seems most reasonable during therapy, to reduce the risk of severe nephrotoxic side effects [99,122–125].

The incidence of central nervous system toxicity induced by ifosfamide has strongly been associated with the degree of dechloroethylation. In particular, the stereoselective dechloroethylation resulting in *R*-2DCE (*R*-2-dechloroethylifosfamide) has been suggested to be a critical parameter for the development of severe neurotoxic side effects. However, routine measurement of this metabolic pattern does not seem to be warranted because the neurotoxic symptoms are generally transient and manageable by the intermittent use of methylene blue [112].

2.1.2.3 Trofosfamide

Trofosfamide (Fig. 1), which is applicable as an oral palliative therapy, is indicated in patients with several forms of lymphomas and hemoblastoses, as well as solid tumors (e.g., ovarian and breast cancer). Like the other oxazaphosphorines, trofosfamide is a prodrug [126]. The toxicity pattern of trofosfamide includes dose-limiting myelosuppression, mild nausea and vomiting, a transient increase of liver enzymes, alopecia, and moderate cystitis.

Trofosfamide is exclusively administered orally (e.g., initial dose: 300–400 mg/d PO; maintenance dose: 50–150 mg/d PO). The drug is rapidly and almost completely absorbed from the GI tract. Indeed, trofosfamide may be metabolized during absorption. The major metabolite detected in serum and urine is ifosfamide, whereas cyclophosphamide is released only to a minor extent. Thus the AUC values for the parent compound, ifosfamide, and cyclophosphamide have recently been recorded to average 4.4, 33.7, and 3.3 nmol $\times$ h/mL, respectively. The β-elimination half-life of trofosfamide approximates 1.5 hours. In contrast, ifosfamide is recovered in the urine as unchanged drug only to a minor extent (about 12% of the delivered dose). It is not yet fully understood why neurotoxic symptoms are very rare after trofosfamide ingestion in spite of extensive metabolic dechloroethylation. However, the amount of chloroacetaldehyde formed may be too low to exert significant neurotoxic side effects, in contrast to the case of high-dose ifosfamide [127].

2.1.3 Monofunctional and Bifunctional Alkylating Agents: Procarbazine, Dacarbazine, Mitomycin C, and Altretamine

Like the oxazaphosphorines, the alkylating agents procarbazine and dacarbazine (DTIC) represent prodrugs that must be activated via cytochrome P450. The corresponding methylazoxy isomer seems to be the most active cytotoxic metabolite of procarbazine, whereas DTIC is converted into an unstable triazene derivative spontaneously decomposing into nitrogen, 5-aminoimidazole carboxamide, and a very reactive methylcarbenium ion. Altretamine (hexamethylmelamine, HMM) is a prodrug, too, which has to be converted by cytochrome P450 into the corresponding *N*-methylol derivative, the precursor of a very reactive immonium intermediate.

Mitomycin C represents a "bioreductive bifunctional alkylating agent," which causes damages to DNA following reduction of the molecule and subsequent release of methanol and carbaminate [1–3].

2.1.3.1 Procarbazine

Procarbazine [*N*-isopropyl-α-(2-methylhydrazine)-*p*-toluamide] is a methylhydrazine derivative with antineoplastic activity against a variety of tumors, especially Hodgkin's disease. The usually recommended dose ranges from

75 to 150 mg/m^2 PO, on days 1–14 [128,129]. It is part of the COPP or MOPP regimen used for Hodgkin's disease [128,129].

The toxicity pattern of procarbazine includes dose-limiting myelosuppression, mild nausea and vomiting, a transient increase of liver enzymes, alopecia, skin disorders, influenza-like symptoms, infertility, and, rarely, CNS toxicity [128,129].

It is rapidly and almost completely absorbed from the GI tract. During the first pass through the liver, the prodrug is rapidly converted via cytochrome P450 into the corresponding azoprocarbazine. This metabolite is further N-oxidized via cytochrome P450 to yield the isomeric methylazoxy and benzylazoxy derivatives. Further oxidation of these azoxy procarbazines to hydroxyazoxy procarbazines results in the formation of the corresponding methyl and benzyl diazonium ions, which are considered to be the most important metabolites in regard to antiproliferative activity (Fig. 8).

The major metabolite in urine, *N*-isopropylterephthalamic acid, is considered to be an inactive oxidative metabolite (Fig. 8): 70% of the dose seems to be eliminated in the urine within 24 hours, mainly as *N*-isopropylterephthalamic acid. Dosage reduction does not seem to be warranted in the presence of impaired renal function [129–132].

2.1.3.2 Dacarbazine (DTIC)

Dacarbazine is used in the treatment of metastatic melanoma and advanced Hodgkin's disease [e.g., 375 mg/m^2 within the ABVD (doxorubicin, bleomycin, vinblastine, and DTIC) regimen]. For the treatment of melanoma, doses of 250 mg/m^2, IV, on days 1–5, every 3 weeks, have been recommended.

The toxicity pattern of DTIC includes dose-limiting myelosuppression, severe nausea and emesis, hepatic dysfunction, alopecia, and skin disorders.

After intravenous administration, DTIC is metabolized via cytochrome P450 to the corresponding hydroxymethyl derivative. Upon release of formaldehyde, the unstable triazene derivative is formed, which decays rapidly into the major metabolite aminoimidazole carboxamide (AIC) as well as nitrogen and a very reactive carbenium ion, which is able to alkylate DNA especially at guanine sites (Fig. 9). The terminal elimination half-life of the parent compound approximates 5 hours [133,134].

DTIC is very unstable after reconstitution and further dilution, particularly when exposed to light, because the toxic degradation product 2-azahypoxanthine (Fig. 9), which enhances the toxic side effects of dacarbazine, is formed rather rapidly. Thus, it is very important to protect DTIC-containing infusion solutions strictly from light exposure [135,136].

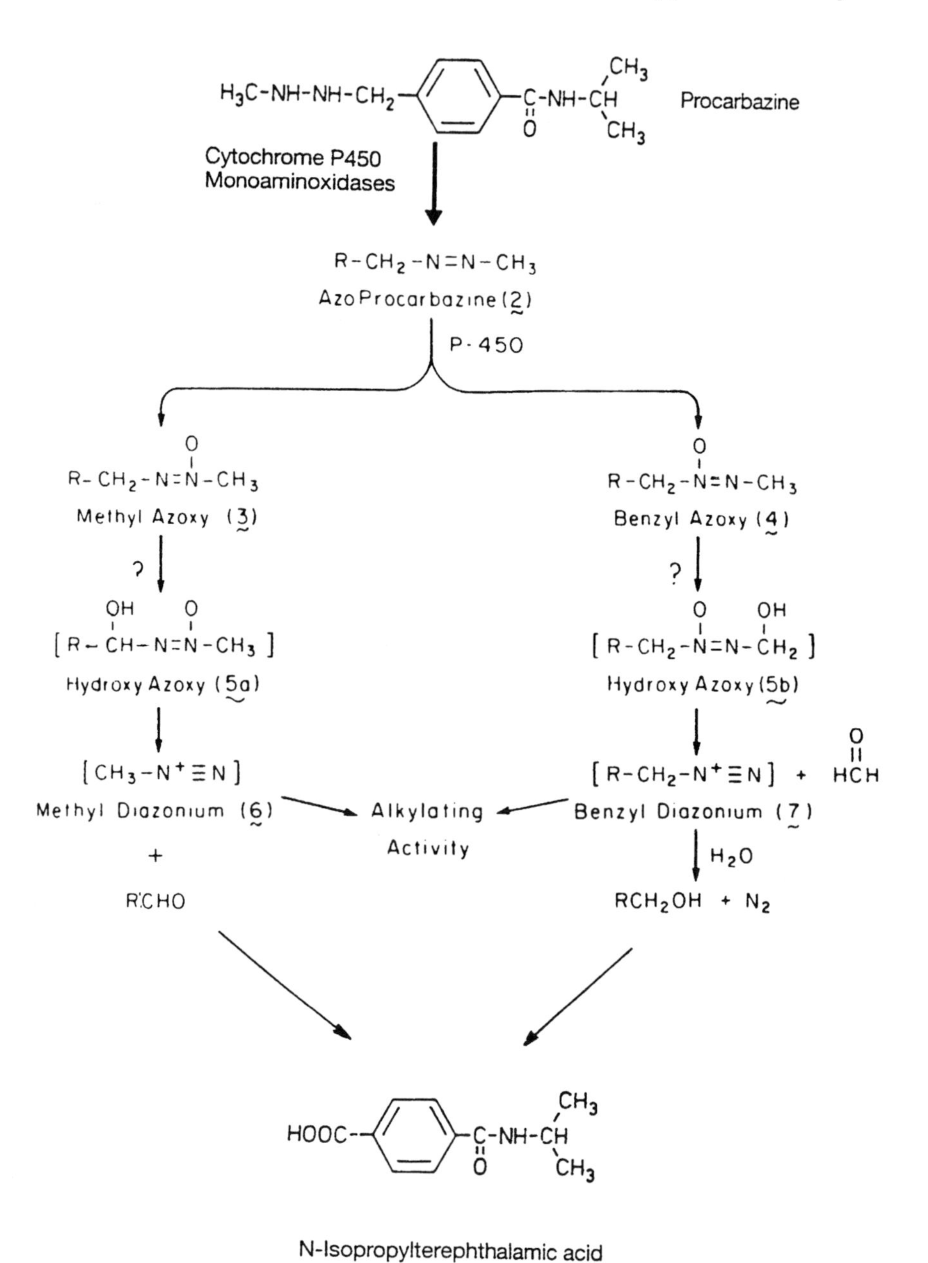

Fig. 8 Cytochrome P450-mediated metabolism of the prodrug procarbazine. Probably the release of alkylating intermediates is mediated by the methyl diazonium and Benzyl diazonium derivatives. (From Ref. 130.)

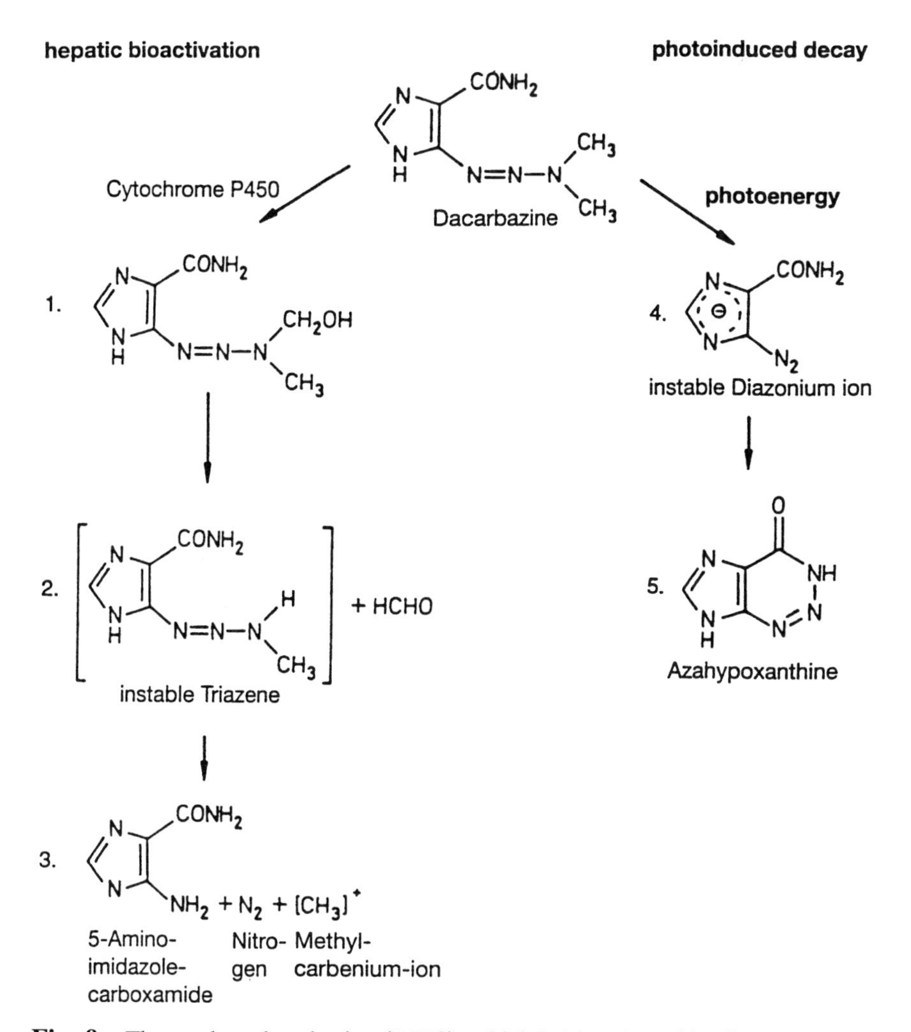

Fig. 9 The prodrug dacarbazine (DTIC), which is bioactivated by liver enzymes, is very sensitive to light, with exposure leading to the release of the highly toxic azahypoxanthine.

2.1.3.3 Mitomycin C

Mitomycin C is used in combination chemotherapy of several solid tumors, including breast, NSCLC, gastrointestinal, and prostate cancer. It is also used for intravesicular administration in superficial bladder cancer. The usually recommended dose for intravenous administration ranges from 10 to 20 mg/m^2 IV, every 4–6 weeks [137–139].

The toxicity pattern of MMC includes cumulative dose-limiting myelosuppression (in particular a prolonged thrombocytopenia), pulmonary fibrosis, alopecia, and, rarely, microangiopathic hemolytic uremia and liver dysfunction [137,138]. There is some evidence that a prolonged infusion of MMC (e.g., 3.6 $mg/m^2/d$ day 1–5) may be more tolerable than a bolus administration in respect to the risk for severe side effects, especially with a concomitant administration of 50 mg oral prednisone.

If accidental extravasation or paravasation of MMC occurs, a rapid therapeutic intervention is necessary in order to avoid severe skin necrosis. There is some evidence that the use of cold compresses, 1% hydrocortisone cream, subcutaneous dexamethasone injections, and topical intermittent massages with undiluted DMSO solutions appears to be most successful as emergency care. (See also chapter 6.)

Mitomycin C is a prodrug that is transformed to the corresponding hydroquinone by the NADPH-dependent cytochrome P450 reductase or the DT diaphorase (Fig. 10). The successive intramolecular release of methanol and carbaminate results in the formation of a bifunctional alkylating agent (Fig. 10).

After i.v. administration, the initial elimination half-life approximates 8 minutes; the terminal half-life has been recorded to range between 30 and 70 minutes.

About 10% of the drug is excreted intact in the urine. Thus far, in patients with impaired renal function, a dosage reduction has not seemed to be warranted. However, it must be kept in mind that the use of mitomycin C (MMC) is associated with a considerable risk of nephrotoxicity (e.g., hemolytic uremic syndrome with azotemia, proteinuria, and microscopic hematuria). As a consequence, MMC may severely worsen preexisting impaired renal function [140–143].

2.1.3.4 Altretamine (Hexamethylmelamine, HMM)

Hexamethylmelamine (HMM) is a prodrug that can be applied as an oral palliative therapy in patients with advanced ovarian or lung cancer and refractory lymphomas. The toxicity pattern of HMM includes mild myelosuppression, and severe nausea and emesis, as well as neurotoxic side effects.

Usually it is administered orally (e.g., 8 mg/kg PO, days 1–21). A parenteral formulation based on Intralipid 20% is under investigation [144–146].

The absolute bioavailability of unchanged HMM is estimated to average 20% because the drug undergoes an extensive first-pass metabolism. Cytochrome P450 isozymes in the liver catalyze the N-demethylation of HMM, which results in the formation of *N*-methylolpentamethylmelamine

(HMPMM). HMPMM may be converted to either the inactive metabolite pentamethylmelamine (PMM) or to a very reactive immonium ion. Probably the latter is important for HMM-induced antineoplastic activity (Fig. 11).

The terminal elimination half-life of HMM has been estimated to be about 3–10 hours; 70–90% of dose is excreted in the urine, however, less than 1% is eliminated as unchanged drug. As a consequence, dosage adjustments do not seem to be warranted in patients with impaired renal function [147–149].

2.1.4 Nitrosoureas

The discovery of nitrosoureas as promising anticancer drugs started with the observation that the compound 1-methyl-l-nitroso-3-nitroso-guanidine demonstrated considerable antitumor activity against murine leukemic cell lines. In the meantime, several nitrosureas are available for cancer chemotherapy. Because of their ability to cross the blood–brain barrier, they represent an important class of drugs used, particularly against cerebral tumors [150].

In common they can spontaneously degrade in aqueous solutions, leading to chloroethyldiazonium hydroxide and the corresponding isocyanate. This degradation process is considerably accelerated by the presence of proteins. As a consequence, the physicochemical half-life of BCNU or CCNU (see Sections 2.1.4.1 and 2.1.4.2) decreases from 50 minutes to 15 minutes and from 60 minutes to 30 minutes in plasma, respectively. A central feature of nitrosourea-mediated antitumoral activity is the release of a reactive carbonium ion, which subsequently alkylates macromolecules within the cell. However, a multiplicity of other alkylating species are formed (Fig. 12) [151].

The toxicity pattern of the nitrosoureas includes a prolonged and cumulative myelosuppression, nausea and emesis (incidence: 60–90%), alopecia, infertility, and a cumulative interstitial pneumonitis, liver, and renal dysfunction.

2.1.4.1 Carmustine [BCNU, Bis(chloroethyl)nitrosourea]

Carmustine is used alone or in combination with appropriate surgical, radiotherapeutic, and/or chemotherapeutic interventions in the palliative treatment of primary and metastatic brain tumors. The drug is also used in combination therapy for the treatment of multiple myeloma and relapsed Hodgkin and non-Hodgkin lymphoma. The recommended dose ranges from 80 and 200 mg/m^2 IV every 6 weeks. High-dose therapy with carmustine (e.g., 300–600 mg/m^2 IV) has been used followed by transplantation of bone

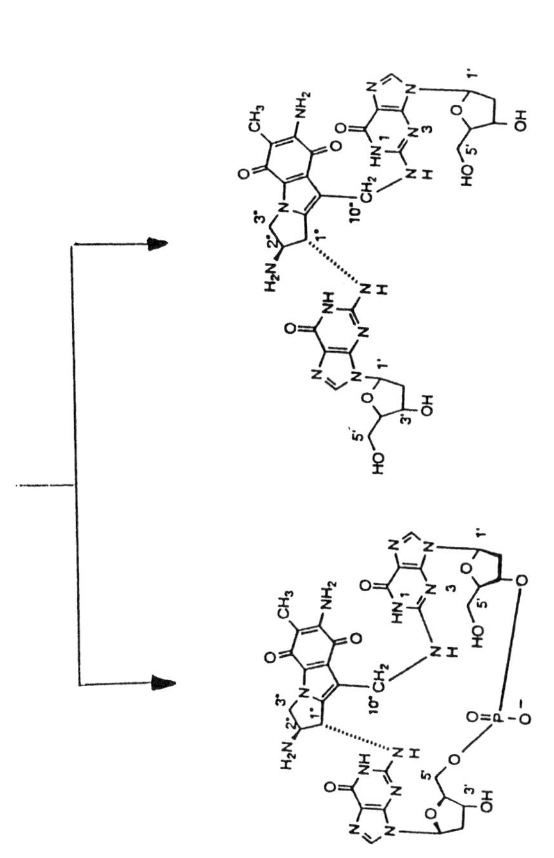

Fig. 10 Metabolic pathways of the prodrug mitomycin C. In contrast to the reduction by the NADPH-dependent cytochrome P450 reductase, which results in the formation of the semiquinone and toxic superoxidase radicals, the reduction to the hydroquinone (mediated by the enzyme DT diaphorase) leads to the bifunctional agent, which is able to mediate DNA cross-links. (From Refs. 140 and 142.)

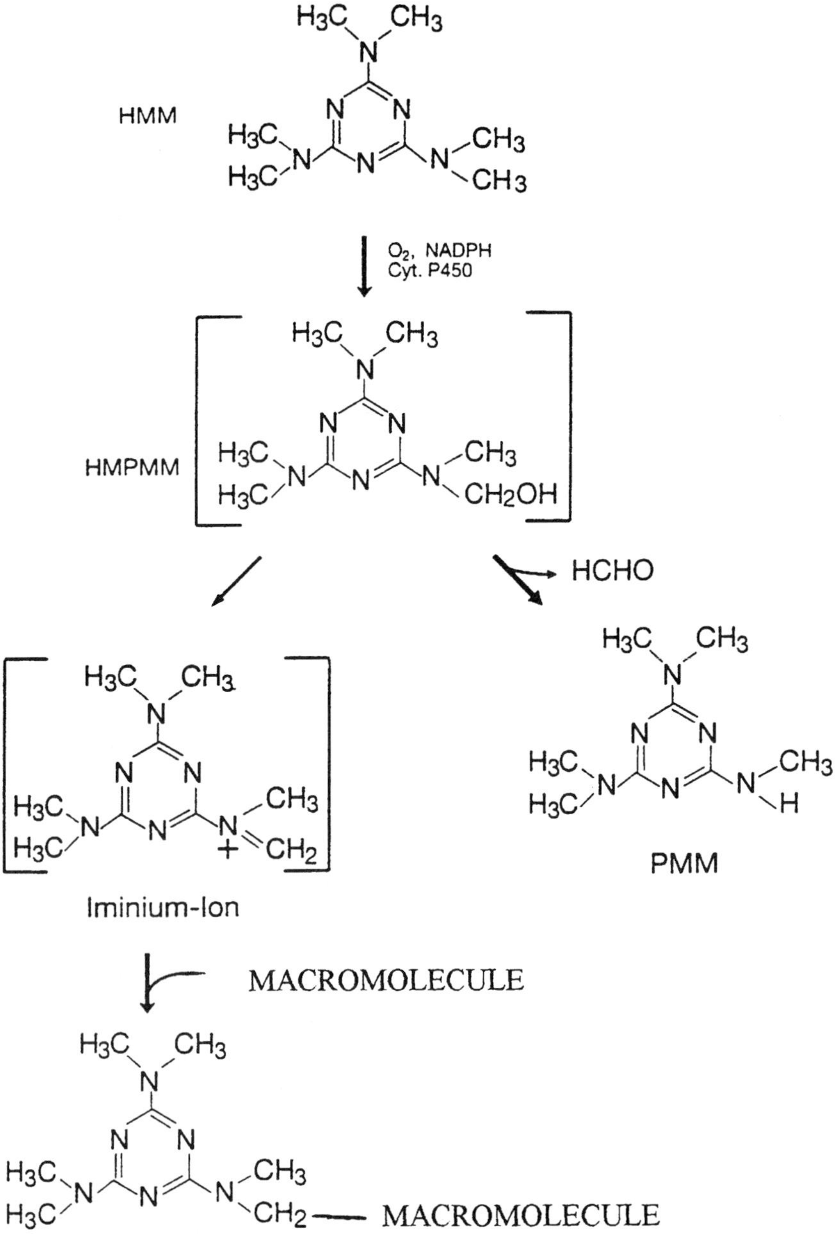

HMM

O_2, NADPH
Cyt. P450

HMPMM

HCHO

Iminium-Ion

PMM

MACROMOLECULE

MACROMOLECULE

Fig. 11 Metabolic pathways of hexamethylmelamine (HMM). The intermediate HMPMM, which is formed by cytochrome P450, decomposes to pentamethylmelamine (PMM) or to the corresponding immonium ion, which appears to be able to bind covalently to macromolecules and to exert antiproliferative activity.

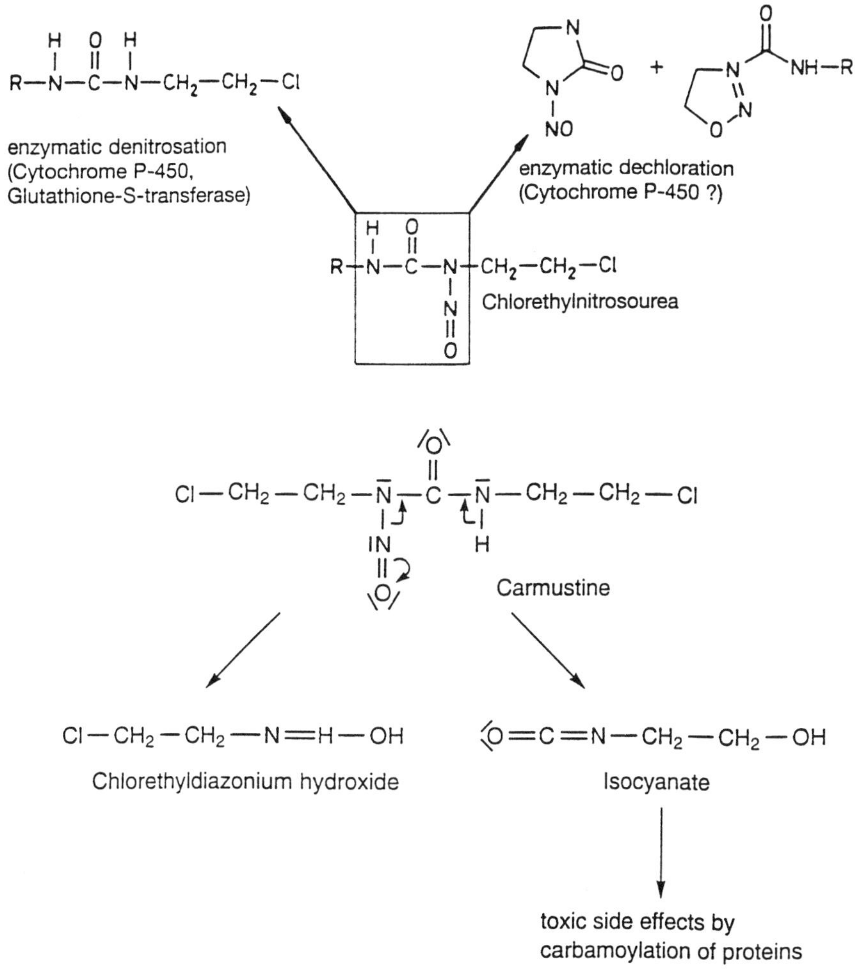
R—N—C—N—CH₂—CH₂—Cl
enzymatic denitrosation
(Cytochrome P-450,
Glutathione-S-transferase)
NO
NH—R
enzymatic dechloration
(Cytochrome P-450 ?)
R—N—C—N—CH₂—CH₂—Cl
Chlorethylnitrosourea
Cl—CH₂—CH₂—N—C—N—CH₂—CH₂—Cl
Carmustine
Cl—CH₂—CH₂—N=H—OH
Chlorethyldiazonium hydroxide
O=C=N—CH₂—CH₂—OH
Isocyanate
toxic side effects by
carbamoylation of proteins

Fig. 12 The enzymatic and chemical degradation of nitrosoureas is rather complex because it leads to a variety of alkylating products and corresponding glutathione adducts.

marrow or peripheral blood progenitor cells particularly in relapsed lymphomas [152,153].

After infusion of 45–170 mg/m^2 BCNU, the initial half-life (distribution half-life) is estimated to be about 6 minutes and the elimination half-life to be about 20 minutes. The latter does not seem to be prolonged if high doses (300–750 mg/m^2) are administered over 2 hours. However, distribution volume (5.1 vs. 3.25 L/kg) as well as the total clearance (77.6 vs. 56 mL/min/kg) appear to be increased during high-dose therapy. About 70% of dose is excreted in urine within 96 hours as metabolites with considerable alkylating activity; about 10% is exhaled as carbon dioxide [151,154,155]. Metabolic inactivation is partially mediated by glutathione-*S*-transferase [151]. If this enzyme is constitutively overexpressed in tumor cells, such tumors may be resistant to BCNU [156].

It has been suggested that the determination of the AUC of BCNU may be useful in high-dose chemotherapy. Jones et al. reported that AUC values greater than 600 μg/mL × min were associated with an increased risk of acute lung toxicity [157]. In spite of these interesting observations, some questions are still unresolved. There is some evidence that some of the formed metabolites, particularly the isocyanates, rather than the parent compound, seem to be responsible for nitrosourea-induced organ toxicity. In conclusion, it is questionable whether the AUC quantification of the parent compound may serve as an appropriate prognostic factor to be used in calculating the risk of BCNU-induced pulmonary toxicity. On the other hand, BCNU is a rather unstable drug. Thus, blood samples must be handled very carefully to avoid artifacts [157–159].

2.1.4.2 Lomustine [CCNU, Chloroethyl(cycohexyl)nitrosourea]

Lomustine is primarily used in the treatment of Hodgkin's disease, as well as primary and secondary brain tumors (e.g., 130 mg/m^2 PO every 6–8 weeks) [160].

Lomustine is almost completely absorbed from the GI tract after oral administration. Like other nitrosoureas, lomustine can decompose rather rapidly under physiological conditions, resulting in the formation of the corresponding alkyldiazonium hydroxide as well as a variety of alkylating products and an alkylisocyanate derivative. Thus it is not surprising that the parent compound is not detectable in urine, feces, or the cerebrospinal fluid [151].

The spontaneous degradation of the alkyldiazonium hydroxide leads to the formation of a chloroethyl alkylating intermediate that is able to react with the O-6 position of guanine in DNA. This reaction results in crosslinking between this purine base and cytosine.

The cyclohexylisocyanate also formed during spontaneous degradation is able to carbamoylate amino or thiol groups of proteins. If these proteins are involved in DNA repair mechanisms, these isocyanates may increase the overall antineoplastic activity. However, if physiological proteins are car-

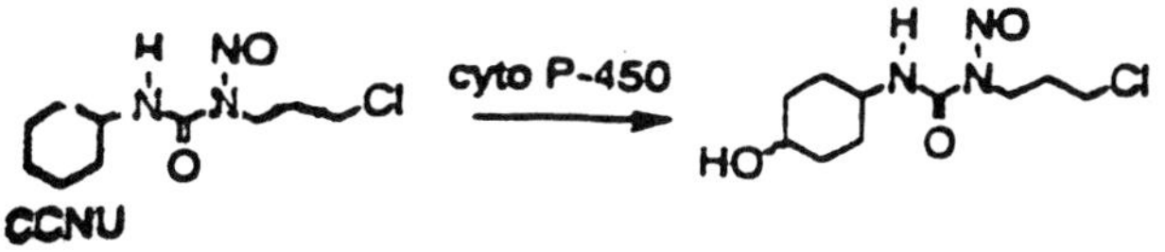

Fig. 13 During first pass, the cyclohexyl moiety of lomustine (CCNU) is hydroxylated by hepatic cytochrome P450 isozymes resulting in the formation of the more active metabolites *trans*-4-H-CCNU and *cis*-4-OH-CCNU.

bamoylated, these isocyanate derivatives may be responsible for organ toxicity, particularly cumulative pulmonary toxicity [161,162].

During first pass, the cyclohexyl moiety is predominantly hydroxylated by hepatic cytochrome P450 isozymes (Fig. 13). The *trans*-4-OH-CCNU and *cis*-4-OH-CCNU may be twice as active as the parent compound. Their half-lives are similar and range from 1 to 3 hours. These metabolites seem to be taken up by tumor tissue rather rapidly, whereas unchanged CCNU is hardly detectable in tissues as well as plasma.

A variety of alkylating metabolites that have not yet been fully characterized, as well as the cyclohexylisocyanate, are excreted in the urine and feces within several days after oral administration of lomustine. Nearly 50% of the dose is excreted in the urine within 24 hours [160–162].

2.1.4.3 Nimustine (ACNU)

ACNU plays a special role in the treatment of primary and secondary brain tumors. The usually recommended dose ranges from 90 to 100 mg/m^2 IV every 6 weeks. The drug is much more water-soluble than BCNU or CCNU [163].

After parenteral administration ACNU is widely distributed in liver, skin, and kidneys, as well as brain tissues. The CSF concentration may reach 0–0.076 μg/mL 30 minutes after the administration of 100–150 mg of ACNU, which correlates with 0–63% of the corresponding plasma concentration. Extraordinarily high ACNU levels were detectable in malignant brain tissues.

ACNU is rapidly hydrolyzed in plasma and extensively metabolized in the liver. The elimination half-life of unchanged ACNU has been recorded to be about 0.6 hour, whereas the half-life of the formed metabolites and hydrolysis products seem to be even longer. The metabolic pathway is similar when the catabolism of ACNU is compared with that of other nitrosoureas. The chloroethyl alkylating intermediate that is formed during chemical degradation seems to react with the O-6 position of guanine, resulting in cross-linking between this purine base and cytosine. It has been reported that core particles, especially, seem to be alkylated by ACNU metabolites. Few data exist regarding the potential organ toxicity induced by the released isocyanate [164].

2.1.4.4 Streptozocin

Streptozocin is primarily used for the treatment of advanced islet cell carcinoma and malignant carcinoids (e.g., 500 mg/m^2 IV on days 1–5, every 6 weeks). Combination with 5-fluorouracil may increase its therapeutic efficacy [165]. Though its toxicity pattern is similar to that of the other nitrosoureas, it may lead to severe subacute nephrotoxic side effects as well as pancreatitis and diabetes [166].

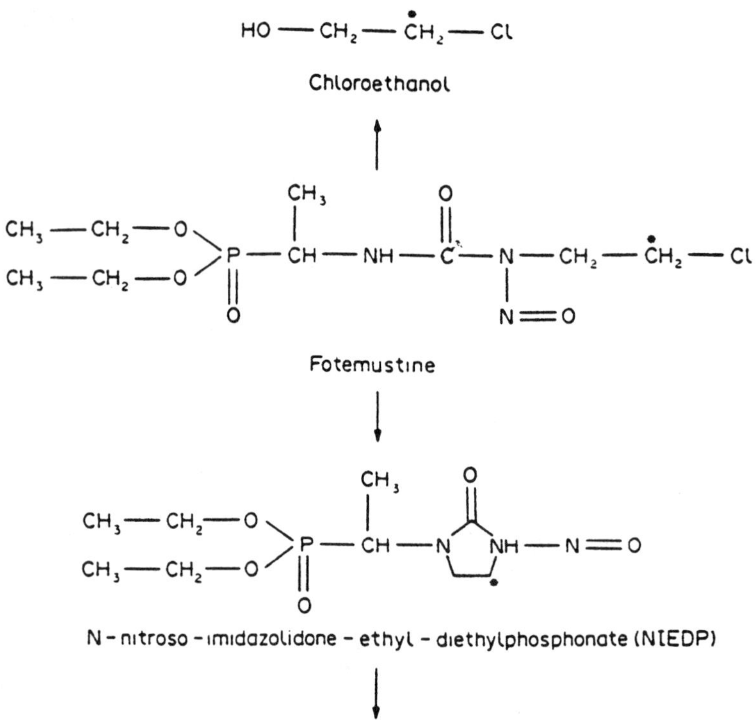

HO—CH$_2$—CH$_2$—Cl

Chloroethanol

Fotemustine

N-nitroso-imidazolidone-ethyl-diethylphosphonate (NIEDP)

Fig. 14 Metabolic pathways of fotemustine in cancer patients. (From Ref. 167.)

CH$_3$—CH$_2$—O / CH$_3$—CH$_2$—O >P(=O)—CH(CH$_3$)—N (imidazolidone ring, C=O, NH, •)

1-imidazolidone-ethyl-diethylphosphonate (IEDP)

↓

CH$_3$—CH$_2$—O / CH$_3$—CH$_2$—O >P(=O)—CH(CH$_3$)—N (hydantoin ring, C=O, NH, O, •)

1-hydantoin-ethyl-diethylphosphonate (HEDP)

↓

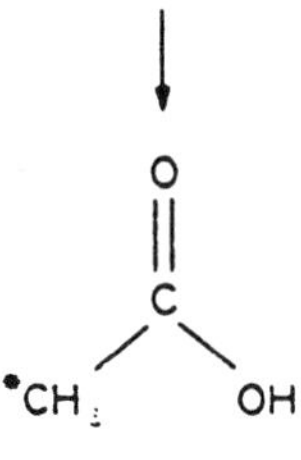

acetic acid

• indicates position of the radiolabel

Fig. 14 *Continued*

The distribution of IV-administered streptozocin has not yet been fully characterized. The drug and its metabolites seem to be rapidly distributed into the liver, pancreas, kidneys, and intestine. Some metabolites seem to be able to pass the blood–brain barrier.

After i.v. administration, the plasma levels of the parent compound decline rather rapidly. The initial half-life has been reported to be about 5 minutes, the second to be about 35–40 minutes. Some of the metabolites reveal longer terminal half-lives of about 40 hours.

About 60–70% of the dose is excreted in the urine within 24 hours; about 10–20% seems to be unchanged drug. Approximately 5% of dose is eliminated in the expired air (as carbon dioxide), and less than 1% is excreted in the feces [151].

Although a definite dosage adjustment for streptozocin does not seem to be warranted in patients with impaired renal function, it must be kept in mind that the use of streptozocin is associated with a considerable high risk for nephrotoxic side effects, which may significantly worsen preexisting impairments in the moderate to severe category [11].

2.1.4.5 Fotemustine

Fotemustine is a novel chloroethylnitrosourea derivative. Its chemical structure is characterized by the addition of an aminophosphonate, a bioisostere of alanine, which is supposed to facilitate higher permeability through cell membranes as well as the blood–brain barrier. Fotemustine is mostly used in the treatment of disseminated malignant melanoma (e.g., 100 mg/m^2/week every 3 weeks) and primary brain tumors [167].

Fotemustine seems to be extremely unstable in solutions, especially upon exposure to light. Thus, it is important that infusion solutions containing fotemustine be protected from light.

About 50–60 and 7% of the dose is excreted in the urine and feces, respectively. The terminal elimination half-life of the parent compound and its metabolites averages 24 minutes and 70–100 hours, respectively. The biotransformation pathways are complex. Besides chloroethanol, another major component in plasma is NIEDP (*N*-nitroso-imidazolidone-ethyl-diethylphosphonate), which is further metabolized by denitrosation, resulting in the release of HEDP (1-hydantoin-ethyl-diethylphosphonate (HEDP)) (Fig. 14). The consequences of renal or hepatic dysfunction on fotemustine pharmacokinetics are not yet fully understood [168,169].

REFERENCES TO SECTION 2.1

1. Farmer PB, Newell DR. Alkylating agents. In: MM Ames, G Powis, JS Kovach, eds. Pharmacokinetics of Anticancer Agents in Humans. New York: Elsevier Science Publishers, 1983, pp. 77–107.
2. Lind MJ, Ardiet C. Pharmacokinetics of alkylating agents. Cancer Surv. 1993: 17:157–188.
3. Newell DR, Gore ME. Toxicity of alkylating agents: Clinical characteristics and pharmacokinetic determinations. In: G. Powis, MP Hacker, eds. The Toxicity of Anticancer Drugs. New York: Pergamon Press, 1991, pp. 44–62.
4. Adair FE, Bagg HJ. Experimental and clinical studies on the treatment of cancer by dichloroethylsulfide (mustard gas). Ann Surg 1931:93:190–199.
5. Gilman A. The initial clinical trials of nitrogen mustard. Am J Surg 1963: 105:574–578.
6. Bosanquet AG. Stability of solutions of antineoplastic agents during preparation and storage for in vitro assays—General considerations, the nitrosoureas and alkylating agents. Cancer Chemother Pharmacol 1985:14:83–95.
7. Kaldor JM, Day NE, Hemmink K. Quantifying the carcinogenicity of antineoplastic drugs. Eur J Cancer Clin Oncol 1988:24:703–711.

8. Boivin J-F. Second cancers and other late side-effects of cancer treatment—A review. Cancer 1990:65:770–775.
9. O'Dwyer PJ, LaCreta F, Engstrom PF, Peter R, et al. Phase I/Pharmacokinetic reevaluation of thioTEPA. Cancer Res 1991:51:3171–3176.
10. Gilam A, Philips FS. The biological actions and therapeutic applications of beta-chloroethyl amines and sulfides. Science 1946:103:409–415.
11. Kintzel PE, Dorr RT. Anticancer drug renal toxicity and elimination: Dosing guidelines for altered renal function. Cancer Treatment Rev 1995:21:33–64.
12. Adair CG, McElnay JC. The effect of dietary amino acids on the gastrointestinal absorption of melphalan and chlorambucil. Cancer Chemother Pharmacol 1987:9:343–346.
13. Alberts DS, Chang SY, Chen HSG, et al. Comparative pharmacokinetics of chlorambucil and melphalan in man. Recent Results Cancer Res 1980:74:124–127.
14. van der Wall E, Beijnen JH, Rodenhuis S. High-dose chemotherapy regimens for solid tumors. Cancer Treatment Rev 1995:21:105–132.
15. Bosanquet AG, Gilby ED. Comparison of the fed and fasting states on the absorption of melphalan in multiple myeloma. Cancer Chemother Pharmacol 1984:12:183–186.
16. Reece PA, Kotasek D, Morris RG, Dale BM, Sage RE. The effect of food on oral melphalan absorption. Cancer Chemother Pharmacol 1986:16:194–197.
17. Gera S, Musch E, Osterheld KO, Loos U. Relevance of the hydrolysis and protein binding of melphalan to the treatment of multiple myeloma. Cancer Chemother Pharmacol 1989:23:76–80.
18. Reece PA, Hill HS, Green RM, et al. Renal clearance and protein binding of melphalan in patients with cancer. Cancer Chemother Pharmacol 1988:22:348–352.
19. Guyette A, Hartmann O, Pico J-L. Pharmacokinetics of high-dose melphalan in children and adults. Cancer Chemother Pharmacol 1986:16:184–189.
20. Samuels BL, Bitran JD. High-dose intravenous melphalan: A review. J Clin Oncol 1995:13:1786–1799.
21. Ploin DY, Tranchard B, Guastalla J-P, Rebattu P, et al. Pharmacokinetically guided dosing for intravenous melphalan: A pilot study in patients with advanced ovarian adenocarcinoma. Eur J Cancer 1992:28A:1311–1315.
22. Taha IA-K, Ahmad RA, Rogers DW, Pritchard J, Rogers HJ. Pharmacokinetics of melphalan in children following high-dose intravenous injection. Cancer Chemother Pharmacol 1983:10:212–216.
23. Pinguet F, Martel P, Fabbro M, et al. Pharmacokinetics of high-dose intravenous melphalan in patients undergoing peripheral blood hematopoietic progenitor-cell transplantation. Anticancer Res 1997:17:605–612.
24. Kergueris MF, Milpied N, Moreau P, et al. Pharmacokinetics of high-dose melphalan in adults: Influence of renal function. Anticancer Res 1994:14:2379–2382.
25. Pinguet F, Martel P, Rouanet P, Fabbro M, Astre C. Effect of sodium chloride concentration and temperature on melphalan stability during storage and use. Am J Hosp Pharm 1994:51:2701–2704.

26. Bolton MG, Hilton J, Robertson KD, et al. Kinetic analysis of the reaction of melphalan with water, phosphate and glutathione. Drug Metab Dispos 1993:21:986–886.
27. Dulik DM, Fenselau C. Conversion of melphalan to 4-(glutathionyl) phenylalanine—A novel mechanism for conjugation by glutathione-*S*-transferases. Drug Metab Dispos 1987:15:195–198.
28. Bleichner F, Mende S. Allergische Reaktion auf Melphalan? Onkologie 1982: 5:195.
29. Cornwell GG, Pajak TF, MyIntyre OR. Hypersensitivity reactions to IV melphalan during treatment of multiple myeloma: Cancer and leukemia group B experience. Cancer Treatment Rep 1979:63:399–403.
30. Hall A, Harris AL, Hickson ID, et al. The involvement of glutathione-*S*-transferase in cellular resistance to nitrogen mustards. In: TJ Mantle, CB Picket, JD Haynes, eds. Glutathione-*S*-Transferases and Carcinogenesis. London: Taylor & Francis, 1987, p. 245.
31. Tranchard B, Ploin Y-D, Minuit M-P, Sapet C, et al. High-dose melphalan dosage adjustment: Possibility of using a test-dose. Cancer Chemother Pharmacol 1989:23:95–100.
32. Preiss R, Sohr R, Matthias M, Brockmann B, Huller H. The pharmacokinetics of Bendamustine (cytostasane) in humans [Untersuchungen zur Pharmakokinetik von Bendamustin (Cytostasan) am Menschen]. Pharmazie 1985: 40(11):782–784.
33. Buggia I, Locatelli F, Regazzi MB, Zecca M. Busulfan. Ann Pharmacother 1994:28:1055–1062.
34. Hassan M, Ljungman P, Bolme P, et al. Busulfan bioavailability. Blood 1994: 84:2144–2150.
35. Hassan M, Fasth A, Gerritsen B, et al. Busulphan kinetics and limited sampling model in children with leukemia and inherited disorders. Bone Marrow Transplant 1996:18:843–850.
36. Grochow LB. Busulfan disposition: The role of therapeutic drug monitoring in bone marrow transplantation induction regimes. Semin Oncol 1993: 20(suppl 4):18–25.
37. Hassan M, Öberg G, Ehrsson H, Ehrnebo M, et al. Pharmacokinetic and metabolic studies of high-dose busulphan in adults. Eur J Clin Pharmacol 1989:36:525–530.
38. Shaw PJ, Scharping CE, Brian R, Earl JW. Busulfan pharmacokinetics using a single daily high-dose regimen in children with acute leukemia. Blood 1994: 84:2357–2362.
39. Hassan M, Ehrsson H. Urinary metabolites of busulfan in the rat. Drug Metab Dispos 1987:15:399–402.
40. Czerwinski M, Gibbs JP, Slattery JT. Busulfan conjugation by glutathione *S*-transferases. Drug Metab Dispos 1996:24:1015–1019.
41. Fitzsimmons WE, Ghalie R, Kaizer H. The effect of hepatic enzyme inducers on busulfan neurotoxicity and myelotoxicity. Cancer Chemother Pharmacol 1990:27:226–228.

42. Schuler U, Schroer S, Kühnle A, Blanz J, et al. Busulfan pharmacokinetics in bone marrow transplant patients: Is drug monitoring warranted? Bone Marrow Transplant 1994:14:759–765.
43. Vassal G, Deroussent A, Hartman O, Challine D, et al. Dose-dependent neurotoxicity of high-dose busulfan in children: A clinical and pharmacological study. Cancer Res 1990:50:6203–6207.
44. Vassal G, Koscielny S, Challine D, Valteau-Couanet D, et al. Busulfan disposition and hepatic veno-occlusive disease in children undergoing bone-marrow transplantation. Cancer Chemother Pharmacol 1996:37:247–253.
45. Dix SP, Wingard JR, Mullins RE, et al. Association of busulfan area under the curve with veno-occlusive disease following BMT. Bone Marrow Transplant 1996:17:225–230.
46. Morgan M, Dodds A, Atkinson K, Szer J, et al. The toxicity of busulphan and cyclophosphamide as the preparative regimen for bone marrow transplantation. Br J of Haematol 1991:77:529–534.
47. Peters WP, Henner WD, Grochow LB, Olsen G, et al. Clinical and pharmacological effects of high-dose single agent busulfan with autologous bone marrow support in the treatment of solid tumors. Cancer Res 1987:47:6402–6406.
48. Slattery JT, Sanders JE, Buckner CD, et al. Graft-rejection and toxicity following bone marrow transplantation in relation to busulfan pharmacokinetics. Bone Marrow Transplant 1995:16:31–42.
49. Chattergoon DS, Saunders EF, Klein J, et al. An improved limited sampling method for individualised busulphan dosing in bone marrow transplantation in children. Bone Marrow Transplant 1997:20:347–354.
50. Rifai N, Sakamoto M, Lafi M, Guinan E. Measurement of plasma busulfan concentration by high-performance liquid chromatography with ultraviolet detection. Ther Drug Monit 1997:19:169–174.
51. Grochow LB, Jones RJ, Brundrett RB, et al. Pharmacokinetics of busulfan: Correlation with veno-occlusive disease in patients undergoing bone marrow transplantation. Cancer Chemother Pharmacol 1989:25:55–61.
52. Hilger RA, Harstrick A, Eberhardt W, et al. Clinical pharmacokinetics of intravenous treosulfan in patients with advanced solid tumors. Cancer Chemother Pharmacol 1998:42:99–104.
53. White WF, Masding JE. Treosulfan chemotherapy in advanced ovarian cancer. A long term evaluation in previously untreated disease. Br J Cancer 1982:46: 491.
54. Cohen BE, Egorin MJ, Kohlhepp EA, Alsner J, Gutierrez PL. Human plasma pharmacokinetics and urinary excretion of thiotepa and its metabolites. Cancer Treat Rep 1986:70:859–864.
55. Strong JM, Collins JM, Lester C, Poplack DG. Pharmacokinetics of intraventricular and intravenous thiotepa in rhesus monkeys and humans. Cancer Res 1986:46:6101–6104.
56. Ackland SP, Choi KE, Ratain MJ, et al. Human plasma pharmacokinetics of thiotepa following administration of high-dose thiotepa and cyclophosphamide. J Clin Oncol 1988:6:1192–1196.

57. Ng Sze-fong, Waxman DJ. Biotransformation of thioTEPA: Oxidative desulfuration to yield TEPA associated with suicide inactivation of a phenobarbital-inducible hepatic P-450 monooxygenase. Cancer Res 1990:50:467–471.
58. Cohen BE, Egorin MJ, Balachandran Nayar MS, Gutierrez PL. Effects of pH and temperature on the stability and decomposition of thioTEPA in urine and buffer. Cancer Res 1984:44:4312–4316.
59. Egorin MJ, Snyder SW, Pan S-S, Daly C. Cellular transport and accumulation of thiotepa. Semin Oncol 1990:17(suppl 3):7–17.
60. Przepiorka D, Madden T, Ippoliti C, Estrov Z, Dimopoulos M. Dosing of thioTEPA for myeloablative therapy. Cancer Chemother Pharmacol 1995:37: 155–160.
61. Xu QA, Trissel LA, Zhang Y, et al. Stability of thiotepa (lyophilized) in 5% dextrose injection at 4 and 23°C. Am J Health Syst Pharm 1996:53:2728–2730.
62. Brock N. Oxazaphosphorine cytostatics: Past—Present—Future. Cancer Res 1989:49:1–7.
63. Struck RF, Schmid SM, Waud WR. Antitumor activity of halogen analogs of phosphoramide, isophosphoramide, and triphosphoramide mustards, the cytotoxic metabolites of cyclophosphamide, ifosfamide, and trofosfamide. Cancer Chemother Pharmacol 1994:34:191–196.
64. Przepiorka D, Ippoliti C, Giralt K, et al. A phase I-II study of high-dose thiotepa, busulfan and cyclophosphamide as a preparative regimen for allogenic marrow transplantation. Bone Marrow Transplant 1994:14:449–453.
65. Grochow LB, Colvin M. Clinical pharmacokinetics of cyclophosphamide. In: MM Ames, G Powis, JS Kovach, eds. Pharmacokinetics of Anticancer Agents in Humans. Amsterdam-Elsevier Science Publishers, 1983, pp. 135–153.
66. Tasso MJ, Boddy AV, Price L, Wyllie RA, Pearson ADJ, Idle JR. Pharmacokinetics and metabolism of cyclophosphamide in paediatric patients. Cancer Chemother Pharmacol 1992:30:207–211.
67. Chang TKH, Weber GF, Crespi CL, Waxman DJ. Differential activation of cyclophosphamide and ifosfamide by cytochromes P-450 2B and 2A in human liver microsomes. Cancer Res 1993:53:5629–5637.
68. Yu L, Waxman DJ. Role of cytochrome P450 in oxazaphosphorine metabolism—Deactivation via N-dechloroethylation and activation via 4-hydroxylation catalyzed by distinct subsets of rat liver cytochromes P450. Drug Metab Dispos 1996:24:1254–1262.
69. Bohnenstengel F, Hofmann U, Eichelbaum M, Kroemer HK. Characterization of the cytochrome P450 involved in side-chain oxidation of cyclophosphamide in humans. Eur J Clin Pharmacol 1996:51:297–301.
70. Stilwell TJ, Benson RC. Cyclophosphamide-induced hemorrhagic cystitis—A review of 100 patients. Cancer 1988:61:451–457.
71. Brock N, Pohl J. The development of mesna for regional detoxification. Cancer Treatment Rev 1983:10(suppl A):33–43.
72. James CA, Mant T, Rogers HJ. Pharmacokinetics of intravenous and oral sodium 2-mercapto-ethane sulphonate (mesna) in normal subjects. Br J Clin Pharmacol 1987:23:561–568.

73. Katz A, Epelman S, Anelli A, et al. A prospective randomized evaluation of three schedules of mesna in patients receiving an ifosfamide-containing chemotherapy regimen: Sustained efficiency and simplified administration. J Cancer Res Clin Oncol 1995:121:128–131.
74. Haselberger TI, Schwinghammer MB. Efficacy of mesna for prevention of hemorrhagic cystitis after high-dose cyclophosphamide therapy. Ann Pharmacother 1995:29:918–921.
75. Hows JM, Mehta A, Ward L, Woods K, Perez R, Gordon MY, et al. Comparison of mesna with forced diuresis to prevent cyclophosphamide induced hemorrhagic cystitis in marrow transplantation: A prospective randomised study. Br J Cancer 1984:50:753–756.
76. Fleming RA, Cruz JM, Webb CB, et al. Urinary elimination of cyclophosphamide alkylating metabolites and free thiols following two administration schedules of high-dose cyclophosphamide and mesna. Bone Marrow Transplant 1996:17:497–501.
77. Hadidi AK, Coulter CE, Idle JR, et al. Phenotypically different urinary elimination of carboxyphosphamide after cyclophosphamide administration to cancer patients. Cancer Res 1988:48:5167–5171.
78. Graham MI, Shaw JC, Souhami RL, Sidau B, et al. Decreased plasma half-life of cyclophosphamide during repeated high-dose administration. Cancer Chemother Pharmacol 1983:10:192–193.
79. Schuler U, Ehninger G, Wagner T. Repeated high-dose cyclophosphamide administration in bone marrow transplantation: Exposure to activated metabolites. Cancer Chemother Pharmacol 1987:20:248–252.
80. Schwinghammer TL, Wiggins LE, Burgunder MR, Michell TE, Bailey WL. Adverse reactions related to i.v. infusion of high-dose cyclophosphamide in bone marrow transplant patients. Am J Hosp Pharm 1994:51:2419–2421.
81. Ayash LJ, Wright JE, Tretyakov O, Gonin R, et al. Cyclophosphamide pharmacokinetics: Correlation with cardiac toxicity and tumor response. J Clin Oncol 1992:10:995–1000.
82. Slattery JT, Kalhorn TF, McDonald GB, et al. Conditioning regimen-dependent disposition of cyclophosphamide and hydroxycyclophosphamide in human marrow transplantation patients. J Clin Oncol 1996:14:1484–1494.
83. Chen T-L, Kennedy MJ, Anderson LW, et al. Nonlinear pharmacokinetics of cyclophosphamide and 4-hydroxycyclophosphamide/aldophosphamide in patients with metastatic breast cancer receiving high-dose chemotherapy followed by autologous bone marrow transplantation. Drug Metab Dispos 1997: 25:544–551.
84. Zalupski M, Baker LH. Ifosfamide. J Natl Cancer Inst 1988:80:556–566.
85. Bokemeyer C. Current trends in chemotherapy for metastatic nonseminomatous testicular germ cell tumors. Oncology 1998:55:177–188.
86. Dechant KL, Brogden RN, Pilkington T, Faulds D. Ifosfamide/mesna—A review of its antineoplastic activity, pharmacokinetic properties and therapeutic efficacy in cancer. Drugs 1991:42(3):428–467.
87. Wagner T. Ifosfamide clinical pharmacokinetics. Clin Pharmacokinet 1994: 26:439–456.

88. Gilard V, Malet-Martino MC, de Forni M, Niemeyer U, Ader JC, Marino R. Determination of the urinary excretion of ifosfamide and its phosphorated metabolites by phosphorus-31 nuclear magnetic resonance spectroscopy. Cancer Chemother Pharmacol 1993:31:387–394.
89. Wainer IW, Ducharme J, Granvil CP, et al. The N-dechloroethylation of ifosfamide: Using stereochemistry to obtain an accurate picture of a clinically relevant metabolic pathway. Cancer Chemother Pharmacol 1996:37:332–336.
90. Walker D, Flinois J-P, Monkman SC, et al. Identification of the major human hepatic cytochrome P450 involved in activation and N-dechlorethylation of ifosfamide. Biochem Pharmacol 1994:47:1157–1163.
91. Kaijser GP, Korst A, Beijnen JH, Bult A, Underberg WJM. The analysis of ifosfamide and its metabolites. Anticancer Res 1993:13:1311–1324.
92. Joqueviel C, Gilard V, Martino R, Malet-Martino M, Niemeyer U. Urinary stability of carboxyphosphamide and carboxyifosfamide, two major metabolites of the anticancer drugs cyclophosphamide and ifosfamide. Cancer Chemother Pharmacol 1997:40:391–399.
93. Lind MJ, Margison JM, Cerny T, Thatcher N, Wilkinson PM. Comparative pharmacokinetics and alkylating activity of fractionated intravenous and oral ifosfamide in patients with bronchogenic carcinoma. Cancer Res 1989:49: 753–757.
94. Schoenike SE, Dana WJ. Ifosfamide and mesna. Clin Pharm 1990:9:179–191.
95. Boddy AV, Cole M, Pearson ADJ, Idle JR. The kinetics of the auto-induction of ifosfamide metabolism during continuous infusion. Cancer Chemother Pharmacol 1995:36:53–60.
96. Lewis LD, Fitzgerald DL, Harper PG, Rogers HJ. Fractionated ifosfamide therapy produces a time-dependent increase in ifosfamide metabolism. Br J Clin Pharmacol 1990:30:725–732.
97. Lind MJ, Margison JM, Cerny T, et al. Prolongation of ifosfamide elimination half-life in obese patients due to altered drug distribution. Cancer Chemother Pharmacol 1989:25:139–142.
98. Garcia AA. Ifosfamide-induced Fanconi syndrome. Ann Pharmacother 1995: 29:590–591.
99. Skinner R, Sharkey IM, Pearson ADJ, Craft AW. Ifosfamide, mesna, and nephrotoxicity in children. J Clin Oncol 1993:11:173–190.
100. MacLean FR, Skinner R, Hall AG, et al. Acute changes in urine protein excretion may predict chronic ifosfamide nephrotoxicity: a preliminary observation. Cancer Chemother Pharmacol 1998:41:413–416.
101. Lewis LD, Meanwell CA. Ifosfamide pharmacokinetics and neurotoxicity. Lancet 1990:335:175–176.
102. Miller LJ, Eaton VE. Ifosfamide-induced neurotoxicity: A case report and review of the literature. Ann Pharmacother 1992:26:183–187.
103. Goren MP, Wright RK, Pratt C, Bell FE. Dechloroethylation of ifosfamide and neurotoxicity. Lancet 1986:II:1219–1230.
104. Granvil CP, Duchrame J, Leyland-Jones B, et al. Stereoselective pharmacokinetics of ifosfamide and its 2- and 3-N-dechloroethylated metabolites in female cancer patients. Cancer Chemother Pharmacol 1996:37:451–456.

105. Wainer IW, Ducharme J, Granvil CP, et al. Ifosfamide stereoselective dechloroethylation and neurotoxicity. Lancet 1994:343:982–983.
106. Kurowski V, Wagner T. Comparative pharmacokinetics of ifosfamide, 4-hydroxyifosfamide, chloroacetaldehyde, and 2- and 3-dechloroethylifosfamide in patients on fractionated intravenous ifosfamide therapy. Cancer Chemother Pharmacol 1993:33:36–42.
107. Wagner T. Mode of action of ifosfamide—New aspects. Onkologie 1998: 21(Suppl. 2):1–4.
108. Highley MS, Momerency G, van Cauwenberghe K, et al. Formation of chloroethylamine and 1,3-oxazolidine-2-one following ifosfamide administration in humans. Drug Metab Dispos 1995:23:433–437.
109. Hofmann U, Eichelbaum M, Seefried S, Meese CO. Identification of thiodiglycolic acid sulfoxide, and (3-carboxymethylthio)lactic acid as major human biotransformation products of *S*-carboxymethyl-L-cysteine. Drug Metab Dispos 1991:19:222–226.
110. Lauterburg BH, Nguyen T, Hartmann B, Junker E, Küpfer A, Cerny T. Depletion of total cysteine, glutathione, and homocysteine in plasma by ifosfamide/mesna therapy. Cancer Chemother Pharmacol 1994:35:132–136.
111. Bhardwaj A, Badesha PS. Ifosfamide-induced nonconvulsive status epilepticus. Ann Pharmacother 1995:29:1237–1239.
112. Aeschlimann C, Cerny T, Küpfer A. Inhibition of (mono)Amine oxidase activity and prevention of ifosfamide encephalopathy by methylene blue. Drug Metabol Dispos 1996:24:1336–1339.
113. Pecci L, Montefoschi G, Fontana M, Cavallini D. Aminoethylcysteine ketimine decarboxylated dimer inhibits mitochondrial respiration by impairing electron transport at complex I level. Biochem Biophys Res Commun 1994:199: 755–760.
114. Cavallini D, Ricci G, Dupré S, et al. Sulfur-containing cyclic ketimines and imino acids. Eur J Biochem 1991:202:217–223.
115. Boddy AV, Yule SM, Wyllie R, et al. Comparison of continuous infusion and bolus administration of ifosfamide in children. Eur J. Cancer 1995:31A:785–790.
116. Boos J, Silies H, Hohenlöchter B, Jürgens H, Blascke G. Short-term versus continuous infusion: No influence on ifosfamide side-chain metabolism. Eur J Cancer 1995:31A:2418–2419.
117. Lewis LD, Fitzgerald DL, Mohan P, Thatcher N, et al. The pharmacokinetics of ifosfamide given as short and long intravenous infusions in cancer patients. Br J Clin Pharmacol 1991:31:77–82.
118. Cerny T, Castiglione M, Brunner K, et al. Ifosfamide by continuous infusion to prevent encephalopathy. Lancet 1990:335:175.
119. Boddy AV, English M, Pearson ADJ, Idle JR, Skinner R. Ifosfamide nephrotoxicity: Limited influence of metabolism and mode of administration during repeated therapy in paediatrics. Eur J Cancer 1996:32A:1179–1184.
120. Wright JE, Elias A, Tretyakov O, Holden S, et al. High-dose ifosfamide, carboplatin and etoposide pharmaco-kinetics: Correlation of plasma drug levels with renal toxicity. Cancer Chemother Pharmacol 1995:36:345–351.

121. Willemse PHB, de Jong PE, Elema JD, Mulder NH. Severe renal failure following high-dose ifosfamide and mesna. Cancer Chemother Pharmacol 1989:23:329–330.
122. Fields KK, Elfenbein GJ, Lazarus HM, et al. Maximum-tolerated dose of ifosfamide, carboplatin, and etoposide given over 6 days followed by autologous stem cell rescue: Toxicity Profile. J Clin Oncol 1995:13:323–332.
123. Le Cesne A, Antoine E, Spielmann M, et al. High-dose ifosfamide: Circumvention of resistance to standard-dose ifosfamide in advanced soft tissue sarcomas. J Clin Oncol 1995:13:1600–1608.
124. Rosen G, Forscher C, Lowenbraun S, et al. Synovial sarcoma. Cancer 1994: 73:2506–2511.
125. Boddy AV, Yule SM, Wyllie R, et al. Intrasubject variation in children of ifosfamide pharmacokinetics and metabolism during repeated administration. Cancer Chemother Pharmacol 1996:38:147–154.
126. Falkson G, Falkson HC. Trofosfamide in the treatment of patients with cancer. S Afr Med J 1987:53:886.
127. Hempel G, Krümpelmann S, May-Manke A, et al. Pharmacokinetics of trofosfamide and its dechloroethylated metabolites. Cancer Chemother Pharmacol 1997:40:45–50.
128. Henry MC, Marlow M. Preclinical toxicologic study of procarbazine. Cancer Chemother Rep 1973:4:97–102.
129. Prough RA, Tweedie DJ. Procarbazine. In: G Powis, RA Prough, eds. Metabolism and Action of Anticancer Drugs. Oxford: Taylor & Francis, 1987, pp. 29–47.
130. Tweedie DJ, Fernandez D, Spearman ME, et al. Metabolism of azoxy derivatives of procarbazine by aldehyde dehydrogenase and xanthine oxidase. Drug Metab Dispos 1991:19:793–803.
131. Goria-Gatti L, Iannone A, Tomasi A, Poli G, Albano E. In vitro and in vivo evidence for the formation of methyl radical from procarbazine: A spin-trapping study. Carcinogenesis 1992:13(5):799–805.
132. Swaffar DS, Harker WG, Pomerantz SC, et al. Isolation, purification and characterization of two new chemical decomposition products of methylazoxyprocarbazine. Drug Metabol Dispos 1992:20(5):632–642.
133. Breithaupt H, Dammann A, Aigner K. Pharmacokinetics of dacarbazine (DTIC) and its metabolite 5-aminoimidazole-4-carboxamide (AIC) following different dose schedules. Cancer Chemother Pharmacol 1982:9:103–109.
134. Chabot GG, Flaherty LE, Valdivieso M, Baker LH. Alteration of dacarbazine pharmacokinetics after interleukin-2 administration in melanoma patients. Cancer Chemother Pharmacol 1990:27(2):157–160.
135. Shuekla S. A device to prevent photodegradation of decarbazine (DTIC). Clin Radiol 1980:31(2):239–240.
136. Kirk B. The evaluation of a light-protecting giving set—The photosensitivity of intravenous dacarbazine solutions. Intensive Ther Clin Monit May/June 1987:78–86.
137. Dennis IF, Ramsay JR, Workman P, Bleehen NM. Pharmacokinetics of BW12C and mitomycin C, given in combination in a phase 1 study in patients

with advanced gastrointestinal cancer. Cancer Chemother Pharmacol 1993:32: 67–72.
138. Tetef M, Margolin K, Ahn C, et al. Mitomycin C and menadione for the treatment of advanced gastrointestinal cancers: A phase II trial. J Cancer Res Clin Oncol 1995:121:103–106.
139. Bachur NR, Gordon SL, Gee MV. A general mechanism for microsomal activation of guinine anticancer agents to free radicals. Cancer Res. 1978:38: 1745–1750.
140. Bizanek R, Chowdary D, Arai H, et al. Adducts of mitomycin C and DNA in EMT6 mouse mammary tumor cells: Effects of hypoxia and dicumarol on adduct pattern. Cancer Res 1993:53:5127–5134.
141. Dorr RT. New findings in the pharmacokinetic, metabolic and drug-resistance aspects of mitomycin C. Semin Oncol 1988:15(suppl 4):32–41.
142. Cummings J, Spanswick VJ, Smyth JF. Reevaluation of the molecular pharmacology of mitomycin C. Eur J Cancer 1995:31A:1928–1933.
143. Hoey BM, Butler J, Swallow AJ. Reductive activation of mitomycin C. Biochemistry 1988:27:2608–2614.
144. Bonomi PD, Mladineo J, Morrin B, et al. Phase-II trial of hexamethylmelamine in ovarian carcinoma resistant to alkylating agents. Cancer Treatment Rep 1979:63:137–138.
145. Foster BJ, Harding BJ, Leyland-Jones B, Hoth D. Hexamethylmelamine: A critical review of an active drug. Cancer Treatment Rev 1986:13:197–217.
146. Ames MM. Hexamethylmelamine: Pharmacology and mechanism of action. Cancer Treatment Rev 1991:18(suppl A):3–14.
147. Ames MM, Richardson RL, Kovach JS, et al. Phase I and clinical pharmacological evaluation of a parenteral hexamethylmelamine formulation. Cancer Res 1990:50:206–210.
148. Ames MM, Sanders ME, Tiede WS. Role of *N*-methylolpentamethylmelamine in the metabolic activation of hexamethylmelamine. Cancer Res 1983:43:500–504.
149. Ames MM, Kovach JS. Parenteral formulation of hexamethylmelamine potentially suitable for use in man. Cancer Treatment Rep 1982:66:1579–1581.
150. Carter SK. An overview of the status of the nitrosoureas in other tumors. Cancer Chemother Rep 1973:4:35–46.
151. Lemoine A, Lucas C, Ings RMJ. Review: Metabolism of the chloroethylnitrosoureas. Xenobiotica 1991:21:775–791.
152. Diksic M, Sako K, Feindel W, Kato AK, et al. Pharmacokinetics of positron-labeled 1,3-bis(2-chloroethyl)-nitrosourea in human brain tumor using positron emission tomography. Cancer Res 1984:44:3120–3124.
153. Phillips GL, Wolff SN, Fay JW, et al. Intensive BCNU chemotherapy and autologous marrow transplantation for malignant glioma. J Clin Oncol 1986: 4:639–645.
154. Reed DJ, May HE, Boose RB, et al. 2-Chloroethanol formation as evidence for a 2-chloroethyl alkylating intermediate during chemical degradation of 1-(2-chloroethyl)-3-cyclohexyl-1-nitrosourea and 1-(2-chloroethyl)-3(*trans*-4-methylcyclohexyl)-1-nitrosourea. Cancer Res 1975:35:568–576.

155. Henner WD, Peters WP, Eder P, et al. Pharmacokinetics and immediate effects of high-dose carmustine in man. Cancer Treatment Rep 1986:70:877–880.
156. Seidegard J, Pero RW, Miller DG, Beattie EJ. A glutathione transferase in human leucocytes as a marker for the susceptibility to lung cancer. Carcinogenesis 1986:7:751–753.
157. Jones RB, Matthes S, Shpall EJ, et al. Acute lung injury following treatment with high-dose cyclophosphamide, cisplatin, and carmustine: Pharmacodynamic evaluation of carmustine. J Natl Cancer Inst 1993:85:640–647.
158. Babson JR, Reed DJ. Inactivation of glutathione reductase by 2-chloroethyl-nitroso-urea derived isocyanates. Biochem Biophys Res Commun 1978:83:754–762.
159. Smith AC, Boyd MR. Preferential effects of 1,3-bis(2-chloroethyl)-1-nitrosourea (BCNU) on pulmonary glutathione reductase and glutathione/glutathione disulfide ratios: Possible implications for lung toxicity. J Pharmacol Exp Ther 1984:229:658–663.
160. Lee FYF, Workman P, Roberts JT, et al. Clinical pharmacokinetics of oral CCNU (lomustine). Cancer Chemother Pharmacol 1985:14:125–131.
161. Borel AG, Abbott FS. Identification of carbamoylated thiol conjugates as metabolites of the antineoplastic 1-(2-chloroethyl)-3-cyclohexyl-1-nitrosourea, in rats and humans. Drug Metab Dispos 1993:21:889–901.
162. Kastirissios H, Chao NJ, Blaschke TF. Pharmacokinetics of high-dose oral CCNU in bone marrow transplant patients. Cancer Chemother Pharmacol 1996:38:425–430.
163. Nishigaka T, Nakamura K, Kinoshita T, et al. Identification of major urinary metabolites of ACNU 3-[4-amino-2-methyl-5-pyrimidinyl)methyl]-1-(2-chloroethyl)-1-nitrosourea hydrochloride in rats. Pharmacobiol Dyn 1985:8:401–408.
164. Harada K, Kiya K, Uozomi T. Pharmacokinetics of a new water-soluble nitrosourea derivative (ACNU) in human gliomas. Surg Neurol 1980:15:410–415.
165. Adolphe AB, Glasofer ED, Troetel WM, et al. Fate of streptozocin (NSC-85998) in patients with advanced cancer. Cancer Chemother Rep 1975:59:547–556.
166. Ferner RE. Drug-induced diabetes. Baillieres Clin Endocrinol Metab 1992:6(4):849–866.
167. Ings RMJ, Gray AJ, Taylor AR, et al. Disposition, pharmacokinetics and metabolism of ^{14}C-fotemustine in cancer patients. Eur J Cancer 1990:26:838–842.
168. Iliadis A, Launay-Iliadis MC, Lucas C, et al. Pharmacokinetics and pharmacodynamics of nitrosourea fotemustine: A French cancer centre multicentric study. Eur J Cancer 1996:32A:455–460.
169. Lee SM, Margison GP, Thatcher N, et al. Formation and loss of *O*6-methyldeoxyguanosine in human leucoyte DNA following sequential DTIC and fotemustine chemotherapy. Br J Cancer 1994:69(5):853–857.

2.2 PLATINUM COMPOUNDS AS ANTICANCER DRUGS

Cisplatin (Fig. 15) is one of the most commonly used drugs in clinical oncology. It is active against solid tumors of several types, particularly head and neck, bladder, ovarian, testicular cancer, SCLC, and NSCLC, but nephrotoxicity and neurotoxicity are often dose-limiting [1–3]. Vigorous hydration as well as accurate osmodiuresis reduce the risk of severe nephrotoxic side effects, although the optimal amounts of hydration and mannitol required for optimal nephroprotection have not yet been clearly defined [4,5]. The outcome of a massive overdose of cisplatin is generally fatal [6].

Carboplatin (Fig. 15) is a second-generation platinum-containing compound with impressive antineoplastic activity, whereas its nephrotoxic, neu-

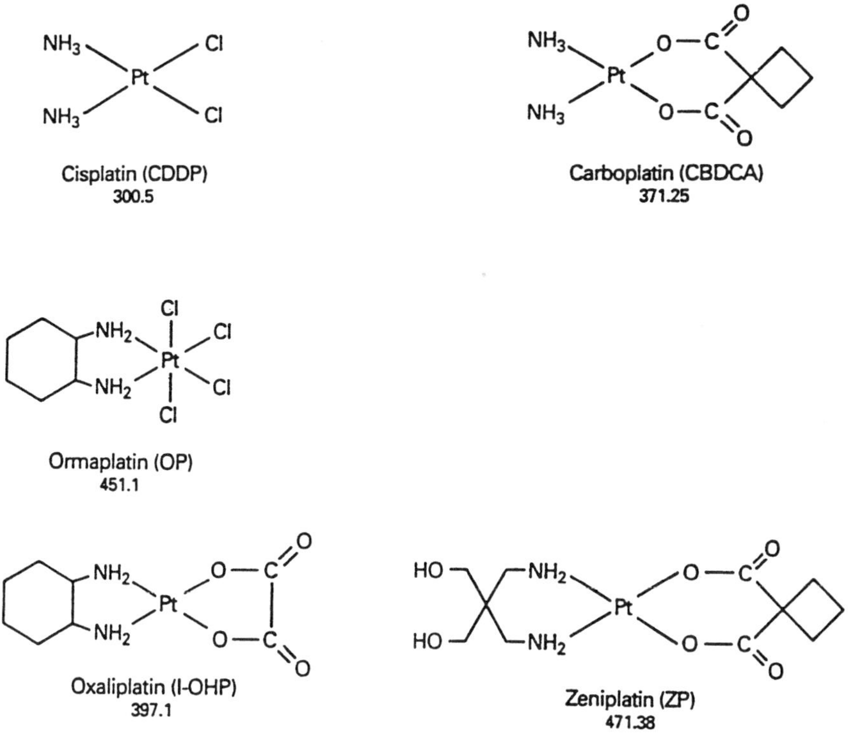

Cisplatin (CDDP)
300.5

Carboplatin (CBDCA)
371.25

Ormaplatin (OP)
451.1

Oxaliplatin (l-OHP)
397.1

Zeniplatin (ZP)
471.38

Fig. 15 Chemical structures of cisplatin, caboplatin, and some newer analogues (and their corresponding molecular weights).

rotoxic, ototoxic, as well as emetogenic potency is less than that of the structurally related cisplatin [7–10]. There is increasing evidence that the level of carboplatin AUC can be closely correlated with the incidence and severity of hematological toxicity and possibly antitumoral efficacy. As a consequence, an individually adapted AUC within a defined therapeutic range (e.g., 4–7.5 mg/mL/min) represents a great step forward in the individualization of cancer chemotherapy [11,12]. Other platinum-compounds, including oxaliplatin and zeniplatin, are currently under investigation [7]. The new diamminocyclohexane derivative oxaliplatin appears to be non-nephrotoxic, is associated with minimal myelosuppressive side effects, and has demonstrated promising activity against colorectal cancer in combination with 5-fluorouracil and folinic acid [7].

2.2.1 Cisplatin

Cisplatin [*cis*-diaminedichloroplatinum(II), CCDP] is a potent anticancer agent for the treatment of a variety of tumors (e.g., testicular, ovarian, bladder, head/neck and esophageal cancer). The usually recommended dose is 100 mg/m^2 1–5, every 3–4 weeks, which may be given once or consecutively on two or five days as 50 mg/m^2 d1 + 2 or 20 mg/m^2 d1–5.

Cisplatin is a square-planar complex consisting of a central platinum atom with two amino and two chloro ligands. Particularly in the cell, where the chloride concentration is lower than in the extracellular medium, the drug undergoes a ligand exchange that results in the formation of an extremely reactive *cis*-diaminediaquoplatinum(II) complex. The displacement of nucleophilic ligands leads to the formation of a variety of macromolecular platinum adducts (Fig. 16). However, the antineoplastic activity of cisplatin appears to be mainly based on the covalent binding of the complex to N-7 atoms of the purine bases guanine and adenine, leading to the formation of intrastrand and interstrand DNS cross-links that cannot be easily repaired [10,13].

The drug is widely distributed into body tissues. High concentrations were recovered in the kidneys, liver, and intestine, whereas penetration into CNS tissue seems to be poor to moderate. The elimination of cisplatin after IV administration is at least triphasic, with an initial half-life about 14–37 minutes and a secondary half-life of about 15–190 hours [14–17]. The terminal elimination half-life is difficult to determine because in cancer patients even after 8 years the urinary platinum excretion may be 40 times higher than the background level (>0.8 vs. 0.02 μg/g creatinine). Within 1 hour after administration of 50 mg cisplatin/m^2, about 15% of the parent compound is supposed to be excreted in the urine [18,19].

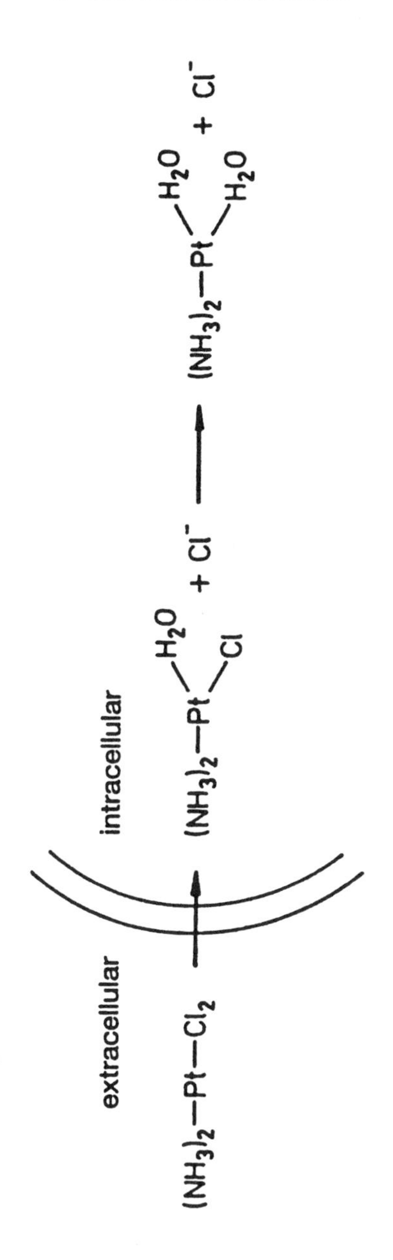

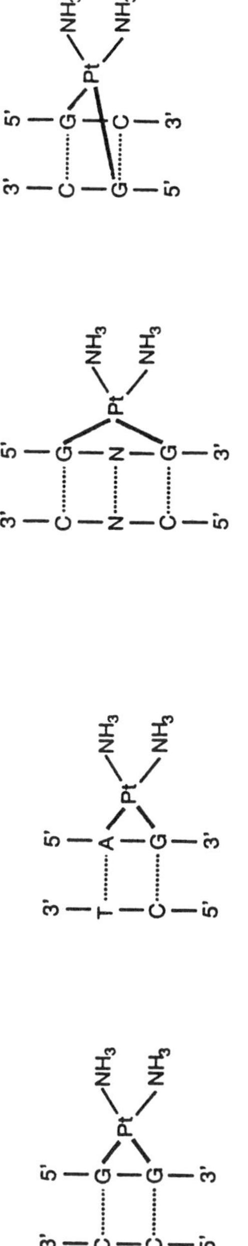

Fig. 16 Within the cell, the platinum compounds undergo a ligand exchange resulting in the corresponding and very reactive diaquoplatinum(II) complexes. As a consequence, a variety of intrastrand and interstrand DNA cross-links are formed.

Cisplatin binds to a very high amount to plasma and tissue proteins, which results in a variety of macromolecular platinum complexes. After 24 hours more than 95% of CDDP dose is bound to plasma proteins and tissues [14–17].

Platinum–protein complexes of low molecular weight may be excreted rather rapidly, whereas complexes of high molecular weight must first undergo enzymatic degradation. These adducts have very long half-lives, which range from several days to years. Because of its very extensive plasma protein binding over time, the drug seems to be dialyzable in significant amounts only within the first 30–60 minutes after administration [20]. If an anephric cancer patient needs CDDP, it is reasonable to determine his or her pharmacokinetic parameters with a CDDP test dose before the full CDDP dose is administered [21].

There is some evidence that liver enzymes, particularly cytochrome P450 isozymes, may form covalent platinum adducts during cisplatin therapy, too, which may explain in part the decreased metabolic clearance of other anticancer drugs (e.g., etoposide, paclitaxel) that is observed shortly after exposure to cisplatin. Additionally cisplatin may impair the renal excretion of other drugs, like topotecan, which explains that topotecan should precede cisplatin administration. Particularly in the case of cisplatin and taxoid combination chemotherapy there is some evidence that intracellular taxoid binding sites may be altered if cisplatin precedes taxoid administra tion. In conclusion, it is generally accepted that cisplatin not precede paclitaxel administration [22,23].

In spite of several controversial discussions the need for dosage adjustments in the presence of renal dysfunction has been generally established. It has been recommended to use only 50% of the usual dose, if the creatinine clearance ranges from 30–60 ml/min. Cisplatin is contraindicant if the creatinine clearance is less than 30 ml/min, because an end-stage renal failure may be provoked [24,25]. According to the results of Thyss et al., moderate CDDP doses (e.g., 60 mg/m^2) may be still applicable without dose reduction to elderly patients having a mean initial creatinine clearance of about 50 mL/min, since renal function appears to be preserved by accurate hydration [26].

The intraperitoneal administration of CDDP has been proposed for patients with histologically proven cancer primarily confined to the peritoneal cavity and refractory to conventional therapy. By this administration route the CDDP dose could be intensified up to 270 mg/m^2, particularly if concomitant sodium thiosulfate (STS) is used as a protectant. If CDDP is distributed into the systemic circulation either via the capillaries of the parietal peritoneal membrane or indirectly via absorption into the portal circulation or into the lymphatics, STS may rapidly inactivate the agent in plasma and kidneys [27–29]. However, this intensified regimen has not been established in clinical practice so far.

2.2.1.1 Clinical Pharmacokinetics Regarding Efficacy and Toxicity

According to several pharmacokinetic studies, there seems to be a close correlation between the severity of CDDP-induced nephrotoxicity or neurotoxicity and cumulative dose of CDDP [30–32]. There is some evidence that cisplatin-induced nephrotoxicity may be associated with high peak plasma concentrations (>6 μg/mL). Thus, the avoidance of short infusion time is recommended during high-dose therapy, inasmuch as several clinical studies have shown that a longer infusion time (e.g., >4–6 h) can reduce the risk of severe nephrotoxic side effects [14,30]. This in accordance with the observation that very high levels of CDDP DNA adducts can be detected in tubular cells within 1 hour of CDDP treatment. The prolongation of infusion time may avoid both the oversaturation of tubular reabsorption processes and potent tissue protection mainly based on glutathione-dependent mechanisms. If further data confirm that efficacy is not impaired by prolonged infusion, it seems reasonable to avoid high cisplatin peak concentrations in plasma and renal tubules [4,5].

There is some evidence that plasma platinum concentrations vary considerably among individuals and indeed may change intraindividually after several courses. For example, peak levels may range from 0.67 to 3.76 μg/mL after 80 mg/m^2 cisplatin among cancer patients. Since cancer patients with peak plasma concentrations or steady-state levels of unchanged cisplatin exceeding 2 μg/mL may be at a higher risk for nephrotoxicity, whereas levels less than 1.5 μg/mL may not provide sufficient antineoplastic activity, it might be prudent to monitor the individual platinum levels more closely with special regard to dose intensification [14,17].

Recently, Lagrange and colleagues measured tumoral platinum concentrations after 5 mg of cisplatin had been infused over 5 days combined with radiotherapy. Biopsy samples were taken from the accessible tumor mass. These authors found a marked variation in tumoral as well as plasma Pt concentrations. Total Pt concentration in plasma as well as in tumoral tissue increased during the treatment cycles. However, the short interval between cisplatin administration and radiotherapy, rather than absolute tissue concentration, may be more critical for arriving at the most effective combination therapy [33].

Usually platinum is quantified by flameless atomic absorption spectrophotometry or HPLC [33–35]. Analysis of total platinum is technically easier to perform than the determination of free platinum levels and appears to be closely correlated with the levels of ultrafilterable platinum [35].

2.2.2 Carboplatin

Carboplatin [*cis*-diammine(1,1-cyclobutanedicarboxylato)platinum(II), CBDCA, JM8; NCS-241240, Paraplatin] is a second-generation platinum compound with proven activity against a range of malignant solid tumors [2,7]. Recently, it has been recommended that a conventional carboplatin dosing be performed according to a target AUC ranging from 4.0 to 7.5 mg × min/ml [11,12]. However, usual dosage recommendations are still based on body surface area ranging from 300 to 400 mg/m^2. High doses of carboplatin (e.g., 1500–2000 mg/m^2 IV in total) have been used in high-dose combination chemotherapy followed by autologous stem cell transplantation [36–38].

Following i.v. administration of carboplatin, the initial half-life (distribution phase) ranges from 6 to 20 minutes and the β-elimination half-life averages 2.5 hours. The systemic clearance approximates 54 mL/min/m^2. Over a dose range of 50–500 mg/m^2 carboplatin, there is a linear relationship between dose, plasma peak level (C_{max}) and the corresponding AUC value. Even at high doses of 1200 mg/m^2, there seems to be close correlation between dose and corresponding AUC. The clinical pharmacokinetics of carboplatin seems to be very similar in adult and pediatric patients.

The drug is widely distributed into body tissues, with highest concentrations in the kidneys, liver, skin, and tumor tissue. Especially after the administration of very high doses, carboplatin is also detectable in the cerebrospinal fluid, in ascites as well as in pleural effusions. The distribution volume averages 16–17 L/m^2.

Within 24 hours about 70% of the dose is excreted in the urine, primarily via glomerular filtration. This in contrast to the structurally related cisplatin, which is eliminated by both glomerular filtration and tubular secretion. The total body clearance of carboplatin approximates 4.4 L/h [39–43].

After glomerular filtration, carboplatin undergoes slow chemical decomposition because the acidic pH of urine facilitates degradation of the intact drug. The chemical half-life of carboplatin in urine at 37°C averages 42 hours. In contrast to cisplatin, the reactivity of carboplatin to proteins in plasma is even less. As a consequence, the elimination half-life of total and unbound (ultrafilterable) platinum is quite similar after 100 minutes of i.v. carboplatin administration. However, the percentage of protein-bound platinum increases over time. During the first 4 hours after administration, about 25% of carboplatin is bound to plasma proteins, whereas after 20 hours more than 85% is protein bound. Like cisplatin, the macromolecular platinum–protein complexes may be decomposed very slowly over time, which may be why the urinary excretion of total platinum increases over a long period of time after treatment [39–43].

2.2.2.1 Clinical Pharmacokinetics Regarding Efficacy and Toxicity

After intravenous administration of carboplatin, about 60–80% of the dose undergoes glomerular filtration as unchanged drug within 24 hours. Because of the underlying high variability of individual glomerular filtration rates (e.g., 10–180 mL/min) the AUC values may range from 2 to 11 mg × min/mL after i.v. administration of 300 mg/m^2 carboplatin (Fig. 17) [44–47].

The results of Jodrell et al. and other study groups however, suggest that AUC values of at least 4 mg × min/mL seem to be necessary to avoid suboptimal effectiveness, whereas AUC values exceeding 7.5 mg × min/mL may be associated with severe myelosuppressive side effects during conventional therapy [11,12,48].

According to the correlation *Dose = AUC × clearance*, Calvert has developed a formula (Table 5) with which a special carboplatin dose (mg) can be calculated to achieve a target AUC value. In his formula [Dose = AUC × (GFR + 25)], the 25 represents the percentage of drug that is not excreted in the urine within 24 hours [49,50].

The AUC values that should be achieved range from 4 to 7 mg × min/mL and are dependent on the therapeutic setting (combination vs. monotherapy) as well as the pretreatment of the patients (Table 6) [11,12,48].

GFR determinations based on the radionuclide [^{51}Cr]EDTA method appear to be most accurate, because those results reflect the real physiologic condition very closely. GFR determinations based on urine collection or on mathematical calculations (according to formula of Jeliffe or Cockcroft-Gault) do not reflect real conditions as closely as the radionuclide method (Table 7) [49,51–53].

The mathematical calculations especially (e.g., according to Cockcroft-Gault) will result in an underestimation of the real GFR value in patients with a constitutive creatinine clearance exceeding 100 mL/min. Additionally, it has been recommended that the mathematical calculation not be performed in patients with massive obesity, hepatic dysfunction (e.g., liver enzymes twice as high as the normal level), or rather unstable serum creatinine values [49,51–53].

Undoubtedly the use of the Calvert formula in adult cancer patients (Table 5) represents great progress in diminishing interindividual variability of carboplatin AUC values. AUC variations of up to 300%, which are com-

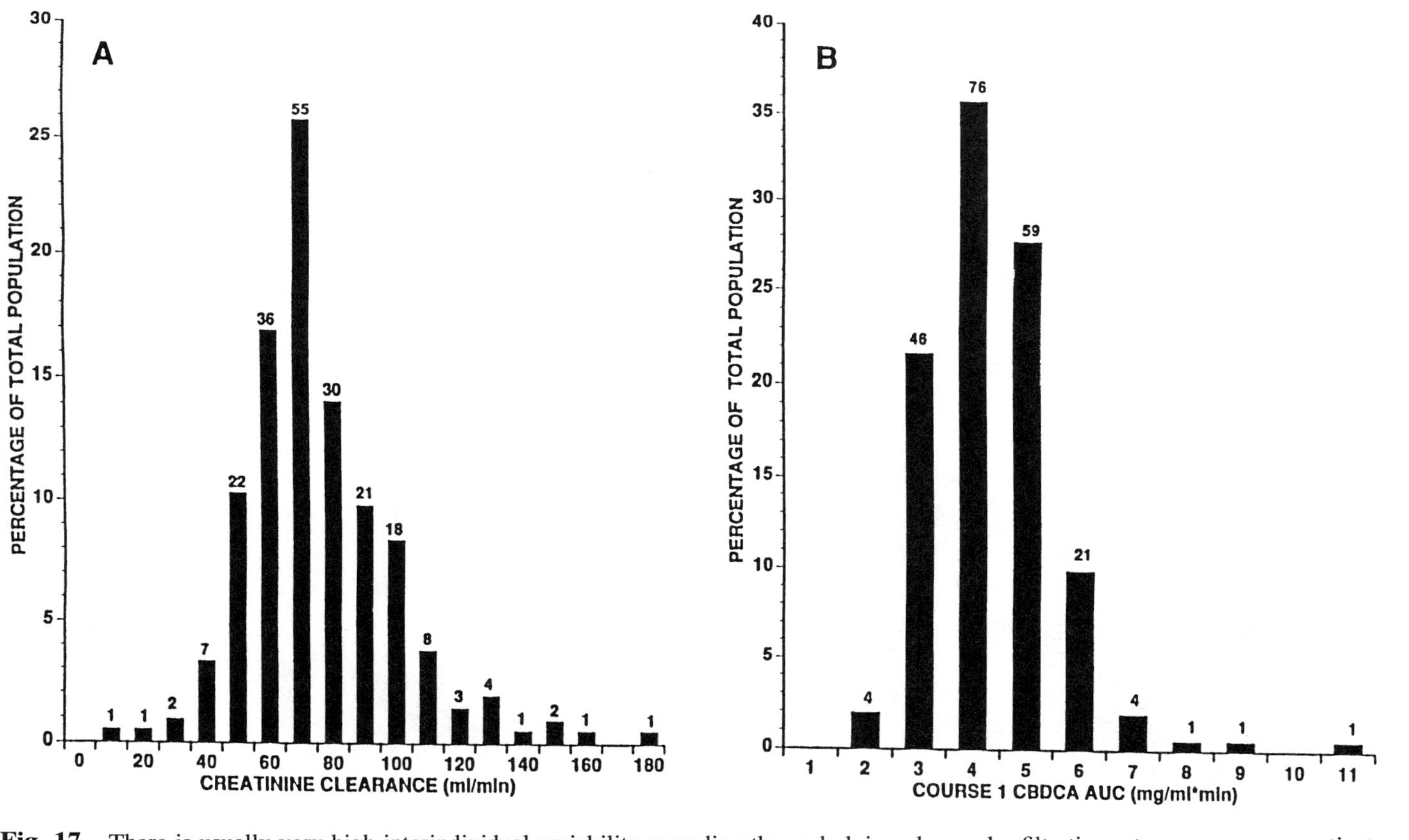

Fig. 17 There is usually very high interindividual variability regarding the underlying glomerular filtration rate among cancer patients. As a consequence, carboplatin AUC values may range from 2 to 11 mg/mL/min, if the drug (e.g., 300 mg/m^2) is given according to body surface area. Data according to the study results of Reyno and colleagues [44].

Table 5 The Formulas of Calvert and Chatelut, with which the Absolute Carboplatin Dose (mg) Can Be Calculated in Adult Cancer Patients

Calvert's formula

$$\text{Carboplatin dose} = \text{target AUC } (\text{GFR} + 25)$$

Chatelut's formula

$$\text{Carboplatin dose} = \text{target AUC} \times \text{carboplatin clearance}$$

Determination of carboplatin clearance (mL/min)[a,b]

$$0.134 \times \text{BW} + \frac{[218 \times \text{BW} \times (1 - 0.00457 \times \text{age})][(1 - 0.314 \times S)]}{\text{serum creatinine } (\mu\text{M})}$$

[a]BW, body weight (kg); age in years; S, sex (male = 0, female = 1).
[b]Serum creatinine (mg/dL) × 88.4 = serum creatinine (μmol/L; i.e., micromolar form).

Table 6 Target Carboplatin AUC Values in Conventional Cancer Chemotherapy

Therapy; pretreatment status	Target AUC
Carboplatin monotherapy	
Not previously treated with cytostatics	5–7
Previously treated with cytostatics	4–6
Combination chemotherapy	
Not previously treated with cytostatics	4–6

Table 7 Calculation According to the Formulas of Cockcroft–Gault and Jeliffe (in modified form) of the Individual Glomerular Filtration Rate Based on the Serum Creatinine Value (mg %)

Cockcroft–Gault formula[a]

$$\text{GFR (mL/min)} = \frac{(140 - \text{age}) \times \text{body weight}}{72 \times \text{serum creatinine (mg/dl)}} \times S$$

Jeliffe formula (modified form)[b]

$$\text{GFR (mL/min)} = \frac{[(98 - 0.8)(\text{Age} - 20)]}{\text{serum creatinine (mg/dl)}} \times \frac{\text{BSA}}{1.73} \times S$$

[a]Age in years; body weight in kilograms; S, sex (male = 1, female = 0.85).
[b]Age in years; body surface area (BSA) in meters squared; S, sex (male = 1, female = 0.9).

mon when carboplatin dosage is based on body surface area, can be impressively diminished to less than 20–40% when the Calvert formula is used (Fig. 18). In conclusion, the simplicity of Calvert's formula is a great advantage in the optimization of cancer chemotherapy [11,54–58].

Recently, another formula for the calculation of carboplatin dose was developed by Chatelut and colleagues (Table 5). Based on a population pharmacokinetic model (**non**linear **m**ixed **e**ffect **m**ode: NONMEM), they developed a formula based on the parameters body weight, sex, age, and serum creatinine. In contrast to the formula of Calvert, the determination of the GFR is not necessary any more [59]. There is some evidence, that the calculated AUC values based on Chatelut's formula are in close accordance

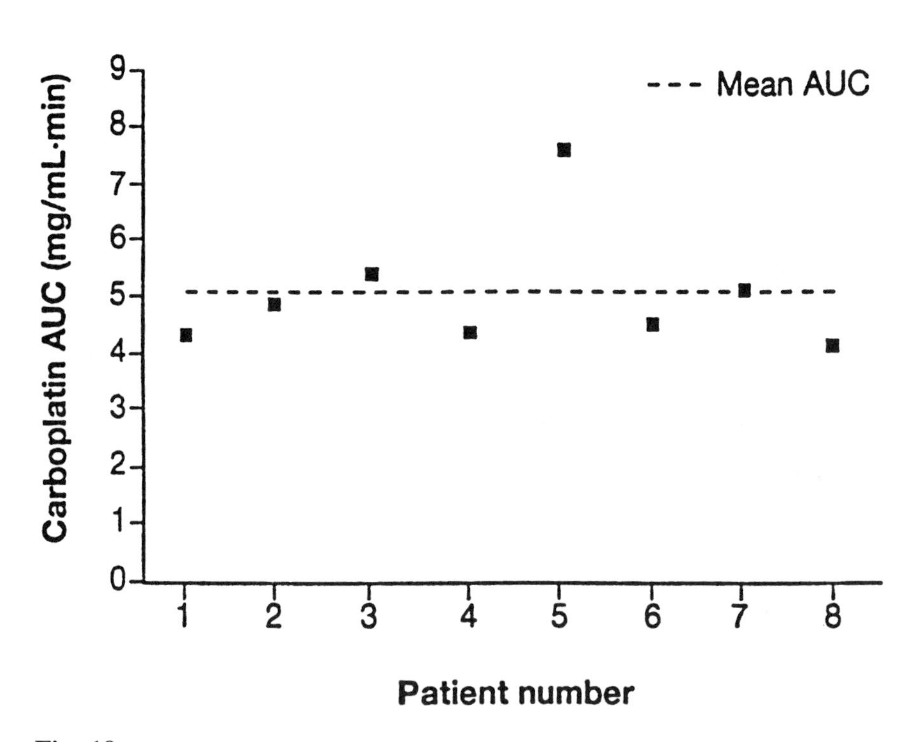

Fig. 18 If carboplatin dose is calculated with a formula (e.g., according to Calvert's formula), the measured AUC values will approximate the target AUC values in the range of 10–20% with very few exceptions. According to the study results of Porter and colleagues [54].

Table 8 Comparison of the Calculated Carboplatin Dose (mg) According to Calvert's Formula (including GFR Determination Based on the Cockcroft–Gault or Jeliffe formula) or Chatelut's Formula to Achieve a Target AUC of 5 mg/mL/min

	Calvert, A[a]	Chatelut	Cockcroft-Gault	Jeliffe
Carboplatin dose (mg) (variation)	595 (285–970)	567 (209–941)	471 (263–727)	472 (317–583)
Coefficient of correlation to A	—	0.75	0.74	0.16
Absolute difference with respect to A				
<20%	—	58%	44%	44%
21–40%	—	39%	48%	29%
>40%	—	2%	7%	26%

[a]Calvert's formula with GFR determination according to the Cr EDTA method as reference; n = 24 patients.
Source: Adapted from Ref. 60.

with the actual AUC values (Table 8). However, more studies seem to be necessary to confirm these preliminary results [60–62]. Particularly, the accuracy of Chatelut's formula in the presence of massive obesity has not been precisely evaluated.

It was shown recently that just one blood sample within 24 hours is sufficient for total carboplatin AUC calculation in clinical practice, a finding that greatly simplified the determination of carboplatin AUC values [63,64].

If calculated AUC values are presented and compared to each other, one must keep in mind that currently four different methods are available. If Calvert's formula is used, it will be feasible to determine GFR by three different procedures: the [^{51}Cr]EDTA method (the most accurate), 24-hour urine collection, or mathematical calculation.

Interestingly, a recently published retrospective analysis of calculated AUC values showed generally higher AUC results when the Calvert formula was used rather than the Chatelut formula. The actually administered carboplatin dose (mg) was well known (according to each patient's body surface area); the underlying GFR was mathematically calculated based on the serum creatinine value. However, the use of retrospective mathematical calculations of GFR results in underestimation of the actual value in patients with constitutively higher GFR values, and thus the corresponding AUC value will be retrospectively overestimated by Calvert's formula in contrast to the Chatelut formula (Table 9) [65].

If the individual creatinine clearance is less than 30 mL/min, the use

Table 9 Retrospective Calculation of AUC Values in Responders and Nonresponders After Treatment of Advanced NSCLC According to Calvert's (based on GFR determination with Cockcroft–Gault's Formula) and Chatelut's Formula

	Median AUC	
Formula	Responders	Nonresponders
Calvert	6.2	4.8
($p = 0.017$)	(Variation: 4.0–7.4)	(Variation: 3.1–7.7)
Chatelut	5.1	3.7
($p = 0.035$)	(Variation: 2.7–5.7)	(Variation: 2.2–6.0)

Source: Adapted from Ref. 65.

of carboplatin is contraindicated irrespective of whether Calvert's or Chatelut's formula is to be used.

For children, a pediatric formula (Newell's formula), which is in close accordance to Calvert's formula, has been established (Table 10) [42]. Comparable to adult patients, a wide range of creatinine clearance can be observed in pediatric cancer patients (e.g., 42–213 mL/min/1.73 m^2). Several data support the validity of the proposed dose equation in comparison with dosing based on surface area, since more than 75% of patients may be within a defined therapeutic AUC range [66]. Recently a limited sampling method was presented for pediatric patients to verify the attainment of the target AUC [66]. Interestingly, a novel formula by Chatelut and colleagues, which

Table 10 The Formula According to Newell (Which Represents a Modified Form of the Calvert's Formula) and the Recently Developed Formula of Chatelut May Be Useful to Calculate the Absolute Dose (mg) of Carboplatin in Pediatric Patients

Newell's formula (for pediatric patients)[a]

Carboplatin dose = target AUC [GFR + (0.6 × BW)]

Chatelut's formula (modified for pediatric patients)

Carboplatin dose = target AUC × carboplatin clearance

Determination of carboplatin clearance (mL/min) in pediatric patients[a,b]

$2.85 \times \text{BW} \times (1 - 0.00357 \times \text{serum creatinine } [\mu\text{M}]) \times (1 - 0.372 \times \text{NP}) + 8.7$

[a]BW, body weight (kg).
[b]NP, nephrectomy (no nephrectomy = 0, unilateral nephrectomy = 1).

does not require estimation of individual GFR, was introduced in clinical oncology very recently (Table 10) [67]. However, the role of this formula in pediatric oncology has not yet been fully established.

According to the data of Newell and colleagues, an AUC of 5 mg/mL × min appears to produce negligible thrombocytopenia, after carboplatin monotherapy whereas 10 mg/mL × min results in a severely decreased platelet count [42]. If carboplatin is combined with other cytostatics (e.g., oxazaphosphorines, etoposide), a target AUC of 6 and 7 mg/mL × min will be reasonable for previously untreated children [68,69].

Higher doses of carboplatin (e.g., 800 mg/m^2) have been used successfully in the treatment of brain metastases or in combination with autologous bone marrow transplantation [38,70]. As mentioned before, if AUC values exceed 7.5 mg/mL × min (equivalent to a median dose of 471 mg/m^2), the use of G-CSF and thrombocyte transfusions will be necessary to overcome overall myelosuppression [71].

As a consequence, if carboplatin doses up to 1500–2000 mg/m^2 are administered per course, AUC values of up to 20–30 mg/mL × min will be achieved [72]. Very recently, Ford et al. suggested that the highest correlation coefficient will be achieved between the predicted and measured AUC values if Chatelut's formula is used during high-dose chemotherapy [73]. However, more data are necessary to define an optimal carboplatin target AUC for high-dose regimens with respect to combination chemotherapy and the type of tumor.

Recently, Chatelut and colleagues suggested that carboplatin can be safely administered to patients with advanced ovarian carcinoma and hemodialysis-dependent renal insufficiency if a dialysis is performed 24 hours after drug administration and if an AUC of 4 or 6 mg/mL × min is achieved in previously platinum-treated or untreated patients, respectively [74].

2.2.3 Oxaliplatin

The diammine cyclohexane platinum complex oxaliplatin which has been approved in France for the treatment of refractory metastatic colorectal cancer represents a new third-generation platinum compound. Usually it is administered intravenously (e.g., 130 mg/m^2) diluted in 25 mL of sterile 5% dextrose solution over 2 hours every 3 weeks. Within other regimens the drug has been applied as a constant-rate or chronomodulated infusion (e.g., 20 mg/m^2/d d1–5) for 5 consecutive days every 16 days. The documented activity of oxaliplatin in combination with 5-fluorouracil and folinic acid or paclitaxel in chemoresistant tumor types, like colorectal or ovarian cancer, may have significant clinical benefits [75–77].

In contrast to cisplatin the novel platinum analogue is neither nephrotoxic nor highly emetogenic, in contrast to carboplatin its myelosuppressive potency is rather low. The dose-limiting toxicity of oxaliplatin appears to be cumulative peripheral neuropathy (dysaesthesia or paraesthesia) [75–77].

There is some evidence that chronomodulation of oxaliplatin administration may ameliorate the risk for neurotoxicity. According to Levi et al. who published a randomised multicenter trial of chronotherapy with oxaliplatin, 5-fluorouracil and folinic acid in metatstatic colorectal cancer, the incidence of peripheral neuropathy was significantly reduced when the amount of oxaliplatin administration was increased during afternoon. Additionally the median time to treatment failure could be prolonged by chronotherapy of these drugs in contrast to constant-rate infusion. In conclusion, circadian scheduling may help to reduce toxicity of oxaliplatin [78,79]. In contrast to cisplatin where chronotherapy had also been associated with reduced organ toxicity, circadian scheduling of carboplatin therapy does not appear to be beneficial [5,80].

Like cisplatin the structurally related oxaliplatin binds also rather rapidly to several proteins in plasma after intravenous administration. It has been suggested that the drug may covalently bind to hemoglobin, the major protein in red blood cells (RBC), which could explain the correlation between RBC platinum concentrations and Hb levels in plasma. Prospective pharmacokinetic studies are under progress [81,82].

2.2.3.1 Amifostine as a Modulator of Cisplatin- and Carboplatin-induced Side Effects

WR2721 [S-2-(3-aminopropylamino)ethylphosphorothioic acid, ethiophos, amifostine, Ethyol] was originally developed by the Walter Reed Army Institute to protect soldiers from radiation in the event of a nuclear war. The thiol compound is a prodrug which is rapidly converted by the enzyme alkaline phosphatase into its active aminothiol form, WR1065 [83,84]. Usually more than 95% of the peak plasma concentration of unchanged drug are removed from plasma within 15 min. WR-1065 is converted to the corresponding disulfide WR-33278, which has some protective properties, too, albeit to a lesser extent than WR 1065, and other disulfides. As compared to the parent drug and its active metabolite the total disulfides are cleared rather slowly from plasma with a final half-life of about 14 hours [85].

This active form is rapidly and preferentially distributed into various tissues such as kidneys, lungs and bone marrow. However, the activation in tumor tissues appears to be marginal because within their membranes the level of alkaline phosphatase is far less than in normal tissues. Within the cell the active drug is able to inactivate radicals and bind covalently to alkylating agents and platinum compounds [86]. Experimental studies indicated that amifostine could protect normal tissues from toxicities induced by alkylating agents and cisplatin without impairing their antineoplastic efficacy. Clinical trials with 740–910 mg/m^2 amifostine and 120 mg/m^2 cisplatin indicated that amifostine protected against long-term renal insufficiency from cumulative doses of cisplatin in patients with metastatic NSCLC. It is important that the administration of amifostine precedes the infusion of any cytotoxic drug to achieve the maximum of tissue protection. For example, amifostine as 15-minute short-time infusion can be started 20 minutes before cisplatin. The recommended dose is 910 mg/m^2 of amifostine. It is currently investigated whether 740 mg/m^2 are as efficacious as 910 mg/m^2 but better tolerable with respect to side effects [87].

In the meantime several studies have been published which indicate that amifostine is able to ameliorate cyclophosphamide-, carboplatin- or mitomycin-induced neutropenia and thrombocytopenia as well as cisplatin-induced nephrotoxicity, neurotoxicity and possibly ototoxicity. One may speculate that the amifostine-related reduction of toxicity may allow dose-intensification of certain cytotoxic drugs in pretreated patients and that the drug may reduce the overall risk for severe late side effects [88–91].

REFERENCES TO SECTION 2.2

1. Reedijk J, Lohman PHM. Cisplatin: Synthesis, antitumor activity, and mechanism of action. Pharm Weekbl Sci 1985:7:173–180.
2. Reed E, Kohn KW. Cisplatin and platinum analogs: In: BA Chabner, J Collins, eds. Cancer chemotherapy: Principles and Practice. Philadelphia: JB Lippincott, 1990, pp 465–490.
3. Ozols RF, Young RC. High dose cisplatin therapy in ovarian cancer. Semin Oncol 1985:12(suppl 6):21–30.
4. Pinzani V, Bressolle F, Haug IJ, et al. Cisplatin-induced renal toxicity and toxicity-modulating strategies: A review. Cancer Chemother Pharmacol 1994: 35:1–9.
5. Anand AJ, Bashey B. Newer insights into cisplatin nephrotoxicity. Ann Pharmacother 1993:27:1519–1525.
6. Chu G, Mantin R, Shen Y-M, et al. Massive cisplatin overdose by accidental substitution for carboplatin. Cancer 1993:72:3707–3714.
7. Christian MC. The current status of new platinum analogs. Semin Oncol 1992: 19:720–733.
8. Doz F, Pinkerton R. What is the place of carboplatin in paediatric oncology? Eur J Cancer Clin Oncol 1994:30A:194–201.
9. Calvert AH, Harland SJ, Newell DR, Siddik ZH, Harrap KR. Phase I studies with carboplatin at the Royal Marsden Hospital. Cancer Treatment Rev 1985: 12(suppl A):51–57.
10. Hacker MP. Toxicity of platinum-based anticancer drugs. In: G Powis, MP Hacker, eds. The Toxicity of Anticancer Drugs. New York: Pergamon Press, 1991, pp 82–105.

11. Bokemeyer C, Lipp H-P. Is there a need for pharmacokinetically guided carboplatin dose schedules? Onkologie 1997:20:343–345.
12. Jodrell DI, Egorin MJ, Canetta RM, Langenberg P, et al. Relationships between carboplatin exposure and tumor response and toxicity in patients with ovarian cancer. J Clin Oncol 1992:10:520–528.
13. Poirier MC, Reed E, Litterst CL, Katz D, Gupta-Burt S. Persistence of platinum–ammine–DNA adducts in gonads and kidneys of rats and multiple tissues from cancer patients. Cancer Res 1992:52:149–153.
14. Johnsson A, Höglund P, Grubb A, Cavallin-Stahl E. Cisplatin pharmacokinetics and pharmacodynamics in patients with squamous-cell carcinoma of the head/neck or esophagus. Cancer Chemother Pharmacol 1996:39:25–33.
15. Reece PA, Stafford I, Gill PG. Nonlinear renal clearance of ultrafiltrable platinum in patients treated with *cis*-dichlordiammineplatinum(II). Cancer Chemother Pharmacol 1985:15:295–299.
16. Belt RJ, Himmelstein KJ, Patton TF, et al. Pharmacokinetics of non–protein bound platinum species following administration of *cis*-diamminedichloroplatinum(II). Cancer Treatment Rep 1979:63:1515.
17. Bin P, Boddy AV, English MW, et al. The comparative pharmacokinetics and pharmacodynamics of cisplatin and carboplatin in paediatric patients: A review. Anticancer Res 1994:14:2279–2284.
18. Schierl R, Roher B, Hohnloser J. Long-term platinum excretion in patients treated with cisplatin. Cancer Chemother Pharmacol 1995:36:75–78.
19. Gamelin E, Allain P, Maillart P, et al. Long-term pharmacokinetics behavior of platinum after cisplatin administration. Cancer Chemother Pharmacol 1995: 37:97–102.
20. Gorodetsky R, Vexler A, Bar-Khaim Y, Biran H. Plasma platinum elimination in a hemodialysis patient treated with cisplatin. Ther Drug Monit 1995:17:203–206.
21. Ribrag V, Droz J-P, Morizet J, et al. Test dose-guided administration of cisplatin in an anephric patient: A case report. Ann Oncol 1993:4:679–682.
22. Vanhoefer U, Harstrick A, Wilke H, et al. Schedule-dependent antagonism of paclitaxel and cisplatin in human gastric and ovarian carcinoma cell lines in vitro. Eur J Cancer 1995:31A:92–97.
23. Jekunen AP, Christen RD, Shalinsky DR, Howell SB. Synergistic interaction between cisplatin and taxol in human ovarian carcinoma cells in vitro. Br J Cancer 1994:69:299–306.
24. Reece PA, Stafford I, Russell J, Gill PG. Reduced ability to clear ultrafiltrable platinum with repeated courses of cisplatin. J Clin Oncol 1986:4:1392–1398.
25. Kintzel PE, Dorr RT. Anticancer drug renal toxicity and elimination: Dosing guidelines for altered renal function. Cancer Treatment Rev 1995:21:33–64.
26. Thyss A, Saudes L, Otto J, et al. Renal toxicity of cisplatin in patients more than 80 years old. J Clin Oncol 1994:12:2121–2125.
27. Abe R, Akiyoshi T, Baba T. Two-route chemotherapy using cisplatin and its neutralizing agent, sodium thiosulfate, for intraperitoneal cancer. Oncology 1990:47:422–426.

28. Guastalla JP, Vermorken JB, Wils JA, et al. Phase II trial for intraperitoneal cisplatin plus intravenous sodium thiosulphate in advanced ovarian carcinoma patients with minimal residual disease after cisplatin-based chemotherapy—A phase II study of the EORTC Gynaecological Cancer Cooperative Group. Eur J Cancer 1994:30A:45–49.
29. Goel R, Cleray SM, Horton C, et al. Effect of sodium thiosulfate on the pharmacokinetics and toxicity of cisplatin. J Natl Cancer Inst 1989:81:1552–1560.
30. Nagai N, Kinoshita M, Ogata H, et al. Relationship between pharmacokinetics of unchanged cisplatin and nephrotoxicity after intravenous infusions of cisplatin to cancer patients. Cancer Chemother Pharmacol 1996:39:131–137.
31. Gregg RW, Molepo JM, Monpetit VJA, et al. Cisplatin neurotoxicity: The relationship between dosage, time, and platinum concentration in neurologic tissues, and morphologic evidence of toxicity. J Clin Oncol 1992:10:795–803.
32. Laurell G, Beskow C, Frankendal B, Borg E. Cisplatin administration to gynecologic cancer patients—long-term effects on hearing. Cancer 1996:78: 1798–1804.
33. Lagrange J-L, Bondiau P-Y, Tessier E, et al. Tumoral platinum concentrations in patients treated with repeated low-dose cisplatin as a radiosensitizer. Int J Cancer 1996:68:452–456.
34. Zieske PA, Koberda M, Hines JL, et al. Characterization of cisplatin degradation as affected by pH and light. Am J Hosp Pharm 1991:48:1500–1506.
35. Desoize B, Berthiot G, Manot L, Coninx P, Dumont P. Evaluation of a prediction model of cisplatin dose based on total platinum plasma concentration. Eur J Cancer 1996:32A:1734–1738.
36. Calvert AH, Harland SJ, Newell DR, Siddik ZH, et al. Early clinical studies with *cis*-diammine-1,1-cyclobutane dicarboxylate platinumII. Cancer Chemother Pharmacol 1982:9:140–147.
37. Wagstaff AJ, Ward A, Benfied P, Heel R. Carboplatin—A preliminary review of its pharmacodynamic and pharmacokinetic properties and therapeutic efficacy in the treatment of cancer. Drugs 1989:37:162–190.
38. van der Wall E, Beijnen JH, Rodenhuis S. High-dose chemotherapy regimes for solid tumors. Cancer Treatment Rev 1995:21:105–132.
39. van der Vigh WJF. Clinical pharmacokinetics of carboplatin. Clin Pharmacokinet 1991:21(4):242–261.
40. Harland SJ, Newell DR, Siddik ZH, et al. Pharmacokinetics of *cis*-diammine-1,1-cyclobutane dicarboxylate platinum(II) in patients with normal and impaired renal function. Cancer Res 1984:44:1693–1697.
41. Shea TC, Flaherty M, Elias A, Eder JP, et al. A phase I clinical and pharmacokinetic study of carboplatin and autologous bone marrow support. J Clin Oncol 1989:7:651–661.
42. Newell DR, Pearson ADJ, Balmanno K, Price L, et al. Carboplatin pharmacokinetics in children: The development of a pediatric dosing formula. J Clin Oncol 1993:11:2314–2323.
43. Newell DR, Siddik ZH, Gumbrell LA, et al. Plasma free platinum pharmacokinetics in patients treated with high dose carboplatin. Eur J Cancer Clin Oncol, 1987:23:1399–1405.

44. Reyno LM, Egorin J, Canetta RM, Jodrell DJ, et al. Impact of cyclophosphamide on relationships between carboplatin exposure and response or toxicity when used in the treatment of advanced ovarian cancer. J Clin Oncol 1993:11: 1156–1164.
45. Madden T, Sunderland M, Santana VM, Rodman JH. The pharmacokinetics of high-dose carboplatin in pediatric patients with cancer. Clin Pharmacol Ther 1992:51:701–707.
46. Calvert AH. Dose optimisation of carboplatin in adults. Anticancer Res 1994: 14:2273–2278.
47. Sorensen BT, Strömgren A, Jakobsen P, Nielsen JT, Andersen LS, Jakobsen A. Renal handling of carboplatin. Cancer Chemother Pharmacol 1992:30:317–320.
48. Alberts DS, Garcia DJ. Total platinum dose versus platinum dose intensification in ovarian cancer treatment. Semin Oncol 1994:21(suppl 2):11–15.
49. Calvert AH, Boddy A, Bailey NP, Siddiqui N, et al. Carboplatin in combination with paclitaxel in advanced ovarian cancer: Dose determination and pharmacokinetic and pharmacodynamic interactions. Semin Oncol 1995:22(suppl 5): 91–98.
50. Calvert AH, Newell DR, Gumbrell LA, O'Reilly S, et al. Carboplatin dosage: Prospective evaluation of a simple formula based on renal function. J Clin Oncol 1989:7:1748–1756.
51. Brown SCW, O'Reilly PH. Glomerular filtration rate measurement: A neglected test in urological practice. Br J Urol 1995:75:296–300.
52. Waller DG, Fleming JS, Ramsay B, Gray J. The accuracy of creatinine clearance with and without urine collection as a measure of glomerular filtration rate. Postgrad Med J 1991:67:42–46.
53. Salazar DE, Corcoran GB. Predicting creatinine clearance and renal drug clearance in obese patients from estimated fat-free body mass. Am J Med 1988:84: 1053–1060.
54. Porter D, Boddy A, Thomas H, et al. Etoposide phosphate infusion with therapeutic drug monitoring in combination with carboplatin dosed by AUC: A cancer research campaign phase I/II committee study. Semin Oncol 1996: 23(suppl 13):34–44.
55. Parsmans M, Sculier JP, Thiriaux J, et al. Carboplatin prescribed in mg/m^2 in patients with advanced NSCLC: Is there an impact of the reached AUC on response, survival and haematological toxicity? Proceedings of the American Society of Clinical Oncology, 1997:vol 16:A716.
56. Sorensen BT, Strömgren A, Jakobsen P, et al. Dose–toxicity relationship of carboplatin in combination with cyclophosphamide in ovarian cancer patients. Cancer Chemother Pharmacol 1991:28:397–401.
57. Jakobsen A, Bertelsen K, Andersen JE, et al. Dose–effect of carboplatin in ovarian cancer: A Danish ovarian cancer group study. J Clin Oncol 1997:15: 193–198.
58. van Warmerdam LJC, Rodenhuis S, ten Bokkel Huinink WW, et al. Evaluation of formulas using the serum creatinine level to calculate the optimal dosage of carboplatin. Cancer Chemother Pharmacol 1996:37:266–270.

59. Chatelut E, Canal P, Brunner V, Chevreau C, et al. Prediction of carboplatin clearance from standard morphological and biological patient characteristics. J Natl Cancer Inst 1995:87:573–580.
60. Izquierdo MA, Sanchez A, Llort G, et al. Comparison of different methods for AUC-dosing of carboplatin (CBCDA). Proceedings of the American Society of Clinical Oncology, 1997:vol 16:A714.
61. Camp MJ, Sencer A, Fanucchi SM. Comparison of Calvert versus Chatelut for dosing carboplatin (CBP) in combination with paclitaxel. Proceedings of the American Society of Clinical Oncology, 1996:vol 15:A1510.
62. Wada T, Nakamura T, Maeda Y, Maruyama H, et al. Actual carboplatin AUC had better correlation with Chatelut's formula using 24-hr creatinine clearance. Proceedings of the American Society of Clinical Oncology, 1996:vol 15: A1503.
63. van Warmerdam LJC, Rodenhuis S, van Tellingen O, et al. Validation of a limited sampling model for carboplatin in a high-dose chemotherapy combination. Cancer Chemother Pharmacol 1994:35:179–181.
64. Ghazal-Aswad S, Calvert AH, Newell DR. A single-sample assay for the estimation of the area under the free carboplatin concentration versus time curve. Cancer Chemother Pharmacol 1996:37:429–434.
65. Morere JF, Piperno-Neumann S, Tete L, et al. Impact of the carboplatin (CBDCA) AUC on the efficacy and tolerance of the CBCDA, taxol association. Proceedings of the American Society of Clinical Oncology, 1997:vol 16: A1712.
66. Peng B, Boddy AV, Cole M, et al. Comparison of methods for the estimation of carboplatin pharmacokinetics in paediatric cancer patients. Eur J Cancer 1995:31A:1804–1810.
67. Chatelut E, Boddy AV, Peng B, Rubie H, et al. Population pharmacokinetics of carboplatin in children. Clin Pharmacol Ther 1996:59:436–443.
68. Marina NM, Rodman J, Shema SJ, et al. Phase I study of escalating targeted doses of carboplatin combined with ifosfamide and etopside in children with relapsed solid tumors. J Clin Oncol 1993:11:554–560.
69. Tonda ME, Heideman RL, Petros WP, et al. Carboplatin pharmacokinetics in young children with brain tumors. Cancer Chemother Pharmacol 1996:38:395–400.
70. Vlasveld LT, Beijnen JH, Boogerd W, et al. Complete remission of brain metastases of ovarian cancer following high-dose carboplatin: A case report and pharmacokinetic study. Cancer Chemother Pharmacol 1990:25:382–383.
71. Bookman MA, McGuire WP, Kilpatrick D, et al. Carboplatin and paclitaxel in ovarian carcinoma: A phase I study of the gynecologic oncology group. J Clin Oncol 1996:14:1895–1902.
72. Johansen MJ, Madden T, Mehra RC, et al. Phase I pharmacokinetic study of multicycle high-dose carboplatin followed by peripheral-blood-stem-cell infusion in patients with cancer. J Clin Oncol 1997:15:1481–1491.
73. Ford C, Reilly W, Spitzer G, Warnick T. Optimal dosing of high-dose carboplatin. Proceedings of the American Society of Clinical Oncology, 1997:vol 16:A834.

74. Chatelut E, Rostaing L, Gualano V, et al. Pharmacokinetics of carboplatin in a patient suffering from advanced ovarian carcinoma with hemodialysis-dependent renal insufficiency. Nephron 1994:66:157–161.
75. Mathé G, Kidani Y, Segiguchi M, et al. Oxalato-platinum or L-OHP, a third-generation platinum complex: an experimental and clinical appraisal and preliminary comparison with cis-platinum and carboplatinum. Biomed Pharmacother 1989:43:237–250.
76. Extra JM, Espie M, Calvo F, et al. Phase I study of oxaliplatin in patients with advanced colorectal cancer. Cancer Chemother Pharmacol 1990:25:299–303.
77. Chollet P, Bensmaine MA, Brienza S, et al. Single agent activity of oxaliplatin in heavily pretreated advanced epithelial ovarian cancer. Ann Oncol 1996:7: 1065–1070.
78. Metzger G, Massari C, Etienne M-C, Comisso M, et al. Spontaneous or imposed circadian changes in plasma concentrations of 5-fluorouracil coadministered with folinic acid and oxaliplatin: relationship with mucosal toxicity in patients with cancer. Clin Pharmacol Ther 1994:56:190–201.
79. Lévi F, Zidani R, Misset J-L, for the International Organization for Cancer Chemotherapy. Randomized multicenter trial of chronotherapy with oxaliplatin, fluorouracil, and folinic acid in metastatic colorectal cancer. Lancet 1997:350: 681–686.
80. Natoli C, Salini V, Irtelli L, et al. A Phase I study of 5-day continuous venous infusion of carboplatin at circadian rhythm-modulated rate compared with constant rate. Anticancer Res 1996:16:1275–1280.
81. Gamelin E, Le Bouil A, Boisdron-Celle M, et al. Cumulative pharmacokinetic study of oxaliplatin, administered every three weeks, combined with 5-fluoroural in colorectal cancer patients. Clinical Cancer Research 1997:3:891–899.
82. Bastian G. Report on the pharmacokinetics of oxaliplatin in patients with normal and impaired renal function. Ann Oncol 1994:5(suppl 5):126.
83. Schuchter L, Glick J. The current status of WR-2721 (amifostine): A chemotherapy and radiation therapy protector. Biol Ther Cancer Update 1993:1:1–10.
84. Treskes M, van der Vijgh WJF. WR2721 as a modulator of cisplatin- and carboplatin-induced side effects in comparison with other chemprotective agents: A molecular approach. Cancer Chemother Pharmacol 1993:33:93–106.
85. Korst AEC, Gall HE, Vermorken JB, van der Vijgh WJF. Pharmacokinetics of amifostine and its metabolites in the plasma and ascites of a cancer patient. Cancer Chemother Pharmacol 1996:39:162–166.
86. Shaw LM, Glover D, Turrisi A, et al. Pharmacokinetics of WR-2721. Pharmacol Ther 1988:39:195–201.
87. Schiller JH, Storer B, Berlin J, et al. Amifostine, Cisplatin and Vonblastine in Metastatic Non–Small-Cell-Lung Cancer: A Report of High Response Rates and Prolonged Survival. J Clin Oncol 1996:14:1913–1921.
88. Kemp G, Rose P, Lurain J, et al. Amifostine pretreatment for protection against cyclophosphamide-induced and cisplatin-induced toxicities: Results of a randomized control trial in patients with advanced ovarian cancer. J Clin Oncol 1996:14:2101–2112.

89. Vermorken JB, Punt CJA, Eeltink CM, et al. Bone marrow protection by amifostine in patients treated with carboplatin: A Phase I study. Eur J Cancer 1995: 30A(suppl 5):S200.
90. Foster-Nora JA, Siden R. Amifostine for protection from antineoplastic drug therapy. Am J Health Syst Pharm 1997:54:787–800.
91. Tannehill SP, Mehta MP. Amifostine and radiation therapy: Past, present and future. Semin Oncol 1996:23(suppl 8):69–77.

2.3 ANTHRACYCLINES AND OTHER INTERCALATING AGENTS

The anthracycline antibiotics doxorubicin (adriamycin), epirubicin, daunorubicin, idarubicin, and aclarubicin are widely used in clinical oncology. They are all red polycyclic substances with some structural similarity to the tetracyclines (Fig. 19) [1,2].

Because of their planar moiety, they are able to intercalate between DNA base pairs (Fig. 20). Additionally, under physiological conditions, their positively charged amino sugar moieties interact with the negatively charged phosphate bridges of DNA, which results in an irreversible change of the tertiary DNA structure. As a consequence, RNA synthesis is blocked and the activity of the DNA topoisomerase II and DNA polymerase is impaired, which results in an inhibition of replication and transcription [1–3]. It has been proposed that the anthracyclines, independent of their DNA-binding affinity, exert their cytotoxic effects partially by a tight binding to cytoplasmic membrane structures, which results in a significant increase of cytoplasmatic membrane permeability [4]. Aclarubicin belongs to the class II anthracyclines because it exerts an additional effect on the synthesis of RNA and proteins [1].

Novel drug developments include the liposomal encapsulation of anthracyclines, which may play a particular role in the treatment of Kaposi's sarcoma, and other substituted derivatives like iododoxorubicin [5,6].

For example, the use of pegylated liposomal doxorubicin (Doxil, Caelyx) has been shown to be active against Kaposi's sarcoma and patients with advanced breast cancer [5]. The sole structural difference of iododoxorubicin is the presence of an iodine atom at the C-4′ position, instead of a hydroxyl group. Preliminary results indicated that iododoxorubicin may be less cardiotoxic than doxorubicin, however, phase II studies had not been full of promise with this agent. Possibly the drug may play a role in the treatment of amyloidosis [6].

All anthracyclines cause dose-limiting myelosuppression, mucositis, cardiotoxicity, and congestive cardiomyopathy. On clinical grounds the 5% probability of developing congestive heart failure differs between anthra-

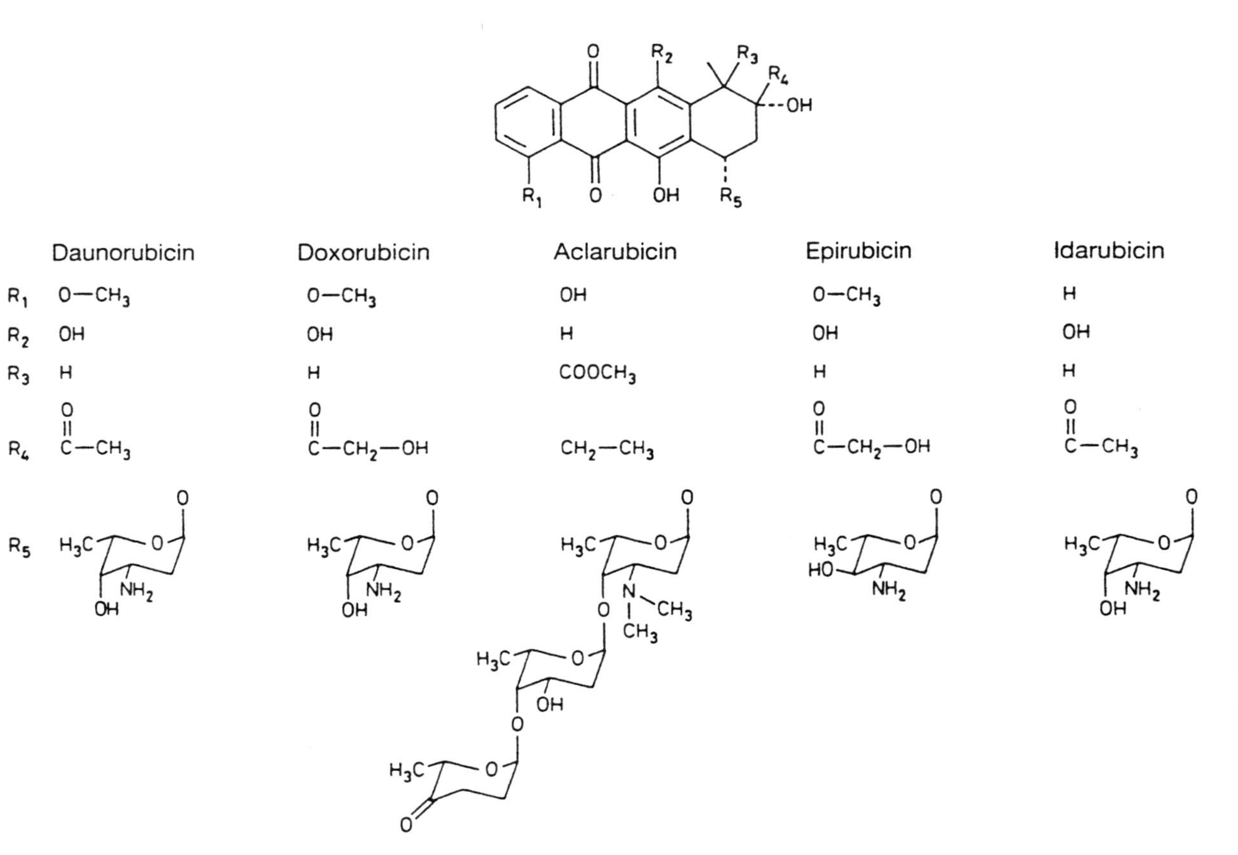

Fig. 19 The chemical structures of the anthracyclines daunorubicin, doxorubicin (Adriamycin), aclarubicin, epirubicin and idarubicin.

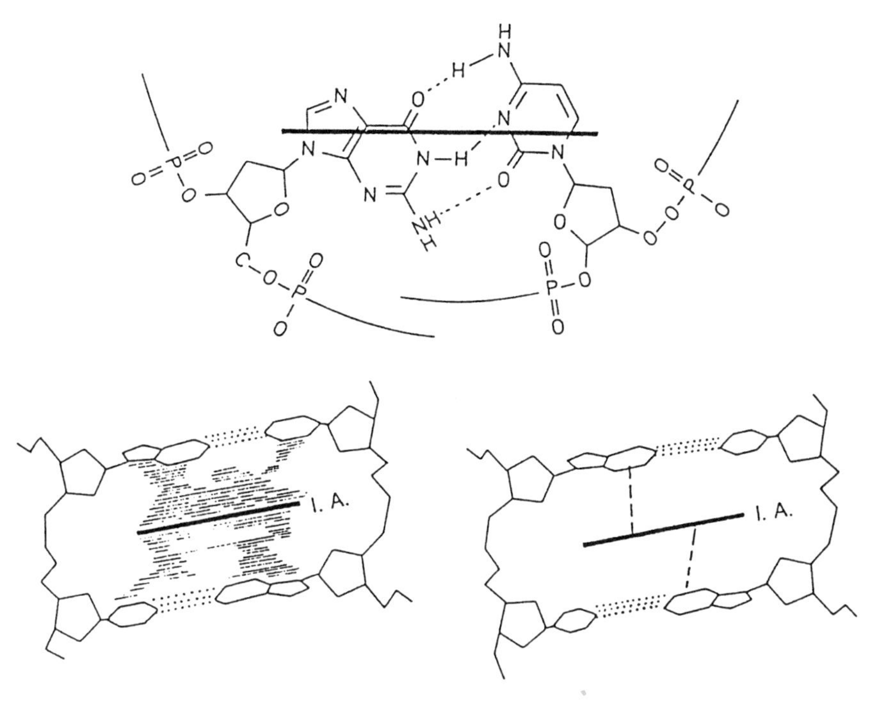

Fig. 20 Anthracycline-induced intercalation. Under physiological conditions, the intercalation is strengthened by the affinity between the positively charged amino sugar moieties of the anthracyclines and the negatively charged DNA phosphate bridges.

cyclines, with a cumulative dose of 450–550 and 800–1000 mg/m^2 for doxorubicin and epirubicin, respectively (Table 11) [1,7–10]. However, there is increasing evidence that the mode of administration plays an important role for cumulative cardiotoxicity. Several data indicate that bolus administration rather than continuous infusion appears to be an important risk factor for anthracycline-induced cardiomyopathy.

Considering the defined cumulative doses (Table 1) it has to be kept in mind that there is a marked interindividual variation in regard to dose-dependent chronic cardiotoxicity. Some patients may develop first signs of congestive cardiomyopathy with less than 300 mg/m^2 Adriamycin, whereas others do not show any cardiotoxic symptoms after cumulative dosages exceeding 1000 mg/m^2 Adriamycin [8]. Several encouraging strategies for the prevention of chronic cardiotoxicity have been presented within the few last years [11,12].

Table 11 Cumulative Anthracycline Dosages That Should Not Be Exceeded in the Interest of Minimizing the Risk of Congestive Cardiomyopathy[a]

Anthracycline	Cumulative total dosage (mg/m^2)	Usual dosage (mg/m^2)
Daunorubicin i.v.	500–600	20–80 q21d
Doxorubicin i.v.	550	60–75 q21d
Epirubicin i.v.	850–1000	50–90 q21d
Idarubicin i.v.	120–(290)	8–12 d1–3 q21d
Idarubicin orally	600–720	15–30 d1–3 q21d
DaunoXome i.v.	>1000	40 q14d
Doxil (Caelyx) i.v.	>860	20 q21d
Mitoxantrone	160–(200)	10–12 d1(–5) q21d
Amsacrine	580–(800)	90–150 d1–5 q7–21d

Notice: It is not recommended to substitute one anthracycline for another when the cumulative dose threshold of one of the drugs has been reached.

[a]There is a strong correlation between the increased risk for congestive cardiomyopathy and the total cumulative dosage of anthracyclines given as bolus applications.

If accidental extravasation or paravasation of anthracyclines or related compounds including amsacrine, mitoxantrone, or actinomycin D has been occurred, a rapid therapeutic intervention is necessary in order to avoid severe skin necrosis. It has been suggested that the use of cold compresses, 1% hydrocortisone cream, subcutaneous dexamethasone injections and topical massages with undiluted dimethyl sulfoxide solutions belong to the most successful strategies to circumvent severe soft tissue injuries [13].

2.3.1 Doxorubicin

Doxorubicin (14-hydroxydaunorubicin) plays an important role in the conventional treatment (e.g., 45–75 mg/m^2 IV every 3 weeks) of a variety of solid tumors, several forms of leukemia and lymphoma, and sarcoma. Doxorubicin is less lipophilic than daunorubicin, which may partially explain its slower accumulation in leukemic cells. However, doxorubicin seems to exert a higher affinity for intracellular DNA than daunorubicin in leukemic and nonleukemic cells. Thus, within the leukemic cells doxorubicin seems to persist for a longer period of time than the corresponding derivative daunorubicin [14,15].

Nonencapsulated (conventional) doxorubicin hydrochloride exhibits linear pharmacokinetics after IV administration. The drug is widely distributed in the plasma and tissues. The volume of distribution is estimated to be about 700–1100 L/m^2. The plasma protein binding ranges from 50 to 85% [1,14,16].

Doxorubicin is extensively metabolized in the liver (Fig. 21) via aldoketoreductase, yielding the corresponding dihydrodiol derivative doxorubicinol, which is still cytotoxic. During metabolism minor amounts of the corresponding aglycones [e.g., doxorubicinone (Adriamycinone) and 7-deoxydoxorubicinone] are released. The cleavage of the amino sugar moiety resulting in the aglycones is catalyzed by the NADPH-dependent cytochrome P450 reductase [16–18]. This enzymatic reduction of doxorubicin, which leads to the 7-deoxyaglycone, may play a considerable role in the cytotoxic effect of anthracyclines because it involves the formation of very toxic and DNA-damaging hydroxyl radicals [19]. In contrast to epirubicin, glucuronidation is of minor importance regarding the metabolic fate of doxorubicin [18].

Unchanged doxorubicin follows a triexponential decay. The initial half-life has been recorded to be about 4.8 minutes, the second half-life about 2.6 hours, and the third half-life about 48 hours in cancer patients (Table 12).

Within 6 days after treatment only about 12% of the doxorubicin dose is recovered in urine. However, already small amounts may impart a red color to the urine. Patients should be advised to expect this phenomenon during therapy [1,14,16].

Biliary elimination and fecal excretion of the parent compound and its metabolites are of major clinical relevance. About 10–20 and 40–50% of the dose is excreted in feces within 24 and 150 hours, respectively. About 50% of biliary eliminated dose seems to be unchanged drug, 23% appears to be doxorubicinol, and the remainder consists of other metabolites.

Considering the important role of hepatic metabolism and biliary excretion in the clinical pharmacokinetics of doxorubicin, a dose reduction in patients with hyperbilirubinemia and elevated liver enzymes has been recommended. If serum bilirubin and SGOT levels range from 1.5 to 3 mg/dl and 60–180 IU/1, respectively, only 50% of planned dose should be given. If serum bilirubin levels range from 3.1 to 5.0 mg/dl and SGOT levels exceed 180 IU/1, only 25% of planned dose should be administered. If serum bilirubin concentrations exceed 5 mg/dl, doxorubicin is contraindicant. In patients with mild hepatic function abnormalities, doxorubicin dosage should not be reduced routinely because there is some evidence that lower peak plasma concentrations may yield a shorter duration of response and survival (Table 13) [20].

7-Deoxyadriamycinone

microsomal Cytochrome-P_{450}-reductase

NADPH

Adriamycin

$H^{\oplus}$

Adriamycinone

Aldo-keto-reductase

NADPH

Aldo-keto-reductase

NADPH

7-Deoxy-adriamycinol-aglycone (dA3)

microsomal Cytochrome-P_{450}-reductase

NADPH

Adriamycinol

$H^{\oplus}$

Adriamycinol-aglycone

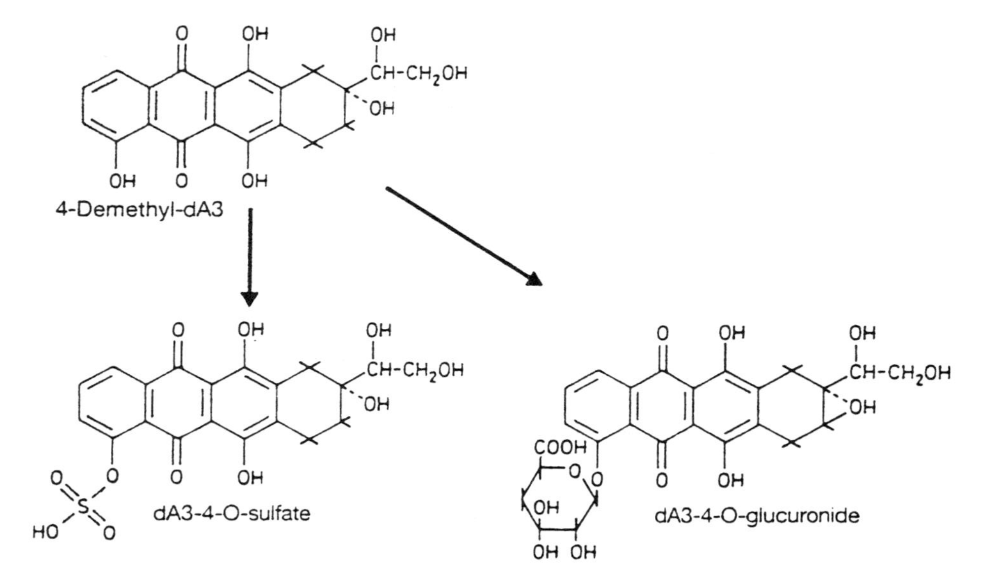

Fig. 21 Metabolic pathways involving doxorubicin. Adriamycinol (doxorubicinol), which is formed by aldoketoreductase, still exerts antineoplastic activity, whereas the aglycones are inactive.

Table 12 Pharmacokinetic Characteristics of Anthracycline Glycosides

	Terminal elimination half-life (h)	Volume of distribution (L/m^2)	Clearance ($L/min \times m^2$)
Doxorubicin	20–70	700–1088	0.3–0.5
Daunorubicin	15–19	1297	0.4–1.8
Epirubicin	18–45	516–794	0.4–0.5
Idarubicin	5–39	2485	1.2
Aclarubicin	2–13	998–2072	2.5–4.0

2.3.1.1 Clinical Pharmacokinetics Regarding Efficacy and Toxicity

It has been reported that doxorubicin-induced cardiomyopathy can be significantly reduced by prolongation of intravenous infusion (e.g., 6 or 24 h). These data indicate that peak plasma levels rather than AUC values may be responsible for the development of chronic cardiotoxicity. However, a prolonged infusion time increases the incidence and severity of mucositis, which then becomes the dose-limiting toxicity [11].

Table 13 Dose Reductions of Anthracyclines in Cancer Patients with Hepatic Dysfunction

Dose reduction (%)	Serum bilirubin (mg/dL)	SGOT
Doxorubicin or Epirubicin		
0	<1.5	<60 IU/l
50	1.5–3.0	60–180 IU/l
75	3.1–5.0	>180 IU/l
contraindicant	>5.0	
Dose reduction (%)	(mg/dl)	SGOT
Daunorubicin		
0	<1.5	<60 IU/l
75	1.5–3.0	60–180 IU/l
50	3.1–5.0	>180 IU/l
contraindicant	>5.0	

It has not yet been precisely established which infusion schedule may result in optimal effectiveness of therapy. There is some evidence that the volume of distribution at steady-state conditions seems to be higher after prolonged infusion. As a consequence, it has been postulated that the prolongation of infusion duration may enhance the uptake of the drug in several tissues, including tumor tissue. Continuous infusion makes a central venous catheter obligatory, however, because of the risk of severe extra- and paravasation [11,21].

Some data indicate that high peak plasma levels of doxorubicin and doxorubicinol 3 hours after the first dose has been administered may be associated with longer remission phases in patients with acute nonlymphocytic leukemia (ANLL) [22,23]. However, the best pharmacokinetic variables for the prediction of doxorubicin-induced myelosuppression after bolus administration have not yet been precisely evaluated.

In clinical practice doxorubicin concentrations are quantified by high-performance liquid chromatography (HPLC) [24]. Recently, a limited sampling method has been presented with which total AUC can be accurately estimated [25].

2.3.2 Epirubicin

Epirubicin plays an important role in the conventional treatment (e.g., 75–90 mg/m^2 IV every 3 weeks; the single dose can be fractionated over 2–3 days) of a variety of solid tumors, especially breast cancer. Several studies indicated that more dose-intensive epirubicin-containing regimens (e.g., 90 mg/m^2 every 3 weeks) seem to be associated with better response rates in advanced breast cancer but not automatically with improved survival. A further dose escalation to 135 mg/m^2 did not seem to show additional benefits [26–29].

Epirubicin is structurally related to doxorubicin. However, on an equimolar basis, epirubicin causes less hematological and cardiac toxicity. The relative myelosuppressive potency of epirubicin has been estimated to be 0.75 in comparison with doxorubicin. Though the cardiac toxicity profiles of epirubicin and doxorubicin are qualitatively similar, a cumulative cardiac toxicity of 450–550 mg/m^2 doxorubicin is comparable to 850–1000 mg/m^2 epirubicin [26]. However, it has not been demonstrated in all tumor systems that equimolar doses of epirubicin and doxorubicin are clinically equieffective.

After bolus intravenous administration, the drug undergoes triphasic elimination from the plasma. Its terminal elimination half-life is estimated to range from 18 to 45 hours (Table 12). Based on its large volume of distribution, epirubicin is widely distributed in a variety of normal tissues, particularly in lymph nodes, liver, stomach, and lung tissue. The drug seems to be concentrated in red blood cells, too.

The drug undergoes extensive hepatic metabolism leading to epirubicinol and glucuronidated metabolites, as well as aglycones. Epirubicinol, which shows an elimination half-life similar to that of the parent drug, is also cytotoxic, but clinically achieved plasma concentrations may be too low for significant antineoplastic activity. The corresponding glucuronides and aglycones lack antiproliferative activity [1,2,30,31].

The main elimination route consists of hepatic metabolism and biliary excretion. About 35% of the dose is excreted in bile and feces. About 6–7% of the dose is excreted in the urine as unchanged drug, 5% is recovered in urine as glucuronides, and only trace amounts are excreted as epirubicinol [32,33]. The pharmacokinetic data of doxorubicin and epirubicin are comparable; because of more extensive glucuronidation, however, the elimination half-life of the latter is somewhat shorter (Fig. 22). Thus, the AUC values of unchanged doxorubicin are higher by a factor of 1.3–1.7 than those of unchanged epirubicin based on equimolar doses [30].

There seems to be a linear relationship between epirubicin dose (12.5–120 mg/m^2) and the corresponding AUC values, indicating that glucuronidation is not oversaturable [34].

Because of extensive hepatic metabolism and biliary excretion of epirubicin and its metabolites, a reduction of the dose in cancer patients with moderate to severe hepatic dysfunction and hyperbilirubinemia is recommended. If serum bilirubin and SGOT levels range from 1.5 to 3 mg/dl and 60–180 IU/1, respectively, only 50% of planned dose should be given. If serum bilirubin levels range from 3.1 to 5.0 mg/dl and SGOT levels exceed 180 IU/1, only 25% of planned dose should be administered. If serum bilirubin concentrations exceed 5 mg/dl, epirubicin is contraindicant. Dosage adjustment in patients with renal dysfunction does not seem to be warranted [32,33].

2.3.2.1 Clinical Pharmacokinetics Regarding Efficacy and Toxicity

There is some evidence that prolonged infusion rather than rapid bolus injection is superior in regard to cardiac tolerability [22].

If 75 mg/m^2 epirubicin is rapidly injected, the peak plasma concentration will average 1.9 μg/mL, whereas levels of 0.04–0.08 μg/mL will be achieved by prolonged epirubicin infusion. Other parameters, such as total plasma clearance, elimination half-life, volume of distribution, and the AUC, do not seem to be significantly changed by the prolongation of parenteral application [34].

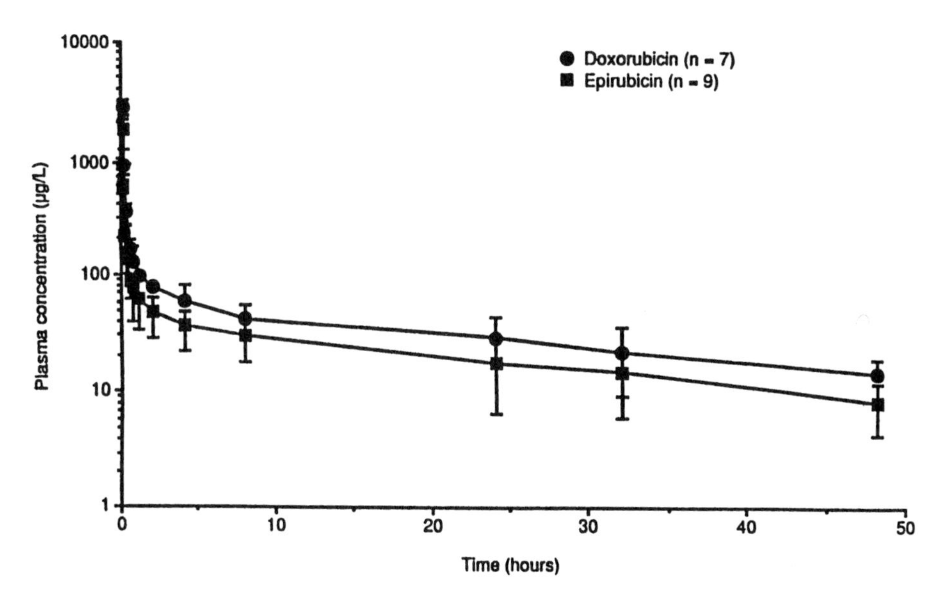

Fig. 22 In contrast to doxorubicin, the structurally related epirubicin shows more extensive glucuronidation. As a consequence, after the same dose (e.g., 50 mg/m^2) the AUC of unchanged epirubicin is somewhat lower than that of unchanged doxorubicin. (From Ref. 31.)

It has been suggested that there may be a particularly strong correlation between epirubicin AUC in plasma with the severity of anthracycline-induced stomatitis, whereas no significant relationship was found between pharmacokinetic parameters and either response to therapy or nausea/vomiting [22].

Because of a large interindividual variation in regard to terminal elimination half-life, AUC, and total plasma clearance, it seems reasonable to determine the individual AUC value (e.g.) on the first day of a treatment course. In the meantime, an analytical method based on limited blood sampling has been presented with which the individual epirubicin AUC can be determined:

$$AUC_{\text{epirubicin}} = 9.44 \times c[2\ \text{h}] + 62.5 \times c[24\ \text{h}] + 157.7$$

where AUC is given in the units ng × h/mL, and c indicates concentration of epirubicin at the indicated number of hours after bolus administration (ng/mL). However, the optimal AUC values in regard to efficacy as well as toxicity have not yet been precisely defined. If concrete target AUC values are defined, the following formula based on the relationship *Dose = AUC*

× *clearance* will be helpful in arriving at doses of epirubicin that are safer in regard to the underlying hepatic function expressed as aspartate aminotransferase (AST) activity if bilirubin levels are within the normal range [27].

$$\text{Dose (mg/m}^2\text{)} = \text{target AUC} \times (97.5 - 34.2 \times \log_{10}\text{AST})$$

Recently, another formula was presented for the selection of cancer patients who may require prophylactic use of hematopoietic growth factors because prolonged and severe leukopenia cannot otherwise be excluded [35]:

$$\log \text{WBC}_{\text{nadir}} = \log \text{WBC}_{\text{pretreatment}} - 0.0073 \times c[6\ \text{h}] - 0.14$$

where

WBC = white blood count
$c[6\ \text{h}]$ = concentration of epirubicin (ng/mL), 6 hours after administration

Generally epirubicin concentrations in plasma are determined by HPLC [36]. In conclusion, therapeutic drug monitoring of epirubicin levels appears to be of great concern, however, more clinical pharmacokinetic studies are still warranted to confirm the existing preliminary data.

2.3.3 Daunorubicin

Daunorubicin is primarily used as an antileukemic agent. The conventional dose ranges from 30 to 60 mg/m^2 IV on days 1–3 every 3 weeks.

Daunorubicin is structurally related to doxorubicin. After IV administration it is widely distributed into tissues. Highest levels were recovered in the spleen, kidney, liver, lung, and heart. The drug passes the blood–brain barrier only to a minimal extent.

Like doxorubicin, daunorubicin and its metabolites decline in a triphasic manner after rapid IV infusion. The plasma half-life of unchanged doxorubicin averages 45 minutes in the initial phase (distribution phase) and 15–18.5 hours in the terminal phase (Table 2).

The major metabolite daunorubicinol is mainly formed by the cytosolic aldoketoreductase. Nearly 40% of the drug in the plasma is present as the corresponding doxorubicinol within 30 minutes after IV administration. After 4 hours it represents 60% of the drug in plasma. Its β-elimination half-life approximates 27 hours.

As in the case of doxorubicin, aglycones can be formed by the NADPH-dependent cytochrome P450 reductase. Other metabolic pathways include demethylation and conjugation reactions.

Urinary excretion of the drug and its metabolites ranges from 14 to 23% of dose within 72 hours, whereas more than 40% of dose is excreted in bile.

Considering the important role of hepatic metabolism and biliary excretion as well as the minor extent of urinary drug elimination, it has been recommended that dose just be reduced, particularly in patients with hyperbilirubinemia. If the serum bilirubin concentrations range from 1.2 to 3 mg/dL, only 75% of the usual dose should be given. If the serum bilirubin levels exceed 3 mg/dL, only 50% of the usual dose should be administered (see Table 13) [1,2,17].

2.3.4 Idarubicin

Idarubicin (4-demethoxydaunorubicin) is a novel anthracycline derivative that has demonstrated an impressive activity in the combination chemotherapy for acute myelogenous leukemia. The usually recommended dose for intravenous use ranges from 8 to 12 mg/m^2 IV on days 1–3 (or 1–5) every 3–4 weeks. In contrast to other anthracyclines, idarubicin can be also given orally (e.g., 45–50 mg/m^2 once or 15 mg/m^2 on days 1–3 every 3 weeks). The oral route offers some advantages particularly in elderly patients with discomfort regarding intravenous access [37–39]. A total dose of at least 120 and 600 mg/m^2 of intravenous and oral idarubicin, respectively should not be exceeded, because otherwise an increased risk of congestive cardiomyopathy cannot be excluded. However, in patients with a myotrophic lateral sclerosis or myelodysplastic syndrome, up to 290 mg/m^2 total dose of idarubicin was administered over 2 years without any signs of idarubicin-induced chronic cardiotoxicity [40].

The chemical structure of idarubicin differs from that of daunorubicin by the lack of the methoxy group in the C-4 position, which may explain its higher uptake into tissues and its higher cytotoxicity at lower concentrations [41].

After oral administration, the peak plasma concentration is achieved in 1–4 hours. The terminal elimination half-life ranges between 5 and 39 hours (medium: 13.7 h) and seems to be independent of application route (Table 12). Based on the parent drug, the oral bioavailability ranges from 18 to 30%. However, since idarubicinol is an equieffective metabolite, it seems reasonable to take its quantity into pharmacological account (Table 14). Considering the sum of idarubicin and idarubicinol, the oral bioavailability is estimated to approximate 28–48% (Fig. 23). Nonfasting conditions may slightly diminish overall absolute bioavailability [42,43]. After oral and intravenous administration of idarubicin, large interindividual variations of pharmacokinetics can be observed in cancer patients.

Table 14 Pharmacokinetic Parameters of Idarubicin in Four Crossover Studies[a]

Number of courses	Dose (mg/m^2)	$t_{1/2}$ (h)	Clearance ($L/h/m^2$)	V_d (l/m^2)	AUC ratio Ida/Ida-ol	Bioavailability (%)	
						Ida	Ida + Ida-ol
5 (IV)	15	34.7	50.8	362	2.3	25	40
5 (PO)	15	20.4	265		5.3		
9 (IV)	8.5–15.6	12.6	46.2		5.1	27	48
9 (PO)	25–45	9.7	218		14.4		
13 (IV)	15	15.5	56	1138	3.0	21	32
13 (PO)	45	11.7	292	1458	5.7		
21 (IV)		16.2	58	955	4.9	25.5	46
21 (PO)	30–35	16.9	406		8.9		

[a]Ida, idarubicin; Ida-ol, idarubicinol.
Source: Ref. 43.

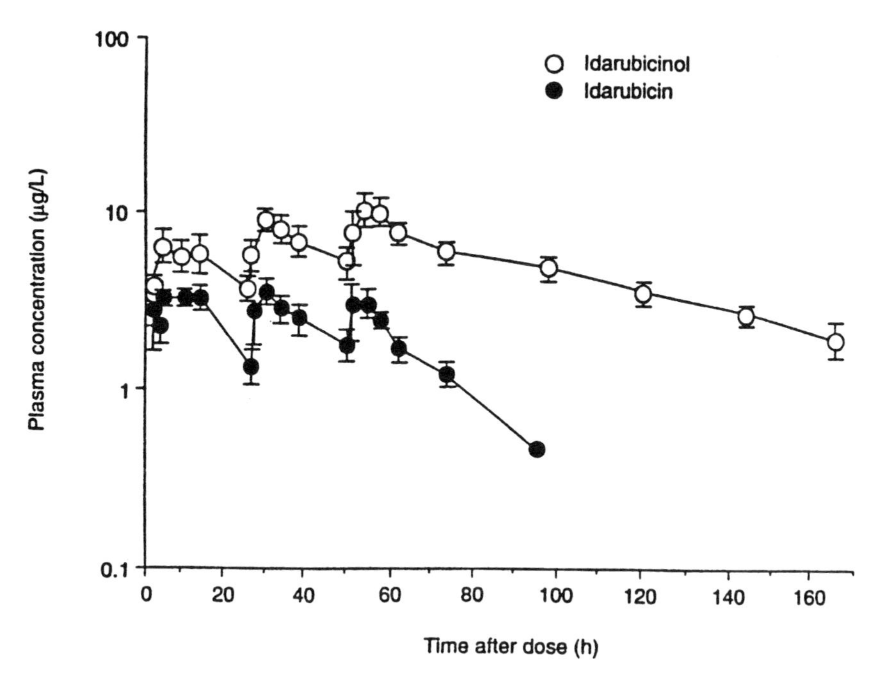

Fig. 23 Representative patterns of the plasma concentration of idarubicin and its active metabolite idarubicinol during and after three consecutive daily oral administrations of 30 mg/m^2. Results are means (± SEM) of the data obtained by the author in patients treated for acute leukemia. (From Ref. 44.)

Like other anthracyclines, idarubicin is extensively metabolized. Similarly the formation of idarubicinol is catalyzed by the cytoplasmic aldoketoreductase. In vitro, this 13-dihydro derivative is nearly as cytotoxic as the parent compound, in contrast to the other corresponding dihydro derivatives of doxorubicin, daunorubicin and epirubicin.

The AUC ratio of metabolites to unchanged drug is nearly twofold higher after oral administration than after IV application, apparently as a result of an extensive first-pass effect in the liver. The terminal elimination half-life of idarubicinol is estimated to be about 46 hours irrespective of administration route. Thus, idarubicinol will slightly accumulate in plasma and tissues when idarubicin is administered once daily for 3–5 days [42,43].

Urinary excretion of the parent compound and its metabolites represents a minor route of elimination, whereas biliary excretion is most predominant. This is in accordance with the pharmacokinetic fate of other anthracyclines. However, it seems reasonable to suggest that in cancer patients with hyperbilirubinemia or severe hepatic dysfunction, the idarubicin dose should be reduced [40].

There is some evidence that idarubicin pharmacokinetics plays a role in the prediction of toxicity. For example, a significant correlation has been recorded to exist between the severity of leukocytopenia and the sum of the AUC of idarubicin and its major metabolite idarubicinol [22]. It has been demonstrated that after oral ingestion of idarubicin a significant correlation between the severity of leukocytopenia and the sum of AUC regarding idarubicinol and the parent compound was detected [44]. As a consequence, one would expect that in cancer patients with even moderate liver dysfunction a routine dosage reduction would be recommended. Since, however, the AUC of idarubicin and idarubicinol also has an important impact regarding clinical efficacy, routine dosage reduction may be associated with a potential undertreatment of cancer patients. In conclusion, clear dosage recommendations for idarubicin in patients with moderate to severe liver dysfunction have not been exactly defined [22,45].

2.3.5 Aclarubicin

Aclarubicin is primarily used for the treatment of hematological malignancies (e.g., acute myelogenous leukemia) and gastrointestinal tumors. In recent clinical trials an oral formulation was presented that appears to be active in the treatment of tumors of the gastrointestinal tract, perhaps because this route of administration provides higher concentrations of the anticancer drug in the stomach tissue [46,47].

Aclarubicin is an anthracycline derivative that differs primarily in its trisaccharide side chain at C-7 and its ethyl side chain at C-9 from other structurally related compounds (Fig. 19).

Its cytotoxic activity is mainly based on the blockage of DNA as well as RNA function and on the inhibition of protein synthesis. Because the drug is able to impair RNA synthesis at very low concentrations, in contrast to the behavior of other anthracyclines, it is classified as class II anthracycline [1,2].

Aclarubicin and its metabolites decline in a triphasic manner after rapid IV infusion. The plasma half-life of unchanged aclarubicin averages 2.5 minutes in the initial phase (distribution phase) and 21 minutes in the second phase. The corresponding metabolites approximate 3 hours in their terminal half-life. These data indicate that aclarubicin and its metabolites, unlike the other anthracyclines, are eliminated rather quickly from the systemic circulation.

Metabolic pathways include the reduction of the keto group within the amino sugar moiety and the successive cleavage of each sugar component.

Like other anthracyclines, the metabolically released aglycone is no longer cytotoxic (Fig. 24). Thus far, only a few data exist regarding the exact quantification of the urinary and biliary excretion pathway [1,2].

2.3.6 Liposomal-Encapsulated Anthracycline Formulations

Recently, several liposomal formulations containing daunorubicin or doxorubicin have been introduced in clinical oncology: pegylated-liposomal doxorubicin hydrochloride (Doxil; Caelyx), liposomal daunorubicin (DaunoXome), and D-99/Lipodox (liposomal doxorubicin).

Although there are some encouraging clinical results regarding the therapeutic efficacy of liposomal anthracyclines, up to now, large randomized prospective trials comparing liposomal with conventional single-agent therapy are still warranted [5,48,49]. Additionally more data are needed to confirm the preliminary hypothesis that liposomal encapsulation may overcome resistance based on the *mdr* gene product (p-glycoprotein) [50].

1. Pegylated-liposomal doxorubicin hydrochloride (Doxil/Caelyx) has been recently introduced in clinical oncology. It is classified as a second-generation, stealth-type formulation because an encapsulation of doxorubicin in conventional liposomes may not favorably influence the intrinsic activity of the anthracycline against systemic malignancies. After intravenous administration of the conventional liposomal form (without further pegylation), a rather rapid uptake of the encapsulated drug by fixed macrophages of the liver can be observed, followed by a slow release of the trapped anthracycline into the systemic circulation. Thus, delivery resembles a sort of prolonged continuous anthracycline infusion by means of which high peak plasma levels are avoided. Whether the accumulation of anthracyclines in tumor tissue can be significantly enhanced in this way has not been precisely examined.

The pegylated form, however, is thought to circulate for a prolonged period of time in the bloodstream without any rapid uptake by liver macrophages. As a consequence, a more selective accumulation into tumor tissue has been postulated based on the observation that the use of Caelyx resulted in encouraging results in the treatment of patients with AIDS-related Kaposi sarcoma (e.g. 20–30 mg/m^2 IV every 2(–3) weeks). In comparison with conventional doxorubicin the incidence and severity of nausea and emesis as well as myocardial damage is lower with Caelyx. The main dose-limiting toxicities associated with this liposomal formulation are mucositis and plantar-palmar erythrodysaesthesia. Phase II data indicate that Caelyx (e.g., 60 mg/m^2 every 3 (–6) weeks) may be a promising tool in combination with taxanes for the treatment of advanced breast or ovarian cancer [51].

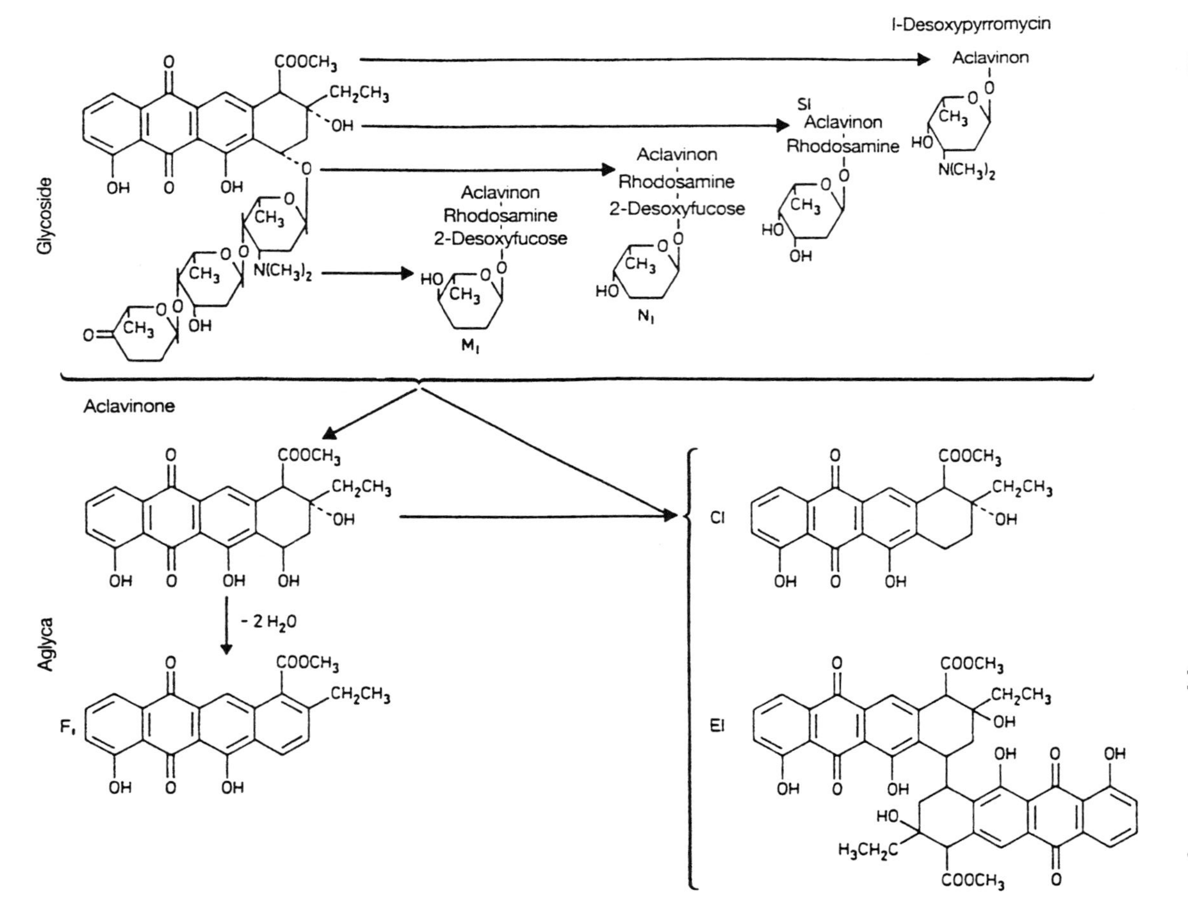

Fig. 24 Metabolic pathways involving aclarubicin.

Pharmacokinetically, Caelyx differs significantly from conventional doxorubicin. The volume of distribution averages 3.3 L/m^2 and the plasma clearance ranges from 0.034 to 0.108 L/h/m^2. Thus, the resulting AUC is about 1000-fold greater than equivalent doses of nonencapsulated doxorubicin. Furthermore, 72 hours after Caelyx administration the doxorubicin peak plasma levels were 5–11 times higher than in patients treated with comparable doses of conventional doxorubicin. In contrast to conventional doxorubicin, the levels of the active metabolite doxorubicinol, which ranges from 40 to 50% of doxorubicin levels after conventional therapy, is very low after Caelyx administration. However, these studies usually do not distinguish among total drug level, the liposomally bound drug amount, and the percentage of the free bioavailable fraction which makes the interpretation of these data in respect to their clinical relevance much more difficult.

The initial half-life of pegylated-liposomal doxorubicin has been estimated to approximate 4 hours. The prolonged terminal elimination half-life averages 52 hours [51,52].

2. In contrast to Doxil, which contains sterically stabilized pegylated liposomes, there is no pegylation of the liposomal structure concerning DaunoXome. The small (60–80 nm) unilamellar liposomes composed of distearoylphosphatidylcholine plus cholesterol are thought to accumulate specifically in tumor tissues. Additionally it has been suggested that DaunoXome may reveal a high degree of serum stability, which minimizes non-specific tissue and protein binding.

The pharmacokinetic profile of DaunoXome is quite different from that of conventionally administered daunorubicin. Peak plasma levels and the half-life at 80 mg/m^2 average 43.6 μg/mL and 5.2 hours, respectively. The mean total body clearance approximates 6.6 mL/min. In conclusion, when DaunoXome is compared with conventional daunorubicin at 80 mg/m^2, the former is associated with much higher peak plasma levels (ratio >100) and AUC values (>35), with a prolonged half-life (ratio >6), and with a highly decreased plasma clearance (6.6 vs. 233 mL/min). However, extended pharmacokinetic data regarding the percentage of the unbound and liposomally bound daunorubicin fraction as well as the quantitative amount of formed daunorubicinol are still lacking [53,54].

The efficacy and safety data of DaunoXome in patients with advanced AIDS-related disease prompted several study groups to give DaunoXome to cancer patients with solid tumors and lymphoma, particularly to investigate the low cardiotoxic risks associated with the use of DaunoXome even at cumulative doses exceeding 1000 mg/m^2. A final assessment of the role of liposomal doxorubicin in the treatment of malignancies other than Kaposi's sarcoma is currently not possible [53,54].

3. D-99/Lipodox is the third liposomal anthracycline that is being evaluated in the treatment of solid tumors. This liposomal preparation seems to induce delayed pyrexia in some patients, possibly as a result of macrophage activation by TLC D-99.

Pharmacokinetic studies suggested that higher and longer lasting plasma levels may be achieved by D-99 than by free doxorubicin. However, pharmacokinetic studies did not distinguish between the encapsulated and free percentage of doxorubicin [55].

2.3.6.1 Clinical Pharmacokinetics Regarding Efficacy and Toxicity of Liposomal Preparations

The encouraging results with pegylated-liposomal doxorubicin notwithstanding, several questions have not yet been satisfactorily answered.

Concerning other liposomal drug preparations, like AmBisome, it has to be questioned whether liposomal encapsulation allows for the retention of potency. For example, a study regarding the antimycotic potency of AmBisome in comparison with the conventional form indicated that the former may be four to eight times less potent than the latter. If this result is confirmed by others, one might speculate that the higher tolerability of liposomal encapsulated drugs may be at least partially due to the lower free bioavailability of the embedded compound. Indeed, pharmacokinetic studies in cancer patients treated with pegylated-liposomal doxorubicin demonstrated that the free drug level in plasma was only in the range of 0.25 to 1.25% of the total measured drug. Thus, more clinical studies concerning the pharmacodynamic consequences based on the different pharmacokinetic behavior of liposomally embedded drugs seem to be warranted [5,48–52, 56]. Additionally, in regard to the role of these liposomal formulations in the treatment of solid tumors, standardized dosage recommendations as well as randomized prospective multicenter trials are still lacking [5,48–52,56].

2.3.7 Mitoxantrone

Mitoxantrone is used as a component of various chemotherapeutic regimens for remission induction in acute leukemia in adults (e.g., 8–12 mg/m^2 IV on days 1–5 every 3 weeks) and in the treatment of low grade NHL. The drug is also used in the palliative treatment of advanced, symptomatic hormone-refractory prostate cancer (e.g., 10–14 mg/m^2 IV every 3–4 weeks) [57]. Mitoxantrone may be useful for dose escalation regimens because it lacks neurotoxic or nephrotoxic side effects, in contrast to a variety of other antileukemic agents. Recently, up to 80 mg/m^2 mitoxantrone was investigated in combination with high-dose cytarabine in patients with acute leukemia [58]. The drug has been successfully used in the management of malignant pleural effusions. By using 30–40 mg mitoxantrone the success rates ranged from 50 to 100% [59].

The toxicity profile of mitoxantrone includes dose-limiting myelosuppression, chronic cardiotoxicity, moderate nausea and emesis, and a transient increase of liver enzymes. A possible advantage of mitoxantrone is the low incidence of alopecia.

Mitoxantrone differs from the common chemical structure of the anthracyclines by the substituted aminoalkylamino groups. Under physiological conditions, these amino groups are positively charged, which facilitates the interaction with the negatively charged phosphate bonds within the DNA. After intercalation, mitoxantrone induces single- and double-strand breaks of DNA, probably via an interaction with the topisomerase II [1]. The exact mechanism of antiproliferative activity is not yet fully understood, but it may include a further oxidation of the molecule to reactive intermediates (Fig. 25) [59].

It has been suggested that in contrast to the anthracyclines, the reduction of the quinone system leading to toxic superoxide radicals may be of minor importance in the case of mitoxantrone-mediated cytotoxicity. However, because mitoxantrone exerts cardiotoxic side effects too, one cannot exclude the possibility that reactive radical species form during mitoxantrone treatment [1,57,58].

After i.v. administration the drug is widely distributed into different tissues. The mean total-body clearance averages 450 mL/min/m^2, and the mean volume of distribution at steady-state conditions has been estimated to range from 270 to 320 L/m^2. About 90% of the dose is bound to plasma proteins. The drug is extensively metabolized in the liver (Fig. 25). The parent drug and its metabolites are primarily excreted in the bile. The terminal elimination half-life has been estimated to be about 37 hours. There is some evidence that mitoxantrone pharmacokinetics is linear with increasing dose. Within 5 hours about 6.5 and 18.3% of the dose is recovered in urine and feces, respectively [60–63]. These data indicate that dosage adjustment is not needed in cancer patients with renal dysfunction. Preliminary data indicate that mitoxantrone does not appear to be extensively eliminated by hemodialysis, thus dosage adjustment does not seem to be warranted in patients undergoing this procedure [64].

The major hepatic biotransformation products, the monocarboxy and dicarboxy acid derivatives, are no longer cytotoxic (Fig. 25) [60–63]. If hepatic function is moderately impaired, a general reduction of dose is not recommended.

2.3.7.1 Clinical Pharmacokinetics Regarding Efficacy and Toxicity

High interindividual variability has been observed with respect to the terminal elimination half-life of mitoxantrone. In some individuals a terminal elimination half-life of up to 215 hours has been reported, which is about five- to sixfold longer than the usual value of about 37 hours [60–63]. This could be of clinical importance regarding the reinfusion of bone marrow or peripheral blood progenitor cells after a few days of high-dose mitoxantrone which has been primarily used in breast cancer patients. However, more clinical data are necessary to establish the relevance of individual clinical pharmacokinetics in high-dose mitoxantrone therapy in combination with PBSCT or BMT [64].

Several data indicate that the intrapleural or intraperitoneal administration of anthracyclines, particularly mitoxantrone, results in high pleural and peritoneal levels, a lower risk of systemic side effects, and an increased quality of life in comparison to other treatment regimens [65–70].

2.3.8 Anthrapyrazole Derivatives

Anthrapyrazole derivatives, like DUP 937, Losoxantrone [biantrazole], and Piroxantrone [oxantrazole], represent a new class of DNA-intercalating agents (Fig. 26). Though the anthrapyrazoles may exert antiproliferative activity comparable to that of the anthracyclines on an equimolar basis, they seem to be far less cardiotoxic. For example, no sign of congestive cardiomyopathy could be detected in cancer patients at cumulative Piroxantrone doses up to 1280 mg/m^2. Because toxicity has mainly been restricted to leukopenia, it has been speculated that these drugs may be very interesting candidates for dose escalation studies with hematopoietic growth factors. Thus, these agents may find an additional role in high-dose combination chemotherapy protocols with transplantation of bone marrow or peripheral blood progenitor cells [71].

Their pharmacokinetic characteristics have not yet been examined in detail. In general, they are highly protein bound and demonstrate a large

Fig. 25 Metabolic pathways of mitoxantrone: (a) oxidation of the hydroxy groups within the side chains, followed by the formation of the corresponding carboxy acids; (b) glucuronidation of these hydroxy groups; (c) oxidation of the hydroquinone system, which may lead to glutathione conjugates or heterocyclic derivatives. The possibility that the third pathway contributes to the overall cytotoxic effects of mitoxantrone cannot be excluded.

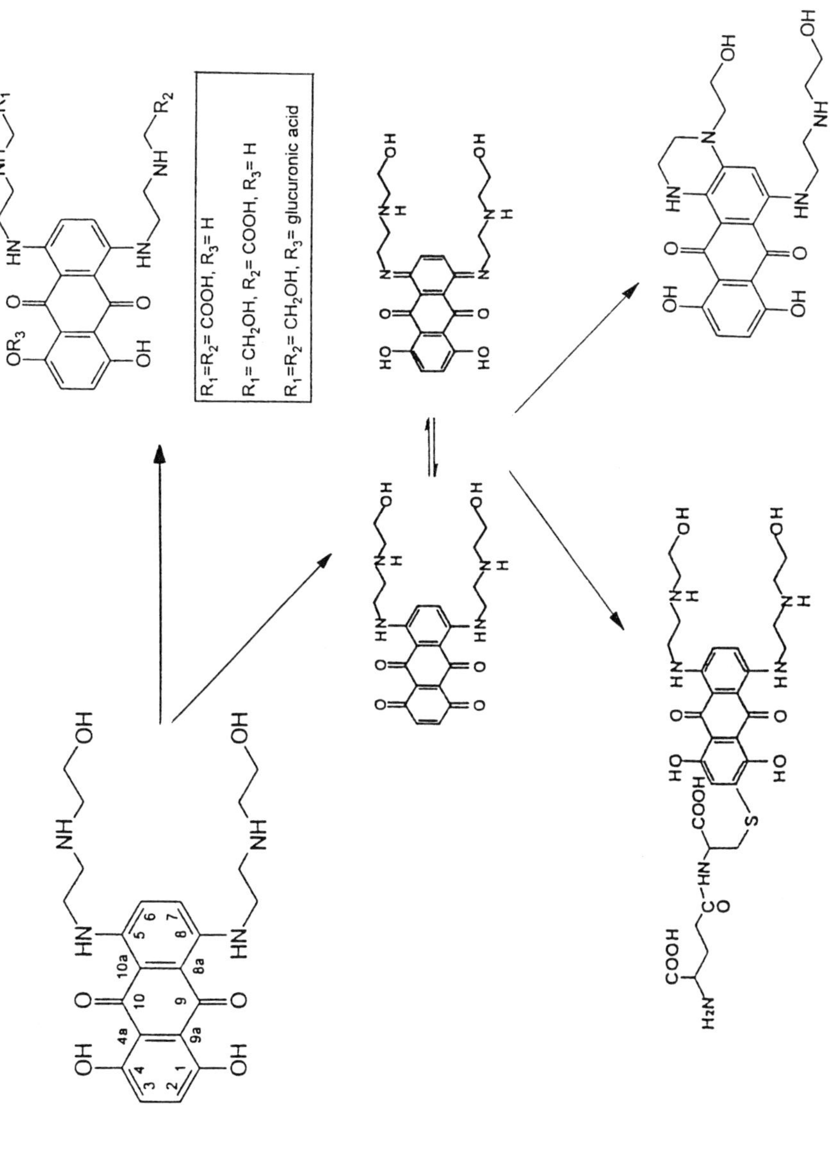

$R_1 = R_2 = COOH$, $R_3 = H$

$R_1 = CH_2OH$, $R_2 = COOH$, $R_3 = H$

$R_1 = R_2 = CH_2OH$, $R_3 =$ glucuronic acid

Fig. 25

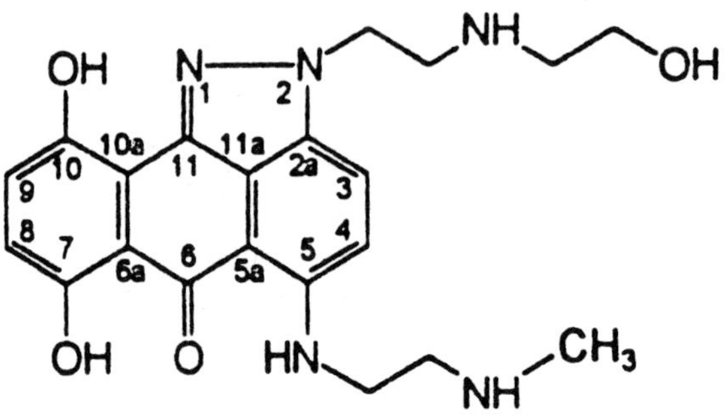

Fig. 26 Common structure of the anthrapyrazoles: the derivatives DUP 937, Losoxantrone, and Piroxantrone represent a new class of DNA intercalating agents that may be even less cardiotoxic.

volume of distribution as well as rather long elimination half-lives. There seems to be some similarity to the biotransformation pathways of mitoxantrone particularly regarding the formation of glutathione conjugates (see Fig. 25).

Despite the structural similarities, some differences regarding clinical pharmacokinetics have been observed. After i.v. administration of DuP 937 (e.g., 22 mg/m^2) the β-elimination half-life seems to approximate 2.8 hours. Because the drug can be detected up to 21 days after administration, the clearance of the drug seems to be extremely prolonged. Phase I studies with Losoxantrone indicate a marked interindividual variability of AUC values that cannot be easily explained by interindividual differences of plasma protein binding or renal and hepatic function. Its elimination half-life has been estimated to be about 14 hours.

In contrast to DUP 937 or Losoxantrone, Piroxantrone appears to have a rather short elimination half-life, approximating 30 minutes [71,72].

2.3.9 Amsacrine

Amsacrine (4′-(9-acridinylamino)-methanesulfonate-*m*-anisidine) exerts considerable antineoplastic activity against a variety of lymphomas and leukemias. It has been used for remission induction in relapsed acute myelogenous leukemia (90 mg/m^2 IV, on days 1–5 every 2–4 weeks). Its cytotoxic effect is mainly based on its ability to intercalate between DNA strands [73–75].

Its toxicity profile includes dose-limiting myelosuppression, cardiotoxic side-effects, gastrointestinal dysfunctions, a transient increase of liver enzymes, alopecia, and skin disorders.

After i.v. administration, about 97% of a dose is bound to plasma proteins. The biexponential elimination curve is characterized by an initial half-life of about 0.6–0.9 hour and a terminal half-life of about 5 hours, which may slightly be prolonged on day 3 of the treatment course. Amsacrine is extensively metabolized in the liver: less than 15% is excreted in the urine as unchanged drug within 72 hours [76,77].

The parent compound and its metabolites are mainly eliminated in the bile and feces. In the liver, amsacrine is very probably oxidized to amsacrine quinone diimine (AQDI) and amsacrine quinone imine (*m*-AQI), which may be transformed either to a glutathione conjugate or to reactive intermediates, which are covalently bound to cellular macromolecules. The *m*-AMSA glutathione conjugate has been identified as major metabolite in rat bile (Fig. 27) [78]. After comparing the metabolism of *m*-AMSA with that of the

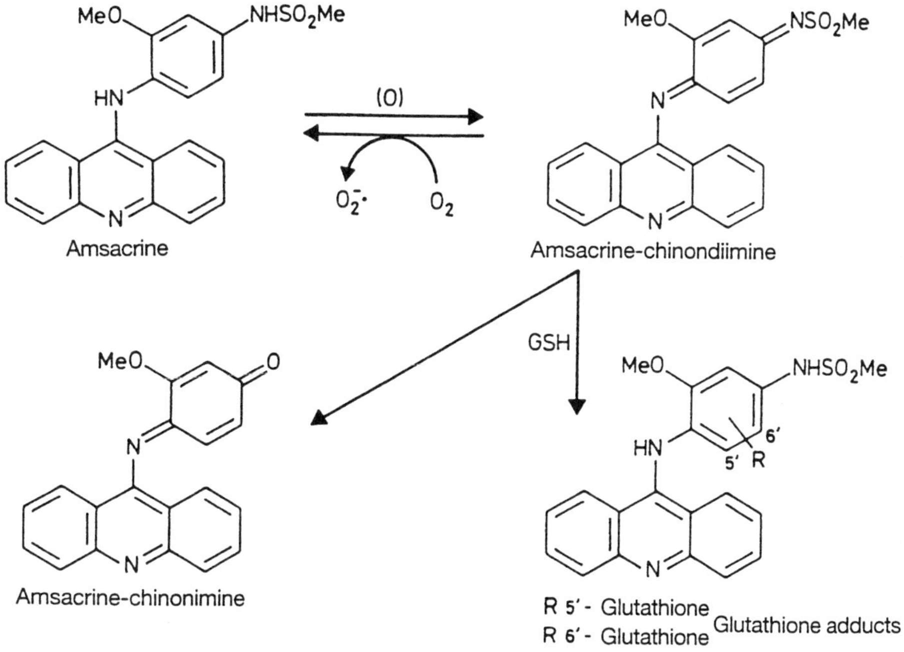

Fig. 27 Biotransformation pathways of amsacrine. The corresponding quinone imine derivative is of major clinical importance. First, if it is reoxidized to amsacrine, very reactive superoxide radicals will be released; second, it is able to bind covalently to a variety of macromolecules. Amsacrine quinone imine, which is released by hydrolysis, appears to be cytotoxic, too, whereas the glutathione conjugates are very probably inactive.

anthracyclines, one cannot exclude the possibility that the release of reactive oxygen radicals during redox cycling is responsible for the cumulative cardiotoxicity of *m*-AMSA [79].

In patients with severe hepatic dysfunction, the plasma clearance of amsacrine may be significantly impaired. In patients with serum bilirubin concentrations exceeding 2 mg/dL, only 75% of the usual dose is recommended [80]. A similar reduction of dose has been recommended in cases of increased serum creatinine concentrations (>1.5 mg/dL). However, the latter recommendation seems to be most reasonable if there is a concomitant marked increase of liver enzyme.

2.3.10 Bleomycin

Bleomycin is often used as part of combination regimens for the treatment of NHL, Hodgkin lymphoma, and testicular germ cell cancer. The usually recommended dose is 10–20 mg/m^2 (10–20 U/m^2) IV once or twice weekly by bolus administration [81,82]. The drug has been successfully used in the management of malignant pleural effusions. By using 60 U of bleomycin the success rates ranged from 63 to 85% [59].

The toxicity profile of bleomycin includes mucositis, alopecia, allergic reactions and skin disorders, influenza-like symptoms, and cumulative interstitial pneumonitis. The myelosuppressive side-effects are generally mild.

Following i.v. administration, bleomycin is widely distributed into the skin, lungs, kidneys, peritoneum, and lymphatic system. The metabolic degradation of bleomycin is catalyzed by the enzyme bleomycin hydrolase (Fig. 28). Constitutive high concentrations of this detoxifying enzyme are found in the bone marrow, whereas very low levels are detectable in lung tissue. The latter may explain the extraordinarily high sensitivity of pulmonary tissues, in contrast to the bone marrow, toward the toxic side effects of the drug [83,84]. Additionally there is some evidence that tumor cells with increased constitutive expression of bleomycin hydrolyase are highly resistant to this anticancer drug [85].

Generally cumulative dosages higher than 360-400 U should be avoided for otherwise the onset of severe and irreversible pulmonary toxicity is more likely irrespective whether the drug has been given as bolus application or continuous infusion [86,87].

About 45–70% of parenterally administered bleomycin is recovered in the urine as unchanged drug. Because of the close correlation between creatinine clearance and bleomycin clearance, it is reasonable to adjust dose according to the individual glomerular filtration rate; otherwise, the probability of bleomycin-induced pneumonitis and pulmonary fibrosis may be severely increased. For creatinine clearances of 60 and 45 mL/min, the rec-

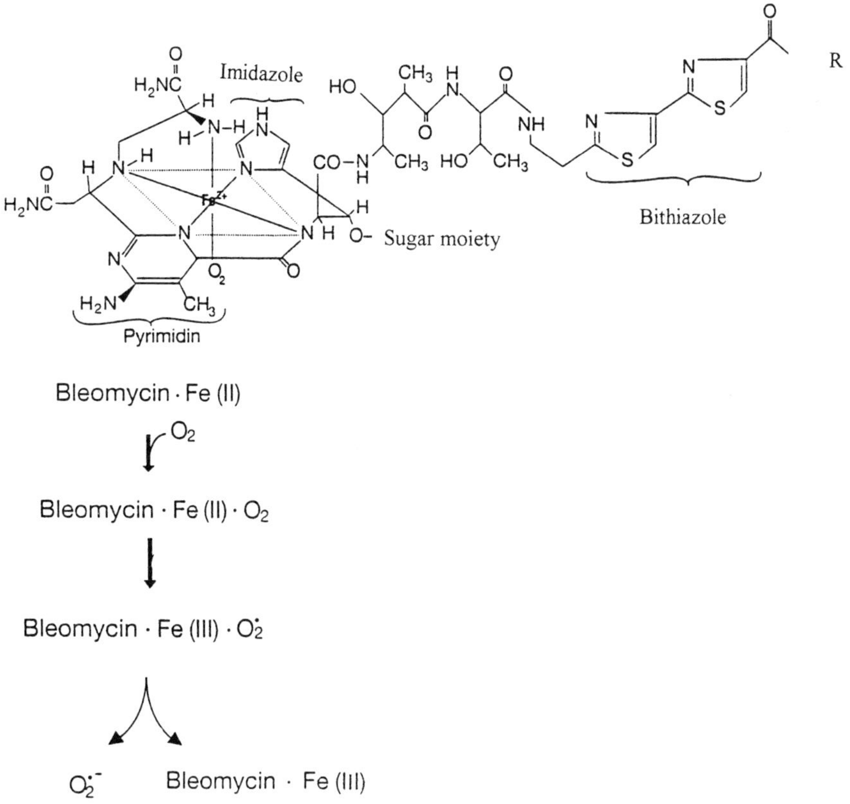

Bleomycin · Fe (II)

↓ O_2

Bleomycin · Fe (II) · O_2

↓

Bleomycin · Fe (III) · $O_2^{\bullet}$

$O_2^{\bullet -}$ Bleomycin · Fe (III)

Fig. 28 Chemical structure of bleomycin sulfate. The drug intercalates into the DNA with its bithiazole moiety. The peptide side chain with its five nitrogen-containing groups forms a chelating complex by binding divalent metal ions, particularly ferrous ions. If oxygen binds as the sixth ligand, very reactive hydroxyl and superoxide anions can be released by an electron transfer.

ommended dose is 70 and 60%, respectively, of the usual amount. The use of bleomycin is contraindicated if the glomular filtration rate is less than 30 mL/min [87].

2.3.11 Actinomycin D

Actinomycin D (Dactinomycin) (Fig. 29) is a component of various chemotherapy regimens in the treatment of localized and metastatic Wilms tumor (nephroblastoma), rhabdomyosarcoma, and Ewing sarcoma in children.

Dactinomycin (Actinomycin D, DACT, ACTD)

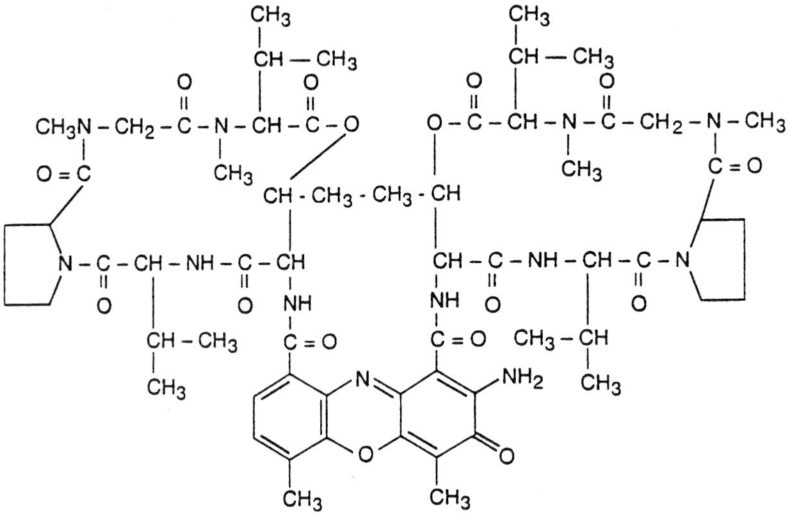

Fig. 29 Chemical structure of actinomycin D.

After i.v. administration, the elimination half-life of actinomycin has been estimated to be about 36 hours. However, within 8 days only 14 or 20% of dose has been recovered in feces or urine, respectively. These data indicate that the drug is not extensively metabolized. As a consequence, if renal or hepatic function is impaired, dosage adjustment does not seem to be warranted [90].

REFERENCES TO SECTION 2.3

1. Powis G. Toxicity of free radical forming anticancer agents. In: G Powis, MP Hacker, eds. The Toxicity of Anticancer Drugs. New York: Pergamon Press, 1991, pp 106–132.
2. Riggs CE, Bachur NR. Clinical pharmacokinetics of anthracycline antibiotics. In: MM Ames, G Powis, JS Kovach, eds. Pharmacokinetics of Anticancer Agents in Humans. New York: Elsevier Science Publishers, 1983, pp 229–277.
3. Foglesong PD, Reckord C, Swink S. Doxorubicin inhibits human DNA topoisomerase I. Cancer Chemother Pharmacol 1992:30:123–125.

4. Goormaghtigh E, Chatelain P, Caspers J, et al. Evidence of a complex between Adriamycin derivatives and cardiolipin: Possible role in cardiotoxicity. Biochem Pharmacol 1980:29:3003–3010.
5. Kim S. Liposomes as carriers of cancer chemotherapy. Drugs 1993:46(4): 618–638.
6. Edwards DMF, Marrari P, Efthymiopoulos C, et al. Pharmacokinetics of iododoxorubicin in the rat, dog and monkey. Drug Metab Dispos 1991:19: 938–945.
7. Brenner DE, Wiernik PH, Wesley M, Bachur NR. Acute doxorubicin toxicity. Cancer 1984:53:1042–1048.
8. Allen A. The cardiotoxicity of chemotherapeutic drugs. Semin Oncol 1992:19: 529–542.
9. Steinherz LJ, Steinherz PG, Tan CTC, Heller G, Murphy ML. Cardiac toxicity 4 to 20 years after completing anthracycline therapy. JAMA 1991:266:1672–1677.
10. Weiss RB. The anthracyclines: Will we ever find a better doxorubicin? Semin Oncol 1992:19:670–686.
11. Basser RL, Green MD. Strategy for prevention of anthracycline cardiotoxicity. Cancer Treatment Rev 1993:19:57–77.
12. Seifert CF, Nesser ME, Thompson DF. Dexroxazone in the prevention of doxorubicin-induced cardiotoxicity. Ann Pharmacother 1994:28:1063–1072.
13. Bertelli G, Gozza A, Forno GB, et al. Topical dimethylsulfoxide for the prevention of soft tissue injury after extravasation of vesicant cytotoxic drugs: a prospective clinical study. J Clin Oncol 1995:13:2851–2855.
14. Ehrke MJ, Mihich E, Berd D, Mastrangelo MJ. Effects of anticancer drugs on the immune system in humans. Semin Oncol 1989:16:230–253.
15. Chassany O, Urien S, Claudepierre P, et al. Comparative serum protein binding of anthracycline derivatives. Cancer Chemother Pharmacol 1996:38:571–573.
16. Benjamin RS, Riggs CE, Bachur NR. Plasma pharmacokinetics of Adriamycin and its metabolites in humans with normal hepatic and renal function. Cancer Res 1977:37:1416–1420.
17. Paul C, Liliemark J, Tidefelt U, Gahrton G, Peterson C. Pharmacokinetics of daunorubicin and doxorubicin in plasma and leukemic cells from patients with acute nonlymphoblastic leukemia. Ther Drug Monit 1989:11:140–148.
18. Launchbury AP, Habboubi N. Epirubicin and doxorubicin: A comparison of their characteristics, therapeutic activity and toxicity. Cancer Treatment Rev 1993:19:197–228.
19. Lown JW, Chen H, Plambeck JA. Further studies on the generation of reactive oxygen species from activated anthracyclines and the relationship to cytotoxic action and cardiotoxic effects. Biochem Pharmacol 1982:31:575–581.
20. Brenner DE, Wiernik PH, Wesley M, Bachur NR. Acute doxorubicin toxicity: Relationship to pretreatment liver function, response and pharmacokinetics in patients with acute nonlymphocytic leukemia. Cancer 1984:53:1042–1048.
21. Sweatman TW, Lokich JJ, Israel M. Clinical pharmacology of continuous infusion doxorubicin. Ther Drug Monit 1989:11:3–9.

22. De Valeriola D. Dose optimization of anthracyclines. Anticancer Res 1994:14: 2307–2314.
23. Preisler HD, Gessner T, Azarnia N, et al. Relationship between plasma Adriamycin levels and the outcome of remission induction therapy for acute nonlymphocytic leukemia. Cancer Chemother Pharmacol 1984:12:125–130.
24. Camaggi CM, Comparsi R, Strocchi E, et al. HPLC analysis of doxorubicin, epirubicin and fluorescent metabolites in biological fluids. Cancer Chemother Pharmacol 1988:21:216–220.
25. Launay MC, Milano G, Iliadis A, Frenay M, Namer N. A limited sampling procedure for estimating Adriamycin pharmacokinetics in cancer patients. Br J Cancer 1989:60:89–92.
26. Biganzoli L, Piccart MJ. The bigger the better? ... or what we know and what we still need to learn about anthracycline dose per course, dose density and cumulative dose in the treatment of breast cancer. Ann Oncol 1997:8:1177–1182.
27. Coukell A, Faulds D. Epirubicin—A review of its pharmacodynamic and pharmacokinetic properties, and therapeutic efficacy in the management of breast cancer. Drugs 1997:53(3):453–482.
28. Bonnadonna G, Gianni L, Santoro A, et al. Drugs ten years later: Epirubicin. Ann Oncol 1993:4:359–369.
29. Bastholt LB, Dalmark M, Gjedde SB, et al. Dose–response relationship of epirubicin in the treatment of postmenopausal patients with metastatic breast cancer: A randomized study of epirubicin at four different dose levels performed by the Danish Breast Cancer Cooperative Group. J Clin Oncol 1996: 14:1146–1155.
30. Camaggi CM, Comparsi R, Strocchi E, et al. Epirubicin and doxorubicin comparative metabolism and pharmacokinetics. Cancer Chemother Pharmacol 1988:21:221–228.
31. Robert J. Epirubicin—Clinical pharmacology and dose–effect relationships. Drugs 1993:45(suppl 2):20–30.
32. Camaggi CM, Strocchi E, Tamassia V, et al. Pharmacokinetic studies of 4′-epi-doxorubicin in cancer patients with normal and impaired renal function and with hepatic metastases. Cancer Treatment Rep 1982:66:1819–1824.
33. Twelves CJ, Dobbs NA, Michael Y, et al. Clinical pharmacokinetics of epirubicin: The importance of liver biochemical tests. Br J Cancer 1992:62:765–769.
34. Mross K, Maessen P, van der Vigjh WJ, Gall H, Bowen E. Pharmacokinetics and metabolism of epidoxorubicin and doxorubicin. J Clin Oncol 1988:6:517.
35. Jakobsen P, Steiness E, Bastholt L, et al. Multiple-dose pharmacokinetics of epirubicin at four different dose levels: Studies in patients with metastatic breast cancer. Cancer Chemother Pharmacol 1991:28:63–68.
36. Deesen PE, Leyland-Jones B. Sensitive and specific determination of the new anthracycline analog 4′-epirubicin and its metabolites by high pressure liquid chromatography. Drug Metab Dispos 1984:12:9–13.
37. Berger DP, Winterhalter BR, Schick U, Höffken K. Idarubicin—Intravenös und oral. Onkologie 1995:1:154–166.

38. Martoni A, Piana E, Guaraldi M, et al. Comparative phase II study of idarubicin versus doxorubicin in advanced breast cancer. Oncology 1990:47:427–432.
39. Lopez M, Contegiacomo A, Vici P, et al. A prospective randomized trial of doxorubicin versus idarubicin in the treatment of advanced breast cancer. Cancer 1989:64:2431–2436.
40. Anderlini P, Benjamin RS, Wong FC, et al. Idarubicin cardiotoxicity: A retrospective study in acute myeloid leukemia and myelodysplasia. J Clin Oncol 1995:13:2827–2834.
41. Speth PAJ, Minderman H, Haanen C. Idarubicin versus daunorubicin: Preclinical and clinical pharmacokinetic studies. Semin Oncol 1989:16(suppl 2):2–9.
42. Goebel M. Oral idarubicin—An anthracycline derivative with unique properties. Ann Hematol 1993:66:33–43.
43. Robert J. Pharmacological properties of oral idarubicin. Clin Drug Invest 1995: 9(suppl 2):1–8.
44. Robert J, Rigal-Huguet F, Huet S, et al. Pharmacokinetics of idarubicin after oral administration in elderly leukemic patients. Leukemia 1990:4:227–229.
45. Sulkes A, Collins JM. Reappraisal of some dosage adjustment guidelines. Cancer Treatment Rep 1987:71:229–233.
46. Mitrou PS, Kuse R, Anger H, et al. Aclarubicin (Aclacinomycin A) in the treatment of relapsing acute leukemias. Eur J Cancer Clin Oncol 1985:21:919–923.
47. Kagawa D, Nakamura T, Ueda T, Domae N, Uchino H. Evaluation of oral aclarubicin treatment for tumors of the gastrointestinal tract. Anticancer Res 1993:13:909–914.
48. Ranson M, Howell A, Cheeseman S, Margison J. Liposomal drug delivery. Cancer Treatment Rev 1996:22:365–379.
49. Gabizon A, Isacson R, Libson E, et al. Clinical studies of liposome-encapsulated doxorubicin. Acta Oncolog 1994:33:779–786.
50. Hu Y-P, Henry-Toulmé N, Robert J. Failure of liposomal encapsulation of doxorubicin to circumvent multidrug resistance in an in vitro model of rat glioblastoma cells. Eur J Cancer 1995:31A:389–394.
51. Muggia FM, Safra T, Jeffers S. Antitumor activity of Doxil (doxorubicin in stealth liposomes) in epithelial ovarian cancer (EOC) or cancers of peritoneal origin. 7th International Congress on Anticancer Treatment, Paris, France, 1997:78 (Abstract 96).
52. Coukell AJ, Spencer CM. Polyethylene glycol-liposomal doxorubicin: A review of its pharmacodynamic and pharmacokinetic properties, and therapeutic efficacy in the management of AIDS-related Kaposi's sarcoma. Drugs 1997:53(3): 520–538.
53. Gill PS, Espina BM, Muggia, F, et al. Phase I/II clinical and pharmacokinetic evaluation of liposomal daunorubicin. J Clin Oncol 1995:13:996–1003.
54. Presant CA, Scolaro M, Kennedy P, et al. Liposomal daunorubicin treatment of HIV-associated Kaposi's sarcoma. Lancet 1993:341:1242–1243.
55. Cowens JW, Creaven PJ, Greco WR, et al. Initial clinical (phase I) trial of TLC D-99 (doxorubicin encapsulated in liposomes). Cancer Res 1993:53: 2796–2802.

56. Pahls S, Schaffner A. Comparison of the activity of free and liposomal amphotericin B in vitro and in a model of systemic and localized murine candidiasis. J Infect Dis 1994:169:1057–1061.
57. Feldman EJ, Alberts DS, Arlin Z, et al. Phase I clinical and pharmacokinetic evaluation of high-dose mitoxantrone in combination with cytarabine in patients with acute leukemia. J Clin Oncol 1993:11:2002–2009.
58. Mewes K, Blanz J, Ehninger G, Gebhardt R, Zeller K-P. Cytochrome P450-induced cytotoxicity of mitoxantrone by formation of electrophilic intermediates. Cancer Res 1993:53:5135–5142.
59. Grossi F, Pennucci MC, Tixi L, et al. Management of malignant pleural effusions. Drugs 1998:55(1):47–58.
60. Schleyer E, Kamischke A, Kaufmann CC, Unterhalt M, Hiddemann W. Mitoxantrone pharmacokinetics. In: T. Büchner et al, eds. Acute Leukemias, Vol IV, Prognostic Factors and Treatment Strategies. Berlin: Springer-Verlag, 1994, pp 221–230.
61. Ehninger G, Schuler U, Proksch B, Zeller KP, Blanz J. Pharmacokinetics and metabolism of mitoxantrone, a review. Clin Pharmacokinet 1990:18(5):365–380.
62. Alberts DS, Peng Y-M, Leigh S, et al. Disposition of mitoxantrone in cancer patients. Cancer Res 1985:45:1879–1884.
63. Schleyer E, Kamischke A, Kaufmann CC, Unterhalt M, Hiddemann W. New aspects on the pharmacokinetics of mitoxantrone and its major metabolites. Leukemia 1994:8:435–440.
64. Boros L, Cacek T, Pine RB, Battaglia AC. Distribution characteristics of mitoxantrone in a patient undergoing hemodialysis. Cancer Chemother Pharmacol 1992:31:57–60.
65. Grant S, Arlin ZA, Gewtiz D, et al. Effect of pharmacologically relevant concentrations of mitoxantrone on the in vitro growth of leukemic blast progenitors. Leukemia 1991:5:336–339.
66. Ozyilkan O, Kars A, Guler N, et al. Intrapleural and intraperitoneal palliative treatment of malignant effusions with mitoxantrone [letter; comment]. Anticancer Drugs 1993:4(1):98–99.
67. Markman H, Hakes T, Reichman B, et al. Salvage intraperitoneal mitoxantrone therapy of ovarian cancer: Influence of increasing the volume of treatment. Gynecol Oncol 1993:49:185–189.
68. Oza M, et al. Phase I/II study of intraperitoneal mitoxantrone in refractory ovarian cancer. Ann Oncol 1994:5:343–347.
69. Alberts DS, Surwit EA, Peng Y-M, et al. Phase I clinical and pharmacokinetic study of mitoxantrone given to patients by intraperitoneal administration. Cancer Res 1988:48:5874–5877.
70. Bjermer L, Gruber A, Sue-Chu M, et al. Effects of intrapleural mitoxantrone and mepacrine on malignant pleural effusion—A randomised study. Eur J Cancer 1995:31A:2203–2208.
71. Judson IR. The anthrapyrazoles: A new class of compounds with clinical activity in breast cancer. Semin Oncol 1992:19:687–694.

72. Renner U, Blanz J, Freund S, et al. Biotransformation of CI-937 in primary cultures of rat hepatocytes. Drug Metab Dispos 1995:23:94–101.
73. van Mouwerik TJ, Caines P, Ballentine R. Amsacrine evaluation. Drug Intell Clin Pharm 1987:21:330–334.
74. De Lena M, Rossi A, Bonnadonna G. Phase II trial of AMSA in patients with refractory breast cancer. Cancer Treatment Rep 1979:63:1961–1964.
75. Isell BF. Amsacrine (AMSA). Cancer Treatment Rev 1980:7:73–83.
76. Jurlina JL, Varcoe AR, Paxton JW. Pharmacokinetics of amsacrine in patients receiving combined chemotherapy for treatment of acute myelogenous leukemia. Cancer Chemother Pharmacol 1985:14(suppl 1):21–25.
77. Rivera G, Evans W, Dahl G, Yee GC, Pratt CB. Phase I clinical and pharmacokinetic study of 4′-(9-acridinylamino)methanesulfan M-anisidine (AMSA) in children with cancer. Cancer Res 1980:40:4250–4253.
78. Lee HH, Palmer D, Denny W. Reactivity of quinone imine and quinone diimine metabolites and the antitumor drug amsacrine and related compounds to nucleophiles. J Org Chem 1988:53:6042–6047.
79. Weiss RB, Grillo-López AJ, Marsoni S, et al. Amsacrine associated cardiotoxicity: Analysis of 82 cases. J Clin Oncol 1986:4:918–928.
80. Mahral PS, Legha SS, Valdiviesa M, Ponds G, Yaffe SM. AMSA toxicity in patients with abnormal liver function. Eur J Cancer Clin Oncol 1981:17: 1343–1348.
81. Dorr RT. Bleomycin pharmacology: Mechanism of action and resistance, and clinical pharmacokinetics. Semin Oncol 1992:9(suppl 5):3–8.
82. Sikic BI. In: BI Sikic, M Rozencweig, SK Carter, eds. Bleomycin Chemotherapy. New York: Academic Press, 1985, pp 247–254.
83. Lazo JS, Sebti SM, Filderman AE. Metabolism of bleomycin and bleomycin-like compounds. In: G Powis, RA Prough, eds. Metabolism and Action of Anticancer Drugs. London: Taylor & Francis, 1987, pp 194–210.
84. Alberts DS, Chen H-S, Liu R, et al. Bleomycin pharmacokinetics in man. I. Intravenous administration. Cancer Chemother Pharmacol 1978:1:177–181.
85. Akiyama S-I, Ikezaki K, Kuramochi H, Takahashi K, Kuwano M. Bleomycin-resistant cells contain increased bleomycin-hydrolase activities. Biochem Biophys Res Commun 1981:101:55–60.
86. Alberts WA. Pulmonary complications of cancer treatment. Curr Opin Oncol 1997:9:161–169.
87. Crooke ST, Comis RL, Einhorn LH, et al. Effects of variations in renal function on the clinical pharmacology of bleomycin administered as an i.v. bolus. Cancer Treatment Rep 1977:61:1631–1636.
88. Kintzel PE, Dorr RT. Anticancer drug renal toxicity and elimination: Dosing guidelines for altered renal function. Cancer Treatment Rev 1995:21:33–64.
89. Tattersall MHN, Sodergren JE, Dengupta SK, et al. Pharmacokinetics of actinomycin D in patients with malignant melanoma. Clin Pharmacol Ther 1975: 17:701–708.

2.4 ANTIMETABOLITES

Antimetabolites are drugs that impair the biosynthesis and function of normal cellular metabolites. In most cases they are structurally related to the antagonized metabolites (Table 15) [1–5].

2.4.1 Folic Acid Antagonists

2.4.1.1 Methotrexate (MTX)

Folic acid and its related derivatives are important cellular cofactors for the biosynthesis of the DNA constituents adenosine, guanosine, and thymidine. *N*-5,10-methylene tetrahydrofolic acid, formed via the enzyme dihydrofolate reductase, is the decisive carbon supplier for the formation of the pyrimidine derivative dTMP (deoxythymidine monophosphate) from dUTP (deoxyuridine triphosphate) (Fig. 30). The competitive inhibition of dihydrofolate reductase (DHFR) by methotrexate (MTX) results in decreased biosynthesis of adenosine, guanosine, and thymidine (Fig. 30) [1–3].

Methotrexate (Fig. 31) belongs to the most widely used group of antineoplastic agents in cancer chemotherapy. It plays an essential role in the treatment of such diverse diseases as acute lymphocytic leukemia, non-Hodgkin lymphoma, osteosarcoma, choriocarcinoma, and bladder cancer, and breast cancer (Table 16). It has also become an important therapeutic alternative in the treatment of psoriasis as well as for rheumatic diseases after primary therapy has failed. It is also used in the prophylaxis and treatment of graft-versus-host disease after allogenic bone marrow transplantation. Leucovorin (syn.: calcium folinate) is used as an antidote at intermediate to high MTX dosages to prevent cell damage of normal tissues [6–10].

In the prevention and treatment of meningeal leukemia, high drug levels in the CSF are necessary to improve the long-term outcome of patients. To circumvent the limited penetration of MTX across the blood-brain-barrier the drug can be administered intrathecally or intraventricularly in order to achieve appropriate CSF MTX levels. Following a 12 mg/m^2 intrathecal dose of MTX, drug elimination is biphasic with half-lives ranging from 4.5 to 14 hours. Generally, the corresponding MTX AUC values in the CSF are highly variable [24].

Leucovorin (Fig. 2) (syn.: Calcium Folinate) is used as an antidote at intermediate-to-high MTX dosages in order to prevent damage of normal tissues [6–10].

Conventional dosages of MTX range from 15 to 50 mg/m^2 intravenously, every 3–4 weeks. Moderate to high-dose MTX therapy (e.g., 100–

Table 15 Pharmacology of Some Antimetabolites

Substance	Pharmacological aspects
Methotrexate	Reversible inhibition of dihydrofolate reductase, the enzyme that reduces folic acid to tetrahydrofolic acid. As a consequence, the availability of one-carbon fragments necessary for purine synthesis as well as for the conversion of deoxyuridylate to thymidylate is limited and DNA synthesis is impaired.
Mercaptopurine	The corresponding ribonucleotide functions as a purine antagonist. As a consequence, the synthesis of RNA and DNA is inhibited. Mercaptopurine is also a powerful immunosuppressant that strongly inhibits the primary immune response, selectively suppressing humoral immunity. The immunosuppressive agent azathioprine is a prodrug of 5-mercaptopurine.
Thioguanine	The corresponding ribonucleotide functions as a purine antagonist. As a consequence, the synthesis of RNA and DNA is inhibited after thioguanine ribonucleotides have been incorporated into DNA and RNA. There is usually complete cross-resistance between thioguanine and 6-mercaptopurine.
Cytarabine (Ara-C)	The synthetic pyrimidine nucleoside Ara-C is converted intracellularly to the nucleotide cytarabine triphosphate (Ara-CTP), which appears to inhibit DNA polymerase, leading to an inhibition of DNA synthesis. Incorporation of the triphosphate into DNA and RNA may also lead to cytarabine-mediated cytotoxicity.
Gemcitabine	Gemcitabine (2′,2′-difluorodeoxycytidine) is phosphorylated sequentially by deoxycytidine kinase to the corresponding monophosphate, which is further converted to the diphosphate (dFdCDP) and triphosphate (dFdCTP) by deoxycytidine monophosphate kinase, and nucleoside diphosphate kinase, respectively. Like cytarabine, gemcitabine inhibits DNA synthesis by competitively inhibiting DNA polymerase and by direct incorporation into replicating DNA.
5-Fluorouracil (5-FU)	The deoxyribonucleotide of the drug (5-fluoro-2′-deoxyuridine-5′-phosphate) inhibits thymidylate synthetase, which leads to a decrease of intracellular thymidylic acid levels. For persistent stable inhibition, the formation of a ternary complex consisting of the deoxyribonucleotide thymidylate synthetase, as well as *N*-5,10-methylentetrahydrofolic acid, is necessary. Cytotoxicity may also be mediated by 5-FU incorporation into RNA, thereby producing a fraudulent RNA.

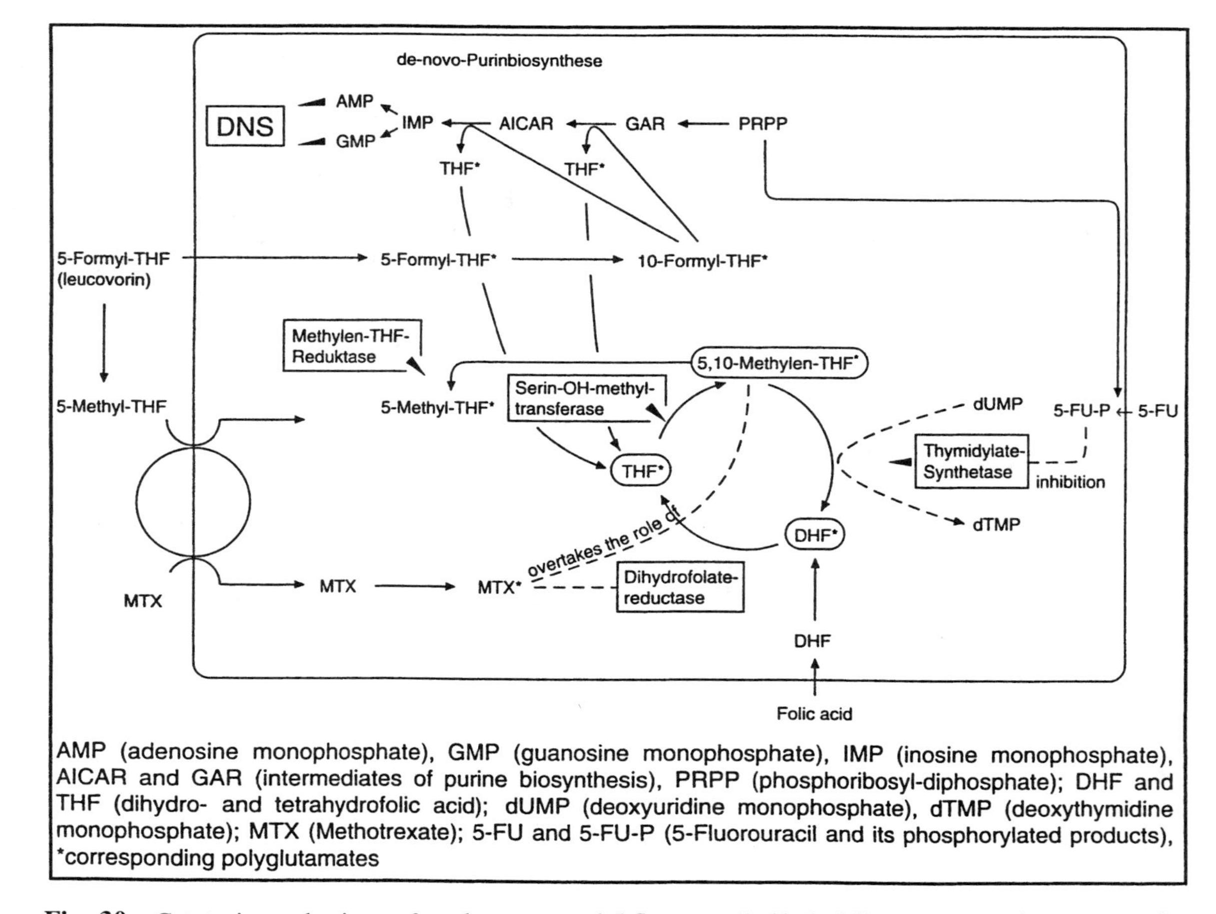

AMP (adenosine monophosphate), GMP (guanosine monophosphate), IMP (inosine monophosphate), AICAR and GAR (intermediates of purine biosynthesis), PRPP (phosphoribosyl-diphosphate); DHF and THF (dihydro- and tetrahydrofolic acid); dUMP (deoxyuridine monophosphate), dTMP (deoxythymidine monophosphate); MTX (Methotrexate); 5-FU and 5-FU-P (5-Fluorouracil and its phosphorylated products), *corresponding polyglutamates

Fig. 30 Cytotoxic mechanisms of methotrexate and 5-fluorouracil (dashed lines represent the corresponding inhibitory pathways).

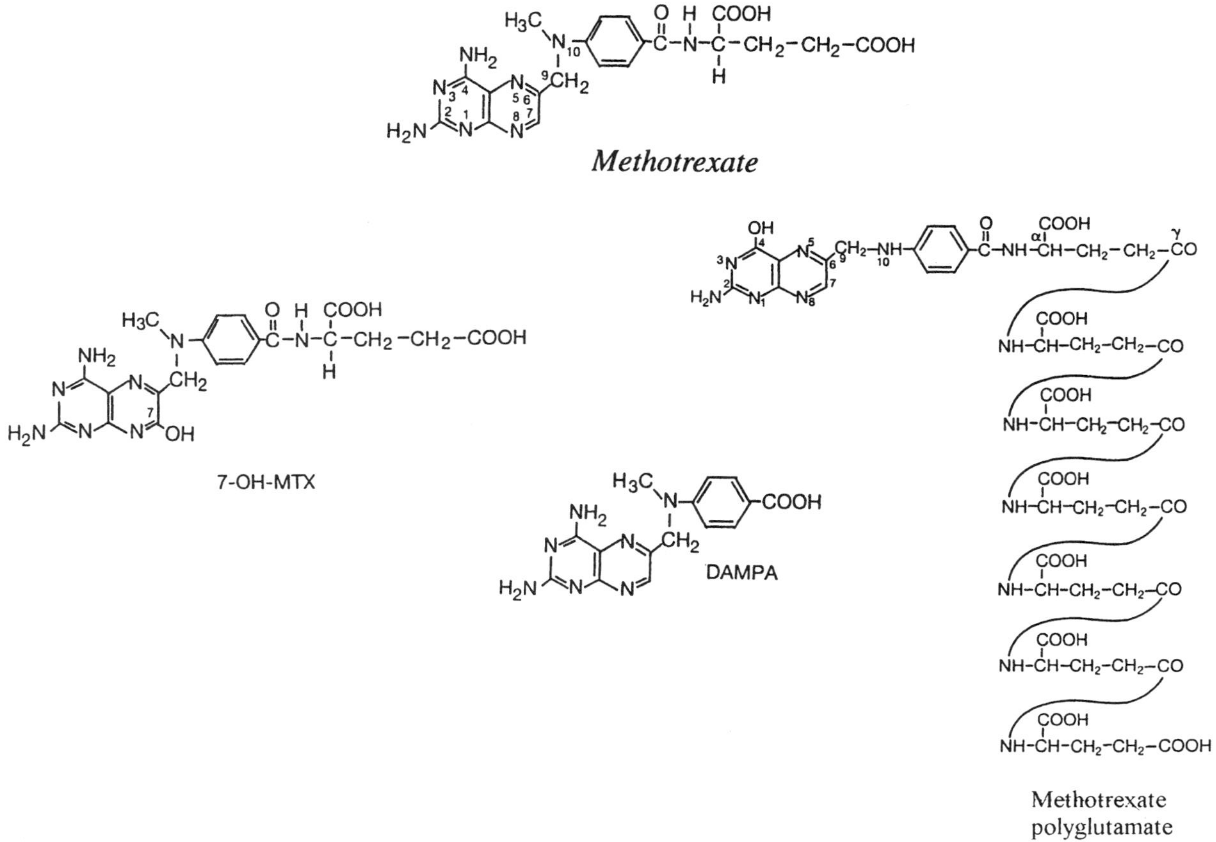

Methotrexate

7-OH-MTX

DAMPA

Methotrexate polyglutamate

Fig. 31 Methotrexate (MTX) and its metabolites 7-hydroxymethotrexate and DAMPA, whose formation is catalyzed by hepatic enzymes and the gut flora, respectively. Their quantitative role is of minor clinical importance. The active metabolite MTX polyglutamate resembles the persistent form of MTX in the cell.

Table 16 Treatment of Neoplastic Diseases with Methotrexate (MTX)

Neoplasm	Treatment regimen[a]
Choriocarcinoma	MTX (plus other drugs)
Lymphoid malignancies	MTX/6-MP; MTX/L-Asp; MTX/Ara-C
Breast cancer	CMF; MTX/5-FU/LV
Osteogenic carcinoma	High-dose MTX
Bladder cancer	M-VAC

[a]6-MP, 6-Mercaptopurine; L-Asp, L-asparaginase; Ara-C, cytarabine; CMF, cyclophosphamide; MTX, methotrexate; 5-FU, 5-fluorouracil; L, Leucovorin; FAMTX, 5-FU + doxorubicin + MTX; M-VAC, MTX + vinblastine + doxorubicin + cisplatin.

1500 mg/m^2) and very intensified MTX therapy (e.g., 8–12 g/m^2) are used for the treatment of leukemia and osteosarcoma, respectively.

The toxicity profile of MTX includes dose-limiting myelosuppression and mucositis, nausea and emesis, acute and chronic liver dysfunction, pulmonary toxicity, skin disorders, CNS side effects, and severe renal dysfunction, which primarily occurs after higher doses and acidic urine pH values.

The maximum tolerated dose (MTD) of MTX in cancer patients varies markedly from 25 to 100 mg/m^2 without Leucovorin rescue and from >100 mg/m^2 up to 20(-50) g/m^2 (and more) with Leucovorin rescue [1–3,6–11]. If doses exceed 100 mg/m^2, serum monitoring of MTX concentrations has been recommended. Leucovorin rescue (usually 12–15 mg/m^2 PO or I.V.) should be started 24 and 42 hours after the beginning of a short-time infusion (e.g., 4 h) and 24-hour continuous infusion, respectively, and should be continued until MTX levels fall below 0.05 μM MTX [12–23].

Although the use of Leucovorin rescue after intrathecal administration of MTX is generally not recommended, it has been suggested that this practice may sometimes be reasonable because marked underlying interindividual variations in delayed MTX kinetics in the cerebrospinal fluid may result in plasma elimination half-lives after redistribution of about 85 hours [24–26].

In plasma, about 43–80% of MTX is bound to proteins. The clinical significance of potential displacement from albumin-binding sites, particularly by drugs like ibuprofen or glibenclamide, has not yet been exactly quantified. The drug is widely distributed in the body tissues, including the CSF. If there are "third spaces" like pleural effusions or ascites, MTX is taken up in significant amounts into those extravascular effusions. This results in a delayed reequilibration of MTX into plasma and a corresponding prolongation of terminal elimination half-life. MTX is contraindicated in those situations and when pleural fluids and ascites must be completely drained before MTX infusion is started [1–3,27].

The elimination kinetics of methotrexate has been demonstrated to be at least triphasic. The initial half-life approximates 2.5 hours, the β-elimination half-life ranges from 8 to 10 hours after conventional dosages (15–50 mg/m^2) and between 8 and 48 hours after high-dose therapy (>1 g/m^2). The terminal elimination half-life is prolonged and approximates several days [1–3,27]. The latter property is based on the slow release of very persistent MTX polyglutamates (Fig. 31), which form intracellularly after MTX uptake [28].

About 70–94% of the dose is excreted in the urine as unchanged drug within 24 hours, whereas the remaining 10% consists of the major metabolite 7-hydroxymethotrexate (7-OH-MTX). Although less cytotoxic than the parent compound, 7-OH-MTX (Fig. 31) contributes significantly to the nephrotoxic side effects [1–3,27,29,30].

MTX is primarily excreted through glomerular filtration and to a lesser extent via tubular secretion. Biliary elimination, which accounts for less than 10% of MTX elimination, may lead to a significant reabsorption of the drug via the enterohepatic circulation. The gut flora may transform some amount to DAMPA (4-amino-4-deoxy-*N*-methylpteroic acid). However, excretion of MTX and DAMPA (Fig. 31) in the feces is generally of minor quantitative importance [1–3,27].

If renal function decreases during therapy (e.g., by means of concomitant diarrhea, emesis without adequate hydration, or the use of indomethacin), MTX will accumulate, and its terminal half-life will be prolonged up to 60 hours and more. The interaction with indomethacin may be based on the inhibition of prostaglandin biosynthesis as well as a competition regarding tubular secretion [22].

If creatinine clearance is already reduced at the start of MTX therapy, it is important to adjust the MTX dose (Fig. 32). If the creatinine clearance approximates 60 or 45 mL/min, it is reasonable to use only 65 or 50% of the usual dose, respectively. If the creatinine clearance is less than 30 mL/min, MTX is generally contraindicated [31].

MTX and 7-OH-MTX are insoluble in acidic solutions. As a consequence, without intensive hydration (e.g., 3 L/m^2/d) and alkalinization (e.g., 40 mmol sodium bicarbonate/L) of the urine before starting moderate to high dose MTX therapy, both substances may precipitate in the distal tubules, causing fatal obstructions and secondary intrarenal uropathy [21,32,33].

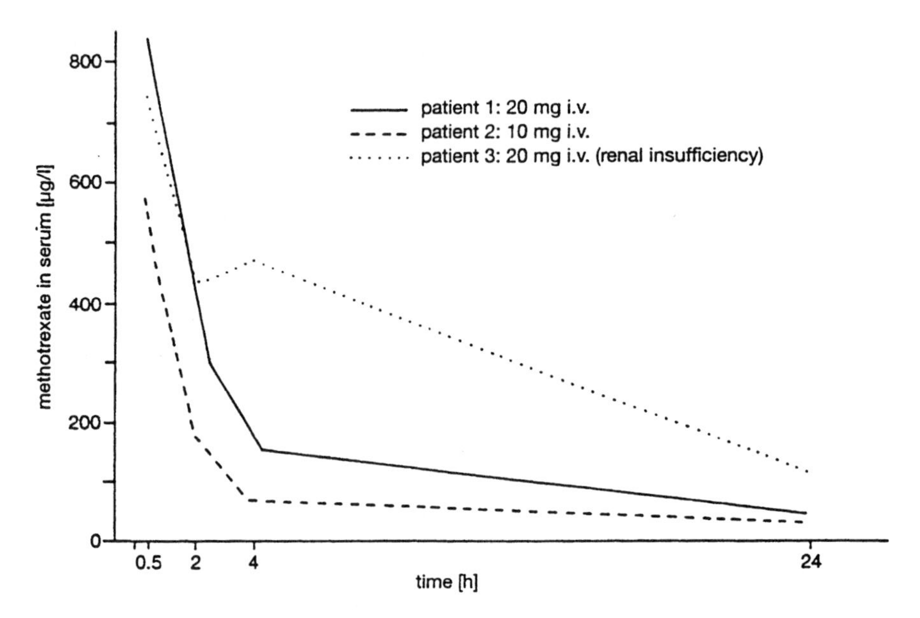

Fig. 32 If renal function is impaired, severe cumulation of MTX is very probable (patient 3). As a consequence, MTX dosage reduction is warranted if individual glomerular filtration rate is decreased.

In patients with severe MTX overdosage or heavily impaired MTX elimination (e.g., because of concomitant acute renal failure), the combined use of hemoperfusion and hemodialysis has been an effective, successful intervention [34–36]. Also in cases of intrathecal MTX overdosage, a strategy for accelerating MTX elimination from the intralumbar space has been presented [37].

Clinical Pharmacokinetics Regarding Efficacy and Toxicity of MTX

MTX blood levels must be measured very accurately during intermediate and high-dose MTX therapy for three important reasons:

1. There are several reports of marked interindividual variability of MTX plasma pharmacokinetics.
2. The MTX plasma clearance may unexpectedly decrease during 96 hours, which significantly elevates the risk of severe side effects.
3. There seems to be a correlation between defined serum concentrations of MTX and the probability of objective responses in patients [8,13,16,19,20,22,26,38].

It has been demonstrated that the toxicity of HD-MTX is directly linked to its exposure time and plasma concentration. However, given the high variability of the underlying individual renal function, usually large variations of inter- and intraindividual MTX kinetics can be observed [1–3,27].

After HD-MTX infusion, peak levels may range from 10 to 1000 μM depending on the dose and the infusion time (Fig. 33). The duration of exposure to MTX in concentrations exceeding 0.05 μM is generally 72–96 hours or more, whereas after a conventional MTX dose (≤40 mg/m^2), the same time is less than 48 hours. It is not possible to predict a delayed MTX excretion by the MTX peak level [22].

The risk of severe mucosal and bone marrow toxicity is increased if MTX serum concentrations exceed 10, 1, 0.1, and 0.05 μM after the start of a 4-hour HD-MTX infusion (8–12 g/m^2) at 24, 48, 72, and 96 hours, respectively (Table 17). Several medical and nursing interventions will be necessary (e.g., intensified hydration and alkalinization) to prevent severe outcome [1–3,6–11]. If MTX levels remain high, Leucovorin rescue must be intensified (Table 17).

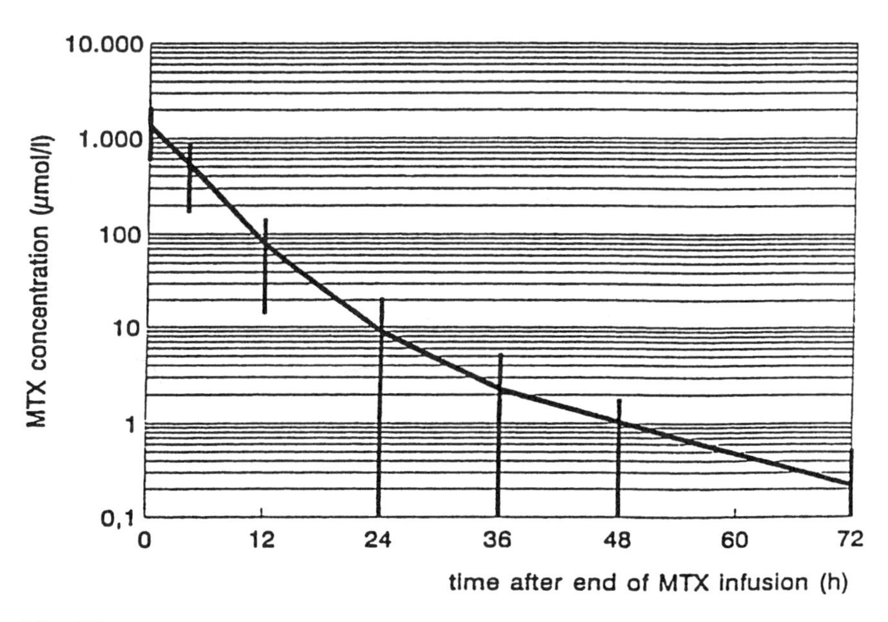

Fig. 33 Usually there is a high variability of MTX pharmacokinetics after high-dose chemotherapy [16]. Thus, it is strongly recommended that MTX plasma levels as well as kidney function be accurately monitored until the MTX levels fall below 0.05 μM. *Source*: Adapted from Ref. 16.

Table 17 Methotrexate Levels Indicating a High Risk of Toxicity[a]

Dosage regimen	MTX level
50–250 mg/kg over 6 h	>0.9 μM 48 h after the start of infusion
50–200 mg/kg over 4 h	>10 μM at 24 h
	>0.5 μM at 48 h
8000 mg/m^2 over 4 h	>10 μM at 24 h
	>1 μM at 48 h
	>0.1 μM at 72 h
1000–1500 mg/m^2 (bolus)	>0.5 μM at 48 h
0.725–15 g/m^2 over 6 h	>5 μM at 24 H

[a]Includes Leucovorin rescue.
Source: Adapted from Ref. 18.

In spite of accurate monitoring of MTX blood levels as well as kidney function, irregular plasma MTX pharmacokinetics may yet occur. The exposure time to MTX concentrations exceeding 0.5 μM seems to be a particularly important prerequisite for the extent of normal tissue damage. MTX plasma clearance may be delayed in spite of accurate alkalinization, hydration and Leucovorin rescue [22]. For example, after 300 mg MTX the measured MTX level may be in the normal range (e.g., 1.3 μM after 48 h), but further decline may be greatly slow. If the MTX level is not measured after 72 hours, the patient may still have MTX concentrations exceeding 1 μM in plasma, a condition that urgently warrants intensified Leucovorin rescue. The background of such an abnormal MTX clearance is not fully understood, but it has been proposed that a sudden decrease in urine volume due to diarrheal episodes, vomiting, or a concomitant therapy with potentially nephrotoxic agents like indomethacin may severely impair the renal clearance of methotrexate [22]. Thus, it is important to monitor MTX blood levels as well as kidney function very accurately until the MTX levels fall below 0.05 (−0.2) μM (Table 17) [15–19].

Regarding pharmacokinetic-pharmacodynamic relationships, Delepine et al. pointed out recently that there may be a threshold MTX serum level of at least 1000 μM which must be achieved for effective treatment of osteosarcoma [39]. Usually only few patients fail to reach this threshold peak level after 12 g MTX/m^2 with concomitant hydration (3 L/m^2/d) and cisplatin therapy.

Regarding the treatment of acute lymphocytic leukemia in children, Evans and colleagues reported that patients who did not achieve defined steady-state concentrations during continuous infusion were seven times more likely to suffer any hematological relapse during therapy. Thus, 1000

mg/m^2 MTX given over 24 hours (once a week for 3 weeks) may be inferior in patients with faster constitutive drug clearance [8]. Very recently they confirmed the importance of individualized chemotherapy for childhood ALL. If a MTX target range from 580 to 980 μM was maintained the outcome in children with B-lineage ALL could be significantly improved in respect to the rate of continuous complete remission at five years [38].

Another example that impressively demonstrates the correlation of defined MTX levels with antitumoral efficacy was recently presented by Comella and colleagues. These researchers suggested that at least 500 mg/m^2 MTX may be necessary to exceed therapeutic serum concentrations of at least 1 μM in the treatment of gastrointestinal malignancies in combination with L-folinic acid and 5-fluorouracil [13].

2.4.1.2 Newer Antifolates in Cancer Chemotherapy

The novel MTX derivative edatrexate (10-EdAM), in which the N^{10}-amine of aminopterin is replaced by a methylene group (Fig. 34), is nearly as effective as MTX in regard to DHFR inhibition. There is some evidence that cellular uptake and intracellular polyglutamation of edatrexate are more prominent in tumor cells than in normal cells. As in the case of MTX, Leucovorin rescue should be initiated 24 hours after edatrexate treatment to reduce the incidence and severity of mucositis.

Trimetrexate and piritrexim (Fig. 34) are more lipophilic than MTX and lack the "classic" terminal glutamic acid residue. Both compounds seem to be very active in a variety of solid tumors. Since these "nonclassic" antifolates cannot be transformed to the corresponding intracellularly persistent polyglutamates, it seems reasonable to attempt to overcome decreased cellular retention by means of prolonged drug exposure rather than bolus administrations. Both compounds may be still active in tumor cells in which resistance to MTX is based on polyglutamation deficiency or impaired MTX transport mechanisms. Trimetrexate and piritrexim have also been shown to be active in the treatment of refractory pneumocystis pneumonia and psoriasis, respectively.

In contrast to MTX, edatrexate, trimetrexate, and piritrexim, the novel MTX derivative ralitrexed (ICI-D1694 Tomudex) and its polyglutamates are very potent non-competitive inhibitors of the enzyme thymidylate synthetase, which catalyzes the methylation of deoxyuridine monophosphate to thymidine monophosphate. Thus, the cytotoxic action of ralitrexed is similar to 5-fluorouracil. It is primarily used in the treatment of advanced colorectal cancer (e.g., 3 mg/m^2 IV q21d). Phase III studies compared the effects of ralitrexed and bolus 5-fluorouracil in patients with colorectal cancer. The toxicity profile of ralitrexed includes dose-limiting myelosuppression, diar-

Structure	Agent

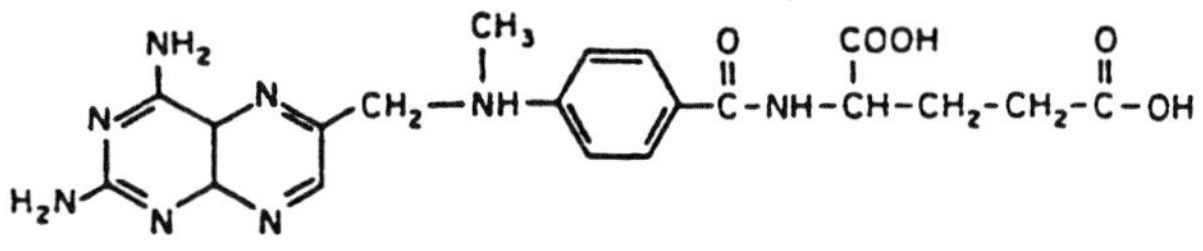

NH2 CH3 O COOH O
N N CH2—NH—C-NH-CH-CH2-CH2-C-OH
H2N N N

Methotrexate

NH2 CH3 OCH3
N CH2—NH— OCH3
H2N N OCH3

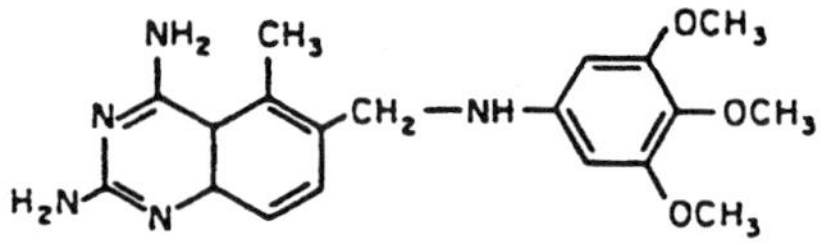

Trimetrexate

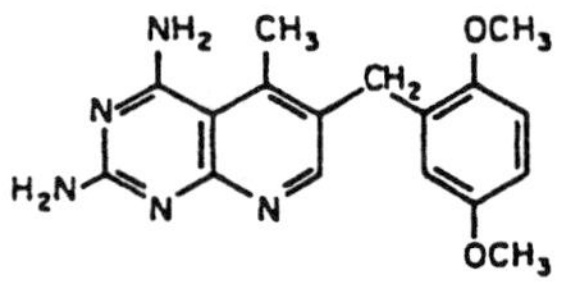

NH2 CH3 OCH3
N CH2
H2N N N
OCH3

Piritrexim

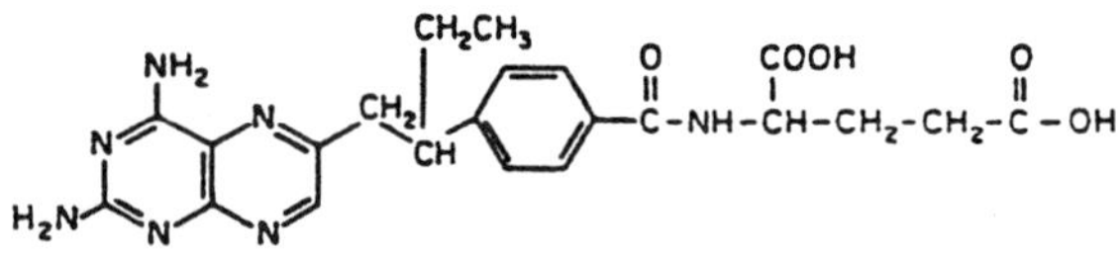

CH2CH3
NH2 O COOH O
N N CH2 C-NH-CH-CH2-CH2-C-OH
CH
H2N N N

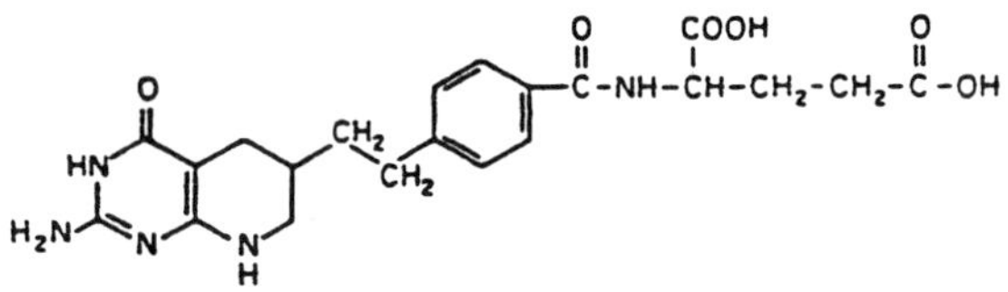

Edatrexate

O COOH O
C-NH-CH-CH2-CH2-C-OH
O
CH2
HN CH2
H2N N N
H

Lometrexol

CH3
O O COOH O
HN CH2N— C-NH-CH-CH2-CH2-C-OH
S
H3C N

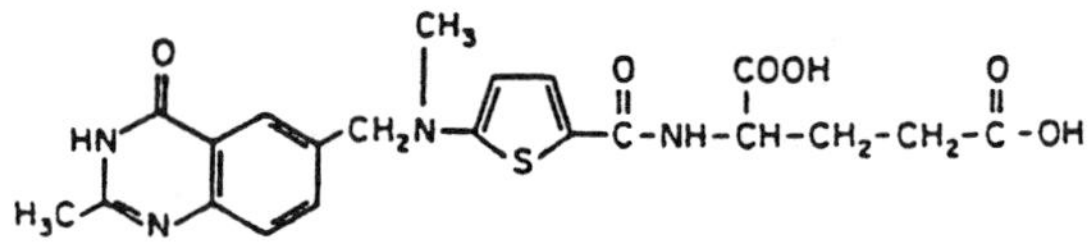

ICI D1694

Fig. 34 Chemical structures of newer antifolates.

rhea, asthenia, a transient increase of liver enzymes, and mild emesis, and has appeared favorable compared to 5-FU in abovementioned studies.

The β-elimination half-life after IV administration approximates 100 min whereas the terminal half-life has been recorded to range from 8 to more than 100 hours. Like MTX, ralitrexed is excreted primarily unchanged in the urine. As a consequence, patients with mild to moderate renal impairment should have a dose reduction of 50% in order to avoid severe leucopenia.

The antineoplastic activity of lometrexol (5,10-dideaza-5,6,7,8-tetrahydrofolic acid) (Fig. 34) is primarily based on the potent inhibition of the enzyme glycinamide ribonucleotide formyltransferase, which mediates the first formyl transfer reaction in de novo purine biosynthesis. This inhibition results in a depletion of cellular pools of adenosine triphosphate (ATP) and guanosine triphosphate (GTP). The corresponding polyglutamates of lometrexol appear to be much more potent than the parent compound. Because of severe hematological and gastrointestinal toxicity during phase I clinical studies, the concomitant oral use of folic acid has been suggested as a possible means of overcoming these toxic side effects [7,40].

The novel pyrrolopyrimidine antifolate LY 231514 which is structurally very similar to lometrexol inhibits thymidylate synthetase. However, there is some evidence that other enzymes in the purine synthesis pathway are inhibited, too, by LY 231514 and its polyglutamates. Thus, the drug represents a multitargeted anti-folate (MTA). Doses of LY 231514 range from 10 to 40 mg/m^2/week in patients with advanced solid tumors, particularly colorectal cancer. Its toxicity profile includes reversible neutropenia, mild-to-moderate fatigue, gastrointestinal disorders, and a reversible increase of liver enzymes [7].

2.4.2 Purine Antimetabolites

2.4.2.1 6-Mercaptopurine

The antimetabolite 6-mercaptopurine (6-MP) constitutes part of the maintenance therapy in ALL. It is administered orally on a daily basis (e.g., 1.5–2.5 mg/kg/d) over a very long period of time. The toxicity profile of 6-MP includes dose-limiting myelosuppression, mild nausea and emesis, and a transient increase of liver enzymes.

The oral administration of the drug is responsible for the large interindividual variations in absolute bioavailability (5–37%) [1–3, 41]. Bioavailability seems to be reduced by about 30% when a dose of 75 mg/m^2 is administered together with a standardized breakfast, compared to fasting conditions. Thus, it has been recommended to administer 6-MP with orange squash after an overnight fast and to give a standard breakfast one hour after

6-MP intake. However, there seems to be a marked day-to-day variation, too, indicating a variable first-pass metabolism in the GI mucosa during absorption [41,42].

Mercaptopurine is an inactive prodrug that must be converted to the corresponding thiopurine nucleotide in the tumor cell to exert its antiproliferative activity. The first step of bioactivation in the cell is the biotransformation to 6-thioinosine-5′-monophosphate (6-thio-IMP) via the enzyme hypoxanthine-guanine phosphoribosyltransferase (HPGRTase). The thioinosinate is further activated by the enzyme IMPD (inosine monophosphate dehydrogenase), yielding 6-thioxanthosine-5′-monophosphate (TXMP) and 6-thioguanosine-5′-monophosphate (Fig. 35) [1–3,43].

Alternatively, the drug can be converted to the inactive *S*-methylmercaptopurine (via thiopurine-*S*-methyltransferase [TPMT]) or deaminated and oxidized to the inactive metabolites 6-thioxanthene and thiouric acid by xanthine oxidase.

The inhibition of xanthine oxidase by other drugs, particularly allopurinol, is of great clinical importance during concomitant 6-MP therapy [1–3,43]. As a consequence the catabolism of 6-MP is severely impaired, which may result in a very severe myelosuppression. Therefore the dose of 6-mercaptopurine must be reduced to one-fourth of the usual dose, if a combination with allopurinol cannot be avoided [44].

TPMT plays a significant role in the metabolic catabolism of 6-mercaptopurine, too. The formed *S*-methyl derivative can be further oxidized, which results in the release of inorganic sulfate [1–3,43].

The elimination half-life of the parent compound ranges from 0.5 to 4 hours. After 8 hours the drug can no longer be detected in serum because it has been modified extensively in the course of its journey on anabolic and catabolic pathways. About 11% of the dose is recovered in the urine within 6 hours. Dose adjustments do not seem to be necessary in the presence of mild to moderate renal dysfunction [1–3].

Clinical Pharmacokinetics Regarding Efficacy and Toxicity

Several reports indicate that there are large interindividual variations in plasma levels of 6-mercaptopurine following oral administration. However, so far, no conclusive evidence has been provided for a correlation between poor availability of oral 6-MP and ALL relapse.

It is of clinical importance that patients with pharmacogenetically based low constitutive thiopurine-*S*-methyltransferase activity (TPMT) expression are at a higher risk for severe and potentially fatal hematopoietic toxicity if they are treated with conventional doses of 6-mercaptopurine or azathioprine. Patients with TPMT deficiency also accumulate higher levels of active thioguanine nucleotides in erythrocytes, which can be closely cor-

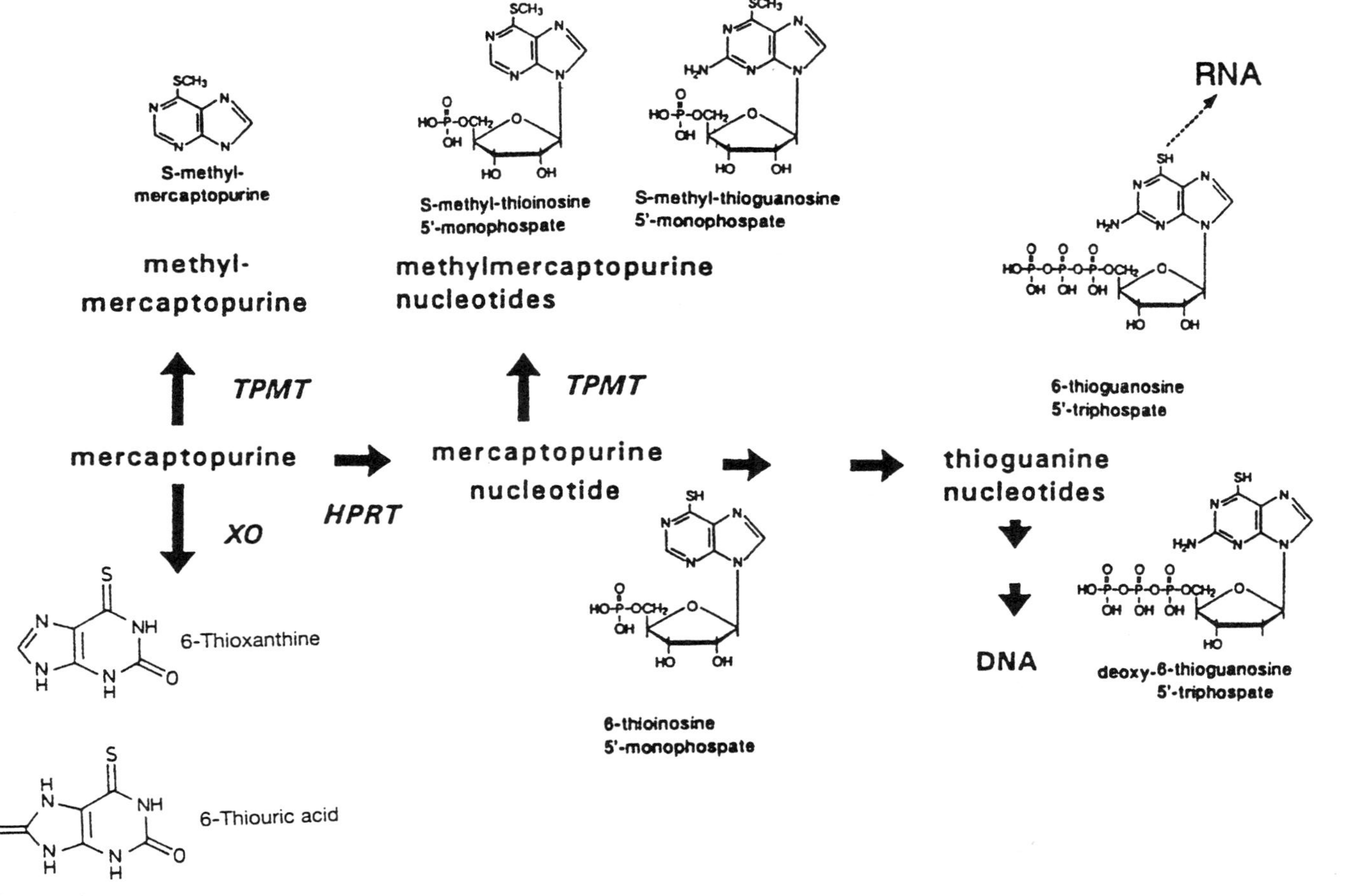

(1) TPMT (Thiopurine-S-methyltransferase); (2) HPRT (Hypoxanthine-guanine-phosphoribosyltransferase); (3) XO (Xanthine oxidase)

Fig. 35 Metabolic pathways of 6-mercaptopurine. (Modified from Ref. 43.)

related with the probability of severe myelosuppression. It has been suggested that those patients need a substantial reduction (about 8- to 15-fold) of the conventional dose [45–47]. About 90 and 10% of the general population express constitutively high (>10 U/mL of packed red blood cells) and intermediate TMPT levels (5–10 U/mL), respectively, whereas about 1 of 300 patients inherits TPMT deficiency (<5 U/mL) as an autosomal recessive trait [45–47]. Very recently, Yates and colleagues presented a novel PCR-based method with which the major nonfunctional mutant alleles can be detected. This genotype method seems to be very sensitive in regard to the identification of TPMT-deficient and heterozygous patients [47]. (See also Chapter 8.3.)

Patients with constitutive high TPMT expression may be at a higher risk for "undertreatment" because their higher level of less active methylated mercaptopurine analogues may be associated with an increased apparent risk for resistance to standard 6-MP-dosages [48].

Welch and colleagues recently published an interesting pharmacokinetic study in which plasma drug as well as red cell metabolite concentrations were measured in children who had received an oral dose. These workers suggested that it could be reasonable to measure methylated mercaptopurine levels in red blood cells because these metabolites appear to be stable for at least 24 hours, which may allow the identification of individuals with too low as well as too high levels based on constitutive high TPMT levels, noncompliance, or genetically low TPMT expression [49].

In conclusion, a more individualized therapy with 6-MP based on therapeutic drug monitoring seems to be a reasonable approach for particularly since it is estimated that about 10% of patients fail to comply fully with their prescribed medication regimen [45–49].

2.4.2.2 Azathioprine

Azathioprine is a well established immunosuppressive agent used to prevent rejection episodes in recipients of solid organ transplants. The initial dose is usually 2 mg/kg mostly combined with cyclosporine 125 mg twice a day, and prednisone [44]. It is also used for immunosuppression in autoimmune diseases. The toxicity profile of azathioprine is very similar to the structurally related 6-mercaptopurine.

In vivo azathioprine is spontaneously converted to 6-mercaptopurine (6-MP) and its corresponding metabolites (Fig. 36). Like 6-MP there is a substantial drug interaction between azathioprine and allopurinol if these drugs are administered concomitantly. Allopurinol is a potent inhibitor of the enzyme xanthine oxidase, which is responsible for the conversion of 6-MP to the inactive metabolite thiouric acid.

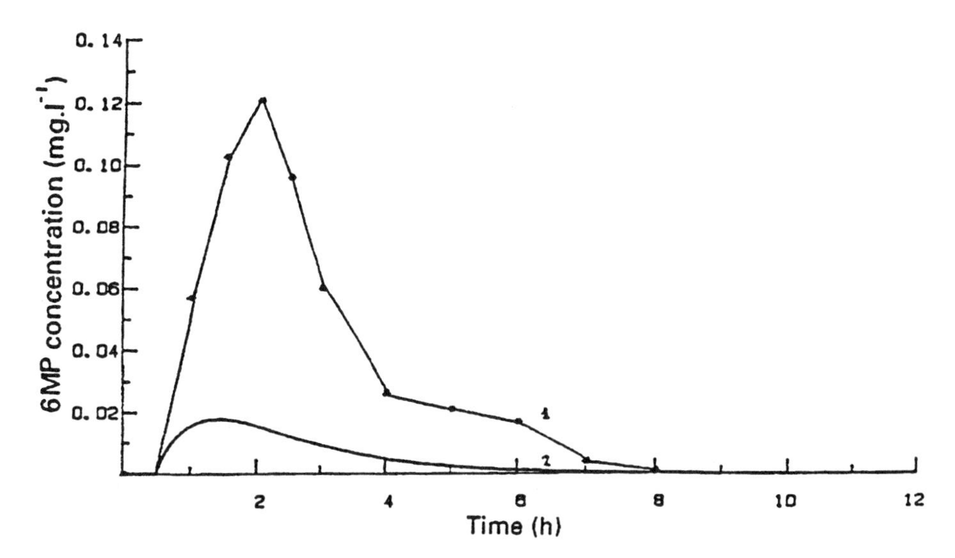

Fig. 36 Comparison of 6-mercaptopurine (6-MP) levels in plasma after a test dose of azathioprine (0.66 mg/kg). Poor metabolizers (curve 1: based on a "poor methylator" phenotype) develop about eightfold higher 6-MP AUC values and sevenfold higher 6-MP peak plasma levels than "normal subjects" (curve 2) [51]. (Adapted from Ref. 51.)

If azathioprine and allopurinol are coadministered orally in conventional dosages, the absolute bioavailability of 6-MP will increase extraordinarily. If this interaction is ignored, the patient will develop severe myelosuppressive side effects, which necessitate an expensive substitution of blood products as well as a prolonged hospital stay [44].

As a consequence, if coadministration is unavoidable, the oral dosage of azathioprine should be reduced by 75–80% during concomitant therapy. Alternatively, it has been suggested that no dosage adjustment would be necessary if azathioprine is administered intravenously, because by this route the first-pass effect is bypassed. It must be kept in mind that xanthine oxidase is found primarily in the liver and the intestinal mucosa [44]. If one wants to circumvent a potential interaction between these two drugs, the use of uricosuric agents rather than allopurinol may be recommended.

As with 6-MP, patients with low constitutive 6-thiopurine methyl transferase (TPMT) activity may develop higher AUC levels of 6-MP than "normal methylators" after conventional azathioprine dosages. If a patient develops unexpected severe leukocytopenia or thrombocytopenia after azathioprine treatment, it is reasonable to measure the 6-MP AUC after a test dose of azathioprine (e.g., 50 mg absolute) or to determine the methylated mercaptopurine concentrations in the red blood cells (RBC). If the AUC and peak levels of 6-MP are nearly tenfold higher than normal, a "poor methylator" phenotype would seem to be the underlying reason for abnormal increased toxicity, especially when the methylated mercaptopurine levels in RBC approximate zero [50–52].

Because only 1–2% of the azathioprine dose is excreted unchanged in the urine, a dosage reduction in patients with renal failure does not seem to be necessary [53].

2.4.3.3 6-Thioguanine

Thioguanine is a component of various chemotherapeutic regimens to induce remission induction and some maintenance schedules in acute myeloid leukemia (AML) and acute nonlymphocytic leukemia (ANLL). It is administered orally on a daily basis (e.g., 60–200 mg/m^2) over a very long period of time. Its toxicity profile includes dose-limiting myelosuppression and moderate nausea and emesis, whereas an increase of liver enzymes is rarely observed in contrast to 6-MP.

As with 6-mercaptopurine (6-MP), the absolute bioavailability of thioguanine is highly variable among individuals and approximates 30% of total dose [1–3].

6-Thioguanine is converted into its corresponding nucleotides, thioguanylic acid and thioguanosine triphosphate, by the enzyme hypoxanthine-guanine phosphoribosyltransferase (HPGRTase). These nucleotides (Fig. 37) are incorporated into the DNA and RNA of bone marrow, thereby replacing the natural purine guanine in DNA [43].

Thioguanine is rapidly and extensively metabolized in the liver and other tissues to the methylated derivative 2-amino-6-methylthiopurine, which is less cytotoxic than the parent compound. Inorganic sulfate will be released by a further oxidation process of this methylated derivative. Additionally, the enzyme guanase catalyzes the inactivation of thioguanine, which results in the formation 6-thioxanthine, which can be further catabolized by xanthine oxidase to the final product, 6-thiouric acid [43].

In contrast to 6-MP, allopurinol can be administered concomitantly with thioguanine without any dosage reduction, since the metabolic step is stopped at the stage of the already inactive metabolite 6-thioxanthine.

In urine, about 75% of the dose is recovered as inactive metabolites, including 6-thioxanthine, *S*-methyl-6-thioxanthine and inorganic sulfate, whereas the parent drug is excreted only in minor amounts.

The terminal elimination half-life averages 11 hours. After 8 hours the parent compound can no longer be detected in serum because the drug has

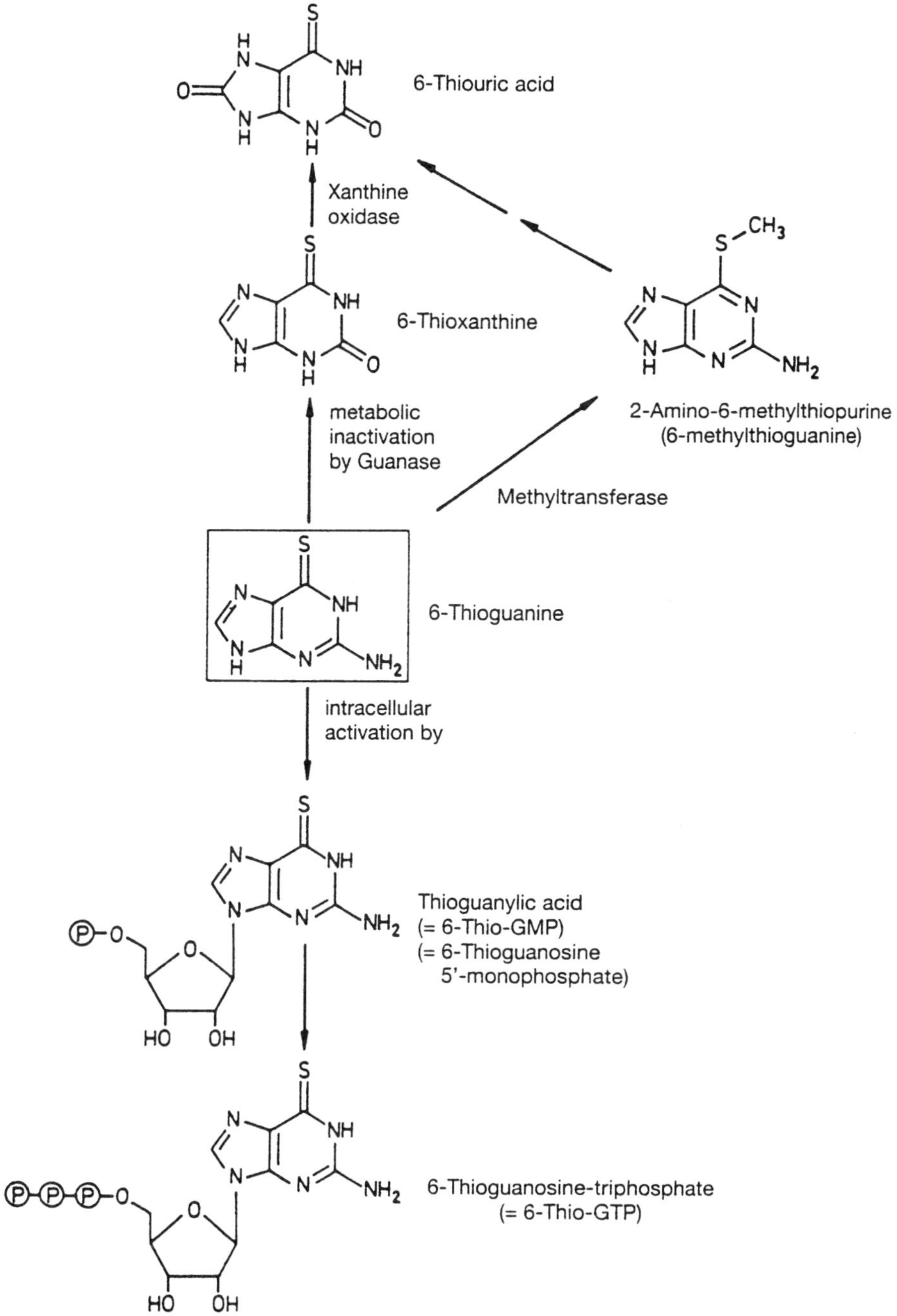

6-Thiouric acid

Xanthine oxidase

6-Thioxanthine

metabolic inactivation by Guanase

2-Amino-6-methylthiopurine (6-methylthioguanine)

Methyltransferase

6-Thioguanine

intracellular activation by

Thioguanylic acid (= 6-Thio-GMP) (= 6-Thioguanosine 5'-monophosphate)

6-Thioguanosine-triphosphate (= 6-Thio-GTP)

Fig. 37 Metabolic pathways of 6-thioguanine.

been processed along extensive anabolic and catabolic pathways. About 11% of the dose is recovered in the urine within 6 hours [1–3].

2.4.3 Pyrimidine- and Pyrimidine Nucleoside Antimetabolites

The pyrimidine analogue cytarabine (Ara-C) was introduced in the treatment of acute leukemia in 1968 and still represents one of the most active agents in this disease. Within the cell it is activated to the corresponding triphosphate Ara-CTP by the enzyme deoxycytidine kinase [1–3]. Gemcitabine, a novel pyrimidine analogue for parenteral use, shows with remarkable activity against a variety of solid tumors. In spite of its structural similarity to Ara-C, gemcitabine is markedly different in its cellular pharmacology and mechanism of action based on its higher affinity to deoxycytidine kinase, which catalyzes phosphorylation to the corresponding nucleotide, and based on the accumulation of the corresponding triphosphate in the tumor cell to higher amounts and for a longer period of time [4].

2.4.3.1 Cytarabine

Cytarabine (Ara-C) is a leading drug for the treatment of hematological malignancies. It is used as a component of various chemotherapeutic regimens to induce remission in AML and ANLL. Conventional doses range from 100 to 200 mg/m^2 IV, on days 1–5 (1–10), whereas doses of 500–3000 mg/m^2/d twice a day on days 1–3 (1–5) are used as high-dose postremission chemotherapy (HD Ara-C) [1–3,54,55]. An oral form of Ara-C, cytarabine ocfosfate (Ara-CMP stearate, YNK01), is under clinical investigation. This derivative may lead to a prolonged exposure of leukemic cells to this anticancer drug and may allow outpatient treatment [56].

The toxicity profile of cytarabine includes dose-limiting myelosuppression, nausea and emesis (incidence: 60–90%), skin disorders, influenza-like symptoms, diarrhea, mucositis and a transient increase of liver-enzymes. Particularly at higher doses peripheral and central nervous system toxicity including keratoconjunctivitis as well as signs of acute pulmonary toxicity can be observed.

After rapid I.V. infusion Ara-C is rapidly and widely distributed: it passes the blood–brain barrier only to a minor extent, however, whereas about 40–60% of the corresponding plasma concentration may reach the CSF by slow continuous I.V. or subcutaneous infusion [57,58].

Higher CSF levels can be achieved by intrathecal administration. Most of the drug received by this route of application diffuses into the systemic circulation, where it is rapidly metabolized. However, because of the low constitutive activity of cytidine deaminase in the central nervous system,

Ara-CTP is cleared rather slowly from the brain and CSF, which may partially explain the neurotoxic side effects of intrathecal administration (e.g., after 50 mg intrathecally on days 1–3) [59,60].

Cytarabine undergoes a biphasic elimination. The initial half-life approximates 10 minutes; the terminal half-life ranges from 110 to 160 minutes [57,58]

The parent compound is rapidly and extensively metabolized in hepatic and extrahepatic tissues by the enzyme cytidine deaminase, which results in the formation of the major metabolite, 1-β-D-arabinofuranosyluracil (Ara-U; uracil arabinoside), which shows an elimination half-life of about 3.8 hours (Fig. 38) [57,58].

In the cell, cytarabine is activated to the corresponding triphosphate, which exerts its antiproliferative activity in different ways. Metabolic catabolism is catalyzed by cytidine deaminase, a pyrimidine nucleoside deami-

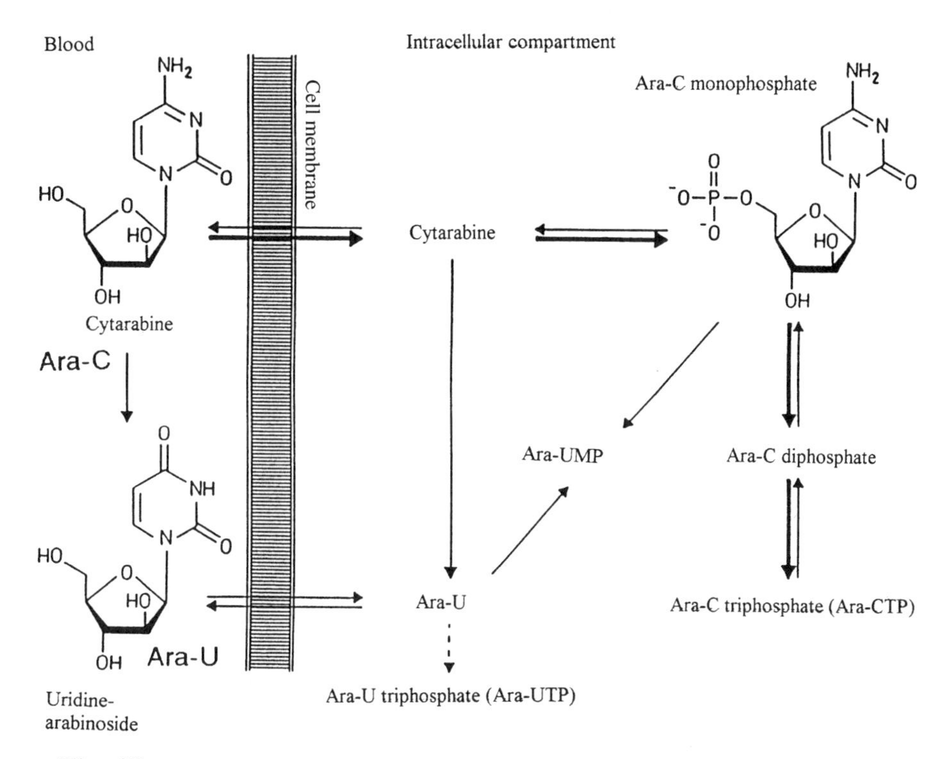

Fig. 38 Metabolic pathways of cytarabine (Ara-C). Inactivation is mediated by the enzyme cytidine deaminase.

nase, resulting in the formation of the corresponding uracil derivative. Both Ara-U and the parent compound are excreted in the urine, with 70–80% of dose recovered in urine within 24 hours (80% Ara-U, and about 10% unchanged drug). Special dosage recommendations in cancer patients with renal or hepatic dysfunction do not seem to be necessary during conventional cytarabine dosages [57,58,61].

However, there seems to be a close correlation between decreased creatinine clearance and the incidence of cytarabine-induced neurotoxicity during high-dose therapy [31,62,63]. The biochemical background is based on the accumulation of the metabolite Ara-U, which is exclusively eliminated by the kidneys. Ara-U, which demonstrates a longer half-life than the parent compound, leads to a dose-dependent inhibition of cytidine deaminase that indirectly results in a higher concentration of Ara-CTP in the central nervous system [62,63]. As a consequence, the use of only 60 and 50% of the original high-dose (1–3 g/m^2) has been recommended for creatinine clearances averaging 60 and 45 mL/min, respectively. Probably the use of HD Ara-C is inadvisable for glomerular filtration rates below 30 mL/min [31].

Clinical Pharmacokinetics Regarding Efficacy and Toxicity

Several pharmacokinetic studies revealed an apparent linear relationship between increasing dose (from 100 mg/m^2 to 3000 mg/m^2) and AUC values, as well as steady-state concentrations. The latter have been reported to be about 4.7 and 13.2 μM after 1 and 3 g/m^2 cytarabine (as a 3-h infusion), respectively.

However, in spite of the close correlation of dose with Ara-C plasma peak levels, plasma levels do not reflect the intracellular Ara-CTP levels. Indeed, there is substantial heterogeneity of intracellular Ara-CTP peak levels among cancer patients after HD Ara-C. This diversity is of clinical importance because intracellular Ara-CTP levels as well as the retention time of active metabolites correlate closely with the likelihood of achieving complete remission and/or the time to progression after HD Ara-C. Thus, a pharmacokinetic and pharmacodynamic optimization of therapy may be based on the achievement of defined Ara-CTP concentrations in leukemic blasts by exceeding 100–150 μM (which corresponds to 185–275 ng/10^7 blasts) over a prolonged period of time.

In conclusion, there is some evidence that certain patients cannot cumulate Ara-CTP in their isolated leukemic blasts in a dose-dependent fashion after application of HD Ara-C. As a consequence, it would be reasonable to determine intracellular Ara-CTP levels in isolated leukemic blasts after the first high dose (Table 18). If there appears to be no evidence of dose-dependent Ara-CTP accumulation, further HD-Ara-C administration may have an unfavorable risk–benefit ratio [64–67].

Table 18 Relationship Among the Dose of Ara-C Administered in Patients with ANLL and Plasma Concentrations of Ara-C and Ara-U, and Leukemic Cell Concentrations of Ara-CTP[a]

	Ara-C[b]		
	100 mg/m^2	2000 mg/m^2	3000 mg/m^2
Ara-C			
μmol/L	0.49 ± 0.41	82.2 ± 55.9	140.6 ± 76.5
range	(0.12–1.2)	(21–214)	(41–362)
Ara-U			
μmol/L	5.88 ± 1.52	264.0 ± 119.6	275.1 ± 131.2
range	(4–8)	(29–411)	(66–555)
Ara-CTP			
pmol/10^7 cells	182.7 ± 148.6	1567 ± 701.7	1225.3 ± 701.7
range	(33–562)	(240–6400)	(260–2900)

[a]Ara-C was either administered by 10 days continuous infusion (100 mg/m^2/d) or by 75 minutes IV infusion (2 and 3 g/m^2).
[b]Plasma steady-state concentration during continuous infusion.
(Adapted from Ref. 67.)

2.4.3.2 Gemcitabine (2′,2′-Difluorodeoxycytidine, dFdC)

Gemcitabine (Fig. 39) is used in the chemotherapy of a variety of solid tumors, like pancreatic carcinoma, NSCLC, breast, ovarian, or bladder cancer. The usually recommended dose ranges from 1000 to 1250 mg/m^2 IV (monotherapy) and 800–1000 mg/m^2 IV (combination chemotherapy) dl, 8, 15 repeating on day 29 [68].

The toxicity profile of dFdC includes dose-limiting myelosuppression, mild nausea and vomiting (incidence: 10–30%), a transient increase of liver enzymes, influenza-like symptoms, and peripheral edema.

After i.v. administration of 1000 mg/m^2 gemcitabine, the maximal plasma concentration ranges from 10 to 40 μg/mL. Like cytarabine (Fig. 39), dFdC is phosphorylated in the cell by deoxycytidine kinase to the corresponding mono-, di-, and triphosphates (dFdCTP). A concentration-dependent insertion of dFdCTP in the DNA may be the most important mechanism of tumor cell apoptosis.

More than 90% of the dose is extensively metabolized in the liver, the kidneys, and the blood to the inactive major metabolite 2′,2′-difluorouro-deoxyuridine (dFdU) by the enzyme cytidine deaminase. The terminal elimination half-life of the parent compound averages 14 hours. Approximately

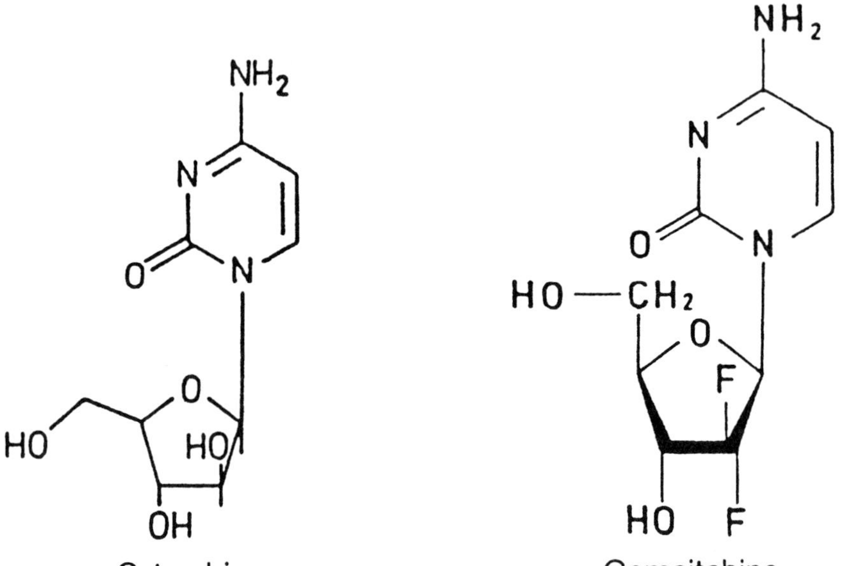

Fig. 39 Chemical structures of cytarabine and gemcitabine.

62% of the dose is recovered in the urine as dFdU; less than 10% is excreted renally as unchanged drug. Dose reduction in the presence of renal dysfunction, therefore, does not appear to be warranted [69–71].

2.4.3.3 5-Fluorouracil

5-Fluorouracil (5-FU) is a fluorinated pyrimidine antimetabolite that blocks the synthesis of the DNA constituent thymidine. For persistent inhibition of thymidine synthesis, a very stable complex between the active 5-FU metabolite, 5-fluorodeoxyuridine monophosphate, the enzyme thymidylate synthetase, and the physiological cofactor *N*-5,10-methylene tetrahydrofolic acid has to be formed (see Fig. 30). Interestingly 5-FU can act synergistically with MTX in spite of an MTX-induced decrease of *N*-5,10-methylene tetrahydrofolic acid in the cell. The proven synergism occurs because MTX polyglutamates, which represent very stable MTX metabolites in the cell, are able to bind very tightly to the thymidylate synthetase. Thus, these MTX polyglutamates overtake the role of the physiological cofactor. Based on this biochemical background, MTX generally is given before 5-FU. The exact time interval between drugs seems to be dependent on the tumor type [1–3].

In clinical oncology 5-FU plays an important role in the treatment of breast cancer and gastrointestinal adenocarcinoma, particularly colorectal cancer. The usually used dosages range from 450 to 550 mg/m^2 IV on days 1–5 (as short-time infusion/bolus application) and 2600 mg/m^2 IV (as 24-h continuous infusion) weekly. However, in the meantime, a multiplicity of different 5-FU dosage regimens exist, particularly for combination chemotherapy and long-term infusion schedules (e.g., with Leucovorin or Levamisole [72–86].

There seems to be an important pharmacodynamic difference between bolus injection and continuous infusion. Whereas the former will primarily induce RNA fraudulence, the latter will mediate its cytotoxicity via thymidilate synthetase inhibition. Hypothetically, combination with Leucovorin, which acts synergistically with 5-FU might be particularly beneficial if IV administration of 5-FU is prolonged [87,88].

The incidence of leukocytopenia and gastrointestinal toxicity seems to be significantly higher in patients receiving bolus injection, whereas stomatitis and dermatitis (e.g., palmar–plantar–erythrodysesthesia syndrome [hand-foot-syndrome]) are more common after prolonged infusion [73,74].

Because of a high first-pass effect, 5-FU monotherapy cannot be given orally. After i.v. administration the plasma levels of 5-fluorouracil decline very rapidly. The terminal elimination half-life ranges from 10 to 30 minutes. The enzymatic inactivation of 5-FU is catalyzed by the enzyme dihydropyrimidine dehydrogenase (DPDH), which is not restricted to the liver. Very recently it has been reported that the combination of oral 5-FU with the oral selective DPDH inhibitor eniluracil (5′-ethinyluracil, 776C85) represents a possibility to achieve 100% oral 5-FU bioavailability [90].

After i.v. administration, about 60–98% of the dose is excreted in the urine; the amount recovered as unchanged drug is less than 5%. Dosage adjustments in the presence of renal or hepatic dysfunction (e.g., bilirubin levels <5 mg/dL) do not seem to be warranted unless the serum bilirubin levels exceed 5 mg/dl or the creatinine clearance falls below 10 mL/min [89,90].

The metabolites dihydrofluorouracil, α-fluoro-β-ureidopropionic acid, and α-fluoro-β-alanine (Fig. 40) are eliminated much more slowly than the parent drug. However, these catabolites do not contribute to the overall antineoplastic activity of 5-FU. Comparing the pharmacokinetics of 5-FU, one finds that the apparent elimination half-lives of the metabolites α-fluoro-β-ureidopropionic acid and α-fluoro-β-alanine are prolonged with values of about 4 and 33 hours, respectively [89].

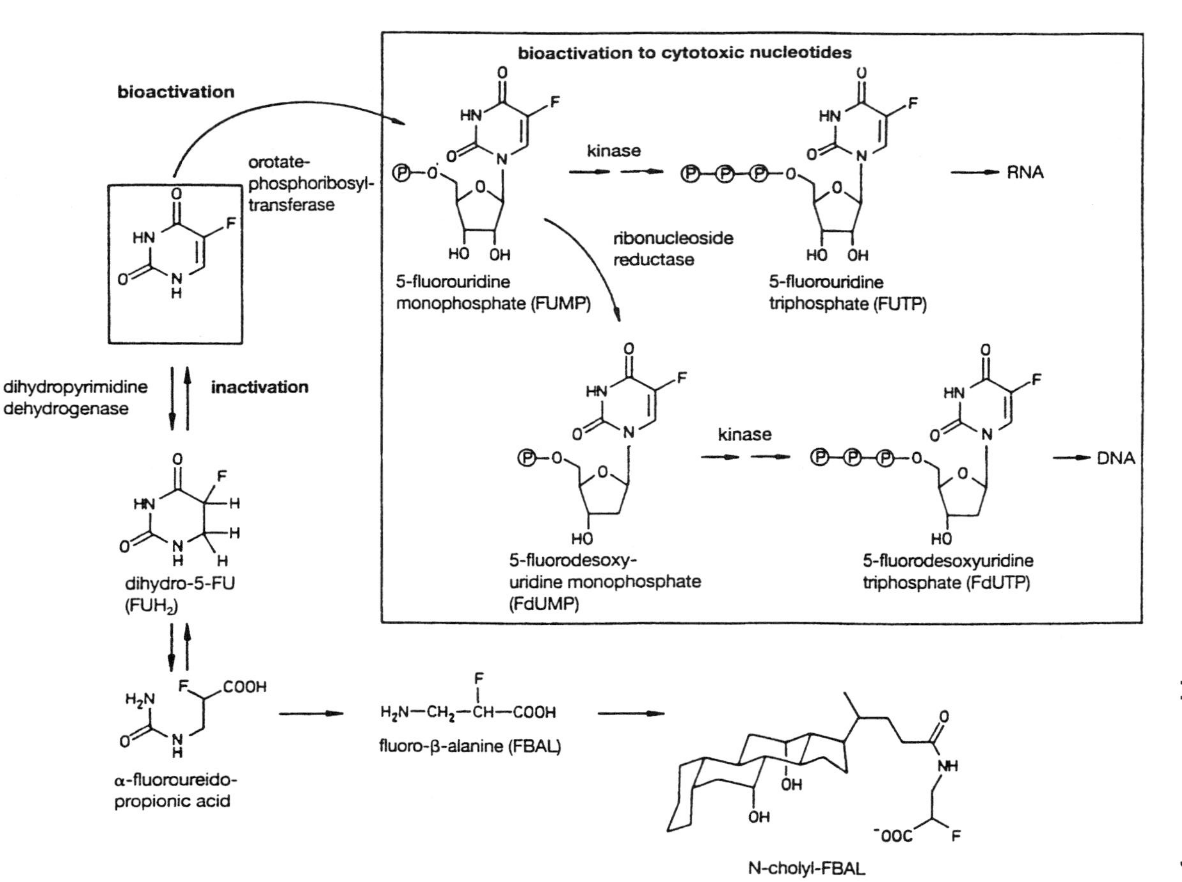

Fig. 40 Enzymatic bioactivation and inactivation pathways of 5-fluorouracil.

Some of the dose (2–3%) may be excreted in the bile, possibly as a conjugate consisting of α-fluoro-β-alanine and a bile acid. It is not fully understood whether this conjugate is responsible for the induction of biliary sclerosis after intra-arterial 5-FU administration; the basis for this hypothesis is the theory that the unphysiological bile acid conjugate may solubilize bile duct cells [91].

Clinical Pharmacokinetics Regarding Efficacy and Toxicity

Some pharmacokinetic studies deal with the possible advantages of individualized therapy with 5-fluorouracil in clinical practice in order to decrease the incidence of toxicity and to optimize the therapeutic outcome [92–96].

It has been recorded that the constitutive activity of the dihydropyrimidine dehydrogenase (DPDH) ranges from 69 to 559 pmol/min per milligram of protein in the peripheral blood mononuclear cells (PBMCs) of cancer patients. Interestingly the DPDH activity appears to be on average 15% lower in women than in men, which is in accordance with the observed lower 5-FU clearance in women. Because 1–3% of patients may demonstrate an almost complete DPDH deficiency (<0.1 nmol/min/mg protein), these patients are at risk for more severe 5-FU-related toxicity after conventional doses [97–99].

There is some evidence that a determination of DPDH activity in blood lymphocytes would be useful in the case of patients who develop unexpected high toxicity, particularly mucositis and myelosuppression, after 500 to 1000 mg/m^2 5-FU; such an investigation would permit the correlation of this phenomenon with an underlying pharmacogenetic disorder (autosomal recessive pattern). However, the quantitative determination of the enzyme has not been shown to be accurate enough for the individual prediction of 5-FU clearance in cancer patients, or to offer any dosage recommendations. The correlation coefficient between 5-FU clearance and PBMC-DPDH activity has been shown to be weak ($p = 0.31$) [97–99].

Consistent with the above-mentioned high interindividual variability of DPDH activity, there is markedly high variability among 5-FU pharmacokinetics, toxicity, and possibly response from cancer patients. Recently a correlation was found between higher 5-FU levels and the severity of drug toxicity, particularly diarrhea and hand–foot syndrome [92,100].

Gamelin et al. recently recorded that during an 8-hour infusion (initial: 1000 mg/m^2 5-FU IV, weekly, with 200 mg/m^2 Leucovorin just before and at the fourth hour of 5-FU infusion), 5-FU levels exceeding 3000 μg/mL were significantly associated with higher toxicity, whereas levels less than 3000 μg/mL were not. This pattern corresponds to an AUC value of about 24 mgxh/L. Others demonstrated a correlation between AUC values exceeding 30 mgxh/L (5-FU therapy without concomitant Leucovorin) and the frequency of cycles with leukopenia, mucositis, and diarrhea [92].

Additionally, for patients whose 5-FU clearance is constitutively high, a conventional dose of 1000 mg/m^2 could be too low to achieve minimal cytotoxic concentrations. Thus, the low systemic 5-FU exposure rather than tumor cell resistance would be the reason for primary therapy failures. A close correlation between 5-FU concentration or 5-FU AUC values in plasma and overall therapeutic outcome has been suggested. For example, in patients with advanced colorectal cancer, a 5-FU concentration exceeding 2000 μg/mL was associated with a higher response rate and a longer time to progression.

Such results emphasize the importance of 5-FU concentrations and 5-FU AUC values as useful predictors for individual toxicity as well as efficacy. However, more studies are needed to define more precisely the range of optimal peak plasma levels or target AUC values by considering tumor type and administration modus, as well as the optimized combination chemotherapy. High 5-FU peak concentrations may be important for incorporation into RNA, whereas long-term exposure might be necessary for persisting thymidilate synthetase inhibition. A combination of a 5-FU bolus dose with continuous infusion and intermittent Leucovorin dosages may result in the most promising outcome. However, 5-FU plasma levels can never reflect the corresponding intracellular concentration of active 5-FU metabolites in the tumor mass [92–96].

More recently, exciting data have been presented concerning the intracellular monitoring of 5-FU in tumor tissue. Presant and colleagues used ^{19}F nuclear magnetic resonance spectroscopy (^{19}F-NMRS) to correlate clinical resistance to 5-FU therapy with failure of tumors to trap 5-FU. Patients whose tumors trapped 5-FU responded to fluorinated pyrimidine chemotherapy (Fig. 41). Although the ^{19}F-NMRS method has been shown to be a promising tool in detecting 5-FU and its metabolites in tumors, it may be inferior to biochemical analysis or positron emission tomography in the area of sensitivity. However, ^{19}F-NMRS as a noninvasive method may help to identify patients who are likely to respond to chemotherapy with 5-FU [101–103].

To increase 5-FU efficacy and decrease 5-FU toxicity, the administration of 5-FU in a circadian periodicity has been suggested. This proposal is based on the observation that there is a circadian rhythm in 5-FU plasma concentrations with peak levels at 11 A.M. and trough levels at 11 P.M. on average, a pattern that seems to be inversely correlated with the circadian profile of DPD activity. However, further studies have demonstrated a marked interindividual variability in the circadian rhythm of PBMC-DPDH activity, particularly with respect to the definite time points of peaks and

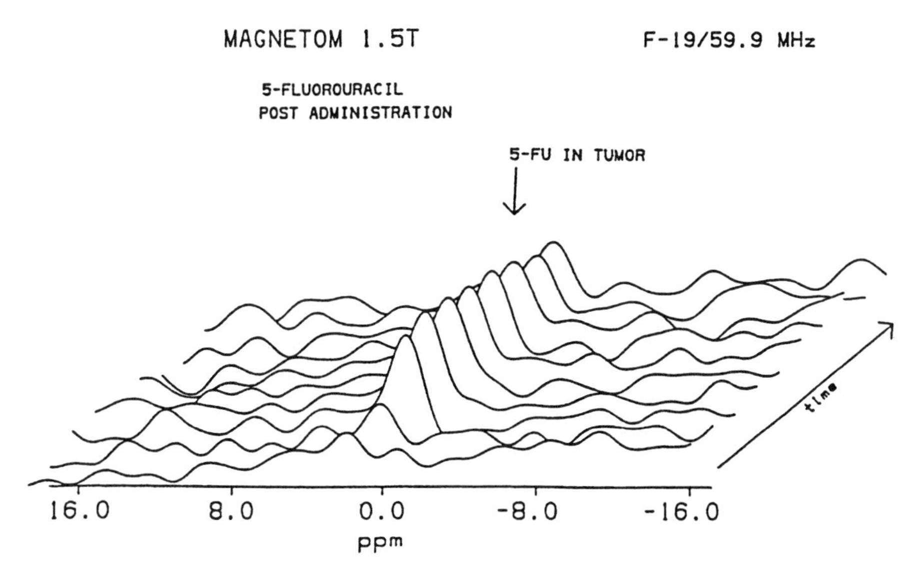

Fig. 41 ^{19}F-NMR spectroscopy: a very interesting, noninvasive method presented by Presant et al. [105] to measure intracellular 5-FU concentration after cancer chemotherapy. Stack plot of 5-minute ^{19}F-NMR spectra of a cervical carcinoma from 0 to 55 minutes after 5-FU treatment. Each spectrum was the result of 256 free induction decays (FIDs) acquired at 10 kHz spectral width with the 90° pulse optimized for 4 cm, at 60.012500 MHz [105]. (Adapted from Ref. 105.)

troughs during a 24-hour period. This aspect makes the routine use of circadian-adapted 5-FU therapy much more difficult [104,105].

2.4.3.4 UFT (Uracil/Tegafur)

Commercially available in Japan and several other countries, UFT is an oral drug formulation that contains uracil and tegafur in a molar ratio of 4:1. Tegafur (Fig. 42) is a prodrug of 5-fluorouracil (5-FU) that is converted to 5-FU by thymidine phosphorylase after oral absorption. However, oral monotherapy with tegafur (e.g., 150 mg/kg/d) was associated with substantial gastrointestinal and CNS toxicity without any obvious therapeutic advantages over i.v. administration of 5-FU [106–108].

Uracil inhibits the enzyme dihydropyrimidine dehydrogenase, which results in an increased 5-FU levels if tegafur is combined with uracil. This property is of special importance because such inhibition may occur predominantly in tumor cells rather than in normal tissue [109].

Recently, it was demonstrated that 300 mg/m^2/d UFT (in 3 daily divided doses) plus oral Leucovorin administered on an empty stomach (no

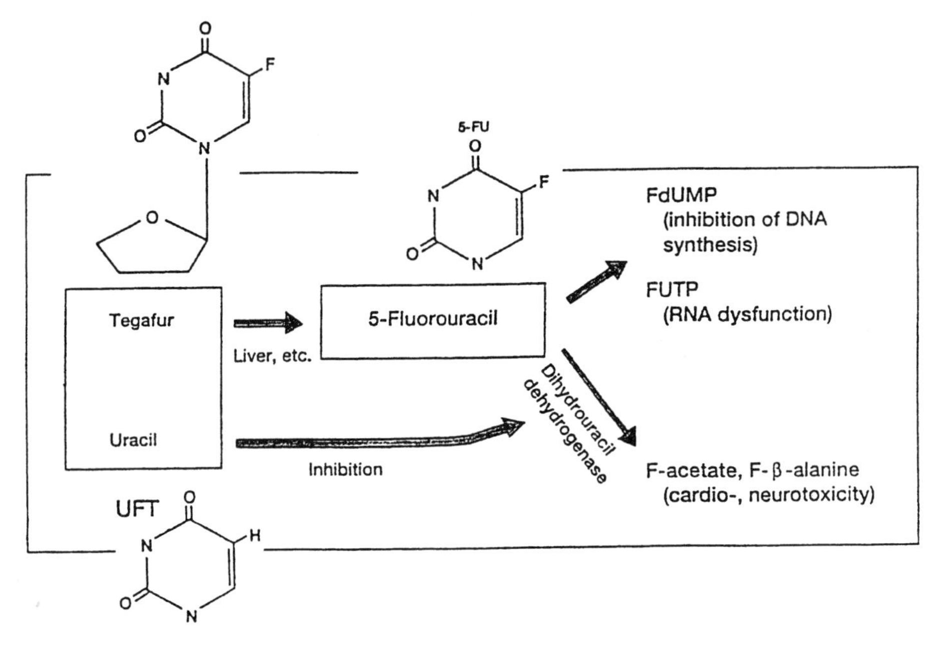

Fig. 42 Metabolic pathways of tegafur, a 5-FU prodrug, and uracil. It has been postulated that the inhibition of 5-FU metabolism by Uracil may occur predominantly in tumor cells. (Adapted from Ref. 109.)

food 1 hour before and after ingestion of the medication) for 28 days exerts significant activity against metastatic colorectal cancer. This oral regimen seems to be well tolerated and is devoid of the significant neutropenia or mucositis that usually complicates intravenous schedules of 5-FU plus Leucovorin.

There is some evidence that UFT alone or in combination with Leucovorin may exert greater antitumor activity than tegafur or 5-FU monotherapy. This observation may reflect the presence of an accumulation of 5-FU in tumor tissue as a result of UFT therapy. Indeed, 5-FU levels in tumor tissues were nearly 5–10 times higher than the corresponding levels in blood [110]. Randomized trials in patients with advanced colorectal cancer comparing oral UFT with parenteral 5-FU-leucovorin combinations are ongoing.

2.4.3.5 Capecitabine

Oral capecitabine has demonstrated antitumor activity in outpatients with advanced taxane-refractory breast cancer and colorectal carcinoma (CRC).

Dosage recommendations range from 1331 mg/m^2/d continuously and 2510 mg/m^2/d intermittently (two weeks on, one week off) or 1657 mg/m^2/d intermittently in combination with oral leucovorin (e.g., 60 mg daily) in the treatment of CRC.

The toxicity profile of capecitabine includes dose-limiting diarrhea, nausea and vomiting and a palmar-plantar-erhythrodysaesthesia (hand-foot-syndrome). Myelosuppressive side effects are uncommon during therapy with capecitabine.

Capecitabine is well and rapidly absorbed from the gastrointestinal tract followed by an extensive enzymatic conversion into 5′-deoxy-5-fluorocytidine (via carboxylesterase) which is further converted into doxifluridine (5′-deoxyfluorouridine) via cytidine deaminase. The metabolic conversion of doxifluridine into the active form 5-FU is catalyzed by the enzyme pyrimidine nucleoside phosphorylase (syn. thymidine phosphorylase, platelet-derived endothelial growth factor, tumor-associated angiogenic factor) which is highly expressed in tumor tissue. More comprehensive pharmacokinetic data are still ongoing [111–113].

2.4.4 Adenosine Deaminase Inhibitors

The cytostatics fludarabine, cladribine, and pentostatin (Fig. 43) represent a new class of anticancer drugs. In spite of their structural similarity to other antimetabolites, their mechanism is mainly based not on DNA incorporation but on the inhibition of adenosine deaminase in lymphocytes, resulting in apoptosis [5].

Unregulated growth or function of lymphoid cells is the background of various diseases like lymphomas, chronic lymphocytic leukemia (CLL), and hairy cell leukemia (HCL), as well as autoimmune disorders.

Since it was known that an accumulation of deoxyribonucleotides in lymphocytes induces their demise, researchers intended to inhibit the physiological enzyme adenosine deaminase (ADA), which prevents this accumulation by catalyzing the deamination of intracellular deoxyadenosine to inosine and deoxyinosine. This enzyme is detectable in virtually all mammalian tissues, but activity is extraordinarily high in the lymphoid system (lymph nodes, spleen, thymus). If ADA activity is congenitally absent, or if it is blocked, the deoxypurine nucleoside adenosine is phosphorylated to its mononucleotide (dAMP) by deoxycytidine kinase. If the activity of deoxycyctidine kinase is high and that of 5′-nucleotidases is low, as is the case in lymphocytes, dAMP, dADP, and particularly dATP accumulate rapidly to lethal concentrations in the lymphocytes, probably inducing apoptosis (Fig. 44).

Additionally, ADA activity is increased at least threefold in the blastic cells acute lymphocytic or myelogenous leukemia.

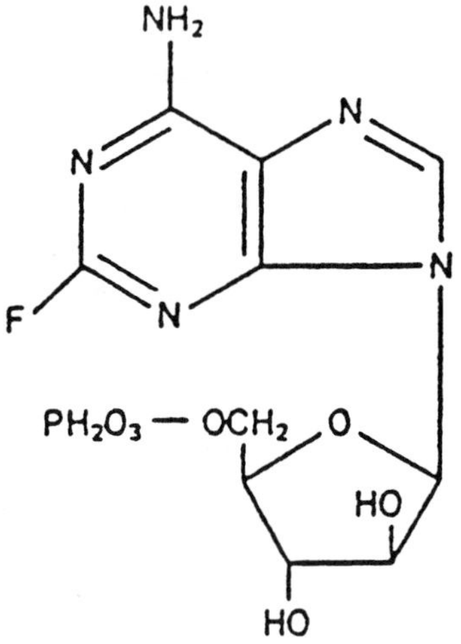

Fludarabine phosphate

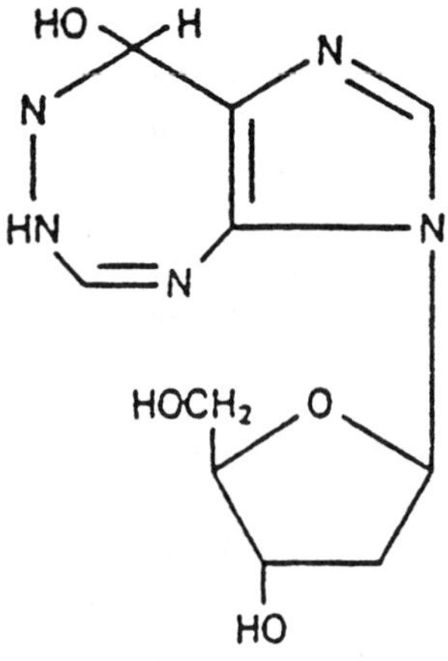

Pentostatin

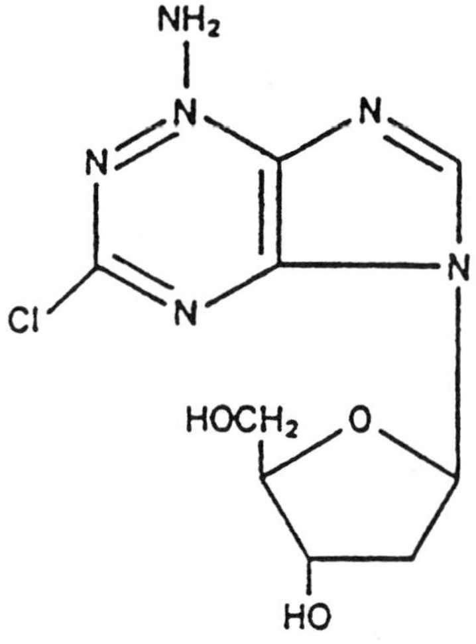

Cladribine

Fig. 43 Chemical structures of the adenosine deaminase inhibitors pentostatin, cladribine and fludarabine monophosphate, which show structural similarity to adenosine.

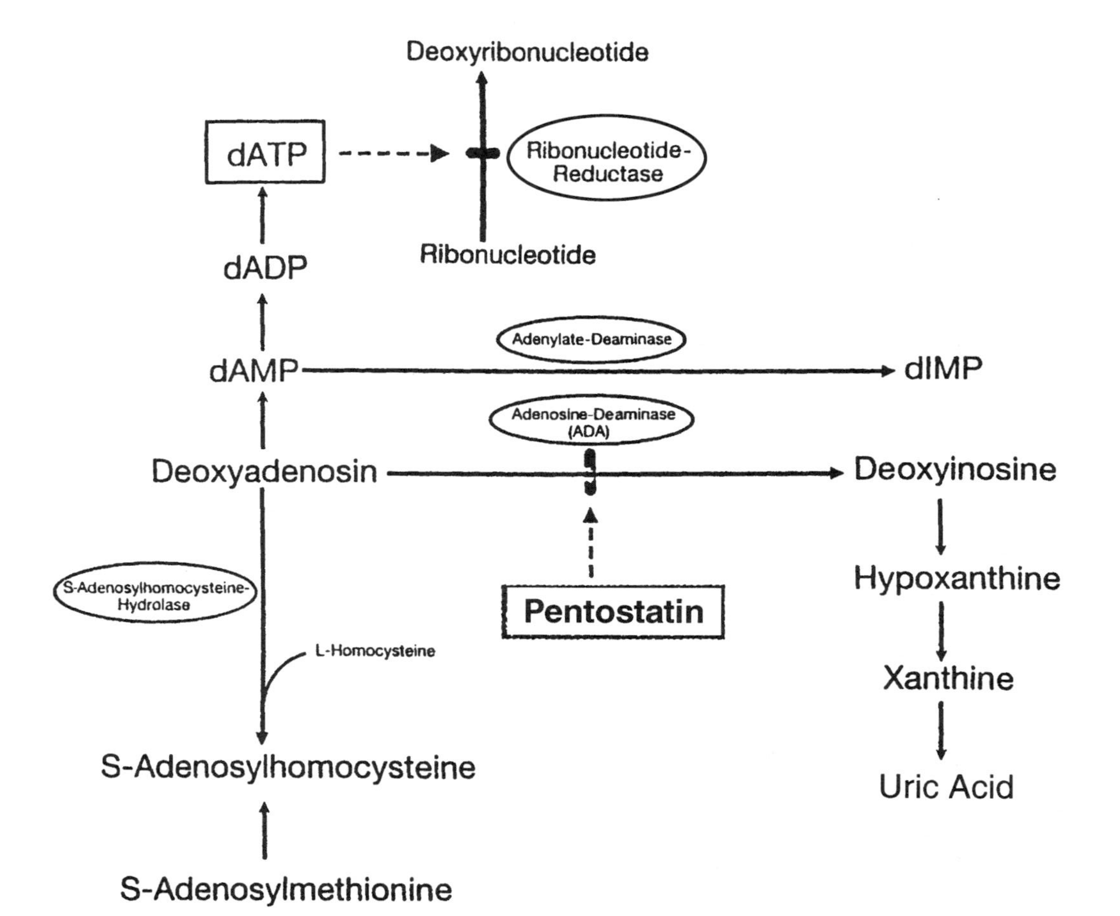

Fig. 44 Cytotoxic mechanism of adenosine deaminase inhibitors in the adenine nucleotide turnover (dashed line indicates inhibition).

Recently, three antimetabolites, pentostatin (2′-deoxycoformycin), cladribine (2-chlorodeoxyadenosine), and fludarabine monophosphate have been demonstrated to exert considerable activity against a variety of indolent lymphoid malignancies. Fludarabine monophosphate is predominantly used in the treatment of alkylator-refractory CLL, while cladribine and pentostatin have been approved for HCL. These three drugs are also active against low grade NHL, Waldenström macroglobulinemia, and cutaneous T-cell lymphoma. By binding to ADA with high affinity, these drugs cause a dose-related inhibition of lymphoblast ADA. As a consequence, intracellular dATP accumulation and lymphoblast lysis can be observed [114,115].

The toxicity profile of adenosine deaminase inhibitors include dose-limiting myelosuppression, mild nausea and vomiting, a transient increase of liver enzymes, peripheral and/or central nervous system toxicity, and immunosuppression related to the drug-induced T cell depletion. Particularly in the case of pentostatin, the risk for severe nephrotoxic side effects is increased especially when the hydration during drug therapy may be inadequate.

2.4.4.1 Pentostatin

Pentostatin was the first adenosine deaminase inhibitor commercially available in several European countries. The drug is particularly effective in the treatment of hairy cell leukemia. Additionally, it has been shown to exert impressive antineoplastic activity in patients with B-cell chronic lymphocytic leukemia, prolymphocytic leukemia, adult T-cell leukemia/lymphoma, and cutaneous T-cell lymphoma refractory to conventional chemotherapy. The usually recommended dose is 4 mg/m^2 IV every 2 weeks. Pentostatin cannot be given orally because of a rapid acid-catalyzed degradation.

Pentostatin has a large volume of distribution (about 42 L). The protein-bound fraction is rather low and ranges from 14 to 28%. The drug can cross the blood–brain barrier. It has been estimated that in the CSF about 10% of the corresponding plasma concentrations 2–4 hours after administration can be achieved.

After intravenous administration the drug displays a biexponential decay curve. The terminal elimination half-life ranges from 3 to 9 hours. Only small amounts of the drug are metabolized. As a consequence, between 50 and 96% of unchanged drug can be recovered in urine within 24 hours (Table 19). Therefore a dosage adjustment is needed in patients with impaired renal function, who otherwise may have a higher risk for CNS and renal toxicity. It has been recommended to use 70 or 60% of the usual dose, if creatinine clearance is about 60 or 45 mL/min, respectively. If the creatinine clearance is less than 30 mL/min, the use of pentostatin is contraindicated [116,117].

Table 19 Pharmacokinetic Comparison of Pentostatin, Cladribine, and Fludarabine Monophosphate

Parameter	Pentostatin, 4 mg/m^2 q14d	Cladribine, 0.14 mg/kg/d	Fludarabine, 18–25 $mg/m^2/d$
Initial half-life	17–85 min	35 min	0.9 h
Terminal half-life	2.6–15 h	6.7 h	9.2 h
Volume of distribution	37–42 L	9.2 L/kg (53.6 L/m^2)	96.2 L/m^2
Metabolism	Only small amounts	Only small amounts	Only small amounts
Clearance	3.1–3.8 $L/h/m^2$	26 $L/h/m^2$	9.1 $L/h/m^2$
Excretion	50–96% of the drug recovered in the urine as unchanged drug on day 1	more than 50% of dose can be excreted in the urine as unchanged drug	31–86% of dose excreted in the urine as dephosphorylated F-Ara-A

2.4.4.2 Cladribine (2-CdA, 2-Chlorodeoxyadenosine)

Cladribine has shown excellent activity in the treatment of hairy cell leukemia (e.g., 0.1 mg/kg/d IV, days 1–7). Impressive response rates were achieved in the treatment of CLL and refractory low- or intermediate-grade non-Hodgkin lymphoma, too.

After a 2-hour intravenous infusion of 2-CdA, the mean maximum plasma concentration ranges from 70 to 381 nmol/L. There does not seem to be a significant difference in AUC values when 2-CdA is given as a 2-hour infusion or as a continuous infusion over 24 hours. In the cerebrospinal fluid, a plasma/CSF ratio of approximately 4 is achievable.

The corresponding nucleotides cladribine monophosphate and triphosphate are rapidly formed inside the cells; their half-lives have been estimated to be about 23 hours. The drug is primarily cleared by the kidneys, possibly via the organic cation carrier system. In plasma the terminal elimination half-life of the parent compound approximates 6.7 hours (Table 19).

Defined dosage recommendation in patients with renal dysfunction have not yet been published so far. However, it may be reasonable to use only 50% of dose, if creatinine clearance ranges from 60 to 30 mL/min.

It has been suggested that cladribine can be given orally (e.g., 0.28 mg/kg/d dissolved in phosphate buffer solution) because its absolute bioavailability appears to average 44%. In the meantime work is in progress on a derivative, 2-chloro-2′-arabino-fluoro-2′-deoxyadenosine, as an orally effective analogue [115,118].

2.4.4.3 Fludarabine Monophosphate

Fludarabine monophosphate has been shown to be very active in chronic lymphatic leukemia and low-grade lymphomas (25–30 mg/m^2 IV, on days 1–5, every 4 weeks).

Following intravenous administration, fludarabine monophosphate is dephosphorylated within minutes in plasma, releasing the active metabolite 9-β-arabinofuranosyl-2-fluoroadenine (F-Ara-A). The F-Ara-A is transported into the cells, where it is rapidly converted into its active mono- and triphosphates.

This adenosine deaminase inhibitor has a rather high volume of distribution (44–96 L/m^2). The initial half-life approximates 9 minutes, the second one 1.7 hours, and the terminal half-life ranges from 7 to 12 hours. Very probably fludarabine may accumulate in third spaces like ascites or pleural effusions, which may partially explain the prolonged and severe neutropenia in patients whose pleural fluid or ascites was not drained before fludarabine treatment.

Fludarabine monophosphate is mainly excreted as F-Ara-A in urine. Urinary excretion of 31–86% of dose has been recovered within 24–72 hours. As a consequence, a dosage reduction should be considered in patients with a glomerular filtration rate below 60 mL/min. If the creatinine clearance ranges from 60 to 30 mL/min, only 50% of the usual dose should be administered to avoid severe side effects, especially granulocytopenia and severe T-cell depletion [119,120].

REFERENCES TO SECTION 2.4

1. Chu E, Takimoto CH, Chabner S. Antimetabolites (Section 4). In: VT DeVita, S Hellman, SA Rosenberg, eds. Cancer: Principles and Practice of Oncology, 4th ed. Philadelphia: Lippincott, 1993, pp 358–374.
2. Lipp H-P. Prevention and Management of Anticancer Drug Toxicity—The Significance of Clinical Pharmacokinetics. Jena: Universität-Verlag, 1995.
3. Sweeny DJ, Diasio RB. Toxicity of antimetabolites. In: G Powis, MP Hacker, eds. The Toxicity of Anticancer Drugs. New York: Pergamon Press, 1991, pp 63–81.
4. Plunkett W, Huang P, Xu Y-Z, Heinemann V, Grunewald R, Gandhi V. Gemcitabine: Metabolism, mechanism of action and self-potentiation. Semin Oncol 1995: 22(suppl 11):3–10.
5. Plankett W, Gandhi V. Evolution of the arabinosides and the pharmacology of fludarabine drugs. 1994:47(suppl 6):30–38.
6. Bertino JR. Ode to methotrexate. J Clin Oncol 1993:11:5–14.
7. Schultz RM. New antifolates in cancer therapy. In: E Jucker, ed. Progress in Drug Research, vol. 44. Basel: Birkhäuser-Verlag, 1995, pp 129–149.

8. Evans WE, Crom WR, Abromowitch M, et al. Clinical pharmacodynamics of high-dose methotrexate in acute lymphocytic leukemia. N Engl J Med 1986: 314:471–477.
9. Frei E, Blum R, Pitman SW, Kirkwood J, Henderson J, Skarin A, Mayer R, Bast R, Garnick M, Parker L, Canellos G. High dose methotrexate with Leucovorin rescue—Rationale and spectrum of antitumor activity. Am J Med 1980:68:370–376.
10. Borsi JD, Sagen E, Romslo I, Moe PJ. Rescue after intermediate and high-dose methotrexate: Background, rationale and current practice. Pediatr Hemato Oncol 1990:7:347–363.
11. Reggev A, Djerassi I. The safety of administration of massive doses of methotrexate (50 g) with equimolar citrovorum factor rescue in adult patients. Cancer 1988:61:2423–2428.
12. Borsi JD, Moe PJ. A comparative study on the pharmacokinetics of MTX in a dose-range of 0.5 g–33.6 g/m^2 in children with acute lymphoblastic leukemia. Cancer 1987:60:5–13.
13. Comella P, Palmieri G, Beneduce G, et al. Significance of methotrexate serum level achieved in patients with gastrointestinal malignancies treated with sequential methotrexate, L-folinic acid and 5-fluorouracil. Oncology 1996:53: 198–203.
14. Teresi ME, Rodman JH. Methotrexate. In: JE Murphy, ed. Clinical Pharmacokinetics Pocket Reference. Bethesda, MD: American Society of Hospital Pharmacists, 19, pp 157–177.
15. Gökbuget N, Hoelzer D. High-dose methotrexate in the treatment of adult acute lymphoblastic leukemia. Ann Hematol 1996:72:194–201.
16. Graf N, Winkler K, Betlemovic M, Fuchs N, Bode U. Methotrexate pharmacokinetics and prognosis in osteosarcoma. J Clin Oncol 1994:12:1443–1451.
17. Isacoff WR, Eilber F, Tabbarah H, et al. Phase II clinical trial with high-dose methotrexate therapy and citrovorum factor rescue. Cancer Treatment Rep 1978:62:1295–1304.
18. Jolivet J, Cowan KH, Curt GA, et al. The pharmacology and clinical use of methotrexate. N Engl J Med 1983:309:1094–1103.
19. Nirenberg A, Mosende C, Mehta BM, Gisolfi AL, Rosen G. High-dose methotrexate with citrovorum factor rescue: Predictive value of serum methotrexate concentrations and corrective measures to avert toxicity. Cancer Treatment Rep 1977:61:779–783.
20. Pignon T, Lacarelle B, Duffaud J, et al. Dosage adjustment of high-dose methotrexate using Bayesian estimation: A comparative study of two different concentrations at the end of 8-h infusions. Ther Drug Monit 1995:17:471–478.
21. Stark AN, Jackson G, Carey PJ, et al. Severe renal failure due to intermediate-dose methotrexate. Cancer Chemother Pharmacol 1989:24:243.
22. Takami M, Kuniyoshi Y, Oomukai T, et al. Severe complications after high-dose methotrexate treatment. Acta Oncol 1995:34:611–612.

23. Wolfram C, Hartmann R, Fengler R, et al. Randomized comparison of 36-hour intermediate-dose versus high-dose methotrexate infusions for remission induction in relapsed childhood acute lymphoblastic leukemia. J Clin Oncol 1993:11:827–833.
24. Blaney SM, Balis FM, Poplack DG. Current pharmacological treatment approaches to central nervous system leukemia. Drugs 1991:41:702–716.
25. Gilchrist NL, Caldwell J, Watson ID, et al. Comparison of serum and cerebrospinal fluid levels of methotrexate in man during high-dose chemotherapy for aggressive non-Hodgkin's lymphoma. Cancer Chemother Pharmacol 1985:15:290–294.
26. Strother DR, Glynn-Barnhart A, Kovnar E, et al. Variability in the disposition of intraventricular methotrexate: A proposal for rational dosing. J Clin Oncol 1989:7:1741–1747.
27. Schilsky RL. Clinical pharmacology of methotrexate. In: MM Ames, G Powis, JS Kovach, eds. Pharmacokinetics of Anticancer Agents in Humans. Amsterdam: Elsevier Science Publishers B V, 1983, pp 187–206.
28. Chabner BA, Allegra CJ, Curt GA, Clendeninn NJ, et al. Polyglutamation of methotrexate—Is methotrexate a prodrug? J Clin Invest 1985:76:907–912.
29. Borsi JD, Sagen E, Romslo I, Slordal L, Moe PJ. 7-Hydroxymethotrexate concentrations in serum and cerebrospinal fluid of children with acute lymphoblastic leukemia. Cancer Chemother Pharmacol 1990:27:164–167.
30. Erttmann R, Bielack S, Landbeck G. Kinetics of 7-hydroxymethotrexate after high-dose methotrexate therapy. Cancer Chemother Pharmacol 1985:15:101–104.
31. Kintzel PE, Dorr RT. Anticancer drug renal toxicity and elimination: Dosing guidelines for altered renal function. Cancer Treatment Rev 1995:21:33–64.
32. Shamash J, Earl H, Souhami R. Acetazolamide for alkalinisation of urine in patients receiving high-dose methotrexate. Cancer Chemother Pharmacol 1991:28:150–151.
33. Freeman-Narrod M, Kim JS, Ohanissian H, et al. The effect of methotrexate on renal tubules as indicated by urinary lysozyme concentration. Cancer 1982: 50:2775–2779.
34. Thomson AH, Daly M, Knepil J, Harden P, Symonds P. Methotrexate removal during hemodialysis in a patient with advanced laryngeal carcinoma. Cancer Chemother Pharmacol 1996:38:566–570.
35. Relling MV, Stapleton B, Ochs J, et al. Removal of methotrexate, Leucovorin and their metabolites by combined hemodialysis and hemoperfusion. Cancer 1988:62:884–888.
36. Molina R, Fabian C, Cowley B. Use of charcoal hemoperfusion with sequential hemodialysis to reduce serum methotrexate levels in a patient with acute renal insufficiency. Am J Med 1987:82:350–352.
37. O'Marcaigh AS, Johnson CM, Smithson WA, et al. Successful treatment of intrathecal methotrexate overdose by using ventricolumbar perfusion and intrathecal instillation of carboxypeptidase G_2. Mayo Clin Proc 1996:71:161–165.

38. Evans WE, Relling MV, Rodman JH, et al. Conventional compared with individualized chemotherapy for childhood acute lymphoblastic leukemia. N Engl J Med 1998:338:499–505.
39. Delepine N, Delepine G, Cornille H, et al. High value of pharmacokinetics adaptation in success of treatment of osteosarcomas by protocols based on high dose methotrexate (HDMTX). Proc Am Soc Clin Oncol 1989:8:319 (Abstr 1240).
40. Fleming GF, Schilsky RL. Antifolates: The next generation. Semin Oncol 1992:19:707–719.
41. Lennard L. Cytotoxic agents; 6-mercaptopurine, 6-thioguanine and related compounds. In: LA Damani, ed. Sulphur-Containing Drugs and Related Organic Compounds. Chemistry, Biochemistry and Toxicology, vol 3: Part B: Metabolism and Pharmacokinetics of Sulphur-Containing Drugs. Chichester: Ellis Horwood, 1989, pp 9–46.
42. Endresen L, Lie SO, Storm-Mathisen I, Rugstad HE, Stokke O. Pharmacokinetics of oral 6-mercaptopurine: Relationship between plasma levels and urine excretion of parent drug. Ther Drug Monit 1990:12:227–234.
43. Krynetski EY, Krynetskaia NF, Yanishevski Y, Evans WE. Methylation of mercaptopurine, thioguanine, and their nucleotide metabolites by heterologously expressed human thiopurine-*S*-methyltransferase. Mol Pharmacol 1995:47:1141–1147.
44. Kennedy DT, Hayney MS, Lake KD. Azathioprine and allopurinol: The price of an avoidable drug interaction. Ann Pharmacother 1996:30:951–954.
45. Weinshilboum RM. Methylation pharmacogenetics: Thiopurine methyltransferase as a model system. Xenobiotica 1992:22:1055–1071.
46. Lennard L, Lilleyman JS. Individualizing therapy with 6-mercaptopurine and 6-thioguanine related to the thiopurine methyltransferase genetic polymorphism. Ther Drug Monit 1996:18:328–334.
47. Yates CR, Krynetski EY, Loennechen T, et al. Molecular diagnosis of thiopurine *S*-methyltransferase deficiency: Genetic basis for azathioprine and mercaptopurine intolerance. Ann Intern Med 1997:126:608–614.
48. Bergan S, Rugstad HE, Bentdal O, et al. Kinetics of mercaptopurine and thioguanine nucleotides in renal transplant recipients during azathioprine treatment. Ther Drug Monit 1994:16:13–20.
49. Welch J, Lennard L, Morton GCA, Lilleyman JS. Pharmacokinetics of mercaptopurine: Plasma drug and red cell metabolite concentrations after an oral dose. Ther Drug Monit 1997:19:382–385.
50. Bergan S, Rugstad HE, Klemetsdal B, et al. Possibilities for therapeutic drug monitoring of azathioprine: 6-Thioguanine nucleotide concentrations and thiopurine methyltransferase activity in red blood cells. Ther Drug Monit 1997: 19:318–326.
51. Escousse A, Rifle G, Sgro C, et al. Azathioprine toxicity, 6-mercaptopurine accumulation and the "poor" 6-thiopurine methylator phenotype. Eur J Clin Pharmacol 1995:48:309–310.
52. Lennard L, Van Loon JA, Weinshilboum RM. Pharmacogenetics of acute

azathioprine toxicity: Relationship to thiopurine methyltransferase genetic polymorphism. Clin Pharmacol Ther. 1989:46:149–154.
53. Bach JF, Dardenne M. The metabolism of azathioprine in renal failure. Transplantation 1971:12:253–259.
54. Kern W, Schleyer E, Unterhalt M, et al. High antileukemic activity of sequential high-dose cytosine arabinoside and mitoxantrone in patients with refractory acute leukemias. Cancer 1997:79:59–68.
55. Capizzi RL, White JC, Powell BL, Perrino F. Effect of dose on the pharmacokinetic and pharmacodynamic effects of cytarabine. Semin Hematol 1991: 28(suppl 4):54–69.
56. Braess J, Kern W, Unterhalt M, et al. Response to cytarabine ocfosfate (YNK01) in a patient with chronic lymphocytic leukemia refractory to treatment with chlorambucil/prednisone, fludarabine and prednimustine/mitoxantrone. Ann Hematol 1996:73:201:204.
57. Ho DHW, Frei E. Clinical pharmacology of 1-β-D-arabinofuranosyl cytosine. Clin Pharmacol Ther 1971:12:944–954.
58. Slevin ML, Piall EM, Aherne GW, et al. The pharmacokinetics of cytosine arabinoside in the plasma and cerebrospinal fluid during conventional and high-dose therapy. Med. Pediatr Oncol 1982:157–168.
59. Crawford SM, Rustin GJS, Bagshawe KD. Acute neurological toxicity of intrathecal cytosine arabinoside—A case report. Cancer Chemother Pharmacol 1986:16:306–307.
60. Resar LMS, Phillips PC, Kastan MB, et al. Acute neurotoxicity after intrathecal cytosine arabinoside in two adolescents with acute lymphoblastic leukemia of B-cell type. Cancer 1993:71:117–123.
61. Damon LE, Plunkett W, Linker CA. Plasma and cerebrospinal fluid pharmacokinetics of 1-β-D-arabinofuranosylcytosine and 1-β-D-arabinofuranosyluracil following the repeated intravenous administration of high- and intermediate dose 1-β-D-arabinofuranosylcytosine. Cancer Res 1991:51:4141–4145.
62. Smith GA, Damon LE, Rugo HS, Ries CA, Linker CA. High-dose cytarabine dose modification reduced the incidence of neurotoxicity in patients with renal insufficiency. J Clin Oncol 1997:15:833–839.
63. Rubin EH, Andersen JW, Berg DT, et al. Risk factors for high-dose cytarabine neurotoxicity: An analysis of a cancer and leukemia group B trial in patients with acute myeloid leukemia. J Clin Oncol 1992:10:948–953.
64. Riva CM, Rustum YM, Preisler HD. Pharmacokinetics and cellular determinants of response to 1-β-D-arabinofuranosylcytosine (Ara-C). Semin Oncol 1985:12(suppl 3):1–8.
65. Plunkett W, Liliemark JO, Adams TM, et al. Saturation of 1-β-D-arabinofuranosylcytosine 5′-triphosphate accumulation in leukemic cells during high-dose 1-β-D-arabinofuranosylcytosine therapy. Cancer Res 1987:47:3005–3011.
66. Hiddemann W, Schleyer E, Unterhalt M, Kern W, Büchner T. Optimizing therapy of acute myeloid leukemia based on differences in intracellular metabolism of cytosine arabinoside between leukemic blasts and normal mononuclear blood cells. Ther Drug Monit 1996:18:341–349.

67. Rustum YM, Riva C, Preisler HD. Pharmacokinetic parameters of Ara-C and their relationship to intracellular metabolism of Ara-C, toxicity and response of patients with acute nonlymphoblastic leukemia treated with conventional and high-dose Ara-C. Semin Oncol 1987:14:141–148.
68. Kaye SB. Gemcitabine: Current status of phase I and phase II trials (Editorial). J Clin Oncol 1994:12:1527–1530.
69. Gandhi V, Mineishi S, Huang P, et al. Difluorodeoxyguanosine: Cytotoxicity, metabolism and actions of DNA synthesis in human leukemia cells. Semin Oncol 1995:22(suppl 11):61–67.
70. Green MR. Gemcitabine safety overview. Semin Oncol 1996:23:32–35.
71. Hui YF, Reitz J. Gemcitabine: A cytidine analogue active against solid tumors. Am J Health-Syst Pharm 1997:54:162–170.
72. Moertel CG. Chemotherapy for colorectal cancer. N Engl J Med 1994:330: 1136–1142.
73. Larsson PA, Carlsson G, Gustavsson B, Graf W, Glimelius B. Different intravenous administration techniques for 5-fluorouracil. Acta Oncol 1996:35: 207–212.
74. Pinedo HM, Peters GJ. 5-Fluorouracil: Biochemistry and pharmacology. J Clin Oncol 1988:6:1653–1664.
75. Diasio RB, Harris BE. Clinical pharmacology of 5-fluorouracil. Clin Pharmacokinet 1989:16(4):215–237.
76. Weh HJ, Wilke HJ, Dierlamm J, Klaasen U, Siegmund R, et al. Weekly therapy with folinic acid (FA) and high-dose 5-fluoro-uracil (5-FU) 24-hour infusion in pretreated patients with metastatic colorectal carcinoma. Ann Oncol 1994:5:233–237.
77. Beerblock K, Rinaldi Y, André T, et al. Bimonthly high dose Leucovorin and 5-fluorouracil 48-hour continuous infusion in patients with advanced colorectal carcinoma. Cancer 1997:79:1100–1105.
78. Leyland-Jones B, O'Dwyer P. Biochemical modulation: Application of laboratory models to the clinic. Cancer Treatment Rep 1986:70:219–229.
79. Marsh JC, Bertino JR, Katz K, Davis C, et al. The influence of drug interval on the effect of methotrexate and fluorouracil in the treatment of advanced colorectal cancer. J Clin Oncol 1991:9:371–380.
80. Peters GJ, van Groeningen CJ. Clinical relevance of biochemical modulation of 5-fluorouracil. Ann Oncol 1991:2:469–480.
81. Poon MA, O'Connell M, Wieland HS, Krook JE, et al. Biochemical modulation of fluorouracil with Leucovorin: Confirmatory evidence of improved therapeutic efficacy in advanced colorectal cancer. J Clin Oncol 1991:9:1967–1972.
82. Scheithauer W, Kornek G, Rosen H, et al. Combined intraperitoneal plus intravenous chemotherapy after curative resection for colonic adenocarcinoma. Eur J Cancer 1995:31A:1981–1986.
83. Schmoll H-J, Köhne C-H, Hossfeld D-K. Zur Therapie kolorektaler Karzinome mit einer Kombination aus 5-Fluorouracil und Folinsäure. Deutsch Ärztebl 1994:91:B-1759–1761.

84. Schöber C, Bokemeyer C, Stahl M, et al. The role of schedule dependency of 5-fluorouracil/Leucovorin combinations in advanced colorectal cancer. Semin Oncol 1992:19:131–135.
85. Rustum YM. Mechanism-based improvement in the therapeutic selectivity of 5-FU prodrug alone and under conditions of metabolic modulation. Oncology 1997:54(suppl 1):7–11.
86. Taguchi T. Clinical application of biochemical modulation in cancer chemotherapy: Biochemical modulation for 5-FU. Oncology 1997:54(suppl 1):12–18.
87. Joulia JM, Pinguet F, Ychou M, et al. Pharmacokinetics of 5-fluorouracil (5-FUra) in patients with metastatic colorectal cancer receiving 5-FUra bolus plus continuous infusion with high dose folinic acid. Anticancer Res 1997:17:2727–2730.
88. Sobrero AF, Aschele C, Bertino JR. Fluorouracil in colorectal cancer—A tale of two drugs: Implications for biochemical modulation. J Clin Oncol 1997:15:368–381.
89. Heggie GD, Sommadossi J-P, Cross DS, Huster WJ, Diasio RB. Clinical pharmacokinetics of 5-fluorouracil and its metabolites in plasma, urine and bile. Cancer Res 1987:47:2203–2206.
90. Schilsky RL, Hohneker J, Ratain MJ, Janisch L, et al. Phase I clinical and pharmacokinetic study of eniluracil plus fluorouracil in patients with advanced cancer. J Clin Oncol 1998:16:1450–1457.
91. Sweeny DJ, Martin M, Diasio RB. *N*-Chenodesoxycholyl-2-fluoro-β-alanine: A biliary metabolite of 5-fluorouracil in humans. Drug Metab Dispos 1988:16:892–894.
92. Gamelin EC, Danquechin-Dorval EM, Dumnesil YF, et al. Relationship between 5-fluorouracil (5-FU) dose intensity and therapeutic response in patients with advanced colorectal cancer receiving infusional therapy containing 5-FU. Cancer 1996:77:441–451.
93. Milano G, Etienne M-C. Individualizing therapy with 5-fluorouracil related to dihydropyrimidine dehydrogenase: Theory and limits. Ther Drug Monit 1996:18:335–340.
94. Poorter RL, Peters GJ, Bakker PJM, et al. Intermittent continuous infusion of 5-fluorouracil and low dose oral Leucovorin in patients with gastrointestinal cancer: Relationship between plasma concentrations and clinical parameters. Eur J Cancer 1995:31A:1465–1470.
95. Barberi-Heyob M, Weber B, Merlin JL, et al. Evaluation of plasma 5-fluorouracil nucleoside levels in patients with metastatic breast cancer: Relationships with toxicities. Cancer Chemother Pharmacol 1995:37:110–116.
96. Presant CA, Wolf W, Waluch V, et al. Association of intratumoral pharmacokinetics of fluorouracil with clinical response. Lancet 1994:343:1184–1187.
97. Etienne MC, Lagrange JL, Dassonville O, et al. Population study of dihydropyrimidine dehydrogenase in cancer patients. J Clin Oncol 1994:12:2248–2253.

98. Diasio RB, Beavers TL, Carpenter JT. Familial deficiency of dihydropyrimidine dehydrogenase. J Clin Invest 1988:81:47–51.
99. Milano G, Etienne M-C. Dihydropyrimidine dehydrogenase (DPD) and clinical pharmacology of 5-fluorouracil. Anticancer Res 1994:14:2295–2298.
100. Santini J, Milano G, Thyss A, et al. 5-FU therapeutic monitoring with dose adjustment leads to an improved therapeutic index in head and neck cancer. Br J Cancer 1989:59:287–290.
101. Martino R, Malet-Martino MC, Vialaneix C, et al. ^{19}F Nuclear magnetic resonance analysis of the carbamate reaction of α-fluoro-β-alanine (FBAL), the major catabolite of fluoropyrimidines. Drug Metab Dispos 1987:15:897–904.
102. Peters GJ, Lankelma J, Kok RM, et al. Prolonged retention of high concentrations of 5-fluorouracil in human and murine tumors as compared with plasma. Cancer Chemother Pharmacol 1993:31:269–276.
103. Presant CA, Wolf W, Albright MJ, et al. Human tumor fluorouracil trapping: Clinical correlations of in vivo ^{19}F nuclear magnetic resonance spectroscopy pharmacokinetics. J Clin Oncol 1990:8:1868–1873.
104. Bjarnason GA, Kerr IG, Doyle N, Macdonald M, Sone M. Phase I study of 5-fluorouracil and Leucovorin by a 14-day circadian infusion in metastatic adenocarcinoma patients. Cancer Chemother Pharmacol 1993:33:221–228.
105. Metzger G, Massari C, Etienne MC, et al. Spontaneous or imposed circadian changes in plasma concentrations of 5-fluorouracil coadministered with folinic acid and oxaliplatin: Relationship with mucosal toxicity in patients with cancer. Clin Pharmacol Ther 1994:56:190–201.
106. Nogue M, Saigi E, Segui MA. Clinical experience with tegafur and low dose oral Leucovorin: A dose-finding study. Oncology 1995:52:167–169.
107. Gonzalez-Baron M, Feliu J, de la Gandara I, et al. Efficacy of oral tegafur modulation by uracil and Leucovorin in advanced colorectal cancer. A phase II study. Eur J Cancer 1995:31:2215–2219.
108. Pazdur R, Lassere Y, Rhodes V, et al. Phase II trial of uracil and tegafur plus oral Leucovorin: An effective oral regimen in the treatment of metastatic colorectal carcinoma. J Clin Oncol 1994:12:2296–2300.
109. Taguchi T. Clinical application of biochemical modulation in cancer chemotherapy: biochemical modulation for 5-FU. Oncology 1997:54(suppl 1):12–18.
110. Okabe H, Toko T, Saito H, et al. Augmentation of the chemotherapeutic effectiveness of UFT, a combination of tegafur with uracil, by oral Leucovorin. Anticancer Res 1997:17:157–164.
111. Bajetta E, Carnaghi C, Somma L, et al. A pilot study of capecitabine, a new fluoropyrimidine, in patients with advanced neoplastic disease. Tumori 1996: 82:450–452.
112. Rustum YM, Harstrick A, Cao S, et al. Thymidylate synthase inhibitors in cancer therapy: direct and indirect inhibitors. J Clin Oncol 1997:15:389–400.
113. Budman DR, Meropol NJ, Reigner B, et al. Preliminary studies of a novel oral fluoropyrimide carbamate: Capecitabine. J Clin Oncol 1998:16:1795–1802.
114. Cheson BD. New antimetabolites in the treatment of human malignancies. Semin Oncol 1992:19:695–706.

115. Beutler E. Cladribine (2-chlorodeoxyadenosine). Lancet 1992:340:952–956.
116. Kane BJ, Kuhn JG, Roush MK. Pentostatine: an adenosine deaminase inhibitor for the treatment of hairy cell leukemia. Annals of Pharma 1992:26: 939–947.
117. Brogden RN, Sorkin EM. Pentostatin: A review of its pharmacodynamic and pharmacokinetic properties, and therapeutic potential in lymphoproliferative disorders. Drugs 1993:46(4):652–677.
118. Bryson HM, Sorkin EM. Cladribine—A review of its pharmacodynamic and pharmacaokinetic properties and therapeutic potential in hematological malignancies. Drugs 1993:46(5):872–894.
119. Spriggs DR, Stopa E, Mayer RJ, Schoene W, Kufe DW. Fludarabine phosphate (NSC 312878) infusions for the treatment of acute leucemia: Phase I and neuropathological study. Cancer Research 1986:46:5953–5958.
120. Ross SR, McTavish D, Faulds D. Fludarabine—A review of its pharmacological properties and therapeutic potential in malignancy. Drugs 1993:45(5): 737–759.

2.5 INHIBITORS OF TOPOISOMERASE I AND II

The enzymes topoisomerase I and II regulate the topology of DNA. However, there are important differences between these two enzymes, particularly with regard to induced strand breaks. Topo-I and Topo-II typically mediate the passage of single and double DNA strands, respectively [1–4].

2.5.1 Topoisomerase II Inhibitors

The enzyme topoisomerase II consists of two homodimers, Topo-IIβ (180 kDa) and Topo-IIα (170 kDa). Topo-IIβ is expressed at low levels throughout the cell cycle, whereas Topo-IIα activity is elevated predominantly during the late S and G_2 phases of the cell cycle during DNA replication. The podophyllotoxin derivatives etoposide (VP-16) and teniposide (VM-26) act as Topo-II poisons (Fig. 45). They form a ternary complex with the enzyme and DNA which inhibits religation of the broken DNA strands. Since Topo-II is maximally active during the S and G_2 phase, exposure to the podophyllotoxin derivatives particularly during this specific phase appears to deliver the optimal antitumoral effect [1].

2.5.1.1 Etoposide and Etoposide Phosphate

The semisynthetic podophyllotoxin derivative etoposide (VP-16) belongs to one of the most commonly used groups of anticancer drugs. It is a component of first-line chemotherapy for a variety of solid tumors, like small-

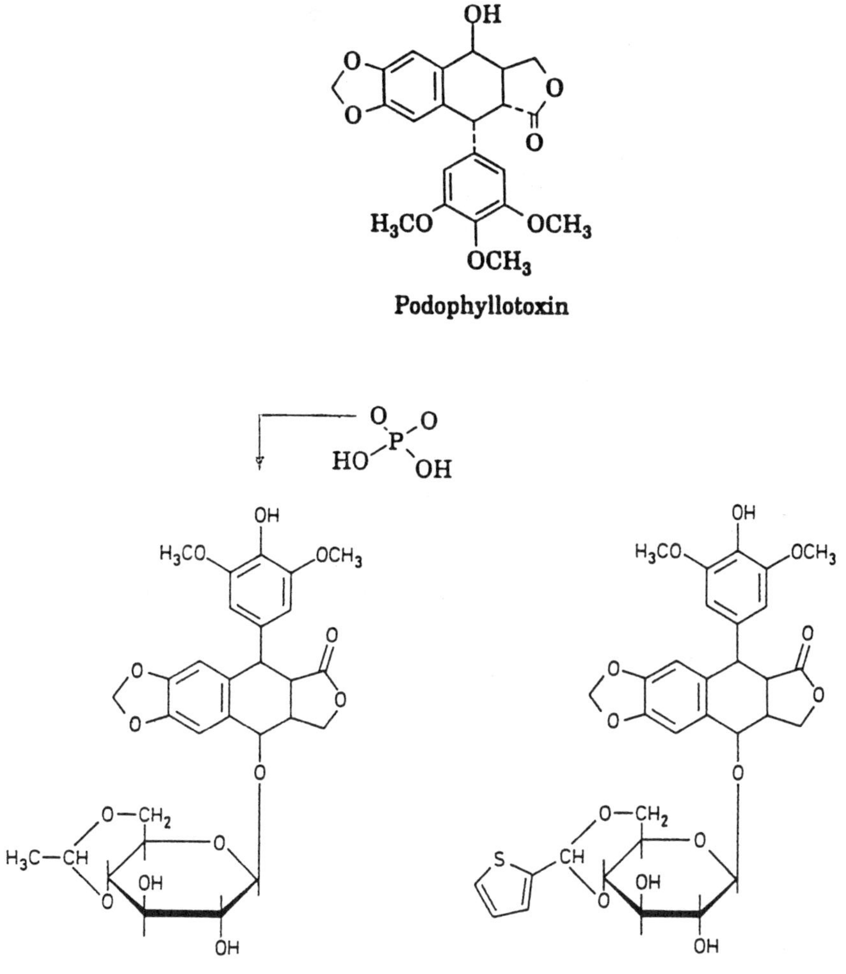

Podophyllotoxin

Etoposide

Teniposide

Fig. 45 The topoisomerase II inhibitor etoposide, its water-soluble derivative etoposide phosphate, and teniposide are semisynthetic derivatives of the natural compound podophyllotoxin.

cell and non-small-cell lung cancer (SCLC, NSCLC), and testicular cancer, as well as high-grade lymphomas and Hodgkin's Disease. Conventional dosages range from 100 to 120 (or 330) mg/m^2 IV on days 1–3 (–5) every 3–4 weeks. Alternatively the drug can be given orally 100 (–200) mg/m^2/d on days 1–5 (–7) every 3–4 weeks. High dose etoposide (e.g., 1200–

1800 mg/m^2 in divided doses administered over 3 to 5 days) has been used in combination high-dose chemotherapy regimens followed by transplantation of bone marrow or peripheral blood progenitor cells [5,6].

The toxicity profile of etoposide includes dose-limiting myelosuppression, mucositis, nausea and vomiting, and a transient increase of liver enzymes. In contrast to formulations which contain the structurally related etoposide phosphate the use of etoposide (e.g., VePesid) may be associated with a higher incidence of allergic reactions and side-effects related to the adjuvants. Several data indicate that there is an increased risk for secondary AML and secondary myelodysplastic syndrome which is related to the use of doses of more than 2000 mg etoposide/m^2 [6].

Etoposide inhibits the enzyme topoisomerase II. The cytotoxic action of etoposide is based on the formation of a ternary complex with the enzyme and DNA, which results in persistent double-stranded breaks. Since the subunit Topo-IIα is maximally active during the S and G_2 phase of the cell cycle, exposure of the drug during this cell cycle phase is required for optimal cytotoxic activity [1].

The drug can be administered intravenously as well as orally. It has been suggested that improved absolute bioavailability may be achieved by smaller oral etoposide doses. There is some evidence that the etoposide transport system in the gut is saturable if absolute doses exceed 300 mg. Thus, about 75% bioavailability may be achieved by doses up to 300 mg, whereas only 50% bioavailability may be the consequence after oral doses exceeding 350 mg [7].

Recently, a novel etoposide analogue, etoposide phosphate, (Etopophos) was introduced for parenteral application [8–11]. In contrast to etoposide, which is part of the conventional formulation VePesid, etoposide phosphate (Fig. 45) is highly soluble in aqueous solutions, thus overcoming several problems of physicochemical instability in infusion solutions [1,12–15]. It is generally accepted that infusion solutions containing VePesid for clinical use should not exceed a final concentration of 400 mg of etoposide in 1000 mL (final concentration: 0.4 mg/mL). However, a recent trial indicated that higher concentrations appear to be more stable than had been commonly assumed [14].

As a consequence, high-dose regimens containing 500–1000 mg etoposide (VePesid) should be infused with concomitant large volumes of fluid (e.g., 2000 mL of sodium chloride 0.9%, or dextrose, 5%) [1,12]. However, in some patients the high saline load associated with the use of more than 1000 mL per day of sodium chloride (0.9%) may contribute to the development of congestive heart failure. The high fluid load may also be a problem in pediatric patients. Thus, if large volumes are contraindicated it is reasonable either to give VePesid (containing etoposide) undiluted or to use the novel formulation Etopophos (containing etoposide phosphate), which can be administered in final concentrations up to 10 (−20) mg/mL [8,16].

Additionally, unlike VePesid, etoposide phosphate does not contain solubilizers like absolute alcohol, polyethylene glycol, and polysorbate, which may explain the lower incidence of hypersensitivity reactions with Etopophos [8–11,17].

Clinical studies did not reveal any significant difference between VePesid and Etopophos in regard to etoposide pharmacokinetics or to clinical efficacy (Fig. 46) when the drugs were administered on an equimolar basis [18]. In plasma the novel analogue is rapidly dephosphorylated (Table 20). Because of the close correlation between etoposide dose and the corresponding AUC up to concentrations of 1400 mg/m^2, it can be concluded that the responsible phosphatases are not oversaturable even at high plasma levels [8–11].

In plasma about 94% of etoposide is highly bound to proteins [19–21]. This is of clinical importance because decreased serum albumin concentrations (<35 g/L) result in an increase of free, biologically active etoposide [22]. The same seems to be true for cancer patients with hyperbilirubinemia, for bilirubin may displace etoposide from its plasma protein binding (Table 21) [23,24]. Etoposide is widely distributed in tissues, especially the liver, spleen, kidneys, and testicles. The volume of distribution ranges from 7 to 17 L/m^2 in adult patients [25–28].

Several studies indicate that etoposide may pass the blood–brain barrier poorly, with CSF levels being less than 10% of the corresponding plasma concentrations. As a consequence, very high doses of etoposide must be administered intravenously to achieve adequate high CSF levels [29,30]. The possibility of intrathecal or intraventricular application may be advantageous in this clinical setting; however, with regard to etoposide these administration routes have not yet been established so far [31].

Hepatic biotransformation of etoposide results in a variety of metabolites. The most important biotransformation pathways are as follows: cleavage of the glycosidic side chain, results in the formation of the corresponding aglycones, the hydrolysis of the lactone ring by which the *cis*- or *trans*-hydroxy acids are released, the glucuronidation and sulfation of the phenolic hydroxy groups, and the *O*-demethylation of the dimethyoxy group in the 4′-position, which results in the release of the corresponding catechol structure (Fig. 47) [25–28]. The latter metabolite appears to exert particularly significant antiproliferative activity, since the catechol moiety can be oxidized to the corresponding *o*-quinone. Within this redox cycle DNA-toxic superoxide radicals are released [32,33].

After IV administration, about 35–50% of the dose is excreted in the urine as unchanged drug; about 20% of this amount has been reported to be

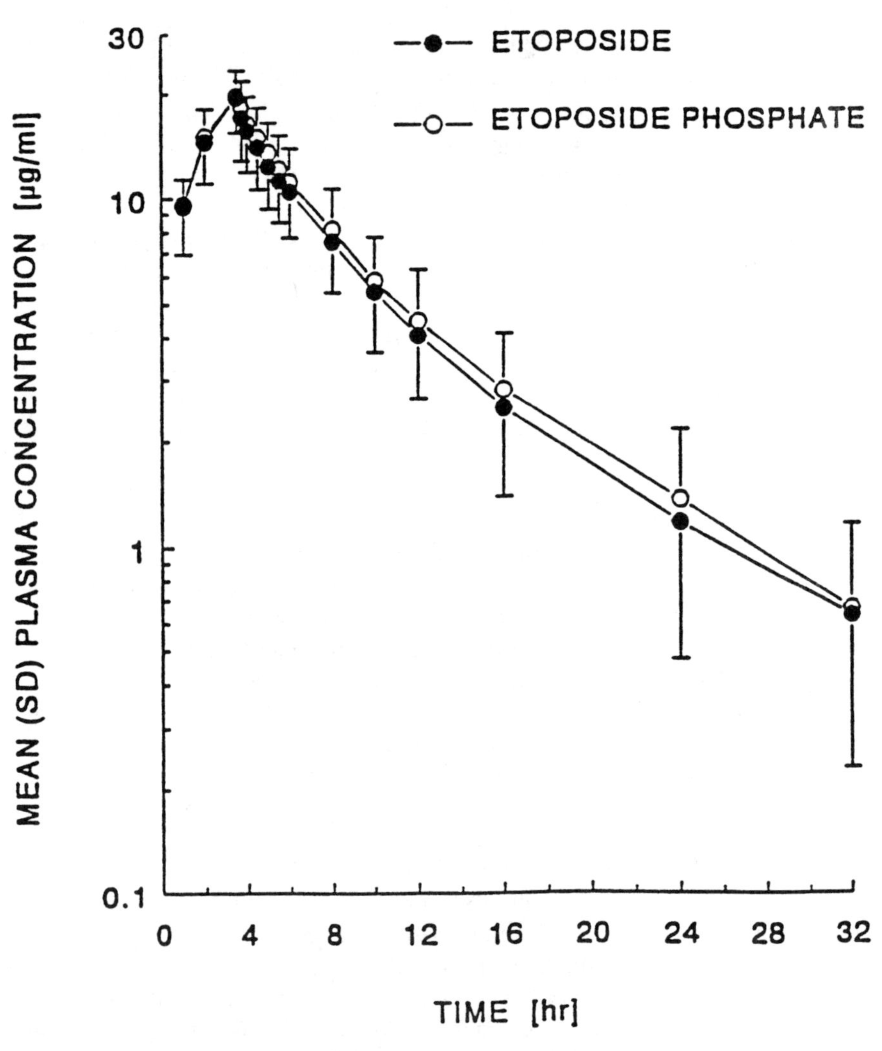

Fig. 46 Mean (SD) plasma concentration–time profiles of etoposide following IV infusion of 150 mg/m^2 dose of etoposide phosphate or etoposide. Dose is expressed as etoposide equivalents. (From Ref. 8).

Table 20 Clinical Pharmacokinetics of Etoposide and Etoposide Phosphate

Parameter	VePesid (etoposide) 150 mg/m^2 in 750 ml* [3.5 h]	Etopophos (etoposide) 150 mg/m^2 in 750 ml* [3.5 h]	Etopophos (etoposide) 150 mg/m^2 undiluted [5 min]	Etopophos (etoposide phosphate) 150 mg/m^2 undiluted [5 min]
^{c}max μg/ml	19.59	19.95	54.93	5.14
^{t}max^{h}	3.7	3.7	0.08	0.08
AUC μgxh/ml	156.7	168.3	164.0	0.39
^{t}1/2^{h}	7.09	7.11	7.24	0.07
Clearance mL/min/m^2	17.5	16.3	15.2	7.5
^{V}dss l/m^2	7.5	7.1	6.8	25.5

*Sodium Chloride 0.9% solution.
Source: Refs. 8, 9.

the glucuronide conjugate, with less than 2% consisting of the hydroxy acid and the aglycone. Etoposide clearance follows a biphasic decline, and the terminal elimination half-life ranges from 4 to 12 hours [25–28]. Recently it was suggested that within 5 days about 56 and 44% of the dose is excreted in urine and in feces (mainly as unchanged etoposide), respectively [25–28]. Thus, renal as well as hepatic dysfunction may impair drug clearance significantly [23,24].

If serum creatinine values exceed 130 μM, if the serum albumin concentration is less than 35 g/L, and if hyperbilirubinemia or severe liver dysfunction are present, only about 70% of the dose should be given to the

Table 21 Mean Etoposide Pharmacokinetic Parameters

Parameter	Total etoposide	Unbound etoposide
Volume of distribution		
V_c (central compartment)	3.4 l/m^2	46.1 l/m^2
V_{ss} (steady state)	11.5 l/m^2	66.7 l/m^2
Clearance half-life	31.8 ml/min/m^2	209.6 ml/min/m^2
Initial half-life	0.7 ± 0.9 h	1.8 ± 0.4 h
β-elimination half-life	7.2 ± 3.7 h	7.1 ± 2.5 h
End-of-infusion-concentration	119.6 μg/ml	22.5 μg/ml
Area-under-the-curve	1273 ± 561 μg/h/ml	168 ± 49 μg/h/ml

Source: Refs. 1, 5.

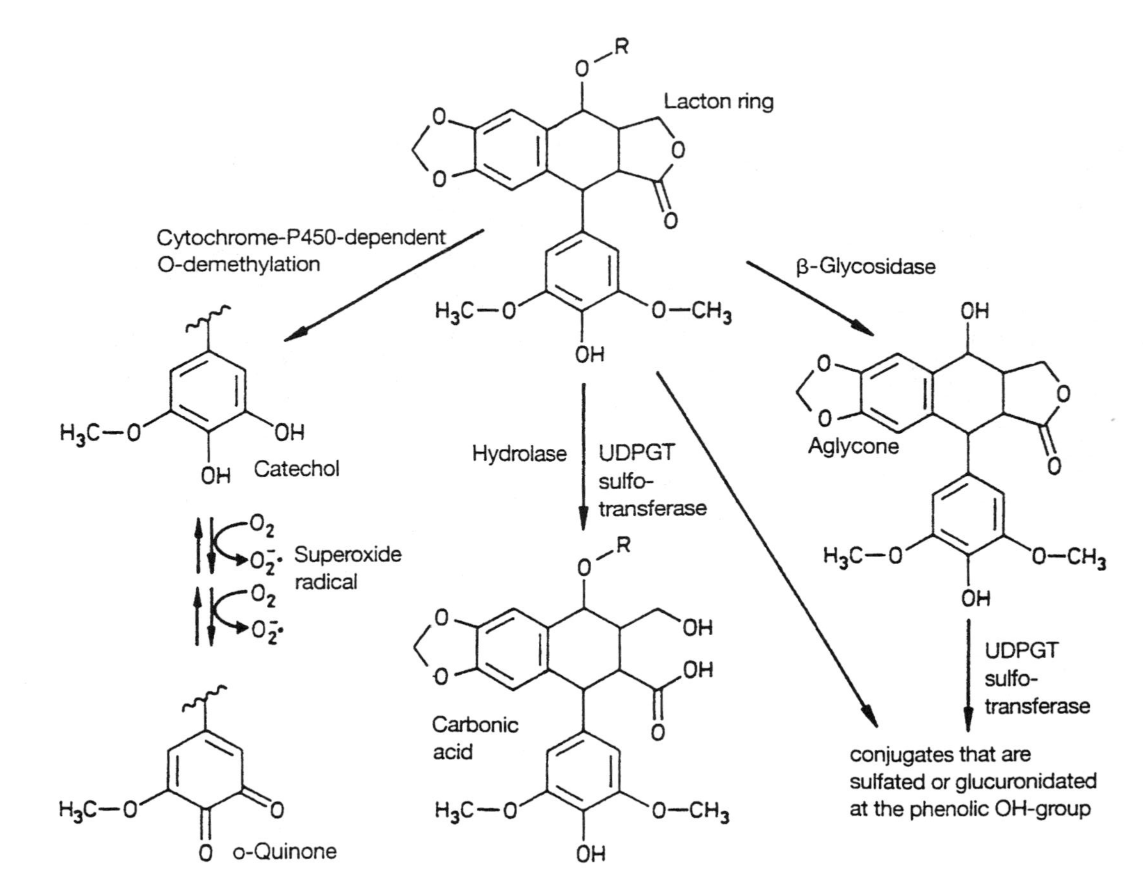

Fig. 47 Metabolic pathways of the semisynthetic podophyllotoxin derivatives etoposide and teniposide.

patient, to prevent the development of high hematological toxicity. If creatinine clearance is decreased without concomitant hepatic dysfunction, the use of 85 and 75% of the usual dose is recommended for a creatinine clearance of about 60 and 30 mL/min, respectively. If the creatinine clearance is less than 10 mL/min, only 50% of the planned dose should be given [1,34].

Although total body clearance of etoposide may be changed in the presence of obstructive jaundice and elevated alanine aminotransferase (ALT) and γ-glutamyl transferase (GGT) levels, a modest increase in renal excretion may compensate a decrease in biliary clearance [1,22]. It has been proposed to use only 75 or 50% of dose, if the serum bilirubin levels range from 1.5 to 3 mg/dl or 3.1 to 5 mg/dl, respectively, or if the SGOT levels range from 60 to 180 IU/l or exceed 180 IU/l, respectively [1,22].

Because of the major role of cytochrome P450 3A4 in the metabolism of etoposide it cannot be excluded that the simultaneous use of Cyp 3A4-inducers (e.g., phenytoin) or inhibitors (e.g., itraconazole) may change etoposide clearance significantly [1,35].

Clinical Pharmacokinetics Regarding Efficacy and Toxicity

Within the last few years numerous studies have been published concerning pharmacokinetic–pharmacodynamic relationships regarding the use of etoposide. Close correlations have been reported between plasma etoposide concentrations and hematologic toxicity (particularly neutropenia) as well as antitumor activity [36]; additionally, high interpatient pharmacokinetic variability may be dramatically reduced if the dose is accurately adapted to a target etoposide concentration [1,37].

For pharmacodynamic evaluation it seems most reasonable to measure the unbound etoposide fraction rather than the total amount in plasma, since only the former plays a bioactive role in clinical oncology (Table 21) [1].

There is some evidence that the nadir white blood cell count will be significantly lower if the percentage of the free fraction exceeds 7.5%. If the level of free etoposide is not measured via ultrafiltration of the sample, it is prudent to use a model for deriving protein binding after total etoposide concentration has been measured [1,38].

Joel and colleagues reported that the total dose of etoposide needed to reach a target level of 3 μg/mL may range from 503 to 1298 mg (with a median value of 675 mg) [37]. One of the major advantages of therapeutic drug monitoring (TDM) is that this pharmacokinetic variability can be reduced, such that pharmacodynamic effects may be more predictable. Even the measurement of unbound plasma etoposide concentrations, however, will not be sufficient to permit the calculation of etoposide pharmacokinetics in tumor tissue [39].

Topoisomerase II inhibition by inhibitors like VP-16 is reversible and very probably is a concentration-dependent effect. When etoposide is removed from the cell environment, the VP-16-induced strand breaks are rapidly resealed, with a half-life of only 6 hours. Thus, theoretically, it should be possible to increase the response rate by means of prolonged exposure to the anticancer drug, since topoisomerase II could be persistently inhibited [1]. As a consequence, a continuous infusion of etoposide (in conventional doses) may be more advantageous for clinical efficacy and toxicity [40–42] although this regimen has not yet been clinically established.

In fact, in vitro pharmacodynamic studies confirmed the hypothesis that the same degree of cell killing can be achieved if cells are exposed to low concentrations (0.5–1 μg/mL) over a long period of time or to very high concentration over a short period of time [1].

Based on clinical results, the same dose (e.g., 500 mg/m^2), appears to have superior clinical efficacy in SCLC if it is given over 5 days continuously rather than 1 day or as intermittent short time infusions. Additionally, it has been suggested that 25–50 mg etoposide/m^2/d (for at least 21 days) may be a rational dose level to maintain tumoricidal etoposide concentrations between 0.5 and 1 μg/mL [40–43].

Regarding toxicity, it has been recorded that higher peak levels are associated with more severe mucositis and myelosuppression. Thus, a lower daily dose given for a prolonged period of time seems to be less myelotoxic than a high-dose intravenous short-time infusion [36,43].

In conclusion, etoposide plasma levels exceeding 3–5 μg/mL appear to be associated with severe myelosuppression and mucositis without any increased probability of clinical response. Thus, daily doses of 30–60 mg etoposide IV for 10–21 days, with the goal of maintaining plasma levels in the range from 0.5–1.5 μg/mL seem to be equieffective and less myelosuppressive than the standard dose of 300–500 mg/m^2 given daily for 3–5 days [1].

Continuous infusion may be preferable to the oral route (e.g., 50 mg etoposide orally twice daily for 14 days) because the former avoids intermittent high peak levels as well as excessively low trough levels (e.g., <0.2 μg/mL) by maintaining rather stable steady-state serum levels (e.g., 0.5–1 μg/mL during 25 mg/m^2 IV, days 1–21). Thus, the former seems to be associated with less myelosuppression [44]. Chronopharmacological aspects do not seem to be of clinical importance concerning continuous infusion of etoposide [45].

Therefore, therapeutic drug monitoring (TDM) of etoposide might help to reduce the high interindividual variability in pharmacokinetics and toxicity, and may improve clinical efficacy, by maintaining plasma levels within a defined therapeutic range.

The most critical parameters influencing the individual VP-16 pharmacokinetics seem to be (a) the constitutive expression of cytochrome P450 3A4, which catalyzes metabolic VP-16 inactivation (with the exception of the corresponding catechol, whose clinical significance is not yet fully understood), (b) the creatinine clearance, since VP-16 is significantly excreted as unchanged drug in the urine, and (c) the albumin concentration, since a decrease will increase the unbound and bioactive fraction of etoposide (Table 22). Thus, TDM allows the timely detection of abnormal and subtherapeutic plasma steady-state levels [1,6].

In the meantime a limited sampling method exists which helps to calculate total AUC with only one to three blood samples and makes TDM management much easier [46].

A new aspect that may strengthen the importance of TDM, particularly regarding high-dose chemotherapy, has been recently reported by Rodman et al. and Mross et al. [47]. According to their results, at the time of reinfusion of bone marrow cells or peripheral stem cells, persistent etoposide levels in plasma may be high enough in some individuals to cause an impaired engraftment (Fig. 48). Rodman et al. suggested that if total etoposide concentration still exceeds 5 mg/L 48 hours after chemotherapy (time of reinfusion), the time to recovery of granulocyte and platelet counts may be significantly prolonged and nearly twice as long as usual [47]. These preliminary results are also very important for pharmacoeconomics, inasmuch as TDM could help to ensure the timely identification of delayed etoposide

Table 22 Clinical Conditions Under Which Etoposide Elimination, Metabolism and/or Protein Binding Are Affected

Excretion (renal)[a]	Metabolism (hepatic)[a]	Reaction of etoposide not bound to proteins	Anticipated pharmacologic effect
Normal	Normal	Increased (e.g., hypoalbuminemia)	None
Decreased	Normal	Normal	Increased
Normal	Decreased	Normal	Increased
Decreased	Normal	Increased (e.g., hypoalbuminemia)	Increased
Normal	Decreased	Increased (e.g., hypoalbuminemia)	None (?)
Decreased	Decreased	Increased	Increased

[a]Renal elimination and metabolism are assumed to remove etoposide from the body. The pharmacological effect is directed against both normal tissue and tumor tissue.
(Adapted from Ref. 24.)

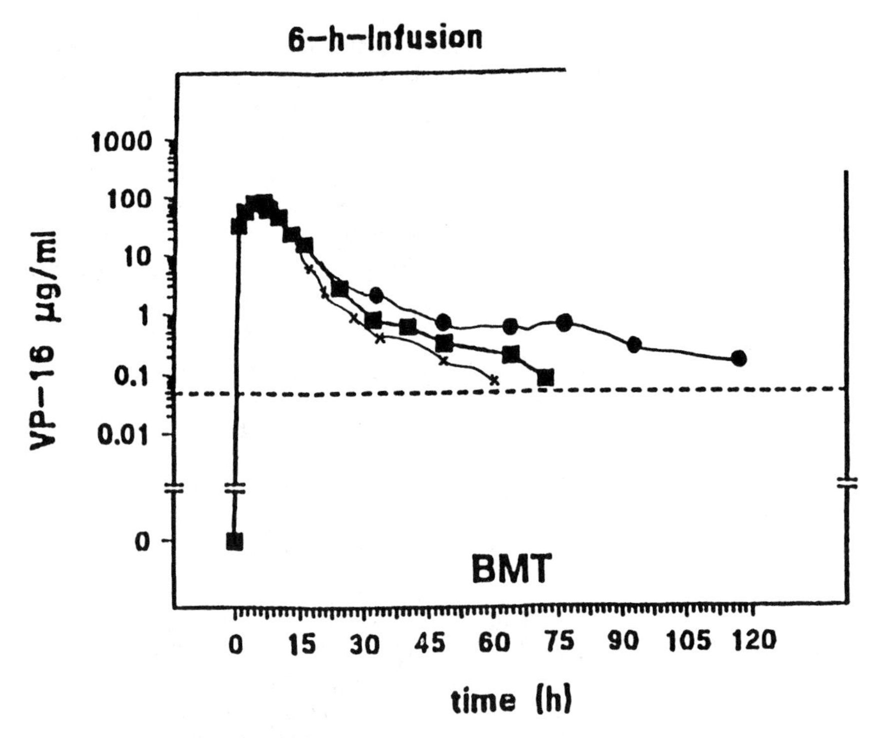

Fig. 48 After the application of high-dose Etoposide the plasma decay of Etoposide is highly variable among cancer patients who receive bone marrow transplants (BMT). Limited data exist indicating that in a few patients, etoposide levels may remain high enough when blood or marrow stem cells are reinfused to impair an engraftment. (Modified from Ref. 16.)

elimination. For the immediate future, however, it appears to be more reasonable to measure the unbound fraction rather than total etoposide.

The potential interactions between etoposide and other anticancer drugs in vivo and in vitro are not fully understood [47–50]. Other drugs, like paclitaxel or ifosfamide, are also metabolized via Cyp 3A4, which might lead to a competitive inhibition of their metabolism. Cisplatin, and possibly high-dose carboplatin and thiotepa, reportedly are able to inhibit Cyp-dependent biotransformation pathways. In conclusion, the possible interactions during combination chemotherapy may be very complex. Regarding transcellular uptake it has been reported that concomitant etoposide administration may impair the uptake of other anticancer drugs, particularly cytarabine and mitoxantrone. Thus, a time interval between the administration of etoposide and those other drugs may circumvent this interaction.

2.5.1.2 Teniposide

Teniposide (VM-26) is structurally related to etoposide. The drug is used for the treatment of pediatric malignancies, including ALL as well as several forms of malignant brain tumors, and in adult Burkitt's lymphoma or B-ALL. The usually recommended dose ranges from 30 mg/m^2 IV on days 1–5 every 5 weeks to 100–130 mg/m^2 IV weekly.

The toxicity profile of teniposide includes dose-limiting myelosuppression, mild nausea and vomiting, infertility, a transient increase of liver enzymes, and allergic reactions.

After i.v. administration, the terminal elimination half-life approximates 7 hours; the plasma clearance averages 10–15 mL/min/m^2. The distribution volume has been calculated to be about 5 L/m^2 [25,26,51].

Teniposide seems to have a longer elimination half-life than etoposide, as well as lower plasma and renal clearance. The protein binding of teniposide is higher than that of etoposide and approximates 99%. Like etoposide, teniposide does not appear to be hemodialyzable, presumably because of the extensive plasma protein binding [52].

The drug is extensively metabolized in the liver to a variety of metabolites with structural similarity to the corresponding etoposide biotransformation products (see Fig. 47). Renal excretion of unchanged teniposide comprises only 5–20% (average 10%). Thus, a dosage reduction of VM-26 in cancer patients with renal dysfunction does not seem to be warranted.

However, concomitant use of potent Cyp 3A inducers (e.g., phenytoin, phenobarbital, carbamazepine, rifampicin) may result in a two- to threefold increase in plasma VM-26 clearance. As a consequence, patients receiving standard fixed doses may be exposed to substantially reduced VM-26 plasma concentrations, which may decrease the likelihood of tumor response. In those patients a higher dosage of teniposide or a change of the anticonvulsant may be necessary [53].

2.5.2 Topoisomerase I Inhibitors

The type I DNA topoisomerase creates transient (reversible) single-strand breaks in double-strand DNA during DNA replication, recombination, or repair processing.

Unlike Topo-IIα, cellular levels of Topo-I in normal tissues are relatively independent of the cell cycle phase. The enzyme is present in normal lymphocytes and in a variety of tissues. In contrast to normal tissues, where the enzyme is only marginally activated during proliferation, there is a significant increase of this enzyme in several tumor tissues [1]. The Topo-I inhibitors topotecan and irinotecan are structurally related to the natural compound camptothecin (Fig. 49) which was isolated from the wood, bark,

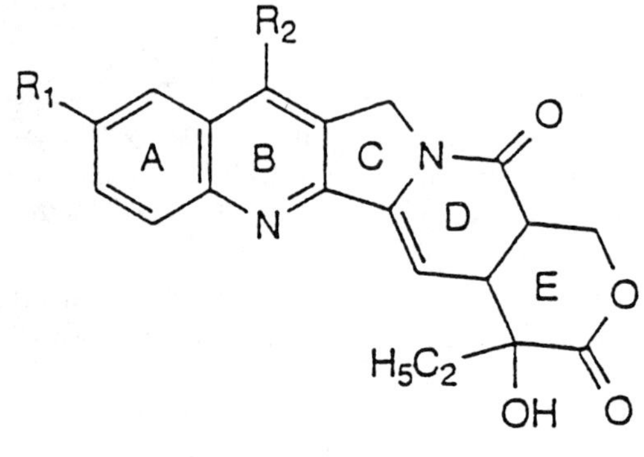

	R_1	R_2
Camptothecin	H	H
Topotecan	OH	$-CH_2-N(CH_3)_2$

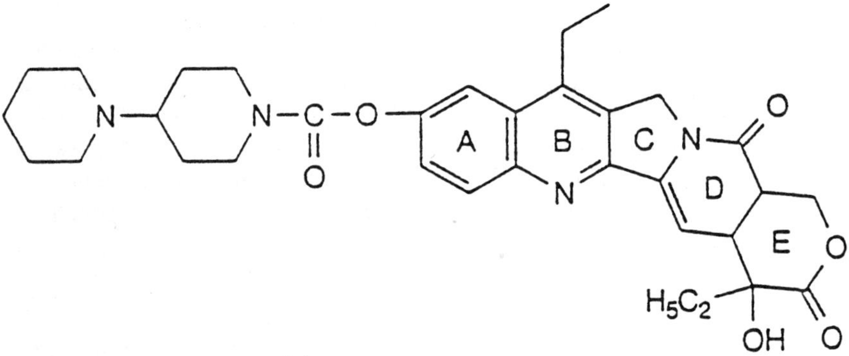

Irinotecan

Fig. 49 Topotecan and irinotecan (CPT-11) resemble a new class of anticancer drugs which are water-soluble derivatives of the natural compound camptothecin.

and fruit of the Oriental tree *Camptotheca acuminata*. Indeed, extracts of this plant have been used in traditional Chinese medicine [3,4]. The natural camptothecin itself is rather unsoluble in aqueous solutions and unfortunately causes dose-limiting hemorrhagic cystitis as well as unpredictable myelosuppression. In contrast to the natural compound, the novel semisynthetic active analogues topotecan and irinotecan (Fig. 49) are water-soluble derivatives, which makes parenteral administration much easier. Both drugs are very potent Topo-I inhibitors. They bind to the enzyme and stabilize a covalent DNA–topoisomerase I complex, which results in DNA single-strand breaks occurring during the action of the replication process [2–4].

There are some important pharmacokinetic and toxicological differences between CPT-11 (irinotecan) and topotecan: in contrast to CPT-11, which is extensively metabolized to its very active metabolite, SN-38, the structurally related lactone topotecan is already the active compound, which is hydrolyzed in plasma nonenzymatically to the rather nonactive open-ring carboxylate form [2–4]. It is of clinical importance that biliary excretion is the major route of CPT-11 elimination, whereas about 40% of topotecan is excreted via the urine in the first 24 hours of treatment [2–4].

Regarding their common toxicity profile dose-limiting myelosuppression, alopecia, mucositis, moderate nausea and emesis (incidence: 30–60%), and skin reactions can be observed. However, the risk for severe acute and subacute diarrheal episodes is especially related to CPT-11.

2.5.2.1 Irinotecan (CPT-11)

Irinotecan (CPT-11, 7-ethyl-10-[4-{1-piperidino}-1-piperidino]carbonyloxy-camptothecin) is a semisynthetic alkaloid derived from *Camptotheca acuminata*. CPT-11 demonstrates remarkable antitumor activity particularly against advanced colorectal cancer, as well as a variety of other solid tumors [54]. The drug has also been used in the treatment of lung cancer and cervix carcinoma. The usually recommended dose is 350 mg/m^2 IV every 3 weeks, or 100–150 mg/m^2 IV weekly.

After i.v. administration, the ester bond of CPT-11 is split rather rapidly by plasma carboxylesterases, causing the formation of the primary metabolite SN-38 (7-ethyl-10-hydroxycamptothecin), which can be further conjugated by UDP-glucuronosyltransferase and leads to the corresponding SN-38 glucuronide (SN-38-G). The active lactone forms of both CPT-11 and SN-38 exist in a pH-dependent equilibrium with their corresponding biologically inactive hydroxy acid derivatives, particularly at more basic pH values (Fig. 50).

SN-38 is about 100-fold more active than CPT-11 in regard to antiproliferative activity as well as toxicity. This is of clinical importance, al-

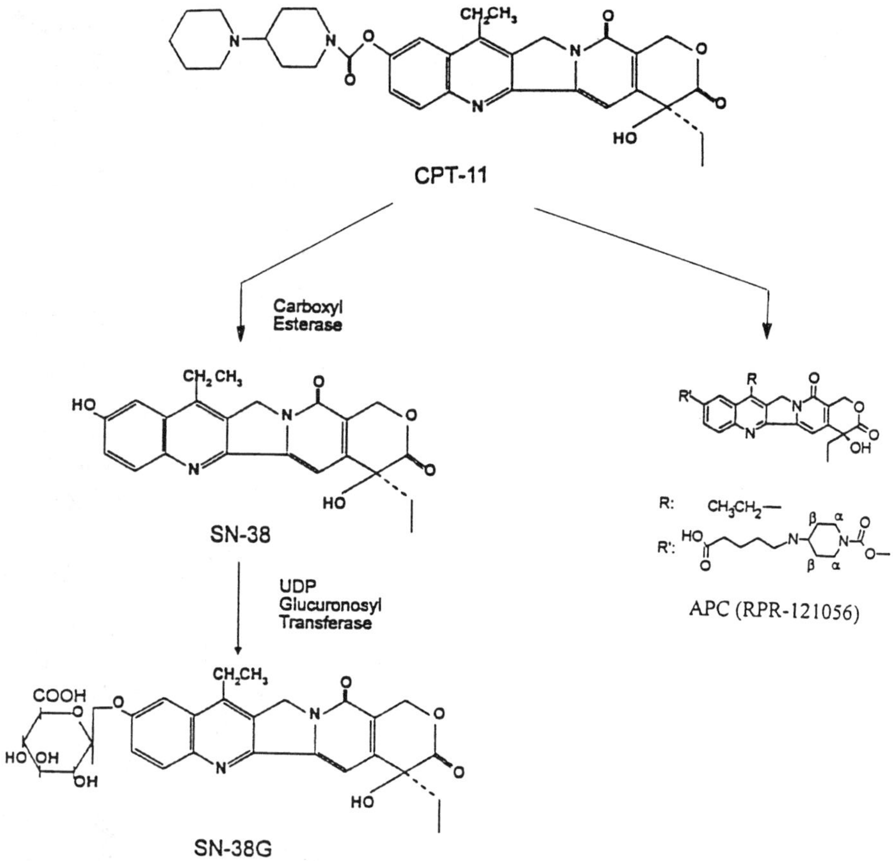

Fig. 50 Metabolic pathways of CPT-11. The much more active metabolite SN-38, which is released via carboxylesterase, can be further converted to the corresponding glucuronide SN-38G via UDPGT. The metabolic pathway leading to APC is of minor clinical importance. (Modified from Ref. 58.)

though the concentration of SN-38 is generally lower than that of unchanged CPT-11 and the corresponding glucuronide SN-38-G. The plasma bioavailabilities of SN-38 and SN-38-G approximate 3 and 10% of the parent drug, respectively.

Recently, a third metabolite that appears to be only a weak inhibitor of topoisomerase I has been isolated: its name is APC (7-ethyl-10-(4-*N*-[5-aminopentanoic acid])-1-piperidino)carbonyloxycamptothecin). However, APC cannot be hydrolyzed to SN-38 and does not seem to contribute significantly to the overall antiproliferative activity and toxicity of CPT-11 in humans.

The terminal elimination half-lives of CPT-11 and SN-38 have been reported to be about 5.5–8.8 and 6.9 hours, respectively. CPT-11 is weakly bound to plasma proteins; its distribution volume at steady-state concentrations approximates 246 L, which indicates substantial tissue distribution.

Urinary recovery of CPT-11, SN-38, and SN-38-G accounts for about 14, 0.2, and 1.1% of the dose, respectively, which explains why renal excretion is not the primary route of CPT-11 elimination. In the bile, however, about 33 to 58% of a CPT-11 dose has been recovered as a mixture of CPT-11, SN-38, and SN-38-G, strongly suggesting that nonrenal excretion is of major quantitative importance [55–59].

High levels of CPT-11 and SN-38 could be identified in the intestine, which indicates a reactivation by gut flora of biliary eliminated SN-38-G to SN-38. In conclusion, a clinically relevant enterohepatic circulation of SN-38 is very probable to occur [58,59]. This phenomenon may be associated with the clinical toxicity of delayed diarrhea occurring in 20–30% of patients.

Clinical Pharmacokinetics Regarding Efficacy and Toxicity

There is some evidence that the neutrophil nadir can be correlated with the AUC of SN-38, the major metabolite in plasma, whereas no correlation could be detected between grade 3 to 4 diarrhea and the individual AUCs of CPT-11 or its metabolites in plasma.

Regarding the incidence of severe gastrointestinal toxicity, experimental data confirm that CPT-11 and SN-38 accumulate in the intestinal mucosa at concentrations four- to sevenfold higher than those found in plasma. Very probably this accumulation is associated with the development of watery diarrhea and sometimes fatal hemorrhagic enterocolitis. It has been hypothesized that patients with a higher plasma SN-38/SN-38G ratio may experience increased intestinal toxicity because they excrete higher levels of the active compound in the intestine. Recently, Gupta and colleagues presented a model for more accurately predicting the severity of intestinal toxicity [58,59].

With a limited sampling method, not only could the respective AUC values of CPT-11, SN-38, and SN-38G be determined, but also a biliary index could be calculated. This limited sampling method is advantageous because it simplifies sample procurement and reduces patient discomfort.

$$\text{Biliary index} = \text{AUC}_{\text{CPT-11}} \times \frac{\text{AUC}_{\text{SN-38}}}{\text{AUC}_{\text{SN-38-G}}}$$

A significantly higher percentage of patients developed dose-limiting grade

3 to 4 diarrhea if their biliary index was determined to exceed 4600 ngxh/mL. According to the formula above, an underlying glucuronidation deficiency will result in a higher incidence of dose-limiting intestinal toxicity. If the predictive role of the Biliary Index as an indicator for individual CPT-11–induced gut toxicity is established by further studies, it may be useful to measure CPT-11 pharmacokinetics in cancer patients [58,59].

2.5.2.2 Topotecan

Topotecan (Fig. 49) has been demonstrated to be clinically active against a variety of tumor types including ovarian carcinoma and SCLC (e.g., 1.5 mg/m^2/d on days 1–5, every 3 weeks). Myelosuppression is the dose-limiting toxicity of topotecan. Topotecan is a semisynthetic derivative of the natural alkaloid camptothecin, structurally very similar to irinotecan. Topotecan and CPT-11 are quite different, however, in their clinical pharmacokinetic behavior [2–4].

Topotecan is rapidly and widely distributed into tissues after administration of 0.5–1.5 mg/m^2. The distribution volume of the parent drug has been estimated to be about 73 L/m^2 at steady-state conditions [60]. Promising data indicate that the drug is able to pass the blood–brain barrier, resulting in concentrations ranging from 30 to 45% of the corresponding plasma levels [61]. As a consequence, this cytotoxic drug appears to be a very useful agent, particularly at higher dosages, for the treatment of small-cell lung cancer, since SCLC is often associated with brain metastasis. However, further studies are required to confirm the special role of topotecan in the treatment of SCLC, especially regarding first-line therapy [62,63].

After IV administration of 1.5 mg/m^2 topotecan, 20–60% of the dose is excreted as unchanged drug in the urine. The β-elimination half-life has been estimated to average 3 hours. Hepatic biotransformation (e.g., hepatic N-demethylation) is only of minor quantitative importance. This is in contrast to CPT-11, where biliary excretion of unchanged drug and the corresponding metabolites is of major quantitative importance. As a consequence, in contrast to CPT-11, hyperbilirubinemia up to 10 mg/dl and impaired liver function does not require need for topotecan dose reductions, whereas in cancer patients with decreased glomerular filtration rates (GFR = 20–39 mL/min), the dose should be reduced about 50%. If the GFR value is less than 20 mL/min, the use of topotecan is generally not recommended.

In aqueous solutions there is an equilibrium between the lactone ring and the ring-opened form (Fig. 51). Lower pH values (e.g., <4.0) favor the biologically active lactone, whereas at physiologic pH and particularly at higher pH values (e.g., >10.0), topotecan exists primarily in the hydrolyzed and biologically inactive ring-opened carboxylate form. As a consequence,

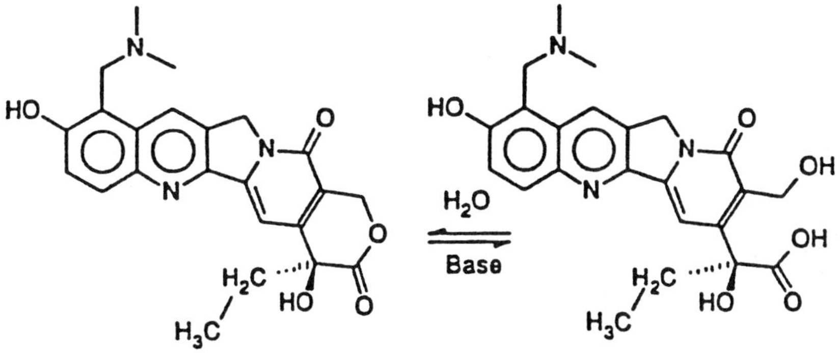

Fig. 51 In aqueous solutions there is an equilibrium between the lactone form of topotecan (biological active) and its corresponding ring-opened form (biological inactive).

it has been recommended that topotecan should be diluted with dextrose 5% (pH 4.0–5.0) rather than 0.9% sodium chloride [2].

Following topotecan bolus administration, the lactone form is rapidly hydrolyzed (about 50% conversion within 15 min), and as a result the parent compound is cleared rather rapidly from plasma. As a consequence, it has not yet been clearly defined whether it is adequate to quantify only total drug concentration (lactone plus open-ring form) if plasma concentrations levels are interpreted in regard to efficacy or toxicity [64].

REFERENCES TO SECTION 2.5

1. Joel SP. The clinical pharmacology of etoposide: An update. Cancer Treatment Rev 1996:22:179–221.
2. Burris HA, Rothenberg ML, Kuhn JG, Von Hoff DD. Clinical trials with topoisomerase I inhibitors. Semin Oncol 1992:19:663–669.
3. Potmesil M. Camphothecins: From bench research to hospital wards. Cancer Res 1994:54:1431–1439.
4. O'Reilly S, Rowinsky EK. The clinical status of irinotecan (CPT-11), a novel water soluble camptothecin analogue: 1996. Crit Rev Oncol Hematol 1996:24: 47–70.
5. Henwood JM, Brogden RN. Etoposide—A review of its pharmacodynamic and pharmacokinetic properties and therapeutic potential in combination chemotherapy of cancer. Drugs 1990:39:438–490.
6. Kollmannsberger C, Hartmann JT, Kanz L, Bokemeyer C. Risk of secondary myeloid leukemia and myelodysplastic syndrome following standard-dose che-

motherapy or high-dose chemotherapy with stem cell support in patients with potentially curable malignancies. J Cancer Res Clin Oncol 1998:124:207–214.
7. Hande KR, Krozely MG, Greco GA, Hainsworth JD, Johnson DH. Bioavailability of low-dose etoposide. J Clin Oncol 1993:11:374–377.
8. Kaul S, Igwemezie LN, Stewart DJ, et al. Pharmacokinetics and bioequivalence of etoposide following intravenous administration of etoposide phosphate and etoposide in patients with solid tumors. J Clin Oncol 1995:13:2835–2841.
9. Budman DR, Igwemezie LM, Kaul S, et al. Phase I evaluation of a water-soluble etoposide prodrug, etoposide phosphate, given as a 5-minute infusion on days 1, 3, and 5 in patients with solid tumors. J Clin Oncol 1994:12:1902–1909.
10. Fields SZ, Budman DR, Young RR, et al. Phase I study of high-dose etoposide phosphate in man. Bone Marrow Transplant 1996:18:851–856.
11. Kreis W, Budman DR, Vinciguerra V, et al. Pharmacokinetic evaluation of high-dose etoposide phosphate after a 2-hour-infusion in patients with solid tumors. Cancer Chemother Pharmacol 1996:38:378–384.
12. Beijnen JH, Beijnen-Bandhoe AU, Dubbelman AC, van Gijn R, Underberg WJM. Chemical and physical stability of etoposide and teniposide in commonly used infusion fluids. J Parent Sci Technol 1991:45:108–112.
13. Holthuis JJM. Etoposide and teniposide—Bioanalysis, metabolism and clinical pharmacokinetics. Pharm Weekbl Sci Ed 1988:10:101–116.
14. Joel SP, Clark PI, Slevin ML. Stability of the i.v. and oral formulations of etoposide in solution. Cancer Chemother Pharmacol 1995:37:117–124.
15. Pearson SD, Trissel LA. Leaching of diethylhexylphthalate from polyvinylchloride containers by selected drugs and formulation components. Am J Hosp Pharm 1993:50:1405–1409.
16. Mross K, Bewermeier P, Krüger W, et al. Pharmacokinetics of undiluted or diluted high-dose etoposide with or without busulfan administration to patients with hematologic malignancies. J Clin Oncol 1994:12:1468–1474.
17. Hoetelmans RMW, Schornagel JH, Hunink WW, Beijnen JH. Hypersensitivity reactions to etoposide. Ann Pharmacother 1996:30:367–371.
18. Hainsworth JD, Levitan N, Wampler GL, et al. Phase II randomzied study of cisplatin plus etoposide phosphate or etoposide in the treatment of small-cell lung cancer. J Clin Oncol 1995:13:1436–1442.
19. Joel SP, Shah R, Clark PI, Slevien ML. Predicting etoposide toxicity: Relationship to organ function and protein binding. J Clin Oncol 1996:14:257–267.
20. Liu B, Earl HM, Poole CJ, Dunn J, Kerr DJ. Etoposide protein binding in cancer patients. Cancer Chemother Pharmacol 1995:36:506–512.
21. Schwinghammer TL, Fleming RA, Rosenfeld CS, et al. Disposition of total and unbound etoposide following high-dose therapy. Cancer Chemother Pharmacol 1993:32:273–278.
22. Stewart CF, Arbuck SG, Fleming RA, Evans WE. Changes in the clearance of total and unbound etoposide in patients with liver dysfunction. J Clin Oncol 1990:8:1874–1879.

23. D'Incalci M, Rossi C, Zucchetti M, Urso R, et al. Pharmacokinetics of etoposide in patients with abnormal renal and hepatic function. Cancer Res 1986: 46:2566–2571.
24. Stewart CF. Use of etoposide in patients with organ dysfunction: Pharmacokinetic and pharmacodynamic considerations. Cancer Chemother Pharmacol 1994:34(suppl):S76–S83.
25. Clark PI, Slevin ML. The clinical pharmacology of etoposide and teniposide. Clin Pharmacokinet 1987:12:223–252.
26. Issell BF. The podophyllotoxin derivatives VP16-213 and VM26. Cancer Chemother Pharmacol 1982:7:73–80.
27. Allen LM, Creaven PJ. Comparison of the human pharmacokinetics of VM26 and VP16, two antineoplastic epipodophyllotoxin glucopyranosides. Eur J Cancer 1975:11:697.
28. Evans WE, Sinkule JA, Crom WR, Dow L, Look T, Rivera G. Pharmacokinetics of teniposide (VM26) and etoposide (VP16-213) in children with cancer. Cancer Chemother Pharmacol 1982:7:147–150.
29. Kiya K, Uozumi T, Ogasawara H, et al. Penetration of etoposide into human malignant brain tumors after intravenous and oral administration. Cancer Chemother Pharmacol 1992:29:339–342.
30. Relling MV, Mahmoud HH, Pui C-H, et al. Etoposide achieves potentially cytotoxic concentrations in CSF of children with acute lymphoblastic leukemia. J Clin Oncol 1996:14:399–404.
31. van der Gaast A, Sonneveld P, Mans DRA, Splinter TAW. Intrathecal administration of etoposide in the treatment of malignant meningitis: Feasibility and pharmacokinetic data. Cancer Chemother Pharmacol 1992:29:335–337.
32. Relling MV, Evans R, Dass C, Desiderio DM, Nemec J. Human cytochrome P450 metabolism of teniposide and etoposide. J Pharmacol Exp Ther 1992: 261:493–496.
33. Relling MV, Nemec J, Schuetz EG, et al. O-Demethylation of epipodophyllotoxins is catalyzed by human cytochrome P450 3A4. Mol Pharmacol 1994: 45:352–358.
34. Kintzel P, Dorr RT. Anticancer drug renal toxicity and elimination: Dosing guidelines for altered renal function. Cancer Treatment Rev 1995:21:33–64.
35. Baker DK, Relling MV, Pui C-H, et al. Increased teniposide clearance with concomitant anticonvulsant therapy. J Clin Oncol 1992:10:311–315.
36. Joel SP, Shah R, Slevin ML. Etoposide dosage and pharmacodynamics. Cancer Chemother Pharmacol 1994:34(suppl):S69–S75.
37. Joel SP, Ellis P, O'Bryne K, et al. Therapeutic monitoring of continuous infusion etoposide in small-cell lung cancer. J Clin Oncol 1996:14:1903–1912.
38. Stewart CF, Arbuck SG, Fleming RA, et al. Relation of systemic exposure to unbound etoposide and hematologic toxicity. Clin Pharmacol Ther 1991:50: 385–393.
39. Millward MJ, Newell DR, Yuen K, et al. Pharmacokinetics and pharmacodynamics of prolonged oral etoposide in women with metastatic breast cancer. Cancer Chemother Pharmacol 1995:37:161–167.

40. Thompson DS, Hainsworth JD, Hande KR, Holzmer MC, Greco FA. Prolonged administration of low-dose infusional etoposide in patients with etoposide-sensitive neoplasms: A phase I/II study. J Clin Oncol 1993:11:1322–1328.
41. Desoize B, Marechal F, Cattan A. Clinical pharmacokinetics of etoposide during 120 hours continuous infusions in solid tumors. Br J Cancer 1990:62:840–841.
42. Perkins JB, Elfenbein J, Fields KK. Analysis of dose–response relationships in the setting of high-dose ifosfamide, carboplatin and etoposide and autologous hematopoietic stem cell transplantation: Implications for the treatment of patients with advanced breast cancer. Semin Oncol 1996:23(suppl 6):42–46.
43. Chatelut E, Chevreau C, Blancy E, Lequelle A, et al. Pharmacokinetics and toxicity of two modalities of etoposide infusion in metastatic non-small-cell-lung carcinoma. Cancer Chemother Pharmacol 1990:26:365–368.
44. Greco FA, Hainsworth JD. Prolonged administration of low-daily-dose etoposide: A superior dosing schedule? Cancer Chemother Pharmacol 1994: 34(suppl):S101–S104.
45. Yamamoto N, Tamura T, Ohe Y, et al. Chronopharmacology of etoposide given by low dose prolonged infusion in lung cancer patients. Anticancer Res 1997: 17:669–672.
46. Strömgren AS, Sorensen BT, Jakobsen P, Jakobsen A. A limited sampling method for estimation of the etoposide area under the curve. Cancer Chemother Pharmacol 1993:32:226–230.
47. Rodman JH, Murry DJ, Madden T, Santana VM. Altered etoposide pharmacokinetics and time to engraftment in pediatric patients undergoing autologous bone marrow transplantation. J Clin Oncol 1994:12:2390–2397.
48. Bonner JA, Kozelsky TF. The significance of the sequence of administration of topotecan and etoposide. Cancer Chemother Pharmacol 1996:39:109–112.
49. Holden SA, Teicher BA, Robinson MF, et al. Antifolates can potentiate topoisomerase II inhibitors in vitro and in vivo. Cancer Chemother Pharmacol 1995: 56:165–171.
50. Ehninger G, Proksch B, Wanner T, et al. Intracellular cytosine arabinoside accumulation and cytosine arabinoside triphosphate formation in leukemic blast cells is inhibited by etoposide and teniposide. Leukemia 1992:6:582–587.
51. Canal P, Bugat R, Michel C, et al. Pharmacokinetics of teniposide (VM26) after IV administration in serum and malignant ascites of patients with ovarian carcinoma. Cancer Chemother Pharmacol 1985:15:149–152.
52. Holthuis JJM, van de Vyver FL, van Oort WJ, et al. Pharmacokinetic evaluation of increasing dosages of etoposide in a chronic hemodialysis patient. Cancer Treatment Rep 1985:69:1279–1282.
53. Rodman JH, Abromowitch M, Sinkule JA, et al. Clinical pharmacodynamics of continuous infusion teniposide: Systemic exposure as a determinant of response in a phase I trial. J Clin Oncol 1987:5:1007–1014.
54. Rougier P, Bugat R, Douillard JY, Culine S, et al. Phase II study of irinotecan in the treatment of advanced colorectal cancer in chemotherapy naive patients and patients pretreated with fluorouracil-based chemotherapy. J Clin Oncol 1997:15:251–260.

55. Lokiec F, Canal P, Gay C, et al. Pharmacokinetics of irinotecan and its metabolites in human blood, bile and urine. Cancer Chemother Pharmacol 1995:36:79–82.
56. Rivory LP, Robert J. Identification and linetics of a β-glucuronide metabolite of SN-38 in human plasma after administration of the camptothecin derivative irinotecan. Cancer Chemother Pharmacol 1995:36:176–179.
57. Rivory LP, Riou J-F, Haaz M-C, et al. Identification and properties of a major plasma metabolite of irinotecan (CPT-11) isolated from the plasma of patients. Cancer Res 1996:56:3689–3694.
58. Gupta E, Mick R, Ramirez J, et al. Pharmacokinetic and pharmacodynamic evaluation of the topoisomerase inhibitor irinotecan in cancer patients. J Clin Oncol 1997:15:1502–1510.
59. Mick R, Gupta E, Vokes EE, Ratain MJ. Limited-sampling models for irinotecan pharmacokinetics–pharmacodynamics: Prediction of biliary index and intestinal toxicity. J Clin Oncol 1996:14:2012–1019.
60. Grochow LB, Rowinsky EK, Johnson R, et al. Pharmacokinetics and pharmacodynamics of topotecan in patients with advanced cancer. Drug Metabol Dispos 1992:20:706–713.
61. Baker SD, Heideman RL, Crom WR, et al. Cerebrospinal fluid pharmacokinetics and penetration of continuous infusion topotecan in children with central nervous system tumors. Cancer Chemother Pharmacol 1996:37:195–202.
62. Rowinsky EK, Grochow LB, Sartorius SE, et al. Phase I and pharmacological study of high doses of the topoisomerase I inhibitor topotecan with granulocyte colony-stimulating factor in patients with solid tumors. J Clin Oncol 1996:14:1224–1235.
63. ten Bokkel Huinink W, Gore M, Carmichael J, et al. Topotecan versus paclitaxel for the treatment of recurrent epithelial ovarian cancer. J Clin Oncol 1997:15:2183–2193.
64. Herben VMM, ten Bokkel Huinink W, Beijnen JH. Clinical pharmacokinetics of topotecan. Clin Pharmacokinet 1996:31(2):85–102.

2.6 MITOTIC INHIBITORS: VINCA ALKALOIDS AND TAXOIDS

More than 30 different alkaloids have been extracted from the periwinkle plant *Vinca rosea*, but only vinblastine and vincristine possess marked antitumor activity [1–4]. Further semisynthetic procedures led to the development of vindesine and vinorelbine [5]. Chemically, these vinca alkaloids have a large dimeric asymmetric structure composed of two heterocyclic nuclei (dihydroindol nucleus for vindoline and indole nucleus for catharanthine) linked by a carbon–carbon bond (Fig. 52) [2,4,5].

The vinca alkaloids act as spindle poisons by arresting cell mitosis at metaphase. Stable vinca alkaloid–tubulin complexes are formed. Preventing tubulin polymerization also prevents the building of a functional active tubular skeleton [2,6].

This mechanism of action is different to those of the taxanes paclitaxel and docetaxel, which are mitotic inhibitors as well. Both drugs enhance rather than inhibit the polymerization of tubulin, which is a protein subunit of the spindle microtubules. As a consequence, very stable, nonfunctional microtubules are formed which cannot be reorganized for cell division [7].

Catharanthine nucleus

6′ 5′ OH
Nb′ 20′
Na′ 15′
H CO2CH3

6′
N
N
CO2CH3

	R_1	R_2	R_3
Vindesine	$-CH_3$	$-CONH_2$	$-OH$
Vincristine	$-CHO$	$-CO_2CH_3$	$-OCOCH_3$
Vinblastine	$-CH_3$	$-CO_2CH_3$	$-OCOCH_3$
Vinorelbine	$-CH_3$	$-CO_2CH_3$	$-OCOCH_3$

Fig. 52 Chemical structures of the commercially available vinca alkaloids vincristine, vindesine, vinblastine, and vinorelbine. (Adapted from Ref. 4.)

The common toxicity profile of vinca alkaloids includes peripheral and autonomic nervous system toxicity, moderate alopecia, and mucositis. Whereas myelosuppression is the dose-limiting side effect if vinblastine, vindesine, or vinorelbine are used, lasting effects on the peripheral and autonomic nervous system limit the use of vincristine.

If accidental extravasation or paravasation of vinca alkaloids occurs, a rapid therapeutic intervention appears to be necessary in order to avoid severe skin necrosis. It has been suggested that the application of warm packs to the affected area and the local infiltration of hyaluronidase are the most successful emergency tools [2]. (See also Chapter 6.)

2.6.1 Vinca Alkaloids

2.6.1.1 Vincristine

The vinca alkaloid vincristine is widely used as a chemotherapeutic agent for the treatment of lymphoma as well as multiple myeloma and for SCLC in combination regimens. The usually recommended dose is 1.4 mg/m^2 IV as bolus administration. Especially in the treatment of plasmocytoma vincristine is administered continuously over 4 days with 0.4 mg/day (VAD regimen).

In adult patients the absolute vincristine dose is generally limited to 2 mg, which is primarily based on the observation that exceeding this limit tends to severely increase peripheral neurotoxicity without any obvious increase in therapeutic benefit [4,8]. However, this strict limitation was questioned very recently because of the underlying high interindividual variability of vincristine pharmacokinetics in cancer patients [9].

Following IV administration, vincristine is widely distributed into body tissues. Since, however, this drug passes the blood–brain barrier only poorly, corresponding concentrations of cerebrospinal fluid do not reach therapeutic levels.

The drug is extensively metabolized in the liver mainly by cytochrome P450 isozymes, particularly Cyp 3A4. This is of clinical importance because concomitant therapy with potent Cyp 3A4 inhibitors, like itraconazole, may significantly impair the metabolic inactivation of vincristine and augment the risk of severe neurotoxicity [10–12].

The elimination of the parent compound and its metabolites appears to decline in a triphasic manner. The terminal elimination half-life of vincristine varies among individuals from 11 to 155 hours. The elimination half-life of vincristine is much longer than that of its structurally related compounds (Table 23). The possibility cannot be excluded that the extraordinarily high neurotoxic potency of vincristine is in part related to its prolonged (compared to other vinca alkaloids) contact with nerve tissues.

Table 23 Comparison of Cytotoxicity and Pharmacokinetic Characteristics of Vinca Alkaloids

Parameter	Vinorelbine (15–30 mg/m^2)	Vinblastine (7–14 mg/m^2)	Vincristine (2 mg/m^2)	Vindesine (1.5–4 mg/m^2)
Cytotoxicity				
IC_{50} values in the NSCLC-N6L2 cell line	1.4	2.6	36	2.8
Pharmacokinetic characteristics				
Initial half-life, h	0.067	0.062	0.077	0.054
β-Half-life, h	1.82	1.64	2.27	1.65
Terminal half-life, h	35.0	24.8	85.0	20.2
V_c, L/kg		0.69	0.33	0.084
Clearance L/h/kg	0.756	0.74	0.106	0.519

(Adapted from Ref. 4.)

Vincristine and its metabolites are primarily excreted in the bile and feces, whereas excretion in the urine is of minor quantitative importance. About 30% of the dose is excreted in the feces within 24 hours and 70% within 72 hours [13–15].

If there is any evidence of hepatic dysfunction (e.g., SGOT levels: 60–180 IU/l) or an increase of serum bilirubin concentration ranging from 1.5 to 3 mg/dl, only 50% of planned dose should be given. If SGOT levels exceed 180 IU/l and if serum bilirubin concentrations range from 3.1 to 5 mg/dl, only 25% of the planned dose should be administered. In patients with bilirubin levels exceeding 5 mg/dl, the drug is contraindicant. No dosage modification appears to be necessary in patients with renal dysfunction [4].

2.6.1.2 Vinblastine (Vinca-Leucoblastine)

Vinblastine sulfate is used alone and in combination regimens in the treatment of disseminated Hodgkin's disease, as well as in non-Hodgkin lymphoma. It is also used in the treatment of a variety of solid tumors, including NSCLC or bladder cancer. The usually recommended dose is 3.7 mg/m^2 IV (up to 18.5 mg/m^2 IV) as monotherapy and 6–8 mg/m^2 IV on day 1 (+2) every 3–4 weeks in combination chemotherapy. Other regimens use 0, 1–0, 15 mg/kg i.v. [1–4].

Following IV administration, vinblastine is widely distributed into body tissues. Since, however, the drug passes the blood–brain barrier only poorly, corresponding concentrations of CSF do not reach therapeutic levels.

The drug is extensively metabolized in the liver. One of these metabolites, deacetylvinblastine (Fig. 53), appears to be at least as active as the parent compound [16].

Vinblastine and its metabolites are primarily excreted in the bile and feces, whereas excretion in the urine is of minor quantitative importance.

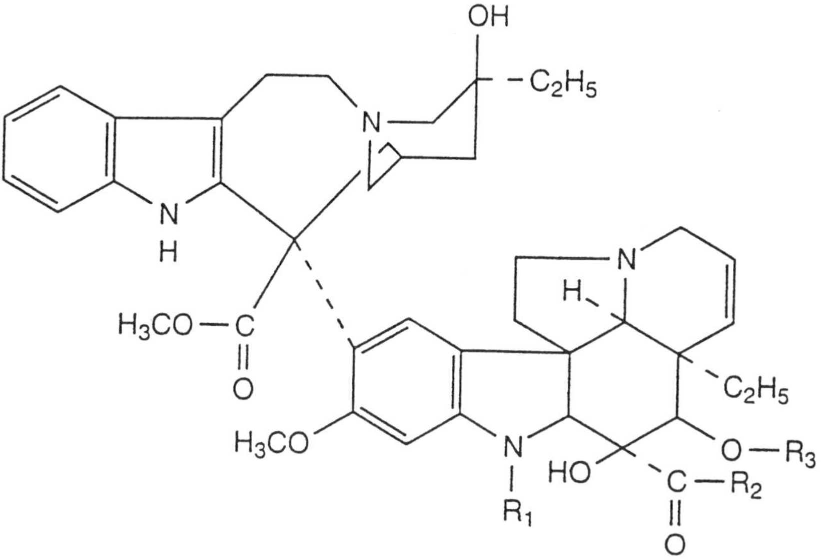

	R_1	R_2	R_3
Vinblastine	$—CH_3$	$—OCH_3$	$—C(=O)—CH_3$
Deacetylvinblastine	$—CH_3$	$—OCH_3$	$—H$

Fig. 53 The metabolite deacetylvinblastine appears to be at least as active as the parent compound.

As a consequence dose reduction is recommended in cancer patients with severe hepatic dysfunction, whereas renal dysfunction does not require dose modifications.

If there is any evidence of hepatic dysfunction (e.g., SGOT levels: 60–180 IU/l) or an increase of serum bilirubin concentration ranging from 1.5 to 3 mg/dl, only 50% of planned dose should be given. If SGOT levels exceed 180 IU/l and if serum bilirubin concentrations range from 3.1 to 5 mg/dl, only 25% of the planned dose should be administered. In patients with bilirubin levels exceeding 5 mg/dl, the drug is contraindicant. No dosage modification appears to be necessary in patients with renal dysfunction [4].

2.6.1.3 Vindesine

Vindesine sulfate is used alone and in combination for the treatment of malignant lymphoma, melanoma, and NSCLC. The recommended dose is 3 mg/m^2 IV weekly.

The pharmacokinetic behavior of vindesine is similar to that of vincristine and vinblastine regarding the α or β half-lives, whereas the terminal elimination half-life is about 24 hours, which is comparable to vinblastine but considerably shorter than those of vinorelbine or vincristine (Table 23). Vindesine and its metabolites are primarily excreted in the bile and feces, whereas excretion in the urine is of minor importance. Thus no dosage reduction is necessary in the presence of renal dysfunction.

If there is any evidence of significant hepatic dysfunction or hyperbilirubinemia, dose modifications (see: Vinblastine or Vincristine) are necessary in order to avoid excessive neurotoxicity [1–4].

2.6.1.4 Vinorelbine

The use of vinorelbine, a novel semisynthetic vinca alkaloid, is rapidly expanding for the treatment of malignant lymphoma, advanced breast cancer, and NSCLC. The usually recommended dose is 30 mg/m^2 IV weekly [4,5].

Vinorelbine differs structurally from the naturally occurring vinca alkaloids vincristine and vinblastine and the semisynthetic vindesine because its catharanthine ring, rather than the vindoline ring, is substituted. Some promising data indicate that vinorelbine can be administered orally because of its considerable absolute bioavailability (approximating 24%). Thus, oral vinorelbine, 100 mg/m^2, seems to provide a similar systemic concentration to that reached by 30 mg/m^2 IV. However, the initial clinical studies using oral vinorelbine were rather disappointing [5,17].

After IV administration the drug is rapidly distributed into the peripheral tissues. The highest concentrations were recovered in spleen, liver, kidneys, and lungs, whereas only minimal concentrations were found in fat, bone marrow, and brain tissue. The extensive distribution into lung tissues may explain the particularly high activity of vinorelbine in NSCLC as a single agent or in combination.

The novel semisynthetic alkaloid vinorelbine is highly bound to various blood components, particularly platelets (about 80%). Total binding in serum has been determined to range from 80 to 90%. Thus, the average unbound fraction approximates 13.5% [18,19]. The terminal elimination half-life of vinorelbine has been recorded to range from 35 to 45 hours, which is considerably longer than those of vinblastine or vindesine, but considerably shorter than that vincristine. One may speculate that the longer the terminal elimination half-life of vinca alkaloids is the higher the risk for peripheral neurotoxicity may be. However, this hypothesis is not valid for vinorelbine because this drug is less neurotoxic than vindesine. There is some evidence that vinorelbine binds with a very low affinity to axonal tubulin.

Renal excretion of the drug approximates 20% of the dose, with about 60–95% being unchanged drug. Fecal excretion of the drug and its metabolites is of major quantitative importance.

So far two metabolites of vinorelbine have been isolated and identified: deacetylvinorelbine and *N*-oxide vinorelbine. The latter does not exert any antiproliferative activity, whereas the former appears to be as active as the parent compound [18,19].

Because the drug and its metabolites undergo extensive biliary excretion, dosage adjustments have been recommended in patients with hyperbilirubinemia and hepatic insufficiency.

If there is any evidence of significant hepatic impairment or an increase of serum bilirubin concentration exceeding 3 mg/dL, a 50% reduction of vinorelbine dose is recommended to avoid severe peripheral neurotoxicity or pronounced myelosuppression. No dosage reduction is necessary in the presence of renal dysfunction [4,5,20].

2.6.2 Taxanes (Diterpenes)

Paclitaxel (Fig. 54) and docetaxel (Fig. 56) are very potent inhibitors of mitosis. Their cytotoxic effect is mediated by a strong stabilization of the microtubule assembly in the tumor cell [7].

Regarding the toxicity profile of paclitaxel and docetaxel there are several similarities and differences. Myelosuppression is the dose-limiting toxicity of both drugs. Additionally, peripheral neuropathy, including arthralgia, alopecia, erythema, an increase of liver enzymes, and gastrointestinal disorders, are common side effects of taxoids. Both drugs are associated

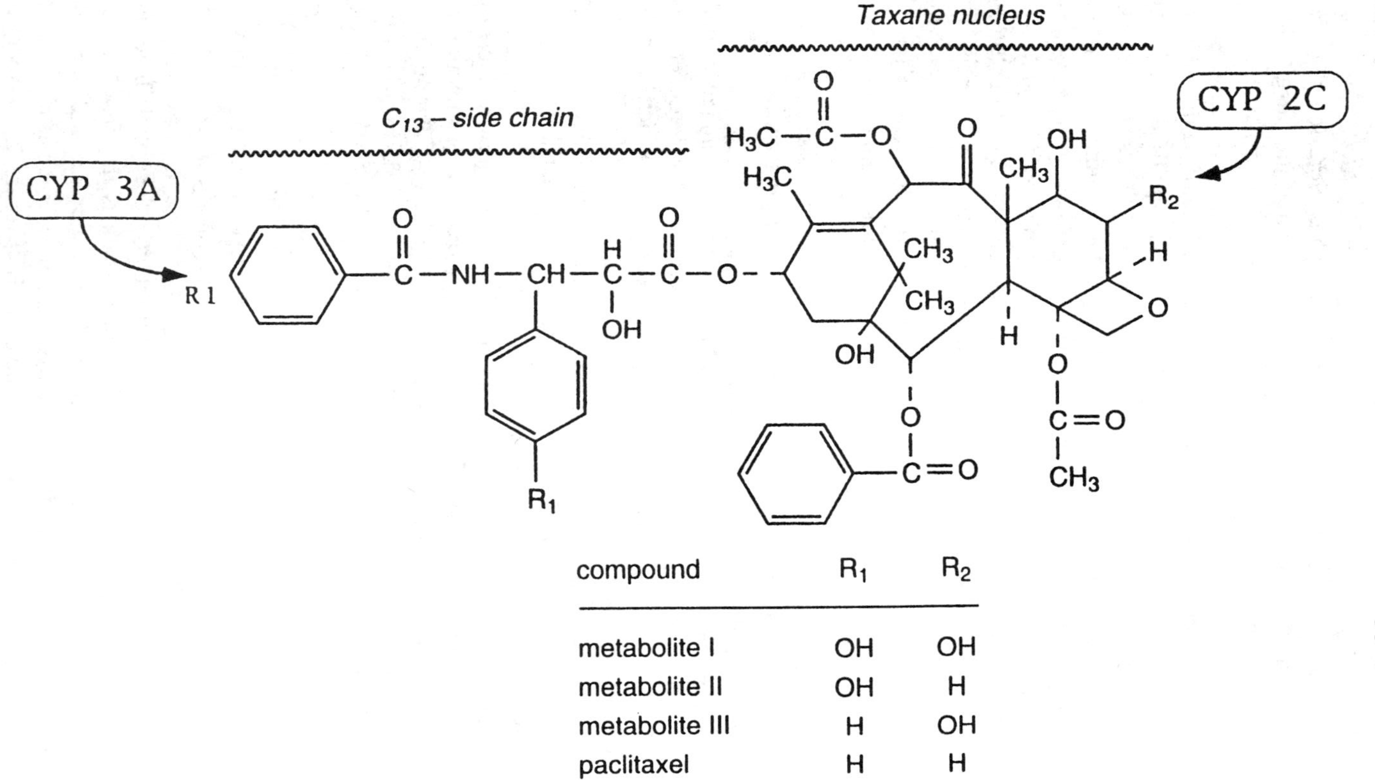

compound	R_1	R_2
metabolite I	OH	OH
metabolite II	OH	H
metabolite III	H	OH
paclitaxel	H	H

Fig. 54 Metabolic pathways of paclitaxel. The biotransformation to the corresponding hydroxy derivative is catalyzed by either Cyp 3A or Cyp 2C. (Modified from Ref. 54.)

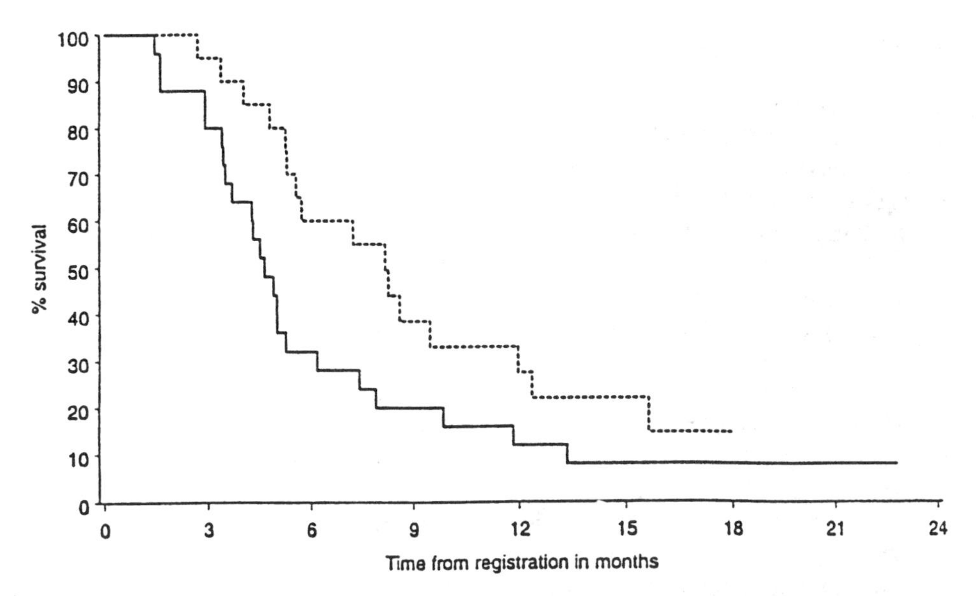

Fig. 55 There seems to be a correlation between the maintenance of defined paclitaxel plasma levels over time (e.g., at least 0.1 μM over 15 h) and improved survival in cancer patients with NSCLC. Solid line: paclitaxel, 0.1 TM <15 h; dashed line, paclitaxel 0.1 TM >15 h. (From Ref 45.)

with an increased risk for severe hypersensitivity reactions including edemas, bronchospasms, or hypotonia. As a consequence, the use of selected premedication regimens as prophylaxis are highly recommended before taxane infusions can be started. However, despite adequate prophylaxis a fluid retention syndrome, or painful onycholysis, can be induced by docetaxel and cardiotoxic side-effects can be induced by paclitaxel, respectively.

Several data indicate that schedule-dependent administration of taxoids with other anticancer drugs may be very important in clinical oncology to achieve synergistic effects or to avoid antagonistic antitumoral effects [21–25]. For example, it has been recommended that anthracyclines be administered before paclitaxel infusion because the other schedule (paclitaxel followed by epirubicin) may result in a higher incidence of severe mucositis [21]. In contrast, platinum compounds, particularly cisplatin, should be administered after paclitaxel has ended. There is evidence that giving platinum compounds before the taxoid derivative not only inhibits the metabolism of paclitaxel but also impairs the cytotoxic effect of the taxane as well, possibly by a platinum-mediated conformational change of binding sites for paclitaxel at the microtubular skeleton [22,24,25].

2.6.2.1 Paclitaxel

With the use of paclitaxel (Taxol), impressive response rates have been achieved in patients with breast, lung, esophageal, head and neck, bladder and ovarian cancer. The usually recommended doses range from 135 to 225 mg/m^2 IV every 3 weeks [26–35]. There is some controversy in regard to the optimal duration of paclitaxel infusion. Several data indicate that the 3-hour infusion of 175 mg/m^2 paclitaxel is safe and less myelosuppressive than the corresponding 24-hour infusion with no obvious compromise in response rate. Recent studies attempted the administration of paclitaxel by 1-hour infusion in an outpatient setting, which avoids the need for hospitalization. However, reducing the infusion duration from 3 hours to 1 hour seems to be accompanied by a significant shift toward neuromuscular toxicity, mainly in the form of peripheral sensorimotor neuropathy and myalgias [36,37].

High-dose paclitaxel, with doses up to 400 and 775 mg/m^2 in combination with other anticancer drugs, has been administered with autologous hematopoietic progenitor cell support in children and adult patients in phase I studies, respectively [38,39]. Intraperitoneal administration of paclitaxel (e.g., 175 mg/m^2 in 2000 mL of normal saline) may represent an encouraging novel application route in gynecologic oncology [40]. Physicochemical stability of such solutions are preserved for at least 24–72 hours [41].

After intravenous administration paclitaxel is widely distributed into body tissues. The volume of distribution (50–100 L/m^2) exceeds total body water despite high protein binding of the drug (93–98%) when the drug is given as a 3- or 6-hour infusion. Higher values (up to 650 L/m^2) are obtained when paclitaxel is administered as a 24-hour infusion. There is no linear correlation between dose intensification and the corresponding AUC values and peak levels. These data clearly indicate that there is a saturable tissue distribution as well as an oversaturation of cytochrome P450 isozymes (Table 24) [42–46].

Paclitaxel has only limited access to the CSF in patients with malignancies of the central nervous system; however, the detected low concentrations of 0.1–8.3% of the corresponding plasma concentrations may be high enough to interact synergistically with the cytotoxic effects of radiation [47]. For example, with concomitant radiotherapy only 45 mg/m^2 paclitaxel/week was administered together with carboplatin (100 mg/m^2/week) for regionally advanced squamous cell carcinoma of the head and neck and for regionally advanced non-small-cell lung cancer [48].

The half-life of unchanged paclitaxel is considered to be about 2.9 hours, whereas the half-life of all metabolites seems to be about 5.6 hours [46].

Table 24 Pharmacokinetic Summary of a Randomized Trial of Paclitaxel in Relapsed Ovarian Cancer: High-Dose Versus Low Dose and Long Versus Short Infusion

	Amsterdam			Milan		
Dose (mg/m^2) schedule (h)	Number of patients	c_{max} (ng/mL)	AUC	Number of patients	c_{max} (ng/mL)	AUC
175/24	4	365	7,993	4	420	7,734
175/3	5	3650	15,007	3	5202	15,048
135/24	2	195	6,300	4	265	5,641
135/3	7	2170	7,952	4	3071	8,604

(Adapted from Refs. 42–44.)

A dose of paclitaxel can be almost completely recovered in the urine and the feces within 36 hours. Renal excretion is of minor quantitative importance for the elimination of unchanged paclitaxel and its metabolites, because only 4.5% of the parent compound can be recovered in urine. Total urinary excretion is estimated to be about 14% of the dose. As a consequence, no dose modification appears to be necessary in the presence of renal dysfunction. In common, about 70% is eliminated via the feces, which indicates that metabolic and biliary clearance is of major quantitative importance [49–53].

Paclitaxel is extensively metabolized in the liver by cytochrome P450 2C8 and 3A4, which results in the formation of 6-α-hydroxypaclitaxel, the main metabolite making up 26% of the dose, and the hydroxyphenyl derivative, respectively (Fig. 54). Both metabolites are less cytotoxic than the parent compound [54].

If the liver enzymes approximate 2.5-fold of the upper limit of normal, it seems to be reasonable to recommend that a dose of 135 mg/m^2 not be exceeded.

Clinical Pharmacokinetics Regarding Efficacy and Toxicity

There are two important pharmacokinetic questions regarding the optimal dose and schedule of paclitaxel in clinical practice [55]:

1. Might therapeutic drug monitoring (TDM) help to reduce the incidence of adverse side effects, particularly myelosuppression and neurotoxicity, as well as mucositis?
2. Might TDM help to improve the therapeutic efficacy of paclitaxel?

Some pharmacokinetic data indicate that maintaining paclitaxel serum concentration above (0.05–)1 μM over several hours may increase the severity of myelosuppressive side effects. As a consequence, by reducing the infusion time, one can decrease the severity of any myelosuppression [42,44].

However, since a threshold paclitaxel level of 0.1 μM seems to be of clinical importance in regard to the persistence of microtubular damage in vitro, longer infusion times might be pharmacodynamically more advantageous in spite of a higher risk of myelosuppression. For example, if 135 mg/m^2 paclitaxel is given as a 3- or 24-hour infusion, as long as 28 and 12 hours will pass before the "critical" concentration of 0.1 μM is exceeded by the latter and the former, respectively.

Previous studies did not reveal a significant advantage for the 24-hour infusion compared to shorter infusion times with respect to the number of complete or partial remissions. Dose reductions and administration delays based on hematological toxicity associated with the 24-hour infusion were more frequent with the prolonged infusion schedule [44].

However, recent data of Huizing and colleagues brought new insights into this discussion, because these investigators demonstrated a correlation between the maintenance of defined paclitaxel levels (at least 0.1 μM over 15 h) in plasma and improved survival in patients with NSCLC (Fig. 55) [45].

There is some evidence that a correlation exists between higher AUC values and the onset of neurologic and musculoskeletal toxicity. For example, children with AUC values exceeding 54 and 71 μmol/L × h experienced significantly more neurotoxicity and myelotoxicity, respectively, than the others [39].

2.6.2.2 Docetaxel

Docetaxel (Taxotere) is a semisynthetic paclitaxel analogue (Fig. 55) based on 10-deacetylbaccatin-III, an inactive precursor isolated from the needles of the European yew tree, *Taxus baccata*. Like paclitaxel, the drug inhibits microtubule depolymerization by forming very stable microtubules.

The drug appears to be clinically effective against a variety of solid tumor types, including ovarian carcinoma, breast cancer, and NSCLC. The usually recommended dose ranges from 70–100 mg/m^2 IV every 3 weeks [56–58]. Recent data indicate that docetaxel is more potent than paclitaxel against some human tumor cell lines and that it may cause less cardiac and bone marrow toxicity.

Docetaxel is extensively metabolized via Cyp 3A, which results in at least four metabolites, M1–M4. In contrast to paclitaxel, cytochrome–P450-

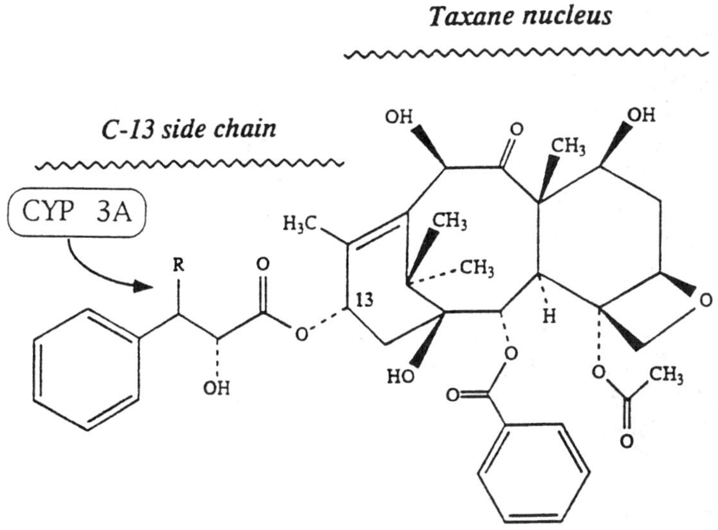

Taxane nucleus

C-13 side chain

CYP 3A

compound	R
docetaxel	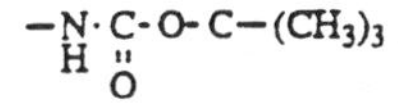 $-NH-C(=O)-O-C-(CH_3)_3$
metabolite M1 & M3	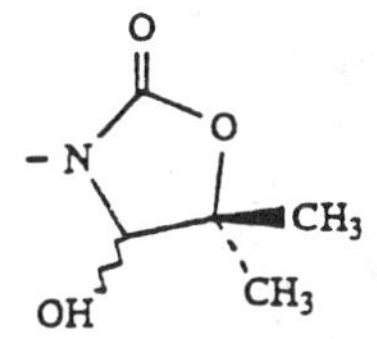
metabolite M2	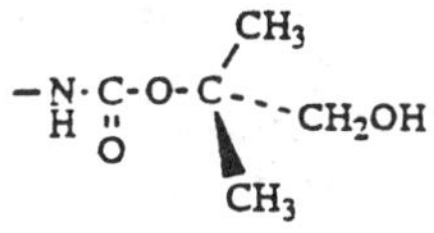 $-NH-C(=O)-O-C(CH_3)(CH_3)-CH_2OH$
metabolite M4	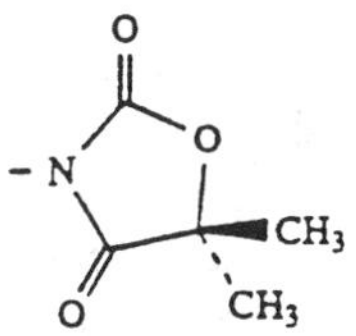

Fig. 56 Metabolic pathways of docetaxel. The corresponding hydroxy derivatives appear to be less cytotoxic than the parent compound. (Adapted from Ref. 51.)

mediated modifications are restricted to the C-13 side chain. Very probably the metabolites do not contribute significantly to the overall antineoplastic activity of the drug (Fig. 56) [59,60].

The initial, second, and terminal half-lives have been recorded to average 4 minutes, 36 minutes, and 11 hours, respectively. Only 5% of the administered dose is excreted in the urine within 24 hours, which indicates that dose modifications do not appear to be necessary in patients with renal insufficiency. However, because of the quantitative importance of the biliary clearance of the drug, limiting the dose of docetaxel to 75 mg/m^2 has been recommended if the aspartate aminotransferase or the alanine aminotransferase (ALT) exceeds 1.5-fold and the alkaline phosphatase exceeds 2.5-fold of upper normal values. If these values are even higher and the serum bilirubin is increased (e.g., >5 mg%), the use of docetaxel does not seem to be reasonable [61,62].

REFERENCES TO SECTION 2.6

1. Budman DR. New vinca alkaloids and related compounds. Semin Oncol 1992: 19:639–645.
2. Summerhayes M. Vindesine: Ten years in the pharmacy. Eur Hosp Pharm 1996: 2:214–221.
3. Van Tellingen O, Sips JHM, Beijnen JH, et al. Pharmacology, bio-analysis and pharmacokinetics of the vinca alkaloids and semi-synthetic derivatives. Anticancer Res 1992:12:1699–1716.
4. Zhou XJ, Rahmani R. Preclinical and clinical pharmacology of vinca alkaloids. Drugs 1992:44(suppl 4):1–16.
5. Toso C, Lindley C. Vinorelbine: A novel alkaloid. Am J Health-Syst Pharm 1995:52:1287–1304.
6. Binet S, Chaineau E, Fellous A, et al. Immunofluorescence study of the action of Navelbine, vincristine and vinblastine on mitotic and axonal microtubules. Int J Cancer 1990:46:262–266.
7. Rowinsky EK, Donehower RC, Jones RJ, et al. Microtubule changes and cytotoxicity in leukemic cells treated with TAXOL. Cancer Res 1988:48:4093–4100.
8. Haim N, Epelbaum R, Ben-Shahar M, et al. Full dose vincristine (without 2-mg dose limit) in the treatment of lymphomas. Cancer 1994:73:2515–2519.
9. McCune J, Lindley C. Appropriateness of maximum-dose guidelines for vincristine. Am J Health-Syst Pharm 1997:54:1755–1758.
10. Nelson RL, Dyke RW, Root MA. Comparative pharmacokinetics of vindesine, vincristine and vinblastine in patients with cancer. Cancer Treatment Rev 1980: 7(suppl):17–24.
11. Ramirez J, Ogan K, Ratain MJ. Determination of vinca alkaloids in human plasma by liquid chromatography/atmospheric pressure chemical ionization mass spectrometry. Cancer Chemother Pharmacol 1997:39:286–290.

12. Rahmani R, Guéritte F, Martin M, Just S, et al. Comparative pharmacokinetics of antitumor vinca alkaloids: Intravenous bolus injections of navelbine and related alkaloids to cancer patients and rats. Cancer Chemother Pharmacol 1986:16:223–228.
13. Jackson DV, Castle MC, Bender RA. Biliary excretion of vincristine. Clin Pharmacol Ther 1978:24:101–107.
14. van den Berg HW, Desai ZR, Wilson R, Bonner L. The pharmacokinetics of vincristine in man: Reduced drug clearance associated with raised serum alkaline phosphatase and dose-limited elimination. Cancer Chemother Pharmacol 1982:8:215–219.
15. Sehti VS, Thimmaiah KN. Structural studies on the degradation products of vincristine dihydrogen sulfate. Cancer Res 1985:45:5386–5389.
16. Zhou-Pan X-R, Sérée E, Zhou X-J, et al. Involvement of human liver cytochrome P450 3A4 in vinblastine metabolism: Drug interactions. Cancer Res 1993:53:5121–5126.
17. Zhou XJ, Bore P, Monjanel S, et al. Pharmacokinetics of Navelbine after oral administration in cancer patients. Cancer Chemother Pharmacol 1991:29:66–70.
18. Wargin WA, Sol Lucas V. The clinical pharmacokinetics of vinorelbine (Navelbine). Semin Oncol 1994:21(suppl 10):21–27.
19. Urein S, Bree F, Breillout F, et al. Vinorelbine high-affinity binding to human platelets and lymphocytes: Distribution in human blood. Cancer Chemother Pharmacol 1993:32:231–234.
20. Robieux I, Sorio R, Borsatti E, et al. Pharmacokinetics of vinorelbine in patients with liver metastases. Clin Pharmacol Ther 1996:59:32–40.
21. Akutsu M, Kano Y, Tsunoda S, et al. Schedule-dependent interaction between paclitaxel and doxorubicin in human cancer cell lines in vitro. Eur J Cancer 1995:31A:2341–2346.
22. Rowinsky EK, Gilbert MR, McGuire WP, et al. Sequences of taxol and cisplatin: A phase I and pharmacologic study. J Clin Oncol 1991:9:1692–1703.
23. Chou T-C, Otter GM, Sirotnak FM. Schedule-dependent synergism of taxol or Taxotere with edatrexate against human breast cancer cells in vitro. Cancer Chemother Pharmacol 1996:37:222–228.
24. Vanhoefer U, Harstrick A, Wilke H, Schleucher N, et al. Schedule-dependent antagonism of paclitaxel and cisplatin in human gastric and ovarian carcinoma cell lines in vitro. Eur J Cancer 1995:31A:92–97.
25. Jekunen AP, Christen RD, Shalinsky DR, Howell SB. Synergistic interaction between cisplatin and taxol in human ovarian carcinoma cells in vitro. Br J Cancer 1994:69:299–306.
26. Donehower RC, Rowinsky EK. An overview of experience with taxol (paclitaxel) in the U.S.A. Cancer Treatment Rev 1993:19(suppl C):63–78.
27. Krämer I, Heuser A. Paclitaxel—Pharmaceutical and pharmacological issues. Eur J Hosp Pharm 1995:1:37–42.
28. Kuhn JG. Pharmacology and pharmacokinetics of paclitaxel. Ann Pharmacother 1994:28:S15–S26.

29. Markman M. Paclitaxel in the management of ovarian cancer: What we know and what we have yet to learn. J Cancer Res Clin Oncol 1996:122:71–73.
30. Pazdur R, Kudelka AP, Kavanagh JJ, Cohen PR, Raber MN. The taxoids: Paclitaxel (taxol) and docetaxel (Taxotere). Cancer Treatment Rev 1993:19: 351–386.
31. Ravdin PM. Taxoids: Effective agents in anthracycline-resistant breast cancer. Semin Oncol 1995:22(suppl 13):29–34.
32. Bokemeyer C, Hartman JT, Kuczyk MA, et al. Recent strategies for the use of paclitaxel in the treatment of urological malignancies. World J Urol 1988:16: 155–162.
33. Runowicz CD, Wiernik PH, Einzig AI, Goldberg GL, Horwitz SB. Taxol in ovarian cancer. Cancer 1993:71:1591–1596.
34. Sledge GW, Robert N, Sparano JA, et al. Paclitaxel (taxol)/doxorubicin combinations in advanced breast cancer: The Eastern Cooperative Oncology Group Experience. Semin Oncol 1994:21(suppl 8):15–18.
35. Vermorken JB, ten Bokkel Huinink WW, Mandjes IAM, et al. High-dose paclitaxel with granulocyte colony stimulating factor in patients with advanced breast cancer refractory to anthracycline therapy: A European cancer center trial. Semin Oncol 1995:22(suppl 8):16–22.
36. Tsavaris N, Polzos A, Kosmas C, et al. A feasibility study of 1-h paclitaxel infusion in patients with solid tumors. Cancer Chemother Pharmacol 1997:40: 353–357.
37. Hainsworth JD, Thompson DS, Greco FA. Paclitaxel by 1-hour infusion: An active drug in metastatic non-small-cell-lung cancer. J Clin Oncol 1995:13: 1609–1614.
38. Stemmer SM, Cagnoni PJ, Shpall EJ, et al. High-dose paclitaxel, cyclophosphamide, and cisplatin with autologous hematopoietic progenitor-cell support: A phase I trial. J Clin Oncol 1996:14:1463–1472.
39. Sonnichsen DS, Hurwitz CA, Pratt CB, et al. Saturable pharmacokinetics and paclitaxel pharmacodynamics in children with solid tumors. J Clin Oncol 1994: 12:532–538.
40. Markman M, Rowinsky E, Hakes T, et al. Phase I trial of intraperitoneal taxol: A gynecologic oncology group study. J Clin Oncol 1992:10:1485–1491.
41. Xu Q, Trissel LA, Martinez JF. Stability of paclitaxel in 5% dextrose or 0.9% sodium chloride injection at 4, 22, or 32°C. Am J Hosp Pharm 1994:51:3058–3060.
42. Beijnen JH, Huizing MT, ten Bokkel Huinink WW, et al. Bioanalysis, pharmacokinetics and pharmacodynamics of the novel anticancer drug paclitaxel (taxol). Semin Oncol 1994:21(suppl 8):53–62.
43. Eisenhauer EA, ten Bokkel Huinink W, Swenerton KD, et al. European–Canadian randomized trial of paclitaxel in relapsed ovarian cancer: High-dose versus low-dose and long versus short infusions. J Clin Oncol 1994:12:2654–2666.
44. Gianni L, Kearns CM, Giani A, Capri G, et al. Nonlinear pharmacokinetics and metabolism of paclitaxel and its pharmacokinetic/pharmacodynamic relationships in humans. J Clin Oncol 1995:13:180–190.

45. Huizing MT, Giaccone G, van Warmerdam LJC, et al. Pharmacokinetics of paclitaxel and carboplatin in a dose-escalation and dose-sequencing study in patients with non-small-cell lung cancer. J Clin Oncol 1997:15:317–329.
46. Sonnichsen DS, Relling MV. Clinical pharmacokinetics of paclitaxel. Clin Pharmacokinet 1994:27(4):256–269.
47. Glantz MJ, Choy H, Kearns CM, Mills PC, et al. Paclitaxel disposition in plasma and central nervous systems of humans and rats with brain tumors. J Natl Cancer Inst 1995:87:1077–1081.
48. Aisner J, Belani CP, Kearns C, et al. Feasibility and pharmacokinetics of paclitaxel, carboplatin, and concurrent radiotherapy for regionally advanced squamous cell carcinoma of the head and neck and for regionally advanced non-small-cell lung cancer. Semin Oncol 1995:22(suppl 12):17–21.
49. Walle T, Walle UK, Kumar GN, Bhalla KN. Taxol metabolism and disposition in cancer patients. Drug Metab Dispos 1995:23:506–512.
50. Andreeva M, Niedmann PD, Binder L, et al. A simple and reliable reverse-phase high-performance liquid chromatographic procedure for determination of paclitaxel (taxol) in human serum. Ther Drug Monit 1997:19:327–332.
51. Sparreboom A, Huizing MT, Boesen JJB, et al. Isolation, purification, and biological activity of mono- and dihydroxylated paclitaxel metabolites from human feces. Cancer Chemother Pharmacol 1995:36:299–304.
52. Berg SL, Cowan KH, Balis FM, et al. Pharmacokinetics of Taxol and doxorubicin administered alone and in combination by continuous 72-hour infusion. J Natl Cancer Inst 1994:86:143–145.
53. Cresteil T, Monsarrat B, Alvinerie P, Treluyer JM, et al. Taxol metabolism by human liver microsomes: Identification of cytochrome P450 isozymes in its biotransformation. Cancer Res 1994:54:386–392.
54. Kumar G, Ray S, Walle T, et al. Comparative in vitro cytotoxic effects of taxol and its major human metabolite 6-α-hydroxypaclitaxel. Cancer Chemother Pharmacol 1995:36:129–135.
55. Kohn EC, Sarosy G, Bicher A, Link C, et al. Dose-intense Taxol: High response rate in patients with platinum-resistant recurrent ovarian cancer. J Natl Cancer Inst 1994:86:18–24.
56. Verweij J. Docetaxel (Taxotere): A new anticancer drug with promising potential? Br J Cancer 1994:70:183–184.
57. Verweij J, Clavel M, Chevalier B. Paclitaxel (taxol) and docetaxel (Taxotere): Not simply two of a kind. Ann Oncol 1994:5:495–505.
58. Piccart MJ, Gore M, ten Bokkel Huinink W, et al. Docetaxel: An active new drug for treatment of advanced epithelial ovarian cancer. J Natl Cancer Inst 1995:87:676–681.
59. Royer I, Monsarrat B, Sonnier M, Wright M, Cresteil T. Metabolism of docetaxel by human cytochrome P450: Interactions with paclitaxel and other antineoplastic drugs. Cancer Res 1996:56:58–65.
60. Sparreboom A, van Tellingen O, Scherrenburg EJ, et al. Isolation, purification and biological activity of major docetaxel metabolites from human feces. Drug Metab Dispos 1996:24:655–658.

61. Extra J-M, Rousseau F, Bruno R, et al. Phase I and pharmacokinetic study of Taxotere (RP 56976; NSC 628503) given as a short intravenous infusion. Cancer Res 1993:53:1037–1042.
62. van Oosterom AT, Schriivers D. Docetaxel (Taxotere), a review of preclinical and clinical experience. Part II: Clinical experience. Anticancer Drugs 1995:6: 356–368.

2.7 OTHER CYTOSTATIC DRUGS: ASPARAGINASE, HYDROXYCARBAMIDE, and *o,p′-DDD*

2.7.1 Asparaginase (ASNase) Preparations as Anticancer Drugs

After intravenous or intramuscular administration, the enzyme asparaginase (isolated from *Escherichia coli*) or the related compounds *Erwinia* asparaginase (erwinase) or pegaspargase, deplete the vascular system completely of asparagine and partially of glutamine. As a consequence, these drugs deprive special forms of leukemic cells of an amino acid that is essential to their survival (Fig. 57).

In the meantime, preparations containing L-asparaginase are part of most chemotherapy regimens for childhood and adult acute lymphatic leukemia (ALL). However, the three commercially available asparaginase preparations differ significantly with respect to their physicochemical characteristics as well as their pharmacokinetic behavior (Table 25). As a consequence, they are not easily interchangeable [1–6].

Liver dysfunction, including elevated liver enzymes, as well as blood coagulation disorders, pancreatitis, neurotoxicity, and allergic reactions, belong to the most prominent side effects related to the use of asparaginase preparations [3,6].

2.7.1.1 Asparaginase Preparations: A Comparison

From the several microbial sources, the bacterium *E. coli* was shown to be a very useful source for clinically active asparaginase (molecular weight 136 kDa). Of the many other species examined, the strain *Erwinia carotovora* (from the National Collection of Plant Pathogenic Bacteria) was selected for further studies (molecular weight 138 kDa). This strain was later reclassified as *Erwinia chrysanthemi*. Recently a novel analogue, pegaspargase, has been approved by the Food and Drug Administration. It resembles a modified form of the enzyme L-asparaginase (*E. coli*) because it is linked to conjugate units of monomethoxypolyethylene glycol (PEG).

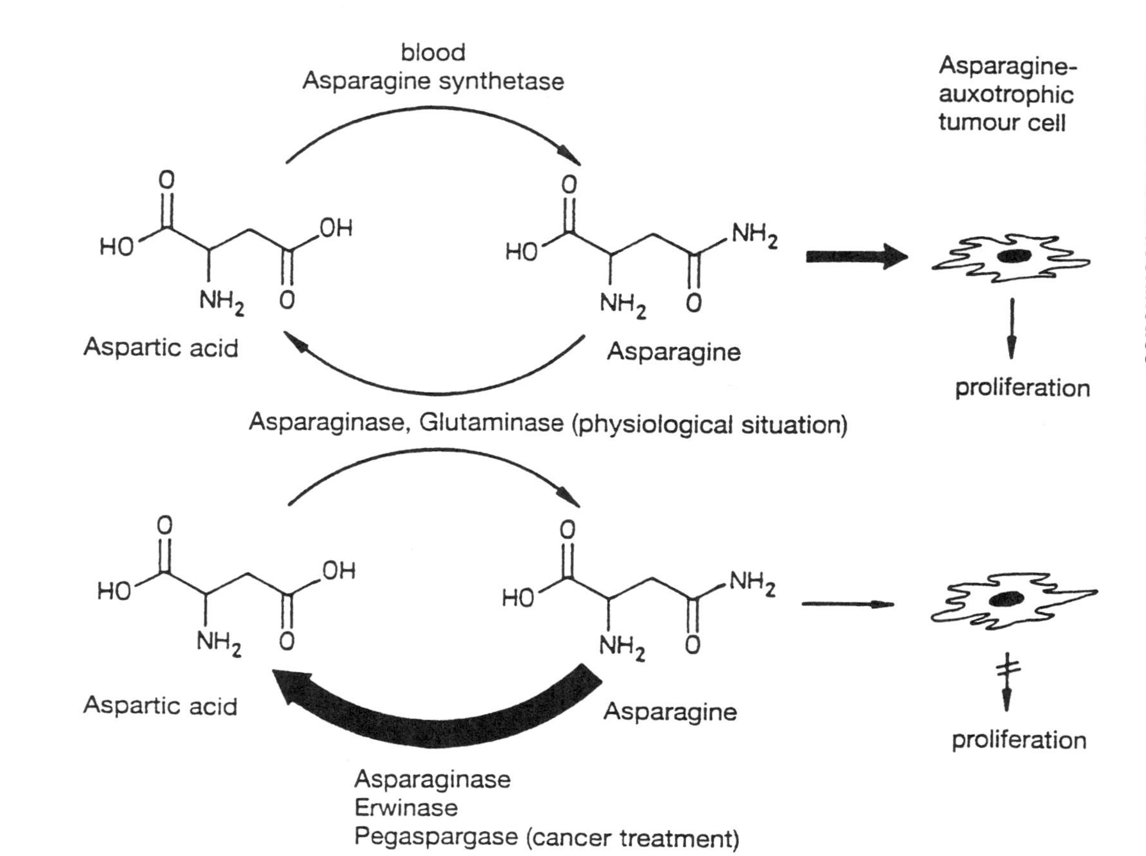

Fig. 57 Pharmacological action of L-asparaginase and the related compounds erwinase and pegaspargase.

Table 25 Pharmacokinetics of Pegaspargase and Asparaginase (*E. coli*, *E. chrysantheius*)

Drug	M weight (kDa)	Activity (IV/mg)[a]	$t_{1/2}$-β (h)	AUC (U/mL/d)	Clearance (mL/m^2/d)
Pegaspargase	141		357 ± 243	10.2	128 ± 74
Asparaginase (*E. chrysanthemi*)	138	350–700	10.5		
Asparaginase (*E. coli*)	136	225	20 ± 6 (8–30)	0.4 ± 0.1	2196 ± 1098

[a]The activity of asparaginase is expressed in international units (IU); 1 IU is the amount of drug required to catalyze the hydrolysis of 1 μmol of ammonia from asparagine in 1 minute under standardized conditions.

About one-quarter of the patients treated with one of these preparations may develop adverse immunological reactions. However, based on serological differences, one can switch over to another preparation to circumvent the increasing severity of allergic reactions [7,8].

The usually recommended doses of these preparations do not appear to be uniform. Usually 6000 IU/m^2 asparaginase (*E. coli* or *E. chrysanthemi*) are recommended for daily administration. However, based on the longer elimination half-life of *E. coli* ASNase (Table 25) it might be reasonable to administer this drug every other day (e.g., 5000 IU every other day for 2 weeks), in contrast to *Erwinia* ASNase (e.g., 5000 IU daily for 2 weeks) to avoid severe hepatotoxic effects that may be related to the extensive systemic aspargine and glutamine depletion [9]. Indeed, Boos et al. recently demonstrated that systemic depletion is quite different after asparaginase (*E. coli*) and after erwinase, lasting about 14 and 3–4 days, respectively (Fig. 58) [2]. Because of its extraordinarily long half-life, pegaspargase is usually administered every 14 days (2000–2500 IU/m^2) as a slow intramuscular injection or intravenous infusion [10]. Based on a pharmacoeconomic evaluation, it has been suggested that the use of pegaspargase may be associated with lower overall costs than ASNase (*E. coli*) because costs of visits to a physician's office, hospitalization fees, and administration and preparation fees may be significantly reduced when pegaspargase (Oncaspar) is used [11].

After intramuscular injection, the plasma concentrations average 10–50% of the corresponding values after IV infusion. Because of their high molecular weights, ASNase preparations cannot diffuse out of the capillaries. Thus, about 80% of the activity remains within the intravascular space. As a consequence, their corresponding distribution volume approximates the intravascular space (e.g., 2–2.3 L/m^2).

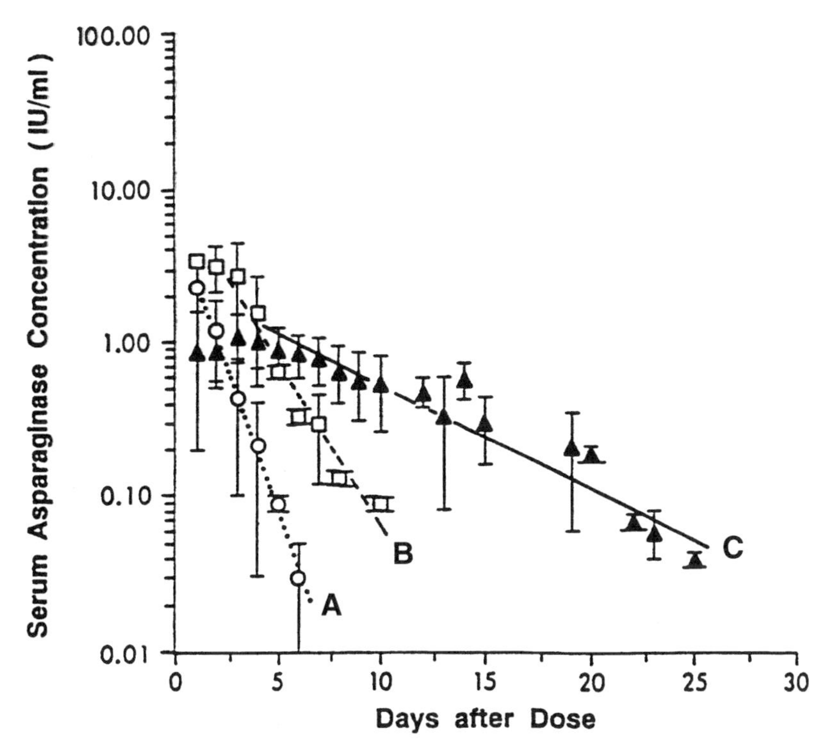

Fig. 58 Plasma decay curves of erwinase (A), L-asparaginase *E. coli* (B), and pegaspargase (C). Based on these pharmacokinetic data, the usually recommended doses are quite different. (After the clinical pharmacokinetic results of Asselin et al. [1].)

Only trace amounts of intact asparaginase (*E. coli*) are excreted in urine. Very few data exist regarding the metabolic fate of asparaginase. It has been postulated that the biological decomposition is primarily mediated by cells of the reticuloendothelial system (RES) [12]. This may explain the very long half-life of pegaspargase, which ranges from 63 to 600 hours, because this molecule may be highly resistant to RES-mediated degradation [3].

The penetration of L-asparaginase through the blood–brain barrier is poor. However, a significant decrease of asparagine and glutamine can be detected in the CSF after IV administration, which may be an indirect consequence of the systemic depletion of the amino acids asparagine and glutamine [13].

2.7.2 Hydroxyurea

Hydroxyurea (HU) (Fig. 59) is primarily used for the treatment of chronic myelogeneous leukemia (CML). The drug inhibits the enzyme ribonucleotide reductase, which leads to a decrease of deoxyribonucleotides in the tumor cells [14–16]. The underlying mechanism of cytotoxicity is not yet fully understood, but it may be based on electron transfer via radicals [17].

After oral administration (20–30 mg/kg/d PO) the drug is almost completely absorbed from the GI tract. Its elimination half-life ranges from 3.5 to 5 hours. HU, which is widely distributed, is able to pass the blood–brain barrier. About 30–60% of the dose is excreted in urine within 24–48, hours mainly as unchanged drug. As a consequence, a dose reduction seems to be reasonable in cancer patients with renal dysfunction. If the creatinine clearance approximates 30 mL/min, only 75% of the usual dose should be administered. In animals HU can be converted to hydroxylamine or urea, whereas this biotransformation pathway has not been proven in humans [15].

2.7.3 Mitotane (*o,p′-DDD*)

Mitotane has been used for the last three decades in the treatment of inoperable or metastatic adrenocortical carcinomas. These tumors are often endocrinologically active and may present as a Cushing-like syndrome. Usually standard oral doses of 2–6 g are given initially in divided doses, 3 to 4 times daily. The dose is commonly titrated upward to 9–10 g daily [18,19].

The exact mechanism of mitotane's antiproliferative action is not fully understood. Possibly it exerts a direct cytotoxic effect mediated through covalent binding of mitotane metabolites to mitochondrial proteins [20].

About 40% of the dose seems to be absorbed by the GI tract, the remaining 60% being excreted in the feces as unchanged drug. Concomitant intake of fat-containing food (e.g., milk) may increase the absolute bioavailability.

Mitotane is metabolized in the liver and other tissues principally to *o,p′*-dichlorodiphenylethene (*o,p′*-DDE) and the acetate derivative [*o,p′*-DDA = 1,1-(*o,p′*-dichlorodiphenyl) acetic acid] (Fig. 60). The elimination of the metabolites proceeds rather slowly, because within 24 hours only 10 and 15% of an oral dose of mitotane has been excreted in the urine and bile, respectively. Plasma elimination half-life has been reported to range from 18 to 159 days. After the discontinuation of therapy, unchanged drug and metabolites can be detected in plasma for as long as 8–18 months.

The drug should be given with caution to patients with liver disease, since their ability to metabolize mitotane may be impaired. However, concrete dosage schedules are not available [21–23].

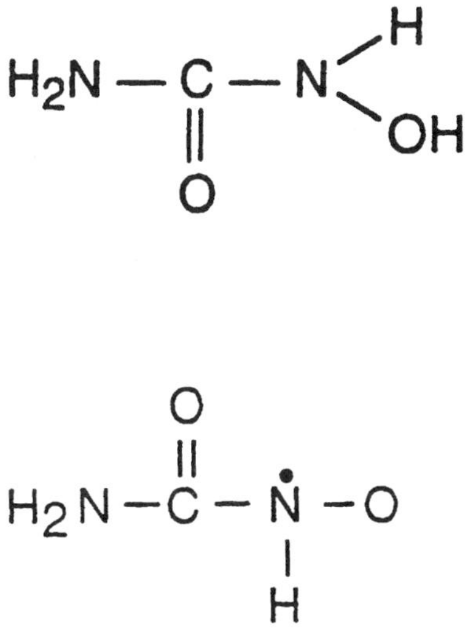

$H_2N-C(=O)-N(H)-OH$

$H_2N-C(=O)-\dot{N}(H)-O$

HU - Radical

Fig. 59 Radical formation may be involved in the cytotoxic mechanism of hydroxyurea (HU, hydroxycarbamide).

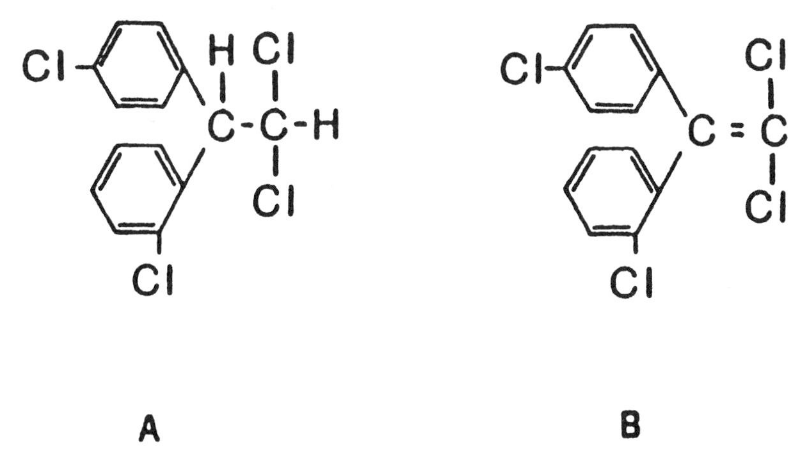

Fig. 60 Chemical structure of *o,p'*-DDD (A) and its major metabolite *o,p'*-DDE (B).

2.7.3.1 Clinical Pharmacokinetics Regarding Efficacy and Toxicity

Recently it has been suggested that therapeutic drug monitoring of *o,p′*-DDD levels might be feasible. There is some evidence that mitotane levels exceeding 14 μg/mL may have a significant and independently favorable influence on patient survival, whereas serum levels below 13 μg/mL may be associated with inadequate tumoricidal efficacy. However, if the values greatly exceed 20 μg/mL, the severity of side effects (e.g., progressive neurological toxicity) may limit compliance. DDE seems to be inactive or at least far less active than DDD; thus its measurement does not seem to be warranted [24].

REFERENCES TO SECTION 2.7

1. Asselin BL, Whitin JC, Cappola DJ, et al. Comparative pharmacokinetic studies of three asparaginase preparations. J Clin Oncol 1993:11:1780–1786.
2. Boos J, Werber G, Ahlke E, et al. Monitoring of asparaginase activity and asparagine levels in children on different asparaginase preparations. Eur J Cancer 1996:32A:1544–1550.
3. Holle LM. Pegaspargase: An alternative? Ann Pharmacother 1997:31:616–624.
4. Koerholz D, Brueck M, Nuernberger W, et al. Chemical and immunological characteristics of four different L-asparaginase preparations. Eur J Hematol 1989:42:417–424.
5. MacEwan E, Rosenthal R, Matus R, et al. A preliminary study on the evaluation of asparaginase. Cancer 1987:59:2011–2015.
6. Haskell CM, Canellos GP, Leventhal BG, et al. L-Asparaginase: Therapeutic and toxic effects in patients with neoplastic disease. N Engl J Med 1969:281: 1028–1034.
7. Ohnuma T, Holland JF, Meyer P. *Erwinia carotovora* asparaginase in patients with prior anaphylaxis to asparaginase from *E. coli*. Cancer 1976:38:1843–1846.
8. Land VJ, Sotow WW, Fernbach DJ, et al. Toxicity of L-asparaginase in children with advanced leukemia. Cancer 1972:40:339–347.
9. Durden DL, Salazar AM, Distasio JA. Kinetic analysis of hepatotoxicity associated with antineoplastic asparaginase. Cancer Res 1983:43:1602–1605.
10. Ettinger LJ, Kurtzberg J, Voute PA, et al. An open-label multicenter study of polyethylene glycol-L-asparaginase for the treatment of acute lymphoblastic leukemia. Cancer 1995:75:1176–1181.
11. Peters BG, Goeckner BJ, Ponzillo JJ, et al. Pegaspargase versus asparaginase in adult ALL: A pharmacoeconomic assessment. Formulary 1995:30(7):338–393.
12. Cooney DA, Capizzi RL, Handschuhmacher RE. Evaluation of L-asparaginase metabolism in animals and man. Cancer Res 1970:30:929–935.

13. Chabner BA, Loo TL. Enzyme therapy: L-Asparaginase. In: BA Chabner, DL Longo, eds. Cancer Chemotherapy and Biotherapy: Principles and Practice. Philadelphia: Lippincott-Raven, 1996, pp 485–492.
14. Hehlmann R, Anger B, Messerer D, Zankovich R, et al. Randomized study on the treatment of CML in chronic phase with busulfan versus hydroxyurea versus interferon alpha. Blut 1988:56:87.
15. Donehower RC. An overview of the clinical experience with hydroxyurea. Semin Oncol 1992:19(suppl 9):11–19.
16. Nocentini G. Ribonucleotide reductase inhibitors: New strategies for cancer chemotherapy. Crit Rev Oncol/Hematol 1996:22:89–126.
17. Reichard D, Ehrenberg A. Ribonucleotide reductase—A radical enzyme. Science 1983:221:514–519.
18. Boven E, Vermorken JB, van Slooten H, Pinedo HM. Complete response of metastasized adrenal cortical carcinoma with *o,p'*-DDD. Cancer 1984:53:26–29.
19. van Slooten H, Moolenaar AJ, van Seters AP, et al. The treatment of adrenocortical carcinoma with *o,p'*-DDD: Prognostic implications of serum level monitoring. Eur J Cancer Clin Oncol 1984:20:47–53.
20. Jönsson CJ, Lund BO. In vitro bioactivation of the environmental pollutant 3-methysulphonyl-2,2-bis(4-chlorophenyl)-1,1-dichloroethene in the human adrenal gland. Toxicol Lett 1994:71:169–175.
21. Benecke R, Keller E, Vetter B, de Zeeuw RA. Plasma level monitoring of mitotane (*o,p'*-DDD) and its metabolite (*o,p'*-DDE) during long-term treatment of Cushing's disease with low doses. Eur J Clin Pharmacol 1991:41:259–261.
22. Benecke R, Vetter B, de Zeeuw RA. Rapid micromethod for the analysis of mitotane and its metabolites in plasma by gas chromatography with electron capture detection. J Chromatogr 1987:417:287–294.
23. Moolenaar AJ, van Slooten H, van Seters AP, Smeenk D. Blood levels of *o,p'*-DDD following administration in various vehicles after a single dose and during long-term treatment. Cancer Chemother Pharmacol 1981:7:51–54.
24. Andersen A, Warren DJ, Nome O, et al. A HPLC method for measuring mitotane and its metabolite in plasma. Ther Drug Monit 1995:17:526–531.

II

TOXICITY OF CYTOSTATICS IN RAPIDLY PROLIFERATING NORMAL CELLS

3

Prophylaxis and Treatment of Neutropenia with Hematopoietic Growth Factors

HARTMUT LINK
Westpfalz-Klinikum Kaiserslautern, Kaiserslautern, Germany

3.1 INTRODUCTION

Granulocytopenia may be caused by primary or secondary bone marrow insufficiency. Since the process of granulopoiesis is very sensitive toward exogenous effects, it is conceivable that granulocytopenia results first, followed by lymphocytopenia, monocytopenia, anemia, or thrombocytopenia. The secondary granulocytopenias are caused by drugs, chemotherapy, radiotherapy, infections, or allergic reactions. Primary causes associated with affected hematopoietic stem or progenitor cells are aplastic anemia, myelodysplastic syndromes, osteomyelofibrosis, paroxysmal nocturnal hemoglobinuria, and some rare bone marrow disorders.

Granulocytopenia increases the risk of infections, when values below 500 neutrophils/μL are reached. Therefore intensive cytostatic chemotherapy can be given only when infections can be treated properly. If the incidence, severity, and duration of neutropenia following chemotherapy could be positively influenced, a major impact on morbidity and mortality should result.

3.1.1 Hematopoietic Growth Factors: Granulocyte Colony-Stimulating Factor (G-CSF) and Granulocyte–Macrophage Colony-Stimulating Factor (GM-CSF)

Since the detection of the colony-stimulating factors G-CSF and GM-CSF as hematopoietic growth factors and their availability by recombinant production technology, a new tool for clinical treatment has been developed [1].

G-CSF and GM-CSF reduce the duration of neutropenia in patients undergoing myelosuppressive chemotherapy for the treatment of malignancies. They effectively mobilize hematopoietic stem cells from the bone marrow into the peripheral blood.

3.1.2 Reasons for Using G-CSF and GM-CSF in Neutropenia

Neutropenia following cytotoxic chemotherapy is associated with a steadily increasing risk of severe infection [2]. Should an infection occur while the patient is neutropenic, there is a significantly increased risk of death if granulocytes fail to recover. In patients with documented bacteremia and a granulocyte count of below 1000/μL, mortality is 20.5%. However, if the granulocyte count increases after onset of the infection, the mortality rate drops to 7.0% ($p < 0.001$), as was shown in the first trial by the Paul Ehrlich Society for Chemotherapy of intervention in neutropenic patients with acute leukemia or malignant lymphoma following intensive chemotherapy [3]. It is assumed that use of G-CSF or GM-CSF would reduce the rate of infection following myelosuppressive chemotherapy by avoiding neutropenia or reducing its duration.

3.2 INDICATIONS FOR THE USE OF G-CSF AND GM-CSF

Indications for the use of growth factors can be set differentially according to the cause of neutropenia, as determined by the American Society of Oncology and in Germany by a group of experts [4–7].

3.2.1 Major Indication for Hematopoietic Growth Factors: Reduction of Morbidity and Mortality Due to Infections in Neutropenic Patients

The prophylactic use of G-CSF and GM-CSF to reduce chemotherapy-induced neutropenia is, without doubt, their most important indication. A generally accepted definition of tolerable neutropenia is 500 neutrophils/μL; however, an increased risk of infection is already apparent when the neutrophil count is between 500 and 1000/μL [2,8]. Individual risk factors have to be taken into consideration (Table 1) [9]. Both the severity and the duration of neutropenia depend on the underlying disease and the type of chemotherapy given, which is in turn based on the biology of the tumor in question. Experience gained with G-CSF or GM-CSF in a certain tumor type therefore cannot be generalized to other malignancies unless dose intensity and the underlying disease are comparable in both cases. Controlled clinical trials are desirable for each of the major tumor types and chemotherapy regimens.

One of the first multicenter, placebo-controlled randomized trials in G-CSF in 211 patients with small-cell lung cancer showed that the rate of infections can be reduced [10]. G-CSF (230 $\mu g/m^2$) was given daily subcutaneously for 14 days following cytotoxic chemotherapy with cyclophosphamide, doxorubicin, and etoposide. The rate of febrile neutropenia, defined as below 500 neutrophils/μL accompanied by fever of exceeding 38.1°C, was significantly reduced. This effect was most pronounced for the first cycle of chemotherapy, where the incidence of febrile neutropenia decreased from 57% to 28% ($p < 0.001$). Subsequent cycles showed a far less significant difference. The duration of febrile neutropenia was also substantially reduced with G-CSF. Similar reductions in the duration of neutropenia and the number of infections have been achieved with GM-CSF [11]. In an outpatient setting chemotherapy-induced neutropenia (i.e., <500/μL) was reduced from 4 days to 2 days, without relevant difference on the incidence of infectious complications or the need for hospitalization [12]. Another trial in children after intensive chemotherapy for acute lymphoblastic leukemia failed to significantly reduce the rate of hospitalization, increase the rate of event-free survival, or decrease the number of severe infections. However G-CSF significantly reduced the duration of hospitalization (from 10 days to 6 days) and halved the number of documented infections [13]. Therefore whether G-CSF should be given remains a matter of debate. If the argument is to reduce the duration of hospitalization and to improve the quality of life at no extra cost, growth factors should be given [13,14]. If the impact on leukemia-free survival is considered, the growth factors may not be useful [5,13].

In three randomized clinical trials CSFs were shown to reduce the incidence of febrile neutropenia by 50% in which the incidence of febrile neutropenia was greater than 40% [15]. Thus the primary use of CSFs should be restricted to those patients.

Table 1 Risk Factors for Febrile Neutropenia and Infection in Malignant Disease

	Impact on risk of infection	
Risk factor[a]	Low	High
Underlying illness	Solid tumor	Acute leukemia, high grade malignant lymphoma
Tumor burden	Small	Large, more advanced disease
Stage of disease	Primary treatment	Treatment of relapse
Age	<60 years	>60 years
Concurrent morbidity	Moderate	Pronounced
Performance status	Good	Poor
Treatment cycle	Subsequent cycle	First cycle
Treatment intervals	>4–5 weeks, and complete regeneration of hematopoiesis	<4 weeks
Cytotoxic dosage per cycle	Standard	High
Cytotoxic agent used	Mildly myelotoxic	Highly myelotoxic
Regimen	Monotherapy	Combination therapy
Mucous membrane toxicity	Low	High
Treatment aim	Palliative without prolongation of life	Cure, adjuvant, palliative with prolongation of life
Tissue infection	None	Active
Open wounds	None	Wound healing impairment
Individual factors:[a]		
Pharmacokinetics of cytotoxic agent		
Bone marrow reserve (e.g., in seminoma: higher toxicity)		
In- versus outpatient treatment		
Knowledge of treating physicians		
Further cellular immune defects (B and T cells)		
Prognosis		
Cumulative toxicity		
Concomitant therapy, etc.		

[a]In deciding whether treatment with G-CSF or GM-CSF is indicated, the cumulative effects of several risk factors should be considered.

3.2.2 Second Major Indication for G-CSF and GM-CSF

CSFs alleviate the mobilization of hematopoietic stem cells from the bone marrow into the peripheral blood, where they are collected by leukapheresis. Although not primarily intended, this strategy proved to be a very effective means of allogeneic and autologous stem cell harvest for transplantation [16,17].

3.2.3 Possible Indication for G-CSF and GM-CSF

3.2.3.1 Full-Dose Chemotherapy as Scheduled Through Reduction in Bone Marrow Toxicity

Standard cytotoxic chemotherapy consists of a combination of effective, non-cross-resistant agents at effective doses. Antitumor response can significantly decrease if the optimal effective dose is not given. In clinical practice, cycles of chemotherapy are often delayed or the dose has to be reduced to avoid the predominantly myelotoxic side effects of treatment. However, dose reduction often leads to only a small decrease in toxicity, but a significant drop in treatment success [18]. Dose modification may be avoided if hematopoiesis can be stimulated and the duration of neutropenia reduced by the use of growth factors [19–21]. This should in turn improve antitumor response [22]. To date, however, there are only little and not convincing data supporting this hypothesis, or in other words, G-CSF or GM-CSF do not seem to increase the antitumor effect of chemotherapy.

3.3 RECOMMENDED USAGE

Indications for G-CSF or GM-CSF can be classified into five categories (Table 2), depending on the strength of the case for their use. These indications are summarized in Table 3.

3.3.1 Prophylaxis of Chemotherapy-Induced Neutropenia

Patients can be subdivided according to the intensity of the cytotoxic chemotherapy regimen used.

3.3.1.1 Intensive Myelotoxic Chemotherapy

G-CSF or GM-CSF should be given following primary and intensive cytotoxic chemotherapy where neutropenia (<500 neutrophils/μL) is expected for at least 7 days. In those patients the risk of febrile neutropenia usually

Table 2 Indications for the Use of G-CSF or GM-CSF

Class	
I	Definite indication; generally accepted, judged of benefit and effective; use recommended
II	Acceptable indication; efficacy documented in several, but not all studies, therefore opinions differ
III	Possible indication; data indicate likely benefit and efficacy
IV	Not sufficiently documented; may be of benefit and is probably not disadvantageous
V	No indication, may be disadvantageous

exceeds 40%. This applies to highly malignant lymphomas [23,24], acute lymphoblastic leukemia [25–27], malignant myeloma, and small-cell lung cancer [10]. Only in the case of intensive therapy or reduced bone marrow reserve is this regimen used to treat testicular cancer, sarcoma, breast, bladder, and ovarian cancer [21,28].

3.3.1.2 Moderately Myelotoxic Chemotherapy

When moderate myelotoxic therapy is called for, current experience suggests that the relatively short duration of neutropenia (5–7 days) can be reduced by 2–3 days with the use of G-CSF or GM-CSF. It is uncertain whether this reduction is clinically relevant. However, the possibility of a reduced hospital stay has to be considered. In the best scenario, cytotoxic chemotherapy would be given on an outpatient basis, enabling better use of beds in hematological and oncological wards. If risk factors are present (Table 1), prophylactic use should be considered.

3.3.2 Secondary Prophylaxis Following Cytostatic Chemotherapy

The severity of chemotherapy-induced neutropenia can vary considerably depending on the factors listed in Table 1. If neutropenia (<500/μL) of less than 7 days duration is expected, prophylactic use of G-CSF or GM-CSF on the first cycle may not be appropriate. However, it can be started following the second cycle of chemotherapy if prolonged neutropenia occurred after the first cycle. This is particularly relevant for standard chemotherapy in the treatment of testicular, breast, ovarian, and bladder carcinoma as well

Table 3 Effect of the Prophylactic Use of G-CSF or GM-CSF on Infection in Chemotherapy in Various Trials

Class I: Recommended indication
- After myeloablative therapy and autologous or allogeneic bone marrow transplantation
- After myeloablative therapy and autologous or allogeneic peripheral blood progenitor cell transplantation
- Mobilization of hematopoietic progenitor cells from bone marrow in the peripheral blood (allogeneic and autologous transplantation)
- Severe chronic neutropenia (NP): idiopathic NP; congenital metabolic disorders with NP; with severe combined immunodeficiency; congenital or cyclic NP without chromosomal aberrations; NP in Gaucher disease

Class II: Acceptable indication
- Initial prophylaxis following intensive myelotoxic cytotoxic chemotherapy, expected duration of neutropenia (<500 neutrophils/μL) of at least 7 days, with risk of neutropenia >40%
- Aplastic anemia
- Acute agranulocytosis
- HIV infection: drug-induced neutropenia [e.g., zidovudine (AZT) or ganciclovir]

Class III: Possible indication
- Initial prophylaxis following moderately myelotoxic cytotoxic chemotherapy
- Expected duration of neutropenia (<500 neutrophils/μL) of at least 5–7 days and presence of risk factors (Table 1); expected risk of febrile neutropenia >40%
- Secondary prophylaxis following cytostatic chemotherapy if neutropenia (<500/μL) occurred for more than 5 days in the first cycle
- Treatment of chemotherapy-induced febrile neutropenia without and with microbiologically or clinically documented infections [be aware of acute respiratory distress syndrome (ARDS)]
- Neutropenia in Felty syndrome and T-γ-lymphoproliferative syndrome, hairy cell leukemia, autoimmune neutropenia
- Mobilization of granulocytes for transfusion

Class IV: Theoretically possible, but not yet sufficiently investigated indications
- Dose increase of cytotoxic chemotherapy without stem cell transplantation
- Prophylaxis of neutropenia during radiation therapy
- Chronic primary HIV-associated neutropenia
- Severe, nonneutropenic infection (e.g., in early stage or prophylaxis of sepsis)
- Severe infections in surgery; severe burns
- Stimulating myeloblasts prior to cytotoxic chemotherapy
- Premature infants with risk of sepsis
- Recurring infections in high-risk patients

Class V: No indication
- Generally if expected neutrophil count of >500/μL following chemotherapy
- GM-CSF in severe congenital or cyclic neutropenia
- Infections without neutropenia

as sarcoma. Nevertheless, it should be noted that neutropenia-associated morbidity is often highest following the first cycle of chemotherapy.

3.3.3 Treatment of Chemotherapy-Induced Febrile Neutropenia

A controlled study was designed to examine whether G-CSF can influence the duration of infection and neutropenia if it is not given until febrile neutropenia has occurred [29]. The duration of neutropenia (<500/μL) and febrile neutropenia were significantly reduced from a median of 4 days to 3 days and from 6 days to 4 days, respectively. These differences are of little clinical relevance. The benefit was more pronounced in patients with solid tumors (i.e., patients undergoing less aggressive treatment) than in patients with malignant lymphoma or acute lymphoblastic leukemia. A positive effect was more likely to be seen in microbiologically or clinically proven infections than in infections manifested only by fever. Furthermore, the effect was seen in patients with short neutropenia with a low risk of severe infections, and a more recent trial supported this observation [30]. If, however, one considers additional aspects, such as reduction of hospital stay and of antibiotic use, at least in pediatric patients, the effect of G-CSF may turn out to be positive [30].

3.3.4 Treatment of Neutropenia in Radiation Therapy

Severe neutropenia can occur following combination of radiotherapy/chemotherapy, and in cases of bone marrow insufficiency due to malignant marrow infiltration. In these cases the use of hematopoietic growth factors can increase the toxicity. Possible side effects such as thrombocytopenia and dyspnea must be considered if G-CSF or GM-CSF is used at the same time as mediastinal radiation. Simultaneous treatment with radiation, chemotherapy, and cytokines is not recommended.

3.3.5 Aplastic Anemia

In aplastic anemia the bone marrow is hypoplastic and there is a deficiency of hematopoietic progenitor cells. Several studies have shown that G-CSF or GM-CSF raises granulocyte counts in cases of moderately severe aplastic anemia [31–33]. However, this effect is only temporary. No effect is to be expected in cases of severe neutropenia [34]. Nevertheless, there are reports that G-CSF or GM-CSF can stimulate granulopoiesis and, possibly also development of other cell lines, following standard immunosuppressive therapy with cyclosporin A, antilymphocyte globulin, and prednisolone [35,36].

G-CSF and GM-CSF can, at present, be recommended as possible treatment options prior to allogeneic bone marrow transplantation of immunosuppressive treatment. They should be given prophylactically to raise granulocyte counts only when granulocytes are below 500/μL.

3.3.6 Acute Agranulocytosis

When there is a deficit or absence of granulocyte precursors in the bone marrow, severe cases of acute agranulocytosis and neutropenia following chemotherapy can lead to severe and life-threatening infections. This situation calls for treatment with G-CSF or GM-CSF [37–39].

3.3.7 Myeloid Malignancies

G-CSF and GM-CSF are myeloid growth factors that act through corresponding receptors. Malignant myeloid cells in acute myeloid leukemia (AML), chronic myeloid leukemia (CML), and myelodysplastic syndrome also contain these receptors. These cells proliferate in vitro when they are incubated with G-CSF and GM-CSF [40] and also may be stimulated to differentiate. Because of this, G-CSF and GM-CSF can be used to achieve differentiation of blasts or to sensitize blasts to chemotherapy by stimulating the cell cycle [41]. However, uncontrolled stimulation of malignant blasts is a possible adverse effect and must be considered.

3.3.7.1 Acute Myeloid Leukemia

Several clinical trials have shown that G-CSF or GM-CSF can be used in vivo in the treatment of AML without an increased risk of blast stimulation [41–45]. To date there is no convincing evidence of clinical advantage in mobilizing blasts with GM-CSF prior to cytotoxic chemotherapy. However, G-CSF can significantly reduce the rate of severe infections following AML therapy [46]. In 55- to 70-year-old patients with AML, the rate of severe infections was significantly reduced following use of GM-CSF. The remissions increased and median survival time was lengthened [47]. Following allogeneic transplantation, certain relapsed AML patients have achieved remission through treatment with G-CSF alone [48].

The use of G-CSF or GM-CSF has no negative influence on the course of the disease, as has been shown by several prospective randomized trials. In two trials with G-CSF [49,50] and one with GM-CSF the prognosis of AML-patients was improved [51]. The majority of trials, however, did not positively influence the course of the disease [44,45,52,53]. In summary G-CSF or GM-CSF can be given safely in AML.

3.3.7.2 Chronic Myeloid Leukemia

Chronic myeloid leukemia (CML) is a malignant disease, characterized by a cell clone carrying the typical reciprocal translocation between chromosomes 9 and 22, the "Philadelphia chromosome." This cell clone can be minimized with myelosuppressive chemotherapy. G-CSF given during neutropenia after chemotherapy can mobilize hematopoietic stem cells, which are Philadelphia chromosome negative. Those cells can be harvested by leukapheresis and used for autologous transplantation following myeloablative chemotherapy [54–56].

3.3.7.3. Myelodysplastic Syndrome (MDS)

Clinical trials in MDS have shown that, in 90% of cases, neutrophil granulocytes increase following G-CSF or GM-CSF administration [57]. Myeloid blasts, however, also increase in 10 to 25% of patients [58,59]. Early mortality due to neutropenia following aggressive chemotherapy can be avoided through the prophylactic use of G-CSF [60].

3.3.8 Neutropenia in HIV-Infected Patients

Neutropenia is a common hematological problem in the care of HIV-infected patients. Several causes of neutropenia must be differentiated.

Clinical observations have shown that T-cell depletion is still dominant even in cases of pronounced neutropenia. Neutropenia in HIV-infected patients can be easily rectified with the use of G-CSF or GM-CSF; however there have been no controlled trials in relation to relevant parameters such as fever, incidence of infections, and survival.

Neither have there been controlled trials with clinical end points to verify whether the (continuous) application of growth factors causes the progression of either HIV infection itself or its complications (such as cytomegalovirus infection). Available in vitro data, and trials in treated patients that have looked at HIV replication, show that GM-CSF can lead to an increase in the p24 antigen titers [61,62]. This effect, however, has not been seen with concurrent AZT therapy [63–65]. GM-CSF should therefore be used concurrently only with AZT.

3.3.8.1 Chronic Neutropenia Linked Primarily to HIV

Chronic neutropenia linked to HIV is generally not a valid indication for treatment with G-CSF or GM-CSF. Long-term use of GM-CSF, in particular, is not to be recommended given the possible effects on HIV replication. Furthermore, there is a lack of clinical trials (as opposed to in vivo experiments) showing the clinical relevance of such treatments.

3.3.8.2 Neutropenia as a Result of Opportunistic Infections such as Cytomegalovirus (CMV), Disseminated Mycobacteriosis or Malignancies Affecting Bone Marrow

Neutropenia caused directly by opportunistic infections might also be treated with G-CSF or GM-CSF. To date, however, no relevant studies have been published.

3.3.8.3 Drug-Induced Neutropenia Following Treatment (e.g., with AZT or Ganciclovir)

If neutropenia occurs following treatment with AZT, the patient should above all be switched to a different dideoxynucleoside analogue (e.g., DDI or DDC). The same applies with ganciclovir therapy for (recurring) CMV infection, relapse, or prophylaxis. If foscarnet intolerance (renal insufficiency) makes such a change impossible, treatment with G-CSF is recommended.

3.3.8.4 Neutropenia as a Result of Treatment of HIV-Associated Tumors with Polychemotherapy, Radiation, and Interferon

Neutropenia occurring during the cytotoxic treatment of HIV-associated tumors can justifiably be treated with G-CSF, as is the case with chemotherapy for other malignant illnesses. Generally both Kaposi sarcoma and malignant lymphomas should be treated within the confines of a clinical trial that also investigates the use of hematopoietic growth factors.

3.3.9 Increasing Dose Intensity of Chemotherapy

In many malignant illnesses, such as malignant lymphoma, acute leukemia, and testicular, breast, ovarian, and small-cell lung cancer, a dose–response relationship has been observed between cytotoxic drugs and their effect on target cells [66,67]. Chemotherapy aims to utilize this effect and eliminate tumor cells as completely as possible. However, the dose of cytotoxic drugs is often limited by bone marrow insufficiency. By administering G-CSF or GM-CSF following chemotherapy, one can often reduce the duration of neutropenia to tolerable lengths despite increased doses of chemotherapy [68–70]. Improved response and cure rates might then possibly be achieved in some malignancies [71]. This applies particularly in the case of chemosensitive tumors, especially in primary therapy and with minimal residual disease. However, increased chemotherapeutic doses lead to higher toxicity for other organ systems, notably thrombocytopoiesis, erythropoiesis, the immune system, the mucous membranes of the oropharynx and gastrointestinal tract, skin, liver, lungs, kidneys, and heart [70]. This toxicity is not decreased through the use of G-CSF or GM-CSF. The concept of intensified conventional cytotoxic chemotherapy without stem cell replacement should therefore be investigated only by experienced hematologists and oncologists within the confines of carefully planned trials [72].

3.3.10 Hematopoietic Stem Cell Transplantation Following High-Dose Myeloablative Therapy

In contrast to intensification of conventional cytotoxic therapy, high-dose myeloablative therapy is myelotoxic to the extent that without bone marrow stem cell transplantation, hematopoietic regeneration would be unlikely or excessively delayed; that is, this therapy is "myeloablative." In addition to myeloablation, there is usually pronounced systemic toxicity. The therapy can be carried out only if autologous stem cells responsible for hematopoiesis (taken from either the bone marrow or blood) are available to regenerate hematopoiesis and the immune system [54]. If allogeneic stem cells are being transplanted, ablation of the marrow also requires that the immune system of the recipient be suppressed, to avoid rejection of the transplanted cells and to encourage their engraftment (conditioning).

3.3.10.1 Allogeneic Bone Marrow or Blood Progenitor Cell Transplantation

Mortality in the first 100 days posttransplantation is 5–20% and depends on the patient's age, stage of disease, and type of conditioning. Early morbidity and mortality relate to complications in the 2- to 4-week period of pancytopenia following transplantation. The question of whether G-CSF and GM-CSF could stimulate hematopoietic regeneration was therefore one of the earliest investigations in bone marrow transplantation (BMT).

G-CSF

Following allogeneic BMT, G-CSF significantly reduces the duration of neutropenia (<500/μL) from 19–21 days to 15–16 days [73–75]. The incidence of acute graft-versus-host disease is not affected; the rate of chronic graft-versus-host disease, however, is reduced [76].

GM-CSF

Reduced duration of neutropenia and number of infections has been reported in only a few studies with GM-CSF. However, in certain studies GM-CSF was administered for only 14 days (i.e., probably for too brief a period of time) [77–79]. Graft-versus-host disease did not appear to be influenced. The theoretically favorable effect on thrombo- and erythrocytopoiesis was not observed. Possible side effects (fever, capillary-leak syndrome) can hinder the process of diagnosing sepsis and graft-versus-host disease.

3.3.10.2 Autologous Bone Marrow Transplantation

Following high-dose myeloablative therapy and autologous BMT, hematopoiesis recurs after 2–4 weeks. The period of pancytopenia is characterized by a high incidence of fever, bacteremia, and fungal and other clinically documented infections. A small but insignificant percentage of patients die as a result. G-CSF and GM-CSF can significantly improve myelopoesis following autologous BMT.

G-CSF

G-CSF reduces the duration of neutropenia to below 14 days. The incidence of febrile neutropenia is not affected, but the number of days with fever and use of antibiotics are reduced [66,80–82]. A randomized study has confirmed these results [83]. Duration of stay in hospital was also significantly reduced [84].

GM-CSF

The biological effect of GM-CSF has been documented in several studies, including placebo-controlled clinical trials [85–87]. The duration of neutropenia is significantly reduced and the incidence of bacterial and documented infections fell in several studies.

3.3.10.3 Hematopoietic Progenitor Cells from Peripheral Blood

For several years, circulating hematopoietic stem and progenitor cells have been used as an alternative to autologous bone marrow cells following myeloablative therapy [88–92]. They have replaced autologous bone marrow transplantations in almost all indications. These cells are characterized by their growth pattern in bone marrow culture and by their expression of CD34 antigen. The use of G-CSF or GM-CSF produces a marked increase in myeloid and other progenitor cells circulating in blood [93–96], following their mobilization from bone marrow. This is best achieved in the regenerative phase following myelosuppressive therapy, but prior myelosuppression is not an absolute necessity [94,97–101]. Hematopoietic progenitor cells can be collected from the blood by leukapheresis and stored in liquid nitrogen. One to three cell separations yield sufficient progenitor cells ($2–4 \times 10^6$ CD34+ cells per kilogram of body weight) to achieve permanent hematopoietic regeneration, even following myeloablative therapy [102]. Peripheral blood progenitor cells (PBPC) also contain pluripotent hematopoietic stem cells [103]. Their use avoids the need for removal of bone marrow and thus the risks associated with general anesthesia. The danger of these progenitor cells being contaminated with malignant cells is probably lower than that incurred when bone marrow from affected patients is used. In addition, the number of progenitor cells can be increased through positive selection. This simultaneously leads to a decrease in unwanted cells [104–106].

After myeloablative therapy, G-CSF-mobilized PBPCs have been reinfused along with autologous bone marrow cells and followed by G-CSF treatment. The duration of neutropenia was 9 and 10 days with and without PBPC, respectively. The duration of thrombocytopenia (<50,000/μL) was 15 and 39 days, respectively ($p < 0.0005$) [107]. Similar results have also been seen with a combination of bone marrow, GM-CSF, and GM-CSF-mobilized PBPC [108,109]. In a prospective comparative trial, PBPC with G-CSF led to a more rapid regeneration of platelets and neutrophils [17]. In conclusion, G-CSF or GM-CSF can increase hematopoietic regeneration following PBPC transfusion [110].

Developments in both autologous and allogeneic stem cell transplantation are leading to greater use of PBPCs, since the collection procedure is technically easier and there is less risk than taking stem cells from the bone marrow. Furthermore, thrombocytopoiesis returns more quickly with PBPC than with use of bone marrow stem cells [111]. During the last few years allogeneic PBPC from HLA-identical sibling donors are increasingly being used in place of bone marrow cells [112]. It is less uncomfortable for the donor than bone marrow harvest.

The stem cells fully engraft and reconstitute hematopoiesis more rapidly than bone marrow cells [113]. If the large amount of T cells is not reduced in the graft, a high rate of chronic graft-versus-host disease occurs. It is not yet clear whether the T cells in the graft should be reduced or modified [113–117a].

3.3.10.4 Treatment of Transplant Failure Following Allogeneic and Autologous Bone Marrow Transplantation

GM-CSF

The effect of GM-CSF was investigated in 15 patients following allogeneic bone marrow transplantation, in 21 patients following autologous BMT, and in a single patient following syngenic BMT [118]. Bone marrow failure was defined as follows: <1000 neutrophils/μL 28 days post-BMT, or 21 days post-BMT in the case of life-threatening infection, or a renewed fall in neutrophils to below 500/μL after counts of more than 500/μL had already been achieved for one week. Within 2 weeks, 21 out of 37 patients had responded to GM-CSF treatment. After 100 days and 1 year, survival rates were 59 and 50%, respectively, compared to 32 and 23% in a series of 155 historic controls. Increases in thrombocytes or reticulocytes were not observed with GM-CSF treatment, but bone marrow cellularity increased in some patients. No increase in graft-versus-host disease was seen.

G-CSF

There have been no studies of the treatment of transplant failure with G-CSF. However, in view of its profile of action, a positive effect on granulopoiesis in pronounced neutropenia is to be expected.

3.3.11 Neutropenia in Felty Syndrome, T-γ-Lymphoproliferative Syndrome

Neutropenia in rheumatoid arthritis (Felty syndrome) leads to an increased risk of infection. This type of neutropenia can be successfully corrected in the short term and up to one year with G-CSF [119–121]. Neutropenia in the course of T-γ-lymphoproliferative syndrome can be treated with either G-CSF or GM-CSF [122]. Since, however, granulopoietic cells can influence pathogenesis, the use of myeloid or monocyte growth factors must be critically evaluated in cases of underlying rheumatoid illnesses.

3.3.12 Congenital, Cyclic, or Chronic Idiopathic Neutropenia

In chronic neutropenia, neutrophil counts drop below 2000/μL for long periods. In cases of severe neutropenia, counts drop below 500/μL and this diminution is accompanied by clinical complications, especially if counts fall below 100/μL. Patients with cyclic, congenital, or chronic idiopathic neutropenia produce insufficient neutrophils. These patients therefore suffer increasingly from inflammation and recurrent bacterial infections [123]. Continuous treatment with G-CSF or GM-CSF stimulates maturation of neutrophils and their production. Accordingly, there is a dramatic clinical improvement in these patients who are often chronically seriously ill [124–127]. Experience in the long-term use of G-CSF and evidence of its excellent tolerability have been gained in these patients. GM-CSF is biologically inappropriate for use in severe congenital neutropenia (Kostman syndrome) and in cyclic neutropenia, since it leads to stimulation of eosinophils and only a marginal rise in neutrophils [128,129]. Chronic autoimmune neutropenia can successfully be treated by G-CSF stimulated granulopoiesis [130,131].

3.3.13 Other Possible Indications

Illnesses leading to a decrease in neutrophils or monocytes or a functional disturbance of these cells can be treated with G-CSF or GM-CSF. These are often rare illnesses such as glycogen storage disease (type 1B) [132,133]. With the possibility of mobilizing large amounts of neutrophils in normal individuals, the interest in granulocyte transfusions for neutropenic infections has been revitalized [134–136]. Definite studies are warranted.

3.3.14 Possible Indications Not Sufficiently Investigated

The effects of G-CSF and GM-CSF could lead to further applications in patients who do not have neutropenia but are suffering from an inadequate rise in granulocytes following infection or from decreased granulocyte function, as in phagocytosis [137]. Possible applications include sepsis of the newborn [138,139], extensive burns [140,141], trauma [142,143], severe postsurgical infection [144,145], the early stages of sepsis [146,147], elderly patients with recurrent infections and inadequate endogenous G-CSF production [148], *Listeria* infection [149], and the prevention of infection in high-risk patients [150].

3.4 RECOMMENDED DOSAGE

Dosage recommendations as given by the drug manufacturers are usually acceptable. However, it is possible that sufficient stimulation of granulopoiesis can be achieved with lower doses. In the case of first-line chemotherapy, for optimal mobilization of hematopoietic stem cells into the blood may necessitate doses of G-CSF or GM-CSF higher than are needed to stimulate hematopoietic regeneration [107,151,152].

3.4.1 Starting Prophylactic Treatment Following Chemotherapy

In most of the reported trials of neutropenia prophylaxis, treatment with G-CSF/GM-CSF was started 24 hours after chemotherapy. According to present studies, similar therapeutic results can be achieved when administration begins on day 4 following chemotherapy, rather than day 1 [153–156]. Following autologous BMT, there are indications that G-CSF prophylaxis starting on days 6–8 posttransplantation will limit the duration of neutropenia ($<500/\mu L$) to 14 days [157,158].

3.5 RECOMMENDED TREATMENT DURATION

Following myelotoxic treatment, the use of G-CSF or GM-CSF to stimulate granulopoiesis can be discontinued if counts of at least 500 neutrophils/μL have been achieved on two consecutive days and in the absence of any severe infection. If the patient develops an infection, a neutrophil count of 1500/μL should be achieved before the growth factor is discontinued.

REFERENCES

1. Welte K, Gabrilove J, Bronchud MH, Platzer E, Morstyn G. Filgrastim (r-metHuG-CSF): The first 10 years. Blood 1996:88:1907.
2. Bodey GP, Buckley M, Sathe YS, Freireich EJ. Quantitative relationships between circulating leukocytes and infection in patients with acute leukemia. Ann Intern Med 1966:64:328.
3. Link H, Maschmeyer G, Meyer P, Hiddemann W, Stille W, Helmerking M, Adam D, for the Study Group of the Paul Ehrlich Society for Chemotherapy: Interventional antimicrobial therapy in febrile neutropenic patients. Ann Hematol 1994:69:231.
4. American Society of Clinical Oncology. American Society of Clinical Oncology recommendations for the use of hematopoietic colony-stimulating factors: Evidence-based, clinical practical guidelines. J Clin Oncol 1994:12: 2471.
5. Hoelzer D. Hematopoietic growth factors—Not whether, but when and where. N Engl J Med 1997:336:1822.
6. Link H, Herrmann F, Welte K, Aulitzky WE, Ganser A, Kern W, Meyer P, Schrappe M, Schmoll HJ, Werdan K, Kern P. Rationale Therapie mit G-CSF and GM-CSF. Med Klin 1994:89:429.
7. Yim JM, Matuszewski KA, Vermeulen LC, Ratko TA, Burnett DA, Vlasses PH. Surveillance of colony-stimulating factor use in U.S. academic health centers. Ann Pharmacother 1995:29:475–481.
8. Maschmeyer G, Link H, Hiddemann W, Meyer P, Helmerking M, Eisenmann E, Schmitt J, Adam D. Empirische antimikrobielle Therapie bei neutropenischen Patienten. Med Klin 1994:89:114.
9. Lyman GH, Lyman CG, Sanderson RA, Balducci L. Decision analysis of hematopoietic growth factor use in patients receiving cancer chemotherapy. J Natl Cancer Inst 1993:85:488.
10. Crawford J, Ozer H, Stoller R, Johnson D, Lyman G, Tabbara I, Kris M, Grous J, Picozzi V, Rausch G, Smith R, Gradishar W, Yahanda A, Vincent M, Stewart M, Glaspy J. Reduction by granulocyte colony-stimulating factor of fever and neutropenia induced by chemotherapy in patients with small cell lung cancer. N Engl J Med 1991:325:164.
11. Mayordomo JI, Rivera F, Diaz-Puente MT, Lianes MP, López-Brea M, López E, Paz-Ares L, Hitt R, Alonso S, Sevilla I, Rivas I, Cortés-Funes H.

Decreasing morbidity and cost of treating febrile neutropenia by adding G-CSF and GM-CSF to standard antibiotic therapy: Results of a randomized trial. Proceedings of the American Society of Clinical Oncology, 1993, vol 12, p 437.

12. Hartmann LC, Tschetter LK, Habermann TM, Ebbert LP, Johnson PS, Mailliard JA, Levitt R, Suman VJ, Witzig TE, Wieand HS, Miller LL, Moertel CG. Granulocyte colony-stimulating factor in severe chemotherapy-induced afebrile neutropenia. N Engl J Med 1997:336:1776.
13. Pui CH, Boyett JM, Hughes WT, Rivera GK, Hancock ML, Sandlund JT, Synold T, Relling MV, Ribeiro RC, Crist WM, Evans WE. Human granulocyte colony-stimulating factor after induction chemotherapy in children with acute lymphoblastic leukemia [see comments]. N Engl J Med 1997: 336:1781.
14. Gupta P. Granulocyte colony-stimulating factor in children with acute lymphoblastic leukemia [letter]. N Engl J Med 1997:337:1320.
15. Anonymous. Update of recommendations for the use of hematopoietic colony stimulating factors: Evidence-based clinical practical guidelines. J Clin Oncol 1996:14:1957.
16. Link H, Arseniev L, Bähre O, Kadar JG, Bernson RJ, Battmer K, Kühl J, Jacobs R, Schubert J, Casper J, Diedrich H. Transplantation of allogeneic peripheral blood and bone marrow CD34+ cells after immunoselection. Exp Hematol 1995:23:855.
17. Schmitz N, Linch DC, Dreger P, Goldstone AH, Boogaerts MA, Ferrant A, Demuynck HMS, Link H, Zander A, Barge A, Borkett KM. Randomized trial of filgrastim-mobilized peripheral blood progenitor cell transplantation versus autologous bone-marrow transplantation in lymphoma patients. Lancet 1996:347:353.
18. Devita VT. Cancer Principles and Practice of Oncology. Philadelphia: Lippincott, 1989.
19. Aglietta M, Monzeglio C, Pasquino P, Carnino F, Stern AC, Gavosto F. Short-term administration of granulocyte–macrophage colony stimulating factor decreases hematopoietic toxicity of cytostatic drugs. Cancer 1993:72: 2970.
20. Jost LM, Pichert G, Stahel RA. Placebo controlled phase I/II study of subcutaneous GM-CSF in patients with germ cell tumors undergoing chemotherapy. Ann Oncol 1990:1:439.
21. Gianni AM, Bregni M, Siena S, Orazi A, Stern AC, Gandola L, Bonadonna G. Recombinant human granulocyte–macrophage colony-stimulating factor reduces hematologic toxicity and widens clinical applicability of high-dose cyclophosphamide treatment in breast cancer and non-Hodgkin's lymphoma [see comments]. J Clin Oncol 1990:8:768.
22. Wolf M, Havermann K. Experience with GM-CSF in the treatment of solid tumors. Infection 1992:20(suppl 2):S111.
23. Hovgaard DJ, Nissen NI. Effect of recombinant human granulocyte–macrophage colony-stimulating factor in patients with Hodgkin's disease: A phase I/II study. J Clin Oncol 1992:10:390.

24. Steinke B, Manegold C, Freund M, Reinold H-M, Fischer JT, Arnold H, Lengfelder E, Lutz M, Zwingers T, Münz A, Hecht T. G-CSF for treatment intensification in high-grade malignant non-Hodgkin's lymphomas. Onkologie 1992:15:46.
25. Hoelzer D, Ottmann O. G-CSF in acute lymphoblastic leukemia. Ann Hermatol 1993:66(suppl II):A81 (Abstr).
26. Kantarjian HM, Talpaz M, Kontoyiannis D, Gutterman J, Keating MJ, Estey EH, O'Brien S, Rios MB, Beran M, Deisseroth A. Treatment of chronic myelogenous leukemia in accelerated and blastic phases with daunorubicin, high-dose cytarabine, and granulocyte-macrophage colony-stimulating factor. J Clin Oncol 1992:10:398.
27. Scherrer R, Geissler K, Kyrle PA, Gisslinger H, Jäger U, Bettelheim P, Laczika K, Locker G, Scholten C, Sillaber C, Schwarzinger I, Thalhammer F, Lechner K. Granulocyte colony-stimulating factor (G-CSF) as an adjunct to induction chemotherapy of adult acute lymphoblastic leukemia (ALL). Ann Hematol 1993:66:283.
28. de Vries EG, Biesma B, Willemse PH, Mulder NH, Stern AC, Aalders JG, Vellenga E. A double-blind placebo-controlled study with granulocyte–macrophage colony-stimulating factor during chemotherapy for ovarian carcinoma. Cancer Res 1991:51:116.
29. Maher DW, Lieschke GJ, Green M, Bishop J, Stuart Harris R, Wolf M, Sheridan WP, Kefford RF, Cebon J, Olver I, et al. Filgrastim in patients with chemotherapy-induced febrile neutropenia. A double-blind, placebo-controlled trial. Ann Intern Med 1994:121:492.
30. Mitchell PL, Morland B, Stevens MC, Dick G, Easlea D, Meyer LC, Pinkerton CR. Granulocyte colony-stimulating factor in established febrile neutropenia: A randomized study of pediatric patients. J Clin Oncol 1997:15: 1163.
31. Antin JH, Smith BR, Holmes W, Rosenthal DS. Phase I/II study of recombinant human granulocyte-macrophage colony stimulating factor in aplastic anemia and myelodysplastic syndrome. Blood 1988:72:705.
32. Shimosaka A. Treatment of aplastic anemia patients with granulocyte colony-stimulating factor, filgrastim: An overview of Japanese experiences. Ann Hematol 1993:66(suppl II):A81 (Abstr).
33. Vadhan-Raj S, Buescher S, Broxmeyer HE, LeMaistre A, Lepe-Zuniga JL, Ventura G, Jeha S, Horwitz LJ, Trujillo JM, Gillis S, Hittelman WN, Gutterman JU. Stimulation of myelopoiesis in patients with aplastic anemia by recombinant human granulocyte–macrophage colony-stimulating factor. N Engl J Med 1988:319:1628.
34. Nissen C, Tichelli A, Gratwohl A, Speck B, Milne A, Gordon-Smith EC, Schaedelin J. Failure of recombinant human granulocyte–macrophage colony stimulating factor therapy in aplastic anemia patients with severe neutropenia. Blood 1988:72:2045.
35. Gordon Smith EC, Yandle A, Milne A, Speck B, Maramont A, Willemze R, Kolb H. Randomised placebo controlled study of RH-GM-CSF following

ALG in the treatment of aplastic anemia. Bone Marrow Transplant 1991: 7(suppl 2):78.
36. Yver A, Tchernia G, Esperou-Bourdeau H, Bertrand Y, Gratwohl A, Gluckman E. rHuG-CSF induced granulopoietic recovery in refractory severe aplastic anemia may be associated with other lineages' recovery. Blood 1991: 78(suppl 1):4a (Abstr).
37. Patton WN, Holyoake TL, Yates JM, Boughton BJ, Franklin IM. Accelerated recovery from drug-induced agranulocytosis following G-CSF therapy. Br J Haematol 1992:80:564.
38. Teitelbaum AH, Bell AJ, Brown SL. Filgrastim (r-metHuG-CSF) reversal of drug-induced agranulocytosis. Am J Med 1993:95:245.
39. Weide R, Koppler H, Heymanns J, Pfluger KH, Havermann K. Successful treatment of clozapine induced agranulocytosis with granulocyte-colony stimulating factor (G-CSF). Br J Haematol 1992:80:557.
40. Löwenberg B, Touw P. Hematopoietic growth factors and their receptors in acute leukemia. Blood 1993:81:281.
41. Bettelheim P, Valent P, Andreef M, Tafuri A, Haimi J, Gorischek C, Muhm M, Sillaber C, Haas O, Vieder L, Maurer D, Schulz G, Speiser W, Geissler K, Kier P, Hinterberger W, Lesche K. Recombinant human macrophage colony-stimulating factor in combination with standard induction chemotherapy in de novo acute myeloid leukemia. Blood 1991:77:700.
42. Büchner T, Hiddemann W, Koenigsmann M, Zuhlsdorf M, Wormann B, Boeckmann A, Freire EA, Innig G, Maschmeyer G, Ludwig WD, et al. Recombinant human granulocyte–macrophage colony-stimulating factor after chemotherapy in patients with acute myeloid leukemia at higher age or after relapse. Blood 1991:78:1190.
43. Estey E, Thall P, Kantarjian H, O'Brien S, Koller C, Freireich E, Keating M. Treatment of newly-diagnosed AML with GM-CSF prior to and during chemotherapy: Comparison to chemotherapy without GM-CSF. Blood 1991: 78(suppl 1):171a (Abstr).
44. Ohno R, Hiraoka A, Tanimoto M, Asou N, Kuriyama K, Kobayashi T, Yoshida M, Teshima H, Saito H, Fujimoto K. No increase of leukemia relapse in newly diagnosed patients with acute myeloid leukemia who received granulocyte colony-stimulating factor for life-threatening infection during remission induction and consolidation therapy. Blood 1993:81:561.
45. Ohno R, Naoe T, Kanamaru A, Yoshida M, Hiraoka A, Kobayashi T, Ueda T, Minami S, Morishima Y, Saito Y, Imai K, Takemota Y, Miura Y, Teshima H, Hamajima N. A double-blind controlled study of granulocyte colony-stimulating factor started two days before induction chemotherapy in refractory acute myeloid leukemia. Blood 1994:83:2086.
46. Ohno R, Tomonaga M, Kobayashi T, Kanamaru A, Shirakawa S, Masaoka T, Omine M, Oh H, Nomura T, Sakai Y, et al. Effect of granulocyte colony-stimulating factor after intensive induction therapy in relapsed or refractory acute leukemia. N Engl J Med 1990:323:871.
47. Rowe JM, Andersen J, Mazza JJ, Paietta E, Bennett JM, Hayes A, Oette D, Wiernik PH. Phase III randomized placebo-controlled study of granulo-

cyte–macrophage colony stimulation factor (GM-CSF) in adult patients (55–70 years) with acute myelogenous leukemia (AML). A study of the Eastern Cooperative Oncology Group (ECOG). Blood 1993:82(suppl 1):329 (Abstr).
48. Giralt S, Escudier S, Kantarjian H, Deisseroth A, Freireich EJ, Andersson BS, O'Brien S, Andreeff M, Fisher H, Cork A, et al. Preliminary results of treatment with filgrastim for relapse of leukemia and myelodysplasia after allogeneic bone marrow transplantation. N Engl J Med 1993:329:757.
49. Dombret H, Chastang C, Fenaux P, Reiffers J, Bordessoule D, Bouabdallah R, Mandelli F, Ferrant A, Auzanneau G, Tilly H, Yver A, Degos L. A controlled study of recombinant human granulocyte colony-stimulating factor in elderly patients after treatment for acute myelogenous leukemia. N Engl J Med 1995:332:1678.
50. Link H, Wandt H, Schönrock-Nabulsi P, Ehninger G, Franke A, Gäckle R, Geer T, Strobel G, Linkesch W, Krieger O, Niederwieser D, Nikiforakis E, Öhl S, Otremba B, Pittermann E, Schmidt H, Tischler J, Weiss J, Wilhelm M, Badri N. G-CSF (Lenograstim) after chemotherapy for acute myeloid leukemia: A placebo controlled trial. Blood 1996:88:666a (Abstr).
51. Rowe JM, Andersen JW, Mazza JJ, Bennett JM, Paietta E, Hayes FA, Oette D, Cassileth PA, Stadtmauer EA, Wiernik PH. A randomized placebo-controlled phase III study of granulocyte-macrophage colony-stimulating factor in adult patients (>55 to 70 years of age) with acute myelogenous leukemia: A study of the Eastern Cooperative Oncology Group (E1490). Blood 1995:86:457.
52. Heil G, Hoelzer D, Sanz G, Lechner K, Yin JAL, Papa G, Noens L, Szer J, Ganser A, O'Brien C, Matcham J, Barge A. A randomized double-blind, placebo-controlled phase III study of filgrastim in remission induction and consolidation therapy for adults with de novo acute myeloid leukemia. Blood 1997:90:4736.
53. Lowenberg B, Suciu S, Archimbaud E, Ossenkoppele G, Verhoef GE, Vellenga E, Wijermans P, Berneman Z, Dekker AW, Stryckmans P, Schouten H, Jehn U, Muus P, Sonneveld P, Dardenne M, Zittoun R. Use of recombinant GM-CSF during and after remission induction chemotherapy in patients aged 61 years and older with acute myeloid leukemia: Final report of AML-11, a phase III randomized study of the Leukemia Cooperative Group of European Organisation for the Research and Treatment of Cancer and the Dutch Belgian Hemato-Oncology Cooperative Group. Blood 1997:90:2952.
54. Boogaerts MA, Brugger W, Carella AM, Cortes-Funes H, Fibbe WE, Hows J, Khayat D, Linch D, Link H, Moore MAS, Testa NG. Peripheral blood progenitor cell transplantation: Where do we stand? Ann Oncol 1996:7(suppl 2):1.
55. Carella AM, Podesta M, Frassoni F, Raffo MR, Pollicardo N, Pungolino E, Vimercati R, Sessarego M, Parodi C, Rabitti C, et al. Collection of "normal" blood repopulating cells during early hematopoietic recovery after intensive conventional chemotherapy in chronic myelogenous leukemia. Bone Marrow Transplant 1993:12:267.

56. Carella AM, Simonsson B, Link H, Proctor SJ, Boogaerts M, Gorin N, Fernandez-Ranada J, Dabouz-Harrouche F, Gautier L. Mobilisation with lenograstim of pH-negative (pH neg) blood progenitor cells (BPC) in patients with chronic myeloid leukemia (CML) not good responders or not tolerant to alpha-interferon (alpha-IFN). Br J Haematol 1998:97.
57. Ganser A, Hoelzer D. Treatment of myelodysplastic syndromes with hematopoietic growth factors. Hematol Oncol Clin North Am 1992:6:633.
58. Herrmann F, Lindemann A, Klein H, Lübbert M, Schulz G, Mertelsmann R. Effect of recombinant human granulocyte-macrophage colony-stimulating factor in patients with myelodysplastic syndrome with excess of blasts. Leukemia 1989:3:335.
59. Vadhan-Raj S, Keating M, LeMaistre A, Hittelman W, McCredie KB, Trujillo JM, Broxmeyer HE, Henney C, Gutterman JU. Effects of recombinant human granulocyte–macrophage colony-stimulating factor in patients with myelodysplastic syndromes. N Engl J Med 1987:317:1545.
60. Ganser A, Heil G, Seipelt G, Fischer JT, Langer G, Brockhaus W, Ittel TH, Fuhr HG, Bergmann L, Hoelzer D. Aggressive induction chemotherapy with idarubicin, Ara-C, VP-16, followed by G-CSF and maintenance immunotherapy with interleukin-2 for high-risk ANLL. Blood 1993:82(suppl 1):128a (Abstr).
61. Kaplan LD, Kahn JO, Crowe S, Northfelt D, Neville P, Grossberg H, Abrams DI, Tracey J, Mills J, Volberding PA. Clinical and virologic effects of recombinant human granulocyte macrophage colony stimulating factor in patients receiving chemotherapy for human immunodeficiency virus-associated non-Hodgkin's lymphoma: Results of a randomized trial. J Clin Oncol 1991:9:929.
62. Perno CF, Yarchoan R, Cooney DA, Hartman NR, Webb DS, Hao Z, Mitsuya H, Johns DG, Broder S. Replication of human immunodeficiency virus in monocytes. Granulocyte/macrophage colony-stimulating factor (GM-CSF) potentiates viral production yet enhances the antiviral effect mediated by 3′-azido-2′3′-dideoxythymidine (AZT) and other dideoxynucleoside congeners of thymidine. J Exp Med 1989:169:933.
63. Davey RT Jr, Davey VJ, Metcalf JA, Zurlo JJ, Kovacs JA, Falloon J, Polis MA, Zunich KM, Masur H, Lane HC. A phase I/II trial of zidovudine, interferon-alpha, and granulocyte-macrophage colony-stimulating factor in the treatment of human immunodeficiency virus type 1 infection. J Infect Dis 1991:164:43.
64. Krown SE, Paredes J, Bundow D, Polsky B, Gold JW, Flomenberg N. Interferon-alpha, zidovudine, and granulocyte–macrophage colony-stimulating factor: A phase I AIDS Clinical Trials Group study in patients with Kaposi's sarcoma associated with AIDS. J Clin Oncol 1992:10:1344.
65. Levine JD, Allan JD, Tessitore JH, Falcone N, Galasso F, Israel RJ, Groopman JE. Recombinant human granulocyte–macrophage colony-stimulating factor ameliorates zidovudine-induced neutropenia in patients with acquired immunodeficiency syndrome (AIDS)/AIDS-related complex. Blood 1991:78:3148.

66. Neidhart J, Mangalik A, Kohler W, Stidley C, Saiki J, Duncan P, Souza L, Downing M. Granulocyte colony-stimulating factor stimulates recovery of granulocytes in patients receiving dose-intensive chemotherapy without bone marrow transplantation. J Clin Oncol 1989:7:1685.
67. Samson MK, Rivkin SE, Jones SE, Costanzi JJ, LoBuglio AF, Stephens RL, Gehan EA, Cummings GD. Dose–response and dose–survival advantage for high versus low-dose cisplatin combined with vinblastine and bleomycin in disseminated testicular cancer. A Southwest Oncology Group study. Cancer 1984:53:1029.
68. Caspar CB, Seger RA, Burger J, Gmur J. Effective stimulation of donors for granulocyte transfusions with recombinant methionyl granulocyte colony-stimulating factor. Blood 1993:81:2866.
69. Lichtman SM, Ratain MJ, Van Echo DA, Rosner G, Egorin MJ, Budman DR, Vogelzang NJ, Norton L, Schilsky RL. Phase I trial of granulocyte–macrophage colony-stimulating factor plus high-dose cyclophosphamide given every 2 weeks: A Cancer and Leukemia Group B study. J Natl Cancer Inst 1993:85:1319.
70. Savarese DM, Denicoff AM, Berg SL, Hillig M, Baker SP, O'Shaughnessy JA, Chow C, Otterson GA, Balis FM, Poplack DG, et al. Phase I study of high-dose piroxantrone with granulocyte colony-stimulating factor. J Clin Oncol 1993:11:1795.
71. Ardizzoni A, Venturini M, Sertoli MR, Giannessi PG, Brema F, Danova M, Testore F, Mariani GL, Pennucci MC, Queirolo P, Silvestro S, Bruzzi P, Lionetto R, Latini F, Rosso R. Granulocyte-machrophage colony-stimulating factor (GM-CSF) allows acceleration and dose intensity increase of CEF chemotherapy: A randomized study in patients with advanced breast cancer. Br J Cancer 1994:69:385.
72. Wandl UB, Niederle N. The concept of dose intensification in the treatment of neoplastic disease. Infection 1992:20(suppl 2):S107.
73. Asano S, Masaoka T, Takaku F, Ogawa N. Placebo controlled double blind trial of recombinant human granulocyte colony-stimulating factor for bone marrow transplantation. Jpn J Med 1990:3:317.
74. Gisselbrecht C, Prentice G, Bacigalupo A, Biron P, Milpied N, Rubie H, Cunningham D, Legros M, Pico JL, Linch DC, Burnett AK, Scarffe JH, Siegert W, Yver A: A phase III randomized placebo-controlled study in 315 pediatric and adult autologous or allogeneic bone marrow transplantation with lenograstim 5 g/kg/day (glycosylated rHu-G-CSF). Blood 1993: 82(suppl 1):455a (Abstr).
75. Schuening FG, Nemunaitis J, Applebaum FR, Storb R. Hematopoietic growth factors after allogeneic marrow transplantation. Bone Marrow Transplantation 1994:14(suppl 4):S74–S77.
76. Asano S, Takahashi S, Okamoto S, Takalu F. Long-term effects of the lenograstim therapies in allogeneic bone marrow transplantation. In: Molecular Biology of Hematopoiesis, 8th Symposium, Basel, 1993 (Abstr).
77. Chap L, Schiller G, Nimer SD. Use of recombinant GM-CSF following allogeneic BMTs for aplastic anemia. Bone Marrow Transplant 1993:12:173.

78. De Witte T, Gratwohl A, Van Der Lely N, Bacigalupo A, Stern AC, Speck B, Schattenberg A, Nissen C, Gluckman E, Fibbe WE. Recombinant human granulocyte-macrophage colony stimulating factor accelerates neutrophil and monocyte recovery after allogeneic T-cell-depleted bone marrow transplantation. Blood 1992:79:1359.
79. Powles R, Smith C, Milan S, Treleaven T, Millar J, McElwain T, Gordon-Smith E, Milliken S, Tiley C. Human recombinant GM-CSF in allogeneic bone-marrow transplantation for leukaemia: Double-blind, placebo controlled trial. Lancet 1990:336:1417.
80. Kodo H, Tajika K, Takahashi S, Ozawa K, Asano S, Takaku F. Acceleration of neutrophilic granulocyte recovery after bone-marrow transplantation by administration of recombinant human granulocyte colony-stimulating factor. Lancet 1988:2:38.
81. Sheridan WP, Morstyn G, Wolf M, Dodds A, Lusk J, Maher D, Layton JE, Green MD, Souza L, Fox RM. Granulocyte colony-stimulating factor and neutrophil recovery after high-dose chemotherapy and autologous bone marrow transplantation. Lancet 1989:2:891.
82. Taylor KM, Jagannath S, Spitzer G, Spinolo JA, Tucker SL, Fogel B, Cabanillas FF, Hagemeister FB, Souza LM. Recombinant human granulocyte colony stimulating factor hastens granulocyte recovery after high-dose chemotherapy and autologous bone marrow transplantation in Hodgkin's disease. J Clin Oncol 1989:7:1791.
83. Stahel RA, Jost LM, Pichert G, Cerny T, Honegger HP, Jacky E, Fey M, Platzer E. Controlled study of filgrastim after high dose chemotherapy and autologous bone marrow transplantation for high risk lymphoma. Abstracts, International Conference on Malignant Lymphoma, Lugano, 1993.
84. Linch DC, Scarffe H, Proctor S, Chopra R, Taylor PR, Morgenstern G, Cunningham D, Burnett AK, Cawley JC, Franklin IM, et al. Randomized vehicle-controlled dose-finding study of glycosylated recombinant human granulocyte colony-stimulating factor after bone marrow transplantation. Bone Marrow Transplant 1993:11:307.
85. Link H, Boogaerts MA, Carella AM, Ferrant A, Gadner H, Gorin NC, Harabacz I, Harousseau JL, Hervé P, Holldack J, Kolb HJ, Krieger O, Labar B, Linkesch W, Mandelli F, Maraninchi D, Naparstek E, Nicolay U, Niederwieser D, Reiffers J, Rizzoli V, Siegert W, Vernant JP, De Witte T. A controlled trial of recombinant human granulocyte–macrophage colony stimulating factor after total body irradiation, high dose chemotherapy and autologous bone marrow transplantation for acute lymphoblastic leukemia or malignant lymphoma. Blood 1992:80:2188.
86. Nemunaitis J, Rabinowe SN, Singer JW, Bierman PJ, Vose JM, Freedman AS, Onetto N, Gillis S, Oette D, Gold M, Buckner D, Hansen JA, Ritz J, Appelbaum FR, Armitage J, Nadler LM. Recombinant granulocyte macrophage colony-stimulating factor after autologous bone marrow transplantation for lymphoid cancer. N Engl J Med 1991:324:1773.
87. Visani G, Gamberi B, Greenberg P, Advani R, Gulati S, Champlin R, Hoglund M, Karanes C, Williams S, Keating A, et al. The use of GM-CSF as

an adjunct to autologous/syngeneic bone marrow transplantation: A prospective randomized controlled trial. Bone Marrow Transplant 1991:7(suppl 2):81.
88. Crown J, Kritz A, Vahdat L, Reich L, Moore M, Hamilton N, Schneider J, Harrison M, Gilewski T, Hudis C, et al. Rapid administration of multiple cycles of high-dose myelosuppressive chemotherapy in patients with metastatic breast cancer. J Clin Oncol 1993:11:1144.
89. Kessinger A, Armitage JO, Smith DM, Landmark JD, Bierman PJ, Weisenburger DD. High-dose therapy and autologous peripheral blood stem cell transplantation for patients with lymphoma. Blood 1989:74:1260.
90. Körbling M, Dörken B, et al. Autologous transplantation of blood-derived hematopoietic stem cells after myeloablative therapy in a patient with Burkitt's lymphoma. Blood 1986:67:529.
91. Reiffers J, Bernard P, David B, Vezon G, Sarrat A, Marit G, Moulinier J, Broustet A. Successful autologous transplantation with peripheral blood hemopoietic cells in a patient with acute leukemia. Exp Hematol 1986:14:312.
92. Tilly H, Bastit D, Lucet JC, Esperou H, Monconduit M, Piguet H. Haematopoietic reconstitution after autologous peripheral blood stem cell transplantation in acute leukaemia. Lancet 1986:II:154.
93. Siena S, Bregni M, Bonsi L, Sklenar I, Bagnara GP, Bonadonna G, Gianni AM. Increase in peripheral blood megakaryocyte progenitors following cancer therapy with high-dose cyclophosophamide and hematopoietic growth factors. Exp Hematol 1993:21:1583.
94. Siena S, Bregni M, Brando B, Belli N, Ravagnani F, Gandola L, Stern AC, Lansdorp PM, Bonadonna G, Gianni AM. Flow cytometry for clinical estimation of circulating hematopoietic progenitors for autologous transplantation in cancer patients. Blood 1991:77:400.
95. Siena S, Bregni M, Brando B, Ravagnani F, Bonadonna G, Gianni AM. Circulation of CD34+ hematopoietic stem cells in the peripheral blood of high-dose cyclophosphamide treated patients: Enhancement by intravenous recombinant human GM-CSF. Blood 1989:74:1905.
96. Socinski MA, Elias A, Schnipper L, Cannistra SA, Antman KS, Griffin JD. Granulocyte–macrophage colony stimulating factor expands the circulating haematopoietic progenitor cell compartment in man. Lancet 1988:1:1194.
97. Antman K, Elias A, Hunt M, Ayash L, Anderson K, Wheeler C, Schwarttz G, Tepler I, Mazanet R, Critchlow J, Schnipper L, Demetri G, Griffin J, Frei E III. GM-CSF potentiated peripheral blood progenitor cell collection and use after high dose chemotherapy. Blood 1990:76(suppl):526a.
98. Gianni AM, Tarella C, Siena S, Bregni M, Boccadoro M, Lombardi F, Bengala C, Bonadonna G, Pileri A. Durable and complete hematopoietic reconstitution after autografting of rhGM-CSF exposed peripheral blood progenitor cells. Bone Marrow Transplant 1990:6:143.
99. Haas R, Ho AD, Bredthauer U, Cayeux S, Egerer G, Knauf W, Hunstein W. Successful autologous transplantation of blood stem cells mobilized with

recombinant human granulocyte-macrophage colony-stimulating factor. Exp Hematol 1990:18:94.

100. Kessinger A, Armitage JO. The evolving role of autologous peripheral stem cell transplantation following high-dose therapy for malignancies [editorial]. Blood 1991:77:211.
101. Peters WP, Ross M, Vredenburgh JJ, Meisenberg B, Marks LB, Winer E, Kurtzberg J, Bast RC Jr, Jones R, Shpall E, et al. High-dose chemotherapy and autologous bone marrow support as consolidation after standard-dose adjuvant therapy for high-risk primary breast cancer. J Clin Oncol 1993:11: 1132.
102. Pettengell R, Testa NG, Swindell R, Crowther D, Dexter TM. Transplantation potential of hematopoietic cells released into the circulation during routine chemotherapy for non-Hodgkin's lymphoma. Blood 1993:82:2239.
103. Neben S, Marcus K, Mauch P. Mobilization of hematopoietic stem and progenitor cell subpopulations from the marrow to the blood of mice following cyclophosphamide and/or granulocyte colony-stimulating factor. Blood 1993:81:1960.
104. Bender JG, Unverzagt KL, Walker DE, Lee W, Lum L, Van Epps DE, Williams SF, To LB. Characterization of CD34+ cells mobilized to the peripheral blood during the recovery from cyclophosphamide chemotherapy. Int J Cell Cloning 1992:10:23.
105. Berenson RJ, Bensinger WI, Hill RS, Andrews RG, Garcia-Lopez J, Kalamasz DF, Still BJ, Spitzer G, Buckner CD, Bernstein ID, Thomas ED. Engraftment after infusion of CD34+ marrow cells in patients with breast cancer or neuroblastoma. Blood 1991:77:1717.
106. Shpall EJ, Jones RB, Franklin W, Curiel T, Bearman SI, Stemmer S, Hami L, Petsche D, Taffs S, Heimfels S, Hallagan J, Berenson RJ. CD34+ marrow and/or PBPCs provide effective haematopoietic reconstitution of breast cancer patients following high-dose chemotherapy with autologous haematopoietic progenitor cell support. Blood 1992:80(suppl 1): 24a (Abstr).
107. Sheridan WP, Begley CG, Juttner CA, Szer J, To LB, Maher D, McGrath K, Morstyn G, Fox RM. Effect of peripheral-blood progenitor cells mobilised by filgrastim (G-CSF) on platelet recovery after high-dose chemotherapy. Lancet 1992:339:640.
108. Elias AD, Ayash L, Anderson KC, Hunt M, Wheeler C, Schwartz G, Tepler I, Mazanet R, Lynch C, Pap S, et al. Mobilization of peripheral blood progenitor cells by chemotherapy and granulocyte–macrophage colony-stimulating factor for hematologic support after high-dose intensification for breast cancer. Blood 1992:79:3036.
109. Gianni AM, Siena S, Bregni M, Tarella C, Stern AC, Pileri A, Bonadonna G. Granulocyte-macrophage colony-stimulating factor to harvest circulating haematopoietic stem cells for autotransplantation. Lancet 1989:2:580.
110. Masaoka T, Takaku F, Kato S, Moriyama Y, Kodera Y, Kamamaru A, Shimosaka A, Shibata H, Nakamura H. Recombinant human granulocyte colony-stimulating factor in allogeneic bone marrow transplantation. Exp Hematol 1989:17:1047.

111. Peters WP, Rosner G, Ross M, Vredenburgh J, Meisenberg B, Gilbert C, Kurtzberg J. Comparative effects of granulocyte-macrophage colony-stimulating factor (GM-CSF) and granulocyte colony-stimulating factor (G-CSF) on priming peripheral blood progenitor cells for use with autologous bone marrow after high-dose chemotherapy. Blood 1993:81:1709.
112. Anderlini P, Korbling M, Dale D, Gratwohl A, Schmitz N, Stroncek D, Howe C, Leitman S, Horowitz M, Gluckman E, Rowley S, Przepiorka D, Champlin R. Allogeneic blood stem cell transplantation: Considerations for donors [editorial]. Blood 1997:90:903.
113. Schmitz N, Dreger P, Suttorp M, Rohwedder EB, Haferlach T, Löffler H, Hunter A, Russell NH. Primary transplantation of allogeneic peripheral blood progenitor cells mobilized by filgrastim (granulocyte colony stimulating factor). Blood 1995:85:1666.
114. Körbling M, Przepiorka D, Van Besien K, Giralt S, Andersson B, Huh YO, Kleine HD, Seong D, Deisseroth AB, Andreeff M, Champlin R. Allogeneic blood stem cell transplantation for refractory leukemia and lymphoma: Potential advantage of blood over marrow allografts. Blood 1995:85:1659.
115. Link H, Arseniev L, Bähre O, Berenson RJ, Battmer K, Kadar J, Jacobs R, Casper J, Kühl J, Schubert J, Diedrich H, Poliwoda H. Combined transplantation of allogeneic bone marrow and CD34+ blood cells. Blood 1995:86:2500.
116. Link H, Arseniev L, Bähre O, Kadar J, Diedrich H, Poliwoda H. Transplantation of allogeneic CD34+ blood cells. Blood 1996:87:4903.
117. Majolino I, Saglio G, Scime R, Serra, Cavallaro AM, Fiandaca T, Vasta S, Pampinella M, Marceno R, Santoro A. High incidence of chronic GVHD after primary allogeneic peripheral blood stem cell (PBSC) transplantation in patients with hematologic malignancies. Blood 1995:86(suppl A):108:A420 (Abstr).
117a. Schmitz N, Gratwohl A, Goldman JM. Allogeneic and autologous transplantation for haematological diseases, solid tumours and immune disorders. Current practice in Europe in 1996 and proposals for an operational classification. Bone Marrow Transplant 1996:17:471.
118. Nemunaitis J, Singer JW, Buckner CD, Durnam D, Epstein C, Hill R, Storb R, Thomas ED, Appelbaum FR. Use of recombinant human granulocyte–macrophage colony-stimulating factor in graft failure after bone marrow transplantation. Blood 1990:76:245.
119. Kaiser U, Klausmann M, Richter G, Pflüger KH. GM-CSF versus G-CSF in the treatment of infectious complication in Felty's syndrome—A case report [letter]. Ann Hematol 1992:64:205.
120. Pixley JS, Yoneda KY, Manalo PB. Sequential administration of cyclophosphamide and granulocyte-colony stimulating factor relieves impaired myeloid maturation in Felty's syndrome. Am J Hematol 1993:43:304.
121. Wandt H, Seifert M, Falge C, Gallmeier WM. Long-term correction of neutropenia in Felty's syndrome with granulocyte colony-stimulating factor. Ann Hematol 1993:66:265.

122. Lang DF, Rosenfeld CS, Diamond HS, Shadduck RK, Zeigler ZR. Successful treatment of T-gamma lymphoproliferative disease with human-recombinant granulocyte colony stimulating factor. Am J Hematol 1992:40:66.
123. Zuelzer WW, Bajoghli M. Chronic granulocytopenia in childhood. Blood 1964:23:359.
124. Bonilla MA, Gillio AP, Ruggeiro M, Kernan NA, Brochstein JA, Abboud M, Fumagalli L, Vincent M, Gabrilove JL, Welte K, Souza LM, O'Reilly RJ. Effects of recombinant human granulocyte colony-stimulating factor on neutropenia in patients with congenital agranulocytosis. N Engl J Med 1989: 320:1574.
125. Ganser A, Ottmann OG, Erdmann H, Schulz G, Hoelzer D. The effect of recombinant human granulocyte–macrophage colony-stimulating factor on neutropenia and related morbidity in chronic severe neutropenia. Ann Intern Med 1989:111:887.
126. Jakubowski AA, Souza L, Kelly F, Fain K, Budman D, Clarkson B, Bonilla MA, Moore MAS, Gabrilove J. Effects of human granulocyte colony stimulating factor in a patient with idiopathic neutropenia. N Engl J Med 1989: 320:38.
127. Zeidler C, Reiter A, Yakisan E, Koci B, Riehm H, Welte K. Langzeitbehandlung mit recombinantem humanen Granulozyten-Kolonien stimulierenden Faktor bei Patienten mit schwerer kongenitaler Neutropenie. Kli Paediatr 1993:205:264.
128. Freund MR, Luft S, Schober C, Heussner P, Schrezenmaier H, Porzsolt F, Welte K. Differential effect of GM-CSF and G-CSF in cyclic neutropenia [letter]. Lancet 1990:336:313.
129. Welte K, Zeidler C, Reiter A, Müller W, Odenwald E, Souza L, Riehm H. Differential effects of granulocyte–macrophage colony-stimulating factor and granulocyte colony-stimulating factor in children with severe congenital neutropenia. Blood 1990:75:1056.
130. Carulli G, Sbrana S, Azzara A, Minnucci S, Angiolini C, Ambrogi F. Reversal of autoimmune phenomena in autoimmune neutropenia after treatment with rhG-CSF: Two additional cases. Br J Haematol 1997:96:877.
131. Kuijpers TW, de Haas M, De Groot CJ, Von dB, Weening RS. The use of rhG-CSF in chronic autoimmune neutropenia: Reversal of autoimmune phenomena, a case history. Br J Haematol 1996:94:464.
132. Hurst D, Kilpatrick L, Becker J, Lipani J, Kleman K, Perrine S, Douglas SD. Recombinant human GM-CSF treatment of neutropenia in glycogen storage disease 1b. Am J Pediatr Hematol Oncol 1993:15:71.
133. Ishiguro A, Nakahata T, Shimbo T, Amano Y, Yasui K, Koike K, Komiyama A. Improvement of neutropenia and neutrophil dysfunction by granulocyte colony-stimulating factor in a patient with glycogen storage disease type Ib. Eur J Pediatr 1993:152:18.
134. Bhatia S, McCullough J, Perry EH, Clay M, Ramsay NK, Neglia JP. Granulocyte transfusions: Efficacy in treating fungal infections in neutropenic patients following bone marrow transplantation. Transfusion 1994:34:226.

135. Dale DC, Liles WC, Price TH. Renewed interest in granulocyte transfusion therapy. Br J Haematol 1997:98:497.
136. Dignani MC, Anaissie EJ, Hester JP, O'Brien S, Vartivarian SE, Rex JH, Kantarjian H, Jendiroba DB, Lichtiger B, Andersson BS, Freireich EJ. Treatment of neutropenia-related fungal infections with granulocyte colony-stimulating factor-elicited white blood cell transfusions: A pilot study. Leukemia 1997:11:1621.
137. Roilides E, Pizzo PA. Modulation of host defenses by cytokines: Evolving adjuncts in prevention and treatment of serious infections in immunocompressed hosts.
138. Cairo MS, Mauss D, Kommareddy S, Norris K, van de Ven C, Modanlou H. Prophylactic or simultaneous administration of recombinant human granulocyte colony stimulating factor in the treatment of group B streptococcal sepsis. Pediatr Res 1992:27:612.
139. Gillan E, Christensen R, Suen Y, Hunter D, van de Ven C, Stringham D, Cairo MS. Results of a phase I/II randomized placebo-controlled trial of recombinant G-CSF in newborns with presumed sepsis. Blood 1992: 80(suppl 1):291a (Abstr).
140. Ono Y, Kunii O, Kobayashi K, Kanegasaki S. Evaluation of opsonophagocytic dysfunctions in severely burned patients by luminol-dependent chemiluminescence. Microbiol Immunol 1993:37:563.
141. Silver GM, Gamelli RL, O'Reilly M. The beneficial effect of granuulocyte colony stimulating factor (G-CSF) in combination with gentamicin on survival after *Pseudomonas* burn wound infection. Surgery 1992:106:452.
142. Anding K, Kropec A, Schmidt-Eisenlohr E, Benzing A, Geiger K, Daschner F. Enhancement of in vitro bactericidal activity of neutrophils from trauma patients in the presence of granulocyte colony-stimulating factor. Eur J Clin Microbiol Infect Dis 1993:12:121.
143. White OC, Hartmann S, Alexander JW, Babcock GF. Reduced PMN beta 2 integrins after trauma: A possible role for colony-stimulating factors. Clin Exp Immunol 1993:92:477.
144. Abraham E, Stevens P. Effects of granulocyte colony-stimulating factor in modifiying mortality from *Pseudomonas aeruginosa* pneumonia after hemorrhage. Crit Care Med 1992:20:1127.
145. O'Reilly M, Silver GM, Greenhalgh DG, Gamelli RL, David JH, Hebert JC. Treatment of intra-abdominal infection with granulocyte colony-stimulating factor. J Trauma 1992:33:679.
146. Gillan EG, Plunkett M, Cario MS. Colony-stimulating factors in the modulation of sepsis. New Horiz 1993:1:96.
147. Gorgen I, Hartung T, Leist M, Niehorster M, Tiegs G, Uhlig S, Weitzel F, Wendel A. Granulocyte colony-stimulating factor treatment protects rodents against lipopolysaccharide-induced toxicity via suppression of systemic tumor necrosis factor-alpha. J Immunol 1992:149:918.
148. Kawakami M, Tsutsumi H, Kumakawa T, Hirai M, Kurosawa S, Mori M, Fukushima M. Serum granulocyte colony-stimulating factor in patients with repeated infections. Am J Hematol 1992:41:190.

149. Serushago BA, Yoshikai Y, Handa T, Mitsuyama M, Muramori K, Nomoto K. Effect of recombinant human granulocyte colony-stimulating factor (rh G-CSF) on murine resistance against *Listeria monocytogenes*. Immunology 1992:75:475.
150. Daley M, Williams T, Coyle P, Furda G, Dougherty R, Hayes P. Prevention and treatment of *Staphylococcus aureus* infections with recombinant cytokines. Cytokine 1993:5:276.
151. Arseniev L, Andres J, Battmer K, Südmeyer I, Könneke A, Zaki M, Bokemeyer C, Klein H-D, Freund M, Link H. Recruitment of peripheral blood stem cells after mobilization with G-CSF alone or following high dose chemotherapy. European Bone Marrow Transplantation Meeting, Garmisch-Partenkirchen, 1993, 102 (Abstr).
152. Link H, Arseniev L, Könneke A, Andres J, Battmer K, Südmeyer I, Poliwoda H. Kinetics of hematopoietic reconstitution after multiple consecutive courses of intensive chemotherapy supported with granulocyte-colony stimulating factor and peripheral blood progenitor cells. Ann Hematol 1993: 67(suppl A):75 (Abstr).
153. Kantarjian HM, Estey E, O'Brien S, Anaissie E, Beran M, Pierce S, Robertson L, Keating MJ. Granulocyte colony-stimulating factor supportive treatment following intensive chemotherapy in acute lymphocytic leukemia in first remission. Cancer 1993:72:2950.
154. Kantarjian HM, Estey EH, O'Brien S, Anaissie E, Beran M, Rios MB, Keating MJ, Gutterman J. Intensive chemotherapy with mitoxantrone and high-dose cytosine arabinoside followed by granulocyte-macrophage colony-stimulating factor in the treatment of patients with acute lymphocytic leukemia. Blood 1992:79:876.
155. Ohno R, Tomonaga M, Ohshima T, Masaoka T, Asou N, Oh H, Nishikawa K, Kanamaru A, Murakami H, Furusawa S, et al. A randomized controlled study of granulocyte colony stimulating factor after intensive induction and consolidation therapy in patients with acute lymphoblastic leukemia. Japan Adulk Leukemia Study Group. Int J Hematol 1993:58:73.
156. Trillet-Lenoir V, Green J, Manegold C, Von Pawel J, Gatzemeier U, Lebeau B, Depierre A, Johnson P, Decoster G, Tomita D, Ewen C. Recombinant granulocyte colony stimulating factor reduces the infectious complications of cytotoxic chemotherapy. Eur J Cancer 1993:29A:319.
157. Faucher C, Le CA, Chabannon C, Novakovitch G, Manonni P, Moatti JP, Nouyrigat P, Maraninchi D, Blaise D. Administration of G-CSF can be delayed after transplantation of autologous G-CSF-primed blood stem cells: A randomized study. Bone Marrow Transplant 1996:17:533.
158. Khwaja A, Mills W, Leveridge K, Goldstone AH, Linch DC. Efficacy of delayed granulocyte colony-stimulating factor after autologous BMT. Bone Marrow Transplant 1993:11:479.

4

Oral and Gastrointestinal Toxicity

CARSTEN BOKEMEYER
University of Tübingen Medical Center, Tübingen, Germany

J.T. HARTMANN
Eberhard-Karls University, Tübingen, Germany

INTRODUCTION

The treatment of malignant diseases with chemotherapeutic agents often markedly affects the gastrointestinal tract in its physiological, structural biochemical, or pharmacological functions, which may contribute to complex symptoms like cachexia, malnutrition, and anorexia. These symptoms may also occur as the presenting features in malignancies for various medical reasons, and they often result in reduced quality of life and increased morbidity. Impairment of the gastrointestinal tract is responsible for a high rate of mortality in patients with advanced disease and, moreover, limits the dose intensity that is appropriate for cancer treatment [1].

Cancer chemotherapy agents have a narrow therapeutic index and poorly discriminate between normal and target tissues in exerting their antiproliferative action. For that reason organs with more rapidly dividing cell systems are generally more vulnerable to cytostatic drugs. Particularly the bone marrow, the spermatogonial hair follicles, and the gastrointestinal epithelium possess a high growth fraction. More than 90% of the cell population of the crypt epithelium in the small intestine consists of principal or undifferentiated cells and goblet cells. Estimations of the generation time and the length of the cell cycle phases in specific regions of the gastrointestinal tract revealed that the esophagus and the rectum developed a completely new epithelium after 2–6 days, whereas the stomach, the jejunum, the ileum, and the mucosa of the colon had renewed themselves after 1–3 days [2].

This chapter discusses common oral and gastrointestinal side effects of cancer chemotherapy, such as nausea and vomiting, mucositis, and motility disorders. Currently approved approaches to supportive management and the prevention of gastrointestinal toxicities are described.

4.1 NAUSEA AND VOMITING

Patients rate chemotherapy-induced nausea and vomiting subjectively among the worst side effects of cancer treatment. Incidence and severity of nausea and vomiting in patients receiving chemotherapy vary depending on the type, dose, and route of chemotherapy and are particularly influenced by several characteristics of the individual patient [3–5]. Considerable progress was made with the identification of benzamides, which prevent the acute nausea and vomiting induced by cancer chemotherapy [6]. However, the most dramatic development in recent years has been the introduction of the antiemetic class of highly selective antagonists of the type III serotonin receptor (5-HT_3), such as ondansetron, dolasetron, granisetron, and tropisetron [7,8]. These antiemetic agents have considerably decreased the incidence and severity of nausea and vomiting induced by chemotherapy compared to the use of the phenothiazines, but they have not totally prevented all problems. Consequences of an unsatisfactory control of nausea and vomiting induced by cancer treatment may lead to medical complications (e.g., failure of patients to comply with further treatment cycles and an at least diminished quality of life).

Besides the prevention of acute emesis, which occurs during the first 24 hours after application of cytotoxic drugs, another major problem is the control of postchemotherapy delayed nausea and vomiting (PCNV) extends beyond the first 24 hours after both moderately emetogenic and high emetogenic chemotherapy [9]. The third emetic syndrome—anticipatory nausea and vomiting, which occurs prior to the application of chemotherapeutic agents—will affect 10–40% of patients and is preferentially prevented by psychological interventions or anxiolytic agents [10,11].

4.1.1 Pathophysiology of Nausea and Vomiting

The precise mechanisms of chemotherapy-induced nausea and vomiting are unknown [12–15]. The vomiting center, localized at the medullary reticular formation, appears to mediate chemotherapy-induced nausea and vomiting [17,18]. It is located close to the chemoreceptor trigger zone (CTZ) in the area postrema of the fourth ventricle. For almost all chemotherapeutic agents, the most common mechanism is thought to be the activation of the CTZ. Other supposed mechanisms by which chemotherapeutic agents cause nausea and vomiting are:

- Peripheral mechanisms
  - Damage of gastrointestinal mucosa
  - Stimulation of gut neurotransmitter receptors
- Cortical mechanisms
  - Direct cerebral activation
  - Indirect/psychogenic activation
- Vestibular mechanisms
- Alterations of taste and smell

Emetogenic chemicals can reach the CTZ via the cerebrospinal fluid or the blood. A variety of neurotransmitters (dopamine, serotonin, histamine, etc.) are supposed to interact between chemotherapy and the CTZ and therefore activate the vomiting center [19–21]. Thus far, dopamine appears to be the neurotransmitter most responsible for chemotherapy-induced nausea and vomiting.

4.1.2 Emetic Syndromes and Patient's Characteristics for Nausea and Vomiting

Chemotherapy-induced acute nausea and vomiting is the most common emetic syndrome that has been characterized in detail. It typically begins 4–8 hours after the intravenous administration of the cytostatic agent and can persist for up to 36 hours. To prevent this side effect appropriately, the emetogenic potency of each agent must be known (see Section 4.1.3 concerning the emetogenicity of cytostatic drugs).

Furthermore, there is wide variation in patients' tolerance for the emetic potency of cytostatic drugs. Studies have identified several patient characteristics and conditions that may affect antiemetic control, such as a history of experience with chemotherapy, alcohol intake history, food intake and amount of sleep before chemotherapy, age and gender, experience of severe emesis during pregnancy, performance status, anxiety, motivation level, and social functioning. The recognition of certain patient factors may help to optimize individualized antiemetic therapy [19–29].

Second, delayed nausea and vomiting is seen in a significant proportion of patients beyond the first 24 hours after both moderately emetogenic and highly emetogenic chemotherapy typically including cisplatin, cyclophosphamide, or an anthracycline-based combination chemotherapy. In a recent study conducted by the National Cancer Institute of Canada Clinical Trials Group and involving more than 1500 patients who received either highly or moderately emetogenic chemotherapy, 75% of patients suffered from postchemotherapy nausea (PCN) and more than 55% from postchemotherapy vomiting (PCV) in the week after chemotherapy despite the use of 5-hydroxytryptamine receptor (5-HT_3) antagonists and dexamethasone during the first 24 hours and several days thereafter [22–24]. This finding is in accordance with other results indicating the difficulty of preventing delayed nausea and vomiting. Recently, Osoba et al. [30] retrospectively analyzed the occurrence of postchemotherapy nausea and vomiting (PCNV) in 832 chemotherapy-naive patients scheduled to receive antiemetic regimens containing 5-HT_3 antagonists with or without dexamethasone for moderately or highly emetogenic chemotherapy. Variables identified as associated with PCNV included low social functioning, prechemotherapy nausea, female gender, highly emetogenic chemotherapy, and the lack of maintenance antiemetics after chemotherapy. A history of low alcohol intake was also associated with postchemotherapy vomiting, whereas increased fatigue and lower performance status were associated with postchemotherapy nausea. In a multivariate risk factor analysis, the incidence of postchemotherapy vomiting increased from 20% in those having no risk factor to 76% in those having any four of the six risk factors. The presence of any six of the seven variables increased the predictive accuracy by about 30% to 97%, but the incidence of any degree of nausea was 67% even in patients having no risk factors. Thus, the predictive power for the occurrence of postchemotherapy nausea was only moderate in the final model compared to postchemotherapy vomiting.

A better recognition of risk factors should lead to modifications in the type and number of antiemetics given prechemotherapy and to the use of more effective maintenance antiemetics treatment after chemotherapy [30]. In summary, about 75% of patients experienced nausea in the week after moderately or highly emetogenic chemotherapy, despite the use of 5-HT_3 antagonists in combination with corticosteroids.

The third emetic syndrome is known as anticipatory emesis, which occurs before the application of cytostatic drugs and is also commonly difficult to treat with antiemetics alone. Main risk factors include bad experience of nausea and vomiting and other side effects during an earlier course of chemotherapy ("classical conditioning"), anxiety, depression, uncommon tastes and odors, history of motion sickness, and age. The prevalence of anticipatory nausea ranges from 14 to 63%, affecting approximately every third patient [26]. As mentioned above, the use of the appropriate antiemetic drugs during an initial course of chemotherapy can often eliminate or significantly reduce the development of anticipatory emesis [27–30]. Additionally, possible interventions such as counseling, cognitive distraction, relaxation training, systematic desensitization hypnosis, and adequate control before chemotherapy of any nausea that may be present may be helpful to prevent all three emetic syndromes [31,32].

4.1.3 Emetogenic Potency of Cytostatic Drugs

The emetogenic properties of chemotherapeutic agents vary greatly and are influenced by dose, schedule, concomitant drugs, and radiation therapy. To use antiemetic agents in an optimal risk-adapted strategy, it is essential to accurately predict the severity of acute nausea and vomiting related to the chosen chemotherapeutic agent. Cytostatic agents are classified differently with respect to emetogenic potency [33–38]. A recently presented classification of the acute emetogenicity of antineoplastic agents (based on an earlier schema of Lindley et al. [39] takes the dose, rate, and route of administration and new available cytotoxic agents into account. Additionally, based on this publication of Hesketh et al. [38], the overall emetogenicity of combination cancer chemotherapy may be more predictable (see Table 1).

The estimation of the emetogenic potency of combination chemotherapy is adapted to the identification of the emetogenic level of the most emetogenic single agent in the combination. For assessing the relative contributions of other agents to the emetogenicity of the combination, the following rules apply: level 1 agents do not contribute; using one or more level 2 agents increases the emetogenicity by one level and level 3 or 4 agents by one level per agent.

However, it must be kept in mind that the single-agent emetogenic classification and the combination classification scheme are partly based on subjective judgments, hence are limited to the clinical experience of the authors. Moreover, the validation of the combination chemotherapy classification is based on fewer than 200 patients, of whom 88% patients are female, and is based on cyclophosphamide-containing protocols only. Nevertheless this scheme represents a progressive connection between the known literature and clinical trial experience, which provides a practical means of classifying the emetogenicity of individual chemotherapy agents and of combination chemotherapy regimens. The guidelines for the management of chemotherapy-induced nausea and vomiting in this chapter are derived from the emetogenicity classification by Hesketh et al. [38].

4.1.4 Antiemetic Agents

The clinical management of chemotherapy-induced nausea and vomiting requires a comprehensive strategy of pharmacologic intervention, patient and family support, and psychological as well as behavioral adjustment. Knowledge of the mechanism of action, routes of administration, and adverse re-

Table 1 Emetogenic Potential of Chemotherapy Agents

Level	Frequency of emesis (%)	Start of emesis (h)	Duration (h)	Agent	Dosing schedule
5	>90	2–4	4–24	Carmustine	>250 mg/m^2
		1–6	24–48	Cisplatin	≥50 mg/m^2
		4–12	4–10	Cyclophosphamide	>1500 mg/m^2
		1–3	1–12	Dacarbazine	
		24	—	Mechlorethamine	
		1–4	12–24	Streptozocin	
4	60–90			Carboplatin	
		2–4	4–24	Carmustine	≤250 mg/m^2
		1–6	24–48	Cisplatin	<50 mg/m^2
		4–12	4–10	Cyclophosphamide	>750 mg/m^2 to ≤1500 mg/m^2
				Cytarabine	>1 g/m^2
		3–6	6–8	Doxorubicin	>60 mg/m^2
				Methotrexate	>1000 mg/m^2
		24–47	Variable	Procarbazine	125 mg/m^2
				Irinotecan (CPT-11)	weekly, or 350 mg/m^2 3–weekly
3	30–60			Cyclophosphamide	<750 mg/m^2
				Cyclophosphamide	(oral)
		4–6	6	Doxorubicin	20–60 mg/m^2
				Epirubicin	≤90 mg/m^2
		3–6		Hexamethylmelamine	(oral)
				Idarubicin	
		1–2	>24	Ifosfamide	
		4–12	3–12	Methotrexate	250–1000 mg/m^2
				Mitoxantrone	<15 mg/m^2
				Topotecan	
2	10–30			Paclitaxel	
				Docetaxel	
		3–8	—	Etoposide	
		3–6	—	5-Fluorouracil	<1000 mg/m^2
				Gemcitabine	
				Methotrexate	>50 mg/m^2 to <250 mg/m^2
		1–4	48–72	Mitomycin	

Table 1 Continued

Level	Frequency of emesis (%)	Start of emesis (h)	Duration (h)	Agent	Dosing schedule
1	<10	3–6	—	Bleomycin	
				Busulfan	
				Chlorambucil	(oral)
				2-Chlorodeoxyadenosine	
				Fludarabine	
		6–12	—	Hydroxyurea	
				Methotrexate	≤50 mg/m^2
				L-Phenylalanine mustard	(oral)
				Thioguanine	(oral)
		4–8	—	Vinblastine	
				Vincristine	
				Vinorelbine	

Source: Modified from Ref. 38.

actions of the various classes of currently available antiemetics is mandatory for effective therapy (Table 2).

4.1.4.1 Moderately Active Antiemetics

The antiemetic potency of phenothiazines, butyrophenones, or cannabinoids is substantially lower than that of the serotonin antagonists or high-dose metoclopramide for highly emetogenic cancer chemotherapy. However, these agents exert considerably anxiolytic and sedative activity. Thus, these drugs may be of particular importance in patients with anticipatory emesis who failed to respond to benzodiazepines (e.g., lorazepam) or cyclopyrrolones (e.g., zopiclone) [40,41].

Corticosteroids like dexamethasone or methylprednisolone are very useful antiemetic drugs in regard to the combination with serotonin antagonists. A single dose of 20 mg dexamethasone has been proven to act synergistically with ondansetron, tropisetron or granisetron for the prevention of high-dose, cisplatin-induced emesis. In a consideration of the prevention of delayed nausea and emesis, corticosteroids were shown to be very effective in combination with conventionally dosed metoclopramide [42–48].

4.1.4.2 Highly Active Antiemetics

The antagonism of the type III serotonin receptor is an important approach to controlling chemotherapy-induced acute emesis that occurs within the first

Table 2 Classes of Commonly Administered Antiemetics and Their Clinical Effectiveness

Effectiveness in monotherapy	Classes of antiemetics	Common side effects
Highly active	$5\text{-}HT_3$ receptor antagonists	Constipation/headaches
	High-dose benzamides	Parkinson-like syndrome,[a] sedation, diarrhea, akathisia
Moderately active	Phenothiazines—dopamine antagonists	Sedation, extrapyramidal symptoms
	Butyrophenones—dopamine antagonists	
	Corticosteroids	Hyperglycemia
Less active	Benzodiazepines, cyclopyrrolones	Sedation
	Antihistaminics	Sedation

[a]Preventable with concomitant application of diphenhydramine or benzodiazepines.

24 hours after drug administration. High-dose metoclopramide, which blocks emesis particularly by the blockage of dopamine receptors (D_2), may also exert some activity by means of antagonizing the $5\text{-}HT_3$ pathway—especially at higher doses [49]. However, higher doses (e.g., 3 mg/kg/day) are associated with considerable side effects, including sedation, diarrhea, akathisia (restlessness), and Parkinson-like symptoms, such as tremor and rigidity and major dystonic reaction. The latter may primarily occur in patients younger than 30 years of age. Some of these effects may be preventable by the concomitant use of diphenhydramine or benzodiazepines. Commonly, metoclopramide (up to 1 mg/kg/d) is preferentially used in conventional doses for the control of acute nausea and emesis induced by moderately emetogenic cancer chemotherapy and for the control of delayed nausea and emesis, particularly in combination with dexamethasone [50].

In contrast to high-dose metoclopramide, the serotonin antagonists are tolerated very well, which makes them the agents of first choice in cancer patients who receive highly emetogenic cancer chemotherapy. Thus, this pharmacological group represents one of the most progressive tools in clinical oncology during the last 10 years [7,8]. In the meantime, numerous studies have investigated ondansteron, granisetron, or tropisetron for efficacy or tolerability [51]. Pharmacological differences are mainly based on receptor binding affinity and pharmacokinetics. Half-lives in serum vary from about 3–5 hours (ondansetron) to more than 10 hours (granisetron). Randomized studies using a variety of doses and schedules have consistently revealed both ondansetron (1–3 × 8 mg/day) and granisetron (1 × 1–3 mg) to be significantly more effective than high-dose/standard-dose metoclopramide-containing regimens for the prevention of acute cisplatin-induced nausea and vomiting [52,53]. Approximately 65–75% of patients obtain major emetic control with either one of these serotonin antagonists. When compared to regimens consisting of metoclopramide plus dexamethasone, the serotonin antagonists generally result in a longer period of time to the first emetic episode, fewer side effects, decreased need of salvage antiemetics, and substantial patient preference. Because the serotonin receptor antagonists are relatively high in cost, different dosing schedules have been evaluated and controversy remains concerning the optimal dose. Most trials have indicated that lower doses are as effective as higher doses. As a general rule, the lowest recommended dose should be assumed to be the best dose for single-agent or combination use (for details see Table 3) [8,54–56]. The Consensus Conference on Antiemetic Therapy in Perugia, Italy (ESMO), suggested the following single dose regimens for the 5-HT_3 antagonists [57].

Ondansetron 8 mg IV
Granisetron 3 mg IV, 2 mg PO
Tropisetron 5 mg IV
Dolasetron 1.8 mg/kg IV

For highly emetogenic cancer chemotherapy, the combination of 5-HT_3 antagonists with a corticosteroid-like dexamethasone, has been recommended to improve antiemetic activity. Generally, the serotonin antagonists are tolerated very well. Common side effects include mild headaches (6–40%) usually not requiring treatment, transient increase of liver enzymes, and mild constipation (3–11%). Table 4 summarizes the practical guidelines for the management of acute nausea and vomiting with respect of emetogenicity of chemotherapy according to Hesketh et al. [38].

4.1.5 Delayed Nausea and Vomiting

Concerning delayed postchemotherapy nausea and vomiting which usually starts 24 h or more after drug administration, no superiority of 5-HT_3 receptor antagonists over substituted benzamides in combination with corticosteroids appears to be proven. As a consequence, the use of substituted benzamides in combination with corticosteroids is currently recommended to prevent delayed emesis after chemotherapy (e.g., dexamethasone ± substituted benzamides: see Table 5). Extrapyramidal symptoms represent rare events during conventional doses of metoclopramide. The mechanisms of delayed emesis and nausea are not fully understood but may include other

Table 3 Classes, Schedules, and Recommended Doses of Commonly Administered Antiemetics

Drug	Application	Dosing schedule
1. $5\text{-}HT_3$ receptor antagonists		
Ondansetron	PO	1–3 × 4–8 mg
	IV	1–3 × 4–8 mg
Granisetron	IV	1 × 1 (−3) mg
	PO	1 × 2 mg
Dolasetron	IV	1 × 1.8 mg/kg
Tropisetron	PO	1 × 5 mg
	IV	1 × 5 mg
2. Substituted benzamides		
Metoclopramide	PO	2–5 × 10–20 mg
	IV (high dose)	2–5 × 100–200 mg
Alizapride	PO	2–5 × 50–100 mg
	IV	2–5 × 50–100 mg
3. Corticosteroids		
Dexamethasone	PO	1–3 × 4–8 mg
	IV	1–3 × 4–8 mg
		1 × 20 mg
4. Benzodiazepine		
Lorazepam	PO	1–2 × 1–2 mg
	IV	1–2 × 1–2 mg
5. Antihistamine		
Dimenhydrinate	PO	3 × 200 mg
	Rectal	3–4 × 150 mg
	IV	3 × 62–124 mg
6. Neuroleptics		
Promethazine	PO	1–3 × 10–25 mg
	IV	1–3 × 25–50 mg
Triflupromazine	Rectal	1–2 × 70 mg
	IV	1–2 × 5–10 mg
Haloperidol	PO	1–3 × 1–3 mg
	IV	1–3 × 1–3 mg

mechanisms than serotonin release such as an enhanced activity of proinflammatory agents (e.g., prostaglandins).

4.1.6 Anticipatory Emesis

There is some evidence that the best prophylaxis of anticipatory emesis is based on the most effective antiemetic control during the first treatment

Table 4 Management of Nausea and Vomiting with Respect of Emetogenicity of Chemotherapy

Level I.	Not emetogenic chemotherapy (= expected incidence <10%) No prophylaxis or Substituted benzamide (e.g., 50–100 mg alizapride PO or IV, 30 min prior to chemotherapy)
Level II.	Low emetogenic chemotherapy (= expected incidence 10–30%) Prophylaxis: substituted benzamide (about 30 min prior to and 4 h after application of chemotherapy, e.g., 50–100 mg alizapride PO or IV) In case of nausea despite prophylaxis: additional application of benzamides combined with corticosteroids In case of insufficient efficacy: application of additional corticosteroid plus benzodiazepine or switch to 5-HT_3 receptor antagonists plus corticosteroid plus benzodiazepine in the next cycle Alternative for a chemotherapy application on an outpatient basis: primary 5-HT_3 receptor antagonists (e.g., ondansetron, 4–8 mg PO)
Level III/IV.	Moderate emetogenic chemotherapy (expected incidence = 30–90%) Prophylaxis: substituted benzamide prior to and 4 hours after treatment (e.g., 100 mg alizapride PO or IV plus corticosteroid) or 5-HT_3 receptor antagonists [e.g., 1–(3) mg granisetrone plus corticosteroid] In case of nausea despite prophylaxis: additional application of benzamide plus corticosteroid or 5-HT_3 receptor antagonists plus corticosteroid In case of insufficient efficacy: application of 5-HT_3 receptor antagonists plus corticosteroid plus benzodiazepine in the next cycle
Level V.	Highly emetogenic chemotherapy or high-dose chemotherapy expected incidence >90%) Prophylaxis: 5-HT_3 receptor antagonists (e.g., 3 mg granisetrone or 3 $\times$ 8 mg ondensatron IV plus corticosteroid, e.g., 20 mg dexamethasone IV or PO with or without benzodiazepine) In case of nausea despite prophylaxis: additional application of a benzodiazepine plus an antihistamine In case of insufficient efficacy: application of a 5-HT_3 receptor antagonists plus corticosteroid plus benzodiazepine plus antihistamine in the next cycle

Source: Adapted from Ref. 38.

Table 5 Antiemetic Regimen for Delayed Emesis

Days 1 and 2:	Metoclopramide[a] (4 × 20 mg PO) + dexamethasone (2 × 20 mg PO) or (5-HT_3 serotonin antagonist)
Days 3 and 4:	Dexamethasone (1–2 × 4 mg PO)

[a]Diphenhydramine in case of extrapyramidal symptoms or prophylactically in patients younger than 30 years.

cycle. If anticipatory emesis is very likely, the use of anxiolytic agents (e.g., 2 × 1–2 mg lorazepam, starting on the day before chemotherapy) appears to be most appropriate [15].

4.2 MUCOSITIS

Approximately 40% of patients undergoing cancer chemotherapy experience acute or chronic oral complications. "Mucositis" is a common term for the oral symptoms the cancer patient may develop during the course of chemotherapy, but mucositis is not simply the result of mucosal ulcerations from cancer chemotherapy or radiation therapy. Oral pain has multiple etiologies arising from dental appliances, soft tissue, or bone. The oral mucosa can be directly damaged by cytoreductive therapies. This disruption in mucosal barrier function in a myelosuppressed cancer patient can lead to systemic infections [58]. Disturbances in salivary gland function can result in increased levels of pathogens colonizing the oral tissues and may contribute to the risk for systemic complications. Despite the biological complexity of oral toxicity of chemotherapy, appropriate oral interventions before myelosuppressive cancer treatment combined with comprehensive care of the oral cavity during or after treatment result in reduced morbidity and mortality.

4.2.1 Oral Management During Cancer Treatment

Chemotherapeutic agents affect rapidly proliferating cells in the oral cavity and the gastrointestinal tract in ways that may lead to severe stomatitis, cheilosis, glossitis, esophagitis, and oral ulcerations, which in common make eating difficult. The frequency and severity of mucositis depends on the particular antineoplastic drug and its dose schedule and regimen (i.e., given alone or in combination with other cytotoxic agents or radiation therapy). Mucositis is commonly caused by methotrexate, the antibiotic antitumor agents (particularly the anthracyclines and actinomycin D), 5-fluorouracil, and the vinca alkaloids (Table 6).

Table 6 Chemotherapeutic Agents Commonly Associated with Mucositis and Oral Complications

Drug	Related factors
Methotrexate	Severe mucositis, especially after prolonged infusions; compromised renal function; insufficient folinic acid rescue Severity is enhanced by irradiation
5-Fluorouracil	Severe with higher doses, frequent schedule, arterial infusion, intravenous bolus injection, and modulation by folinic acid
Actinomycin D	May impair oral alimentation; enhanced by irradiation
Doxorubicin/daunorubicin	May be severe and ulcerative; increased with liver disease; enhanced by irradiation
Bleomycin	Often severe and ulcerative
Vinblastine	Frequently ulcerative
Miscellaneous	Amsacrine, cyclophosphamide, cytarabine, mercaptopurine, mitomycin, nitrosoureas, procarbazine

The severity of methotrexate-induced side effects on the oral cavity and the gastrointestinal epithelium (and other normal tissues) has been shown to depend on the duration of drug exposure in the plasma over time rather than peak levels [59]. Disappearance of methotrexate (MTX) from plasma following an intravenous injection is a three-phase process [60,61]. The terminal half-life ranges from 6 to 24 hours after intravenous administration of conventional doses and 30–48 hours after high-dose therapy. The severity of mucosal toxicity and myelosuppression can be diminished by calcium folinate (Leucovorin) [59]. The close-meshed monitoring of MTX plasma concentrations is warranted after moderate to high-dose chemotherapy to avoid the risk of increased MTX toxicity (see also Section 2.4.1.1) [62–65].

Stomatitis caused by 5-fluorouracil (5-FU) may be associated with bloody diarrhea whose severity appears to be dependent on dose, duration of injection, route of administration, and biochemical parameters such as inborn defect of the enzyme dihydropyrimidine dehydrogenase and simultaneous modulation of 5-FU activity by folinic acid. Profound mucositis is more likely to occur with higher doses, shorter infusion time, intra-arterial infusion (e.g., via the hepatic artery for local chemotherapy of liver metastases), and the addition of biochemical modulators.

However, patients differ markedly in their ability to tolerate a given chemotherapy regimen. Patients who developed oral toxicity within the first course of therapy often show similar side effects during subsequent courses unless the doses are decreased or the drugs are changed. State of oral health, performance status, and age are critical factors for the risk of complications. There is some evidence that young patients may experience more mucocutaneous toxicity than older patients [66]. Patients suffering from mucositis often describe a burning sensation in the mouth within 3–10 days after the initiation of chemotherapy. This symptom frequently precedes objective signs and should alert the clinician to the possibility of problems. Any of the mucosal surfaces may then develop erythema and progress to erosion and ulceration over the next 3–5 days. Intense pain, inability to handle secretions, and severe reduction of oral intake may occur. These forms of damages tend to be reversible, with self-healing occurring over the next 1–2 weeks following completion of therapy. However, infections may further complicate mucositis [67]. Multiple pathogens, including *Pseudomonas aeruginosa, Staphylococcus aureus,* and *Escherichia coli,* can be isolated from the oral cavity while the patient is hospitalized. Recent reports have also identified *viridans* streptococci as important pathogens in immunocompromised cancer patient [67,68].

Oral fungal infections in neutropenic patients are usually caused by *Candida spp.* [69]. The typical loci of oral candidiasis are the sides and top of the tongue, the buccal and gingival mucosa, and the commissures of the lips. Fungal infections manifest as painless, wide, raised strands or patches. Forcible removal of the plaque reveals an erythematous or ulcerated mucosal surface. Diagnoses should be made by microscopic evaluation and tissue cultures.

Herpes simplex virus (HSV type I) and varicella zoster are the two most common viral pathogens causing oral infection in immunocompromized patients. The majority of HSV infections are due to a reactivation of latent primary infections. The characteristic vesicular lesions usually rupture within a day, resulting in a diffuse ulceration. Diagnostic tests with viral cultures reveal characteristic intranuclear inclusions in the epithelial cells of stained smears.

4.2.2 Prevention and Treatment of Mucositis

A variety of methods and agents presented in the last two decades appear to prevent or decrease the severity of mucositis in cancer patients. Approved treatments include stimulation of epithelial proliferation, surface protection of the mucosa, and growth inhibition of potential pathogens. Unfortunately, the efficacy and safety of most regimens have not been clearly validated. In conclusion, there does not appear to be standard regimen for the prevention or management of chemotherapy-induced mucositis. Indeed, larger clinical trials could not confirm promising preliminary results with sucralfate, chamomile extracts, or prostaglandins [69–71]. Thus, patients may develop severe mucositis in spite of the use of selected mucosal protectants. Since well-established antidotes have not yet been established for most regimens, the use of local anesthetics like benzocaine or lidocaine appears to be most preferable because these agents at least offer an improved level of temporary pain relief [72].

4.2.2.1 Oral Decontamination Regimens

Chlorhexidine

Chlorhexidine digluconate (e.g., 0.12 or 0.2%), which reveals particular activity against gram-positive bacteria, is often used as a mucosal protectant. For example, cancer patients are instructed to rinse with 15 mL of chlorhexidine solution for 30 seconds four times daily during and until 2 weeks after the course of chemotherapy or irradiation. However, the degree of mucositis does not appear to be lessened significantly by the drug. On the contrary, patients often complain about altered taste, staining of the teeth, and mouthwash discomfort. Additionally, it cannot be excluded that the prolonged use of chlorhexidine digluconate may predispose patients undergoing bone marrow transplantation to an extended oral colonization by gram-negative bacilli [69,73].

A variety of other topical disinfectants exist, including hydrogen peroxide 3%, polyvidone iodine, and iodinated glycerol. However, their particular role as mucosal protectants has not been fully evaluated [69]. The same is true for the use of the caustic agent silver nitrate (e.g., brushing with 2% $AgNO_3$ three times daily for 5 days), which has also been reported to shorten the duration of mucositis [70].

PTA Lozenges

Lozenges containing polymyxin E, tobramycin, and amphotericin B (PTA) have been used to suppress oral and pharyngeal infections in cancer patients. According to the study results of Kaanders et al., antibiotic-antifungal lozenges successfully reduced the degree and duration of mucositis in some patients with cancer of the oral cavity, whereas no similar effects were observed in patients with cancers of the oropharynx [74]. More recent data confirm that these lozenges containing nonabsorbable antibiotics may, in particular, decrease radiation-induced oral mucositis to a modest degree.

Controversy remains, however, as to whether these lozenges should be part of standard practice [75].

4.2.2.2 Local Vasoconstriction and Inhibition of Salivary Secretion

Oral Cryotherapy

Randomized clinical trials demonstrated that 30 minutes of oral cryotherapy, given at approximately the same time as the cytostatic injection of 5-fluorouracil or high-dose melphalan, can significantly inhibit the subsequent development of oral mucositis. The intraoral use of ice chips induces local vasoconstriction, which results in a selective reduction of drug distribution into the mucosal epithelium. This method appears to be particularly effective if drugs with a short elimination half-life are used as bolus injections [76–78].

Propantheline

Very recently Oblon et al. [79] reported that the prolonged administration of the anticholinergic drug propantheline (e.g., 30–60 mg every 6 h) appears to be safe and effective for the protection of the oral cavity after high-dose chemotherapy, particularly for regimens containing high-dose etoposide. According to these study results, the protective effect of propantheline is restricted to the oral mucosa, whereas the severity of esophagitis and enteritis does not appear to be influenced by this drug. The underlying mechanism of propantheline-mediated mucosal protection may be based on the decreased secretion of etoposide in saliva (via reduced saliva production), which results in lower local drug concentrations in the oral cavity. The authors conclude that propantheline may be a promising candidate for supportive care in etoposide-containing regimens [79].

4.2.2.3 Chemical Protection of the Mucosal Epithelium

Amifostine

Among the sulfhydryl compounds, the prodrug amifostine appears to be the most promising agent for the prevention of radiation-induced mucositis. The prodrug amifostine (WR-2721, *S*-2[3-aminopropylamino]-ethylphosphorothioic acid) is dephosphorylated by alkaline phosphatase, resulting in the formation of the active metabolite WR-1065, which is thought to exert its protective role by scavenging free radicals or by direct inactivation of antineoplastic agents, particularly platinum compounds and alkylating agents.

Its protective role appears to be restricted to normal cells. First, there is a preferential uptake of amifostine in normal cells; second, tumor tissue mostly lacks the bioactivating enzyme. Amifostine is an approved protectant for the reduction of cisplatin-induced nephrotoxicity and cisplatin/cyclophosphamide-induced myelosuppression. Clinical studies regarding the protective effects of WR-2721 on oral and pharyngeal mucosa in patients receiving cancer chemotherapy are ongoing [80].

Granulocyte Colony-Stimulating Factor (G-CSF)

G-CSF is a well-established protectant, administered to mitigate the severity and duration of chemotherapy-induced neutropenia. Based on an open label, phase I/II study, Gabrilove et al. [81] suggested that the use of G-CSF results in less severe mucositis in patients undergoing myelosuppressive chemotherapy for bladder cancer. However, it has not been proven if G-CSF is an effective agent for preventing mucositis [82]. Therefore this question needs to be more carefully addressed in the future, before G-CSF can be recommended for this purpose.

Sucralfate

Sucralfate is a basic albumin salt of sucrose octasulfate that has been approved by the FDA for the treatment of duodenal ulcers. The drug forms a protective coat adhering to exposed proteins in inflamed gastroduodenal mucosa. Additionally, the local production of cytoprotective prostaglandins appears to be enhanced by sucralfate. Whereas previous data suggested that sucralfate (e.g., 1 g of sucralfate suspension 4 times daily as a mouth rinse for 14 days) may be beneficial in the treatment of chemotherapy-induced mucositis, a recent trial could not confirm the influence of the drug on the severity of chemotherapy-induced stomatitis [83–85].

Allopurinol

Clark and Slevin [86] were among the first to report that an allopurinol mouthwash might be advantageous in achieving the reduction of the severity of 5-fluorouracil-induced mucositis. They speculated that the metabolite oxypurinol might be able to impair the bioactivation of the cytotoxic drug to the corresponding phosphorylated metabolites in the mucosae. However, Loprinzi and colleagues [87] could not confirm the preliminary results favoring the use of allopurinol as a mucosal protectant. No substantial difference in mucositis severity and frequency was found to be attributable to the allopurinol-containing mouthwash. As a consequence, allopurinol cannot be recommended as mucosal protectant in cancer patients who receive a bolus injection of 5-fluorouracil [87].

Prostaglandins: Dinoprostone (Prostaglandin E_2) and Misoprostol (PGE_1)

Kührer et al. suggested that topical dinoprostone might alleviate chemotherapy-induced oral mucositis [88]. Indeed, subsequent trials confirmed the special role of dinoprostone as a mucosal protectant [89]. However, these study results were not gained under double-blind, placebo-controlled conditions. The use of prostaglandins is still rather controversial because recent clinical data failed to confirm the promising preliminary results and suggested that a more extensive oral reactivation of HSV infections in prostaglandin-treated cancer patients may occur [90].

Plant Extracts (e.g., Chamomile Mouthwash)

The chamomile plant, containing many different anti-inflammatory, antibacterial, and spasmolytic substances including chamazulene, bisabolole, spiroethers, and flavonoids, has been used for medical purposes for centuries. It has been suggested that diluted chamomile extracts (e.g., 30 drops of a concentrate in 100 mL of water) might be helpful in preventing chemotherapy-induced mucositis. However, the preliminary results of Fidler and colleagues indicate that the use of diluted chemomile extracts does not decrease the severity of 5-fluorouracil-induced stomatitis [91].

In clinical praxis, sage tea and diluted tormentil or myrrh tincture are often recommended for the prophylaxis of chemotherapy- or radiation-induced mucositis. In some cases these solutions may be beneficial for the patient; however, they represent so far untested topical solutions.

Vitamins

Mills was among the first to report that the administration of α-carotene (250 mg/d for the first 3 weeks and 75 mg/d for the next 5 weeks) as a dietary supplement might be useful in decreasing the risk of grade 3 to 4 mucositis [92]. Wadleigh et al. recorded that the topical application of one milliliter of vitamin E oil (400 mg/mL) to oral lesions (e.g., twice a day for 5 days) may result in a more rapid and complete resolution of mucosal lesions [93]. However, in both cases double-blind, placebo-controlled trials are still lacking.

4.3 DIARRHEA AND CONSTIPATION

4.3.1 Diarrhea

Chemotherapy-induced diarrhea results from a direct toxic effect on the rapidly proliferating mucosal cells of the small and large intestine, but it may also be related to gastrointestinal infection, malabsorption, mechanical obstruction, or concomitant drug therapy, particulary antibiotics. Antimetabolites are the most common class of cytotoxic drugs causing diarrhea. Bloody diarrhea accompanying mucositis was most often seen after high-dose 5-fluorouracil (5-FU) regimens containing cisplatin and may be associated with an increased mortality rate [94]. Between 25 and 65% of patients with metastic colon cancer experience some degree of diarrhea associated with 5-FU. Hitherto, there has not appeared to be a significant difference between bolus administration or continuous infusion at comparable doses with respect to the incidence of severity of 5-FU-induced diarrhea. However, the addition of folinic acid or other biomodulators to 5-FU appeared to result in increased frequency and severity of diarrhea in a number of randomized trials. Especially in elderly patients, chemotherapy-induced diarrhea may be severe, causing fatal toxicity. The combination of nausea, vomiting, and profuse diarrhea can lead to profound dehydration and hypotension. Disruption of the integrity of the gut lining may permit access for enteric organisms into the bloodstream, possibly resulting in sepsis, particularly in neutropenic patients with diarrhea. As a consequence, 5-FU treatment should be stopped in the presence of ongoing mucositis or mild diarrhea, and subsequent doses should be reduced when the patient has fully recovered [95].

In patients with severe diarrhea, after the administration of 5-fluorouracil or cisplatin the synthetic polypeptide analogue of somatostatin, octreotide, has proven to be safe and effective [95,96]. In a randomized study, this drug revealed superiority over loperamide in patients with severe diarrhea induced by 5-fluorouracil [97]. Very recently this drug has also been proven to be very effective in patients who develop hematopoietic support-dependent, high-dose chemotherapy-related diarrhea. Dosage recommendations for subcutaneous administration range from 0.1 to 0.5 mg three times daily. However, randomized trials are needed to confirm the superior role of octreotide acetate in chemotherapy-induced severe diarrhea and to establish the optimal dose.

For the topoisomerase l- inhibitor irinotecan (CPT 11), diarrhea represents a dose-limiting toxicity. Two types of diarrhea are associated with the use of this agent. The first type has an early onset, during or immediately after the application of irinotecan (early cholinergic syndrome); the second type has a delayed onset, which may occur in up to 87% of patients. Undoubtedly, patients with concomitant severe diarrhea and myelosuppression are at a higher risk of developing severe infectious complications.

CPT-11-induced acute diarrhea is often accompanied by diaphoresis, abdominal cramps, and facial flushing. There is no evidence that the severity of this type of diarrhea can be effectively prevented or controlled by a prolonged infusion time (e.g., extension to 90 or 180 minutes), but the use of a parasympatholytic agent (e.g., 0.25 mg atropine sulfate IV) might be helpful.

The delayed type of diarrhea may begin several days after drug administration with a median duration of about 5 days (range: 1–34). Several risk factors have been identified for the frequency and severity of this side effect, including age (e.g., patients older than 65 years), previous abdominal/pelvic radiation therapy, and a high biliary index [99–103]. An intensified loperamide-containing regimen (e.g., 2 mg every 2 h) is highly recommended when the first loose stool is observed [104]. Very recently it has been suggested that the combination of a new enkephalinase inhibitor (Tiorfan) and high-dose loperamide may achieve the cessation of delayed diarrhea [105].

If there is any sign of infectious diarrhea, the oral use of sulfamethoxazole plus trimethoprim while awaiting the results of a stool culture may be useful. In patients with a manifest *Clostridium difficile*–associated colitis, the use of oral vancomycin (e.g., 125 mg four times daily for 10 days) appears to be most active. However, because this glycopeptide is far more expensive than metronidazole, it appears to be reasonable to use the latter as first-line therapy and to use the former in patients who fail to respond after 3 days of metronidazole therapy [95].

4.3.2 Constipation

The differential diagnosis of constipation in patients with cancer is diverse. Subacute constipation may be multifactorial, resulting from alterations in diet, decreased fluid intake, physical inactivity, and the use of narcotics or drugs with anticholinergic action (antidepressants). Constipation may also be induced by complications related to the tumor type, hypercalcemia, intestinal obstruction or spinal cord compression, and the use of anticholinergic drugs or opioids.

Autonomic nerve dysfunction manifesting as abdominal pain, constipation, or adynamic ileus has been reported in patients receiving vinca alkaloids like vincristine and vinblastine. The incidence of vincristine-induced constipation approximates 30–50% (see also Chapter 9, on neurotoxicity) [106,107]. The first symptoms are evident within a few days, which may make them particularly difficult to differentiate from acute gastrointestinal obstruction. With conservative treatment, the symptoms usually resolve after 1 or 2 weeks. To avoid constipation in patients receiving opioids and vinca alkaloids, the use of mild laxatives and stool softeners has been recommended.

REFERENCES

1. Schein PS, Macdonald JS, Waters C, Haidak D. Nutritional complications of cancer and its treatment. Semin Oncol 1975:2:337–347.
2. Deschner E, Lipkin M. Proliferation and differentiation of gastrointestinal cells in relation to therapy. Med Clin North Am 1971:55:601–612.
3. D'Acquisto R, Tyson LB, Gralla RJ, et al. The influence of chronic high alcohol intake on chemotherapy-induced nausea and vomiting. Proc Am Soc Clin Oncol 5:257:1986 (Abstr).
4. Hesketh PJ, Plagge P, Bryson JC. Single-dose ondensatron for prevention of acute cisplatin-induced emesis: Analysis of efficacy and prognostic factors. In : AL Bianci, L Grelot, AD Miller, et al, eds. Mechanism and Control of Emesis. London: Libbey, 1992, pp 25–26.
5. Tonato M, Roila F, Del Favero A. Methodology of antiemetic trials: A review. Ann Oncol 1991:2:107–114.
6. Grunberg SM, Hesketh PJ. Control of chemotherapy-induced emesis. N Engl J Med 1993:329:1790–1796.
7. Hesketh PJ. Treatment of chemotherapy-induced emesis in the 1990s: Impact of the 5-HT_3 receptor antagonists. Support Care Cancer 1994:2:286–292.
8. Perez EA. Review of the preclinical pharmacology and comparative efficacy of 5-hydroxytryptamine-3 receptor antagonists for chemotherapy-induced emesis. J Clin Oncol 1995:13:1036–1043.
9. Osoba D, Zee B, Pater J, Warr D, Latreille J, Kaizer L. Determinants of postchemotherapy nausea and vomiting in patients with cancer. Quality of Life and Symptom Control Committee of the National Cancer Institute of Canada Clinical Trials Group. J Clin Oncol 1997:15:116–123.
10. Carey MP, Burish TG. Anxiety as a predictor of behavioral therapy outcome for cancer chemotherapy patients. J Consult Clin Psychol 1985:53:860–865.
11. Wilcox PM, Fetting JH, Nettesheim KM, Abeloff MD. Anticipatory vomiting in women receiving cyclophosphamide, methotrexate, and 5-FU (CMF) adjuvant chemotherapy for breast carcinoma. Cancer Treatment Rep 1982:66: 1601–1604.
12. Wampler G. The pharmacology and clinical effectiveness of phenothiazines and related drugs for managing chemotherapy-induced emesis. Drugs 1983: 25(suppl 1):35–51.
13. Borison HL, McCarthy LE. Neuropharmacology of chemotherapy-induced emesis. Drugs 1983:25(suppl 1):8–17.
14. Akwari OE. The gastrointestinal tract in chemotherapy-induced emesis. A final common pathway. Drugs 1983:25(suppl 1):18–34.
15. Ison PJ, Peroutka SJ. Neurotransmitter receptor binding studies predict antiemetic efficacy and side effects. Cancer Treatment Rep 1986:70:637–641.
16. Stewart DJ. Nausea and vomiting in cancer patients. In: J Kuchaczyk, DJ Stewart, AD Miller, eds. Nausea and Vomiting: Recent Research in Clinical Advances. Boca Raton, FL: CRC Press, 1991, p 177.

17. Borison HL, Wang WC. Physiology and pharmacology of vomiting. Pharmacol Rev 1953:5:193–230.
18. Borison HL. Area postrema: Chemoreceptor trigger zone for vomiting: Is that all? Life Sci 1974:14:1807–1817.
19. Young RW. Mechanisms in treatment of radiation-induced nausea and vomiting. In: CJ David, GV Lake-Bakaar, DG Graham-Smith, eds. Nausea and Vomiting: Mechanisms and Treatment. Berlin: Springer-Verlag, 1986, p 94.
20. Dodds LJ. The control of cancer therapy-induced nausea and vomiting. J Clin Hosp Pharm 1985:10:143–166.
21. Seigel LJ, Longo DL. The control of chemotherapy-induced emesis. Ann Intern Med 1981:955:352–359.
22. Kaizer L, Warr D, Hoskins P, et al. The effect of schedule and maintenance on the antiemetic efficacy of ondansetron combined with dexamethasone in acute and delayed nausea and emesis in patients receiving moderately emetogenic chemotherapy: A phase III trial by the National Cancer Institute of Canada Clinical Trials Group. J Clin Oncol 1994:12:1050–1057.
23. Warr D, Willan AR, Fine S, et al. A double-blind comparison of granisetron with dexamethasone plus prochlorperazine for the prevention of nausea and emesis due to moderately emetogenic chemotherapy. J Natl Cancer Inst 1991: 83:1169–1173.
24. Latreille J, Stewart D, Laberge F, et al. Dexamethasone improves the efficacy of granisetron in the first 24 h following high-dose cisplatin chemotherapy. Support Care Cancer 1995:3:307–312.
25. Morrow GR, Dobkin PL. Anticipatory nausea and vomiting in cancer patients undergoing chemotherapy treatment: Prevalence, etiology, and behavioral interventions. Clin Psychol Rev 1988:8:517.
26. D'Acquisto RW, Tyson LB, et al. Antiemetic trials to control delayed vomiting following high-dose cisplatin. Proc Am Soc Clin Oncol 1986:5:257.
27. Holland JF, Frey E III, eds. Cancer Medicine, 2nd ed. Philadelphia: Lea & Febiger, 1982, p 2332.
28. Stewart DJ. Nausea and vomiting in cancer patients. In J Kochaczyk, DJ Stewart, AD Miller, eds. Nausea and Vomiting: Recent Research and Clinical Advances. Boca Raton, FL: CRC Press, 1991, p 177.
29. Martin M, Diaz-Rubio E. Emesis during pregnancy: A new prognostic factor in chemotherapy-induced emesis. Ann Oncol 1990:1:152–153.
30. Osoba D, Zee B, Pater J, Warr D, Latreille J, Kaizer L. Determinants of postchemotherapy nausea and vomiting in patients with cancer. Quality of Life and Symptom Control Committees of the National Cancer Institute of Canada Clinical Trials Group. J Clin Oncol 1997:15:116–123.
31. Morrow GR, Hickok JT. Behavioral treatment of chemotherapy-induced nausea and vomiting. Oncology 1993:7:83–89.
32. Burish TG, Tope DM. Psychological techniques for controlling the adverse side effects of cancer chemotherapy: Findings from a decade of research. J Pain Symptom Manage 1992:7:287–301.

33. Laszlo J. Treatment of nausea and vomiting caused by cancer chemotherapy. Cancer Treatment Rev 1982:9:3–9.
34. Strum SB, McDermed JE, Pileggi J, Riech LP, Whitaker H. Intravenous metoclopramide: Prevention of chemotherapy-induced nausea and vomiting. A preliminary evaluation. Cancer 1984:53:1432–1439.
35. Craig JB, Powell BL. Review: The management of nausea and vomiting in clinical oncology. Am J Med Sci 1987:293:34–44.
36. Lindley JM, Bernhard S, Fields SM. Incidence and duration of chemotherapy-induced nausea and vomiting in the outpatient oncology population. J Clin Oncol 1989:7:1142–1149.
37. Aapro MS. Methodological issues in antiemetic studies. Invest New Drugs 1993:11:243–253.
38. Hesketh PJ, Kris MG, Grunberg SM, Beck T, Hainsworth JD, Harker G, Aapro MS, Gandara D, Lindley CM. Proposal for classifying the acute emetogenicity of cancer chemotherapy. J Clin Oncol 1997:1:103–109.
39. Lindley CM, Bernard S, Fields SM. Incidence and duration of chemotherapy-induced nausea and vomiting in the outpatient oncology population. J Clin Oncol 1989:7:1142–1149.
40. Gralla RJ, Itri LM, Pisko SE, Squillante AE, Kelsen DP, Braun DW Jr, Bordin LA, Braun TJ, Young CW. Antiemetic efficacy of high-dose metoclopramide: Randomized trials with placebo and prochlorperazine in patients with chemotherapy-induced nausea and vomiting. N Engl J Med 1981:305:905–909.
41. Laszlo J, Clark RA, Hanson DC, Tyson L, Crumpler L, Gralla R. Lorazepam in cancer patients treated with cisplatin: A drug having antiemetic, amnesic, and anxiolytic effects. J Clin Oncol 1985:3:864–869.
42. Kris MG, Gralla RJ, Tyson LB, Clark RA, Kelsen DP, Reilly LK, Groshen S, Bosl GJ, Kalman LA. Improved control of cisplatin-induced emesis with high-dose metoclopramide and with combinations of metoclopramide, dexamethasone, and diphenhydramine. Results of consecutive trials in 255 patients. Cancer 1985:55:527–534.
43. Kris MG, Gralla RJ, Tyson LB, Clark RA, Cirrincione C, Groshen S. Controlling delayed vomiting: Double-blind, randomized trial comparing placebo, dexamethasone alone, and metoclopramide plus dexamethasone in patients receiving cisplatin. J Clin Oncol 1989:7:108–114.
44. Rittenberg CN, Gralla RJ, Lettow LA, Cronin MD, Kardinal CG. New approaches in preventing delayed emesis: Altering the time of regimen initiation and use of combination chemotherapy in 109 patient trials. Proc Am Soc Oncol 1995:14:526 (Abstr).
45. Roila F, DeAngelis V, Cognetti F, et al. Ondensatron vs. granisetron, both combined with dexamethasone in the prevention of cisplatin-induced emesis: Italian Group for Antiemetic Research. Proc Am Soc Oncol 1995:14:523 (Abstr).
46. Kris MG, Gralla RJ, Tyson LB, Clark RA, Cirrincione C, Groshen S. Controlling delayed vomiting: double-blind, randomized trial comparing placebo,

dexamethasone alone, and metoclopramide plus dexamethasone in patients receiving cisplatin. J Clin Oncol 1989:7:108–114.
47. Dilly SG, Freidman C, Yocom K. Contribution of dexamethasone to antiemetic control with granisetron is greatest in patients at high risk of emesis. Proc Am Soc Oncol 1994:13:436 (Abstr).
48. Casper J, Casper S. Köhne-Wömpner CH, Bokemeyer C, Hecker H, Schmoll H-J. 5-HT_3 antagonist ondansetron for the treatment of chemotherapy-induced nausea and vomiting in an outpatient population. Int J Oncol 1994:4: 1283–1289.
49. Gralla RJ, Itri LM, Pisko SE, Squillante AE, Kelsen DP, Braun DW Jr, Brodin LA, Braun TJ, Young CW. Antiemetic efficacy of high-dose metocloramide: Randomized trials with placebo and prochlorperazine in patients with chemotherapy-induced nausea and vomiting. N Engl J Med 1981:305: 905–909.
50. De Mulder PH, Seynaeve C, Vermorken JB, van Liessum PA, Mols Jevdevic S, Allman EL, Beranek P, Verweij J. Ondansetron compared with high-dose metoclopramide in prophylaxis of acute and delayed cisplatin-induced nausea and vomiting. A multicenter, randomized, double-blind, crossover study. Ann Intern Med 1990:113:834–840.
51. Roila F, Ballatori E, Tonato M, Del Favero A. 5-HT_3 receptor antagonists: Differences and similarities. Eur J Cancer 1997:9:1364–1370.
52. Marty M, Pouillart P, Scholl S, Droz JP, Azab M, Brion N, Pujade Lauraine E, Paule B, Paes D, Bons J. Comparison of the 5-hydroxytryptamine-3 (serotonin) antagonist ondansetron (GR 38032F) with high-dose metoclopramide in the control of cisplatin-induced emesis. N Engl J Med 1990:322: 816–821.
53. Hainsworth J, Harvey W, Pendergrass K, Kasimis B, Oblon D, Monaghan G, Gandara D, Hesketh P, Khojasteh A, Harker G, et al. A single-blind comparison of intravenous ondansetron, a selective serotonin antagonist, with intravenous metoclopramide in the prevention of nausea and vomiting associated with high-dose cisplatin chemotherapy. J Clin Oncol 1991:9:721–728.
54. Kamanabrou D. Intravenous granisetron—Establishing the optimal dose. The Granisetron Study Group. Eur J Cancer 1992:28A(suppl):S6-11.
55. Morrow GR, Hickok JT, Rosenthal SN. Progress in reducing nausea and emesis. Comparisons of ondansetron (Zofran), granisetron (Kytril), and tropisetron (Navoban). Cancer 1995:76:343–357.
56. Navari R, Gandara D. Hesketh P, Hall S, Mailliard J, Ritter H, Friedman C, Fitts D. Comparative clinical trial of granisetron and ondansetron in the prophylaxis of cisplatin-induced emesis. The Granisetron Study Group. J Clin Oncol 1995:13:1242–1248.
57. The Consensus Conference on Antiemetic Therapy in Perugia, Italy, April 28–29, 1997.
58. Sonis ST. Epidemiology, frequency, distribution, mechanism and histopathology. In: DE Petersen, ST Sonis, eds. Oral Complications of Cancer Chemotherapy. The Hague: Nijhoff, 1983, pp 1–2.

59. Bleyer WA. The clinical pharmacology of methotrexate: New applications of an old drug. Cancer 1978:41:36–51.
60. Young RC, Chabner BA. An in vivo method for determining differential effects of chemotherapy on target tissues in animals and men. Correlation with plasmopharmacokinetics. J Clin Invest 1973:52:92 (Abstr).
61. Stoller RG, Jacobs SA, Draik JC, et al. Pharmacokinetics of high-dose methotrexate (NSC-47). Cancer Chemother Rep 1975:6:19–24.
62. Stoller RG, Hande KR, Jacobs SA, Rosenberg SA, Chabner BA. Use of plasma pharmacokinetics to predict and prevent methotrexate toxicity. N Engl J Med 1977:297:630–634.
63. Schappner BA, Jones DG, Bertiono JR. Enzymatic clevage of methotrexate provides a method for prevention of drug toxicity. Nature 1972:239:395–397.
64. Jacobs WA. Clinical pharmacology; current status and therapeutic guidelines. Cancer Treatment Rev 1977:4:87–101.
65. Jacobs SA, Bleyer WA, Chabner BA, Johns DG. Altered plasma pharmacokinetics of methotrexate administered intrathecally. Lancet 1977:1:455–456.
66. Schubert MM, Sullivan KM, Truelove EL. Head and neck complications of bone marrow transplantation. In: DE Petersen, EG Elias, ST Sonis, eds. Head and Neck Management of the Cancer Patient. Boston: Nijhoff, 1986, pp 401–427.
67. Schimpff SC. Infections in patients with cancer: Overview and epidemiology. In: AR Moossa, SC Schimpff, MC Roxen, eds. Comprehensive Textbook of Oncology, 2nd ed. Baltimore: Williams & Wilkens, 1991, pp 1720–1732.
68. Wingard JR. Infectious and non-infectious systemic consequences. NCI Monogr 1990:9:21–26.
69. Peterson DE. Oral toxicity of chemotherapeutic agents. Semin Oncol 1992: 19:478–491.
70. Verdi CJ. Cancer therapy and oral mucositis. Drug Safety 1993:9(3):185–195.
71. Marks JE. Mucosal protectants and their application for head and neck chemoirradiation. Curr Opin Oncol 1997:9:267–273.
72. LeVegue FG, Parzuchowski JB, Farinacci GC, et al. Clinical evaluation of MGI 209, an anesthetic, film-forming agent for relief from painful oral ulcers associated with chemotherapy. J Clin Oncol 1992:10:1963–1968.
73. Foote RL, Loprinzi CL, Frank AR, et al. Randomized trial of a chlorhexidine mouthwash for alleviation of radiation-induced mucositis. J Clin Oncol 1994: 12:2630–2633.
74. Kaanders JHAM, Pop LAM, Uitterhoeve RJ, van Daal WAJ. Prevention of irradiation mucositis in the oral cavity and oropharynx by PTA-lozenges. Int J Radiat Oncol Biol Phys 1993:27(suppl 1):253 (Abstr).
75. Okuno SH, Foote RL, Loprinzi CL, et al. A randomized trial of a nonabsorbable antibiotic lozenge given to alleviate radiation-induced mucositis. Cancer 1997:79:2193–2199.
76. Dumontet C, Sonnet A, Bastion Y, et al. Prevention of high-dose L-PAM-induced mucositis by cryotherapy. Bone Marrow Transplant 1994:14:492–494.

77. Loprinzi CL, Foote RL, Michalak J. Alleviation of cytotoxic therapy-induced normal tissue damage. Semin Oncol 1995:22(suppl 3):95–97.
78. Rocke LK, Loprinzi CL, Lee JK, et al. A randomized clinical trial of two different durations of oral cryotherapy for prevention of 5-fluorouracil-related stomatitis. Cancer 1993:72:2234–2238.
79. Oblon DJ, Paul SR, Oblon MB, Malik S. Propantheline protects the oral mucosa after high-dose ifosfamide, carboplatin, etoposide and autologous stem cell transplantation. Bone Marrow Transplant 1997:20:961–963.
80. Foster-Nora J, Siden R. Amifostine for protection from antineoplastic drug toxicity. Am J Health-Syst Pharm 1997:54:787–800.
81. Gabrilove JL, Jakubowski A, Scher H, et al. Effect of G-CSF on neutropenia and associated morbidity due to chemotherapy for transitional-cell carcinoma of the urothelium. N Engl J Med 1988:318:1414–1422.
82. Pettengell R, Gurney H, Radford JA, et al. G-CSF to prevent dose-limiting neutropenia in non-Hodgkin's lymphoma: A randomized controlled trial. Blood 1992:80:1430–1436.
83. Pfeiffer P, Madsen EL, Hansen O, May O. Effect of prophylactic sucralfate suspension on stomatitis induced by cancer chemotherapy: A randomized, double-blind, cross-over study. Acta Oncol 1990:29:171–173.
84. McGinnis WL, Loprinzi CL, Buskirk SJ, et al. Placebo-controlled trial of sucralfate for inhibitin radiation-induced esophagitis. J Clin Oncol 1997:15: 1239–1243.
85. Loprinzi CL, Ghosh C, Comoriano J, et al. Phase III controlled evaluation of sucralfate to alleviate stomatitis in patients receiving fluorouracil-based chemotherapy. J Clin Oncol 1997:15:1235–1238.
86. Clark PI, Slevin ML. Allopurinol mouthwash and 5-fluorouracil-induced oral toxicity. Eur J Surg Oncol 1985:11:267–268.
87. Loprinzi CL, Cianflone SG, Dose AM, et al. A controlled evaluation of an allopurinol mouthwash as prophylaxis against 5-fluorouracil-induced stomatitis. Cancer 1990:65:1879–1882.
88. Kührer I, Kuzmits R, Linkesch W, Ludwig H. Topical PGE_2 enhances healing of chemotherapy-associated mucosal lesions. Lancet 1986:1:623.
89. Porteder H, Rausch E, Kent G, et al. Local prostaglandin E_2 in patients with oral malignancies undergoing chemo- and radiotherapy. Cranio-Maxill Facial Surg 1988:16:371–374.
90. Labar B, Mrsic M, Pavletic Z, et al. Prostaglandin E_2 for prophylaxis of oral mucositis following bone marrow transplantation. Bone Marrow Transplant 1993:11:379–382.
91. Fidler P, Loprinzi CL, O'Fallon JR, et al. Prospective evaluation of a chamomille mouthwash for prevention of 5-FU-induced oral mucositis. Cancer 1996:77:522–525.
92. Mills EED. The modifying effect of beta-carotene on radiation and chemotherapy induced oral mucositis. Br J Cancer 1988:57:416–417.
93. Wadleigh RG, Redman RS, Graham ML, et al. Vitamin E in the treatment of chemotherapy-induced mucositis. Am J Med 1992:92:481–484.

94. Sherlock P, ed. Effect of cancer treatment on nutrition and gastrointestinal function. Clin Bull 1979:9:136–145.
95. Cascinu S. Management of diarrhea induced by tumours of cancer therapy. Curr Opin Oncol 1995:7:325–329.
96. Cascinu S, Fedeli A, Luzi Fedeli SF, et al. Control of chemotherapy-induced diarrhea with octreotide: A randomized trial with placebo in patients receiving cisplatin. Oncology 1994:51:70–73.
97. Cascinu S, Fedeli A, Fedeli SL, Catalano G. Octreotide versus loperamide in the treatment of fluorouracil-induced diarrhea: A randomized trial. J Clin Oncol 1993:11:148–155.
98. Wasserman EI, Hidalgo M, Hornedo J, Cortés-Funes H. Octreotide (SMS 201-995) for hematopoietic support-dependent high-dose chemotherapy (HSD-HDC)-related diarrhea: Dose finding study and evaluation of efficacy. Bone Marrow Transplant 1997:20:711–714.
99. Rougier P, Bugat R, Douillard JY, Culine S, SUC E, et al. Phase II study of irinotecan in the treatment of advanced colorectal cancer in chemotherapy-naive patients and patients pretreated with fluorouracil-based chemotherapy. J Clin Oncol 1997:15:251–260.
100. Abigerges D, Armand JP, Chabot GG, et al. Irinotecan (CPT-11) high-dose escalation using intensive high-dose loperamide to control diarrhea. J Natl Cancer Inst 1994:86:446–449.
101. Mick R, Gupta E, Vokes EE, Ratain MJ. Limited sampling models for irinotecan pharmacokinetics-pharmacodynamics: Prediction of biliary index and intestinal toxicity. J Clin Oncol 1996:14:2012–2019.
102. Gandia D, Abigterges D, Armand JP. CPT-11 induced cholinergic effects in cancer patients. J Clin Oncol 1993:11:196–197.
103. Gupta E, Lestingi TM, Mick R, et al. Metabolic fate of irinotecan (CPT-11) in humans: Correlation of glucuronidation with diarrhea. Cancer Res 1994: 54:3723–3725.
104. Ikuno N, Soda H, Wantanabe M, et al. Irinotecan (CPT-11) and characteristic mucosal changes in the mouse ileum and cecum. Natl Cancer Inst 1995:84: 697–702.
105. Bleiberg H, Cvitkovic E. Characterisation and clinical management of CPT-11-induced adverse events: The European perspective. Eur J Cancer 1996: 32A(suppl 3):S18–S23.
106. Holland JF, Scharlau C, Gailani S, et al. Vincristin treatment of advanced cancer: A cooperative study of 392 cases. Cancer Res 1973:33:1258–1264.
107. Sandler SG, Topin W, Henderson ES. Vincristine induced neuropathy: A clinical study of 50 leukemia patients. Neurology (MINN) 1969:19:367–374.

5

Dermatological Toxicity and Hypersensitivity Reactions Associated with the Use of Cytostatics

HANS-PETER LIPP
University of Tübingen, Tübingen, Germany

5.1 INTRODUCTION

The onset of dermatological complications during or after cancer therapy can be related to many factors: it may be an early sign of radiation injury or a result of infection, metastatic infiltrates, or graft-versus-host disease.

Skin reactions directly associated with the use of special cytostatic drugs (Table 1) may be the result of enhanced cutaneous accumulation (e.g., after high-dose thiotepa) or direct toxic reactions toward keratinocytes, melanocytes, or lymphocytes. The latter may be synergistically influenced by concomitant exposure to UV light. Clinical symptoms of drug-induced skin toxicity include sclerodermoid reactions, acral erythema, severe sunburnlike reactions, and pigmentation or nail disorders. Erythemas based on hypersensitivity reactions might be the result of an immunization reaction that is enforced by allergizing adjuvants, particularly Cremophor EL or Polysorbate 80 (Table 2), or by the chemical reactivity of the cytostatic drug itself against physiological constituents [1,2].

However, for many patients the loss of hair is the most unpleasant dermatological and overall side effect of cancer chemotherapy, because it shows everybody that there is "something wrong." Hair bulb cells divide every 12 to 24 hours, which makes them very sensitive to the antiproliferative effect of antineoplastic agents. The loss of hair begins usually 7–10

Table 1 Dermatologic Toxicities of Cytostatics

Effect	Drugs
Alopecia	Actinomycin D, amsacrine, BCNU, bleomycin, cyclophosphamide, cytarabine, daunorubicin, docetaxel, doxorubicin, etoposide, 5-fluorouracil, hydroxyurea, ifosfamide, mechlorethamine, methotrexate, paclitaxel, thiotepa, vincristine, vindesine, vinblastine
Pigmentation disorders	Diffuse: busulfan, cyclophosphamide, actinomycin D, 5-fluorouracil, hydroxyurea, methotrexate
Radiation enhancement reactions	Actinomycin D, bleomycin, doxorubicin 5-fluorouracil, hydroxyurea, methotrexate
Radiation recall reactions	Actinomycin D, bleomycin, doxorubicin, etoposide, hydroxyurea, methotrexate, trimetrexate, vinblastine
Reactions associated with ultraviolet light	Phototoxic: dacarbazine, 5-fluorouracil, thioguanine, vinblastine Reaction of sunburn: methotrexate
Acral erythema	Cyclophosphamide, cytarabine, doxorubicin, 5-fluorouracil, hydroxyurea, methotrexate, mitotane, 6-mercaptopurine

days after the start of chemotherapy and proceeds over 1–2 months. After 6 weeks alopecia is generally reversible, although in individual cases, structure and color of hair may be changed [3,4].

5.1.1 Alopecia

For many cancer patients alopecia is one of the most distressing side effects of cancer chemotherapy or radiotherapy. One study showed that more than 85% of the women who were treated preoperatively with antineoplastic agents considered the loss of hair the most burdensome aspect of treatment [3]. As a consequence, alopecia induces a negative body image and may alter interpersonal relationships and generate noncompliance regarding further treatment cycles. Since, however, alopecia is not life-threatening compared to pancytopenia or severe stomatitis, it should not be prevented by dosage reduction or early discontinuation of therapy, particularly if therapy is curative. During palliative treatment it may be reasonable to use anticancer drugs like gemcitabine, vinorelbine, and mitoxantrone, which induce only mild alopecia.

Other drugs like the oxazaphosphorines, the anthracyclines, bleomycin, amsacrine, and actinomycin D, the taxanes, etoposide, and methotrexate gen-

Table 2 Allergizing Adjuvants and Preservatives Commonly Used in Commercially Available Preparations Containing Cytostatics

Solubilizing adjuvants
Polyoxyethylated castor oil (Cremophor EL)
Polysorbate 80
Poly(1-vinyl-2-pyrrolidone)
Propylene glycol
N,N-Dimethylacetamide
Macrogol 300
Benzyl alcohol
Preservatives
Methylparaben and propylparaben (methyl- and propylhydroxy benzoate)
Sodium bisulfite

erally induce reversible alopecia [1]. Some authors suggest that the use of cold caps may be effective in the prevention of cytostatic-induced alopecia. Based on transient hypothermia, cutaneous vasoconstriction is induced which decreases local blood flow as well as the amount of drug level reaching the hair follicles. Additionally, the metabolism to active intermediates may be impaired by lower temperatures [5]. Clinical experience demonstrates that hair preservation is improved if a cap temperature of about −25°C is achieved by maintaining the cap for at least 12 hours in a freezer. Most studies use a postinjection cooling time of 30 minutes (15–60 min). It has been suggested that about 85% hair preservation may be achievable if scalp hypothermia is initiated [6].

The criticism has been advanced that cold caps may favor the development of scalp metastases, particularly in hematological malignancies, if tumor cells had spread to the scalp before chemotherapy. However, several studies indicate that there is no fear of increased scalp metastases after local hypothermia. In conclusion, the use of cold caps during palliative therapy may be helpful to increase patients' quality of life during the treatment with taxanes or anthracyclines. The routine use of cold caps in patients who are treated curatively cannot be widely recommended as long as further studies are lacking, however.

Generally, the cold caps are well tolerated, headaches and unpleasant cold sensations being the most prominent side effects. If the safe use of cold caps is confirmed by further studies, this supportive care may be recommended during therapy with taxanes, anthracyclines, and other antineoplastic agents [7,8]. A supportive strategy based on the topical use of minoxidil cannot be recommended at the present time because there is a lack of proven efficacy as well as the risk of severe hypotonia [9].

5.1.2 Hypersensitivity Reactions

Allergic and anaphylactoid reactions are generally rare during treatment with cytotoxic drugs [2]. As in the case of VePesid, which contains considerable amounts of Polysorbate 80, suddenly a coarse, spotted, reddish-purple exanthema may develop. In more severe cases respiratory problems (e.g., dyspnea, bronchospasms, cyanosis) may develop as well as changes in blood pressure and tachycardia may be observed. If these effects are observed, the infusion should be stopped and diphenhydramine as well as hydrocortisone should be administered. If symptoms are more severe, the use of epinephrine will be unavoidable (Table 3) [2,10,11].

The development of hypersensitivity reactions is mainly based on (a) preparations containing high amounts of potentially sensitizing adjuvants (Table 2), (b) the use of unphysiological high molecular weight proteins, particularly asparaginase preparations, or (c) drugs that act as haptens based on their high reactivity against physiological macromolecules, resulting in the development of more or less active immunogens [2,12,13]. Sometimes a preceding therapy with cytokines, (e.g., interleukin-2) may accelerate the onset of hypersensitivity reaction [14].

5.1.2.1 Hypersensitivity Reactions Primarily Based on Adjuvants

Undoubtedly the sort and amount of adjuvants or preservatives used in commercially available preparations plays an important role in the development

Table 3 Recommendations for Managing Acute Hypersensitivity Reactions

1. Interrupt the intravenous application immediately.
2. Inject epinephrine (0.35–0.5 mL, 1:1000, IV), eventually every 15–20 minutes, until reactions resolve (no more than 6 doses).
3. Inject an H_1 antihistaminic agent (e.g., diphenhydramine, 50 mg).
4. If hypotension persists after the maximum recommended amount of epinephrine has been given, the use of plasma volume expanders is recommended.
5. Oral inhalation of synthetic sympathomimetic amines (e.g., terbutaline) or glucocorticoids (e.g., beclomethasone) is indicated for bronchospasms.
6. The prophylactic use of glucocorticoids (e.g., methylprednisolone 125 mg IV) prevents delayed-type hypersensitivity.

of hypersensitivity reactions [2,13]. Some antineoplastic agents that are almost insoluble in aqueous solutions must be mixed with solubilizers or stabilizers to permit parenteral application [15,16]. However adjuvants like Cremophor EL or Polysorbate 80, which are still used in several preparations, are responsible for an unusually high incidence of anaphylactoid reactions that sometimes are potentially life threatening. In a recent comparison of the commercially available preparations VePesid and Etopophos, it was demonstrated that the risk of allergic reactions can be diminished if highly allergic adjuvants are avoided [17].

The Semisynthetic Polophyllotoxin Derivatives Etoposide (VePesid and Etopophos) and Teniposide (Vumon)

Chills, fever, bronchospasms, dyspnea, and tachycardia, as well as hypotension, have been reported in 0.7–2% of cancer patients after the IV administration of VePesid. These symptoms closely resemble an allergic or anaphylactoid reaction and may occur during or shortly after the first infusion of the etoposide-containing preparation VePesid [10,11].

There seems to be a strong relationship between the development of allergic reactions and the amount of adjuvants in commercially available etoposide preparations that contain considerable amounts of ethanol, benzyl alcohol, and polysorbate, as well as polyethylene glycol. This assumption is strengthened by the fact that a novel analogue, etoposide phosphate, which is highly soluble in aqueous solutions and no longer needs those adjuvants for solubilization, is associated with a much lower incidence of hypersensitivity reactions than VePesid. However, it cannot be excluded that very rare cases of allergic and anaphylactoid reactions may be mediated by the drug itself [18,19].

The commercially available preparation of the structurally related teniposide contains considerable amounts of adjuvants, too. As mentioned before, Polyoxyl 35 castor oil (Cremophor EL, polyoxyethylated castor oil) has been reported to possess an extraordinarily high allergic potency [16]. Some data suggest that the overall frequency of hypersensitivity reactions may be as high as 50% if Cremophor EL is infused intravenously. Patients who have experienced rather severe allergic or anaphylactoid reactions should receive further infusions with extreme caution after consideration of the risk–benefit ratio [20].

Paclitaxel (Taxol)

A well-known example of the phenomenon of adjuvants being highly responsible for the development of allergic and anaphylactoid reactions is Taxol: The commercial preparation contains high amounts of ethanol and

Cremophor EL for solubilization of the rather water-insoluble paclitaxel [15].

It has been long known that this solubilizer causes severe allergic reactions. Prophylaxis with H_1- and H_2-antihistaminics and with glucocorticoids is therefore warranted before Taxol is applied (Fig. 1). Previously it had been suggested that a single intravenous application of a corticosteroid (e.g., 20 mg dexamethasone IV 30 min before Taxol administration) in combination with antihistaminic agents may be sufficient to avoid the occurrence of life-threatening hypersensitivity reactions [21–23]. In some cases mild allergic reactions (flushing, rash, dyspnea) may occur in spite of an adequate premedication regimen. However, in clinical trials thus far, none of these mild reactions required interruption of therapy [24].

It cannot be excluded that an improper admixing of Taxol concentrates may result in an inhomogeneous dispersion of Cremophor EL in the infusion bottle. As a consequence, an initial bolus infusion of highly concentrated Cremophor EL could facilitate the onset of anaphylactoid-like reactions [20].

The structurally related docetaxel, which is commercially available as Taxotere, is solubilized not with Cremophor EL but with Polysorbate 80%. However, the use of Taxotere is also associated with the development of severe skin reactions (e.g., erythema, desquamation, exfoliation, peripheral edemas, nail toxicity, and particularly painful oncholysis). As a consequence, at least one day before, on the day of treatment, as well as on the following day, prophylactic administration of corticosteroids (e.g., 8 mg dexamethasone PO twice daily) is highly recommended to minimize the risk of severe skin toxicity. It cannot be excluded that the taxane structure itself may exert some antigenic features, too [25].

5.1.2.2 Hypersensitivity Reactions Based on the Cytotoxic Drug Itself

Most cases of hypersensitivity reactions induced by cytostatic drugs have been associated with the use of melphalan, platinum compounds, and L-asparaginase [26–28]. Sometimes, after the use of dacarbazine, severe skin reactions have been observed, which seem to be due mainly to increased photosensitivity [29,30].

Melphalan

Melphalan is a bifunctional alkylating agent, used primarily for the treatment of multiple myeloma, ovarian carcinoma, and primary amyloidosis [31].

Skin hypersensitivity, allergic reactions, pruritus, rash, edema, tachycardia, and bronchospasms, as well as hypotension, have been observed in

requesting ward	telefone	date	time
patient No.:			

EBERHARD-KARLS-UNIVERSITY TÜBINGEN

PROTOCOL OF CHEMOTHERAPY

height: cm

weight: kg

surface: 2,0 m^2

medical clinic and policlinic

diagnosis:	**protocol:**
breast cancer (previously treated with cisplatin)	Paclitaxel-monotherapy

chemotherapy month: cycle day: day:

drug (INN)	mg/m²	dose, mg	mode of appl.[1]	carrier[2]	final volume	duration of inf.
Paclitaxel	175	350	i.v.	NaCl 0.9%	~500 ml	3 h

remarks:
use IVEX-HP-in-line filter (pore size < 0.22 μm)

supportive measures

cycle day	drug/infusion	dose	mode of appl.[1]	carrier[2]	duration of inf.	ml/hr	−4	−2	0	2	4	6	8	10	12	¼
1	Dexamethasone	20 mg	p.o./i.v.	12 hr and 6 hr before Paclitaxel												
1	Diphenhydramine	50 mg	i.v.	30 min. before Paclitaxel												
1	Ranitidine	50 mg	i.v.	30 min. before Paclitaxel												
1	Alizapride	100 mg	i.v.	15 min. before Paclitaxel												

1) bolus, infusion, perfusor, s.c., i.th., i.m., p.o.
2) NaCl 0.9%, glucose 5%, undiluted

date signature of clinician

Fig. 1 Generally recommended premedications to avoid severe hypersensitivity reactions during or after administration of Taxol.

about 2% of patients who received melphalan intravenously [26,31,32]. In several patients oral melphalan induced signs of allergy, too. However, the incidence will be increased if several courses of melphalan are administered.

The direct reactivity against a variety of natural proteins containing functional groups (e.g., SH groups) may be responsible for the development of both the immunogenic effect of melphalan and the hypersensitivity reactions [33,34].

L-Asparaginase and Related Compounds

Up to 40% of cancer patients treated with asparaginase-containing preparations may develop IgE-mediated allergic reactions, especially if the doses are as high as 5000 U/m^2 or more, applied IV three times per week, continued over several weeks [2,35,36].

If L-asparaginase is combined with other cytostatics or if it is administered intramuscularly, the incidence rate appears to be lower. The clinical manifestation of the hypersensitivity reaction is characterized by reddenings of the skin, urticaria, and a swelling at the injection site. In the advanced stage an anaphylactic shock cannot be excluded.

To identify predisposed patients in timely fashion, the patient's reaction can be tested on 2 U of asparaginase in 0.1 mL of sodium chloride 0.9% with an intradermal injection. If urticaria or erythema around the injection site appears within an hour, an allergic predisposition is highly probable. However, the reliability of this test is still a matter of controversy because some evidence indicates that it may lead to false positive and false negative results [2].

Generally, patients who show an allergic reaction to L-asparaginase isolated from *Escherichia coli* may tolerate L-asparaginase from *Erwinia chrysanthemi* (=erwinase) or pegaspargase, in which the original protein is linked to polyethylene glycol. These latter preparations, being structurally dissimilar to asparaginase (*E. coli*), seem to possess different antigenic epitopes [37].

Platinum Compounds

The possible onset of hypersensitivity reactions in patients who receive repeated courses containing platinum compounds like cisplatin or carboplatin is well established. The incidence of allergic reactions (e.g., facial swelling, flushing, wheezing or respiratory difficulties, tachycardia, hypotension) ranges from 5 to 20%. The onset of symptoms may be evident within a few minutes after IV administration and has been observed in children as well as adult cancer patients [38].

Premedication with steroids and antihistamines may successfully prevent the onset of allergic symptoms in some but not all patients.

It has been proposed that the allergic reactions are primarily based on the high reactivity of platinum compounds, particularly cisplatin, to physiological macromolecules and that an immunization against these unphysiological macromolecular platinum-containing adducts then results [39–42].

Dacarbazine (DTIC)

It has been long known that dacarbazine undergoes photodegradation under light exposure. This property is of clinical importance because the degradation product azahypoxanthine appears to be very toxic [43,44]. As a consequence, skin manifestations (e.g., pruritus, erythema, edema) are based on increased photosensitivity reactions occurring exclusively on sun-exposed skin. As a consequence, the wearing of protective clothing for a few hours after DTIC infusion has been recommended to avoid sunlight-induced dermatological toxicity [29,30].

5.2 FOCAL AND DIFFUSE SKIN REACTIONS NOT BASED ON HYPERSENSITIVITY REACTIONS

Cutaneous hyperpigmentation disorders have been observed after the administration of alkylating agents like busulfan, cyclophosphamide, and thiotepa. Photoaccentuated pigmentation disorders have been demonstrated after the use of methotrexate, 5-fluorouracil, and actinomycin D [1].

In the case of high-dose thiotepa, the secretion of the drug via sweat may be responsible for the development of skin reactions [45]. As a consequence, it is recommended that patients shower thoroughly twice daily on the days high-dose thiotepa is administered, to ensure prompt removal of the drug from the skin [46]. The pigmentation disorder may be caused by a direct toxic effect of cutaneously accumulated thiotepa [47].

Radiation recall reactions are observed if treatment with x-rays precedes the therapy with cytostatics. Later during the course of radiotherapy, the epidermis may show signs of dry desquamation because of the failure of the basal layer to produce new cells. The skin reaction will last for 7–14 days after the radiation is stopped. As a consequence, the concomitant use of antiproliferatively acting cytostatics may amplify the complex nature of radiodermatitis. It has thus far been very difficult to recommend any special topical treatment (e.g., Bepanthen Cream) to prevent such skin reactions [48].

Acral erythemas not primarily due to hypersensitivity reactions have been associated with the use of 5-fluorouracil, cytarabine, and doxorubicin, particularly after high-dose chemotherapy or prolonged infusion [1].

In the case of 5-fluorouracil (5-FU) the development of a palmar–plantar erythrodysesthesia syndrome (PPES), or hand–foot syndrome, has been well established. The syndrome is characterized by erythematous, scanty eruptions affecting the soles, toes, and palms, as well as a tingling sensation in the palms and soles, progressing to frank pain in a few days. Previously underestimated, the incidence of this condition is estimated to approximate 7%. The etiopathogenesis of this skin reaction is not fully understood. Indeed, the possibility that it is due to an idiosyncratic reaction or a cutaneous drug accumulation cannot be excluded. Vitamin B_6 up to 150 mg daily has been successfully used to reverse or prevent PPES. However, further clinical trials are warranted before the routine use of vitamin B_6 can be recommended for the prevention of 5-FU-induced PPES [49–51].

Some patients may develop a cytarabine syndrome 6–12 hours after administration of the antimetabolite. This syndrome is characterized by symptoms like high fever, rigor, diaphoresis, myalgia, keratoconjunctivitis, and maculopapular rashes. Because most patients considered in one study had been treated with cytarabine it has been suggested that the cytarabine syndrome may be a result of an immunologic reaction and vasculitis [52]. If symptoms require treatment, administration of corticosteroids should be considered, as well as discontinuation of cytarabine therapy [53–55].

REFERENCES

1. DeSpain JD. Dermatological toxicity of chemotherapy. Semin Oncol 1992:19: 501–507.
2. Weiss RB. Hypersensitivity reactions. Semin Oncol 1992:19:458–477.
3. Kiebert GM, de Haes JCJM, Kievit J, et al. Effect of preoperative chemotherapy on the quality of life of patients with early breast cancer. Eur J Cancer 1990:26:1038–1042.
4. Loureiro C, Gill PS, Rarick M, et al. Red hair and hyperpigmentation in a black man after chemotherapy. J Clin Oncol 1987:5:1705–1706.
5. Bulow J, Friberg L, Gaardsting O, Hansen M. Frontal subcutaneous blood flow, and epi- and subcutaneous temperatures during scalp cooling in normal man. Scand J Clin Lab Invest 1985:45:505–508.
6. Lemenager M, Lecomte S, Bonneterre ME, et al. Effectiveness of cold cap in the prevention of docetaxel-induced alopecia. Eur J Cancer 1997:33:297–300.
7. Anderson JE, Hunt JM, Smith JE. Prevention of doxorubicin-induced alopecia by scalp cooling in patients with advanced breast cancer. Br Med J 1981:282: 423–424.
8. Satterwhite B, Zimm S. The use of scalp hypothermia in the prevention of doxorubicin-induced hair loss. Cancer 1984:54:34–37.
9. Rodriguez R, Machiavelli M, Leone B, et al. Minoxidil as a prophylaxis of doxorubicin-induced alopecia. Ann Oncol 1994:5:769–770.

10. Hoetelmans RMW, Schornagel JH, ten Bokkel Huinink WW, Beijnen JH. Hypersensitivity reactions to etoposide. Ann Pharmacother 1996:30:367–371.
11. Hudson MM, Weinstein HJ, Donaldson SS, et al. Acute hypersensitivity reactions to etoposide in a VEPA regimen for Hodgkin's disease. J Clin Oncol 1993:11:1080–1084.
12. Weiss RB, Donehower RC, Wiernik PH, et al. Hypersensitivity reactions from Taxol. J Clin Oncol 1990:8:1263–1268.
13. Wilson JP, Solimando DA, Edwards MS. Parenteral benzyl alcohol–induced hypersensitivity reaction. Drug Intell Clin Pharm 1986:20:689–691.
14. Heywood GR, Rosenberg SA, Weber S. Hypersensitivity reactions to chemotherapy agents in patients receiving chemoimmunotherapy with high-dose interleukin-2. J Natl Cancer Inst 1995:87:915–922.
15. Krämer I, Heuser A. Paclitaxel—Pharmaceutical and pharmacological issues. Eur J Hosp Pharm 1995:1:37–42.
16. Beijnen JH, Beijnen-Bandhoe AU, Dubbelman AC, van Gijn R, Underberg WJM. Chemical and physical stability of etoposide and teniposide in commonly used infusion fluids. J Parent Sci Technol 1991:45:108–112.
17. Joel SP. The clinical pharmacology of etoposide: An update. Cancer Treatment Rev 1996:22:179–221.
18. Brooks DJ, Srinivas NR, Alberts DS, et al. Phase I and pharmacokinetic study of etoposide phosphate. Anticancer Drugs 1995:6:637–644.
19. Kaul S, Igwemezie LN, Stewart DJ, et al. Pharmacokinetics and bioequivalence of etoposide following intravenous administrations of etoposide phosphate and etoposide in patients with solid tumors. J Clin Oncol 1995:13:2835–2841.
20. Theis JGW, Liau-Chu M, Chan HSL, et al. Anaphylactoid reactions in children receiving high-dose intravenous cyclosporine for reversal of tumor resistance: The causative role of improper dissolution of Cremophor EL. J Clin Oncol 1995:13:2508–2516.
21. Weiss RB, Donehower RC, Wiernik PH, et al. Hypersensitivity reactions from Taxol. J Clin Oncol 1990:8:1263–1268.
22. Lubejiko BG, Sartorius SE. Nursing considerations in paclitaxel (Taxol) administration. Semin Oncol 1993:20(suppl 3):26–30.
23. Boehm DK, Maksymiuk AW. Paclitaxel premedication regimens. J Natl Cancer Inst 1996:88:463–465.
24. Del-Priore G, Smith P, Warshal DP, et al. Paclitaxel-associated hypersensitivity reaction despite high-dose steroids and prolonged infusion. Gynecol Oncol 1995:56:316–318.
25. Verweij J. Docetaxel (Taxotere): A new anticancer drug with promising potential? Br J Cancer 1994:70:183–184.
26. Bleichner F, Mende S. Allergische Reaktion auf Melphalan? Onkologie 1982: 5:195.
27. Weidmann B, Mülleneisen N, Bojko P, Niederle N. Hypersensitivity reactions to carboplatin: Report of two patients, review of the literature and discussion of diagnostic procedures and management. Cancer 1994:73:2218–2222.

28. Koerholz D, Brueck M, Nuernberger W, et al. Chemical and immunological characteristics of four different L-asparaginase preparations. Eur J Hematol 1989:42:417–424.
29. Serrano G, Aliaga A, Febrer I, et al. Dacarbazine-induced photosensitivity. Photodermatology 1989:6:140–141.
30. Beck TM, Hart NE, Smith CE. Photosensitivity reaction following DTIC administration. Report of two cases. Cancer Treatment Rep 1980:64:725–726.
31. Farmer PB, Newell DR. Alkylating agents. In: MM Ames, G Powis, JS Kovach, eds. Pharmacokinetics of anticancer agents in humans. Amsterdam: Elsevier, 1983:pp 187–206.
32. Bolton MG, Hilton J, Robertson KD, et al. Kinetic analysis of the reaction of melphalan with water, phosphate and glutathione. Drug Metab Dispos 1993: 21:986–996.
33. Samuels BL, Bitran JD. High-dose intravenous melphalan—A review. J Clin Oncol 1995:13:1786–1789.
34. Cornwell GG, Pajak TF, MyIntyre OR. Hypersensitivity reactions to IV melphalan during treatment of multiple myeloma: Cancer and leukemia group B experience. Cancer Treatment Rep 1979:63:399–403.
35. Haskell CM, Canellos GP, Leventhal BG, et al. L-Asparaginase: Therapeutic and toxic effects in patients with neoplastic disease. N Engl J Med 1969:281: 1028–1034.
36. Land VJ, Sotow WW, Fernbach DJ, et al. Toxicity of L-asparaginase in children with advanced leukemia. Cancer 1972:40:339–347.
37. Holle LM. Pegaspargase: An alternative? Ann Pharmacother 1997:31:616–624.
38. Saunders MP, Denton CP, O'Brien MER, et al. Hypersensitivity reactions to cisplatin and carboplatin—A report on six cases. Ann Oncol 1992:3:574–576.
39. Chang SM, Fryberger S, Crouse V, et al. Carboplatin hypersensitivity in children. Cancer 1995:75:1171–1175.
40. Cleare MJ, Hughes EG, Jacoby B, Pepys J. Immediate (type I) allergic responses to platinum compounds. Clin Allergy 1976:6:183–195.
41. Hendrick AM, Simmons D, Cantwell BMJ. Allergic reactions to carboplatin. Ann Oncol 1992:3:239–240.
42. Tonkins KS, Rubin P, Levin L. Carboplatin hypersensitivity: Case reports and review of the literature. Eur J Cancer 1993:29A:1356–1357.
43. Kirk B. The evaluation of a light-protecting giving set—The photosensitivity of intravenous dacarbazine solutions. Intensive Ther Clin Monit May/June 1987, pp 78–86.
44. Shuekla S. A device to prevent photodegradation of dacarbazine (DTIC). Clin Radiol 1980:31(2):239–240.
45. O'Dwyer PJ, LaCreta F, Engstrom PF, Peter R, et al. Phase I/Pharmacokinetic reevaluation of ThioTEPA. Cancer Res 1991:51:3171–3176.
46. Przepiorka D, Ippoliti C, Giralt S, et al. A phase I-II study of high-dose thiotepa, busulfan and cyclophosphamide as a preparative regimen for allogenic marrow transplantation. Bone Marrow Transplant 1994:14:449–453.

47. Horn TD, Beveridge RA, Egorin MJ, et al. Observations and proposed mechanism of *N,N′,N″*-triethylenethiophosphoramide (thiotepa)-induced hyperpigmentation. Arch Dermatol 1989:125:524–527.
48. Lokkevik E, Skovlund E, Reitan JB, et al. Skin treatment with Bepanthen Cream versus no cream during radiotherapy. Acta Oncol 1996:35:1021–1026.
49. Comandone A, Bretti S, La Grotta G, et al. Palmar–plantar erythrodysesthesia-syndrome associated with 5-fluorouracil treatment. Anticancer Res 1993:13: 1781–1784.
50. Feldamn LD, Ajani JA. Fluorouracil-associated dermatitis of the hands and feet. JAMA 1985:254:3479.
51. Curran CF, Luce JK. Fluorouracil and palmar–plantar erythrodysesthesia. Ann Intern Med 1989:111:858.
52. Doll DC, Yarbro JW. Vascular toxicity associated with antineoplastic agents. Semin Oncol 1992:19:580–596.
53. Castleberry RP, Crist WM, Holbrook T, et al. The cytosine arabinoside (AraC) syndrome. Med Pediatr Oncol 1981:9:257–264.
54. Manoharan A. The cytarabine syndrome in adults. Aust NZ J Med 1985:15: 451–452.
55. Williams SF, Larson RA. Hypersensitivity reaction to high-dose cytarabine. Br J Haematol 1989:73:274–275.

III

EXTRAVASATION AND PARAVASATION

6

Managing Extravasations of Vesicant Chemotherapy Drugs

ROBERT T. DORR
College of Medicine, Arizona Cancer Center, The University of Arizona, Tucson, Arizona

6.1 INTRODUCTION

Although infrequent, extravasation of irritating or ulcerogenic (vesicant) cancer chemotherapeutic agents is a severely distressing complication. Since such vesicant extravasations tend to produce long-standing ulceration and occasionally loss of function and physical disfigurement, their prevention of extravasation remains of upmost importance. The term "extravasation" generally implies the inadvertent delivery of an irritating or ulcerogenic agent outside the vein. This can occur with infusions using peripheral veins and, as explained later, rarely, through implanted or exited central vascular access devices. Fortunately, most chemotherapeutic agents are nonvesicants and do not produce soft tissue damage when delivered outside the vein (Table 1) [1–57]. On the other hand, although the vesicants are relatively few in number, they comprise some of the most commonly used anticancer agents, as outlined in Table 1. Nonetheless, even with a known vesicant agent, the likelihood of an extravasation causing soft tissue damage has been estimated at less than one-third incidence [58]. This means that there is a 67% likelihood that an extravasation of a known vesicant agent will not result in severe soft tissue damage. At this time, however, it is impossible to accurately predict which of the patients who experience an extravasation of a vesicant agent will develop a serious lesion. Therefore, prevention and treatment are important components in managing this complication.

Table 1 List of Vesicant Irritant and Nonvesicant Anticancer Agents

Vesicants	Irritants (may cause irritation, rarely necrosis)	Nonvesicants
Doxorubicin [1–8]	Plicamycin [32]	Liposomal doxorubicin [51,52]
Daunorubicin [9–13]	Mitoxantrone [33–37]	Liposomal daunorubicin [53,54]
Dactinomycin [14 16]	Cisplatin [15,36,38–40]	Etoposide [8,55]
Epirubicin [8,17]	Fluorouracil [41–43]	Bleomycin [8,43]
Esorubicin [18–21]	Topotecan [44]	Melphalan [36]
Mechlorethamine [22]	Paclitaxel [45–48]	Carmustine [55]
Mitomycin C [23–25]	Docetaxel [49,50]	Dacarbazine [56]
Vinblastine [26,27]	Etoposides [8,161]	Cytarabine
Vincristine [26,28]		Methotrexate
Vinorelbine [29,30]		Teniposide [161]
Vindesine [8,26,31]		Fludarabine
		Pentostatin
		Cladrabine
		Irinotecan [57]

This chapter does not review all of the nursing administration guidelines for the prevention of extravasation. However, prevention remains the single best defense for this complication. A common mistake that is often noted in extravasation instances include continued administration of the drug via peripheral vein or vascular access device after there has been some indication of a potential problem. In the case of extravasation, the early symptoms include pain, localized swelling, and obvious physical difficulty in administering fluid. All these conditions require immediate cessation of the attempted infusion for evaluation of the venipuncture or vascular access device. Nonirritating isotonic fluids can be used to challenge vein patency. Therefore, blood withdrawal apparatus should be tested and nonirritating test infusions substituted at the earliest sign of physical discomfort or physical change in the administration site or apparatus. If extravasation is suspected at peripheral veins, a new site should be immediately selected and the suspected site closely evaluated for possible treatment. Management of suspected infiltration from implanted devices is discussed later; overall, such management should include careful notation of any complications. The elicitation of the patient's participation in monitoring his or her infusion is also vital to ensure that problems can be addressed at the earliest possible time. Even with these practices, and in the best of circumstances, some venous extravasations of potentially vesicant agents will occur, and therefore, treatment becomes of paramount importance.

The remainder of this chapter deals with the pharmacologic approaches to this treatment, keeping in mind that surgical excision of documented severe extravasation ulcers remains the single best method for resolving large lesions. In the case of certain anthracycline drugs such as doxorubicin, surgery can both debride the nonviable tissue and remove locally entrapped drug, which otherwise would expand the area of ulceration [59–61]. Similar expansive ulcerations have been described for alkylating agents such as nitrogen mustard and mitomycin C, and with these more severe vesicants, surgical debridement at the earliest possible time may ultimately limit the depth and extent of the subsequent necrotic process. In an attempt to prevent serious ulcerations from developing, a variety of pharmacologic antidotes and local treatments using topical agents or heating and cooling have been advocated. The remainder of this chapter describes these experiments, with recommendations for clinical treatment of the major classes of known vesicant anticancer drugs.

6.2 EXTRAVASATION FROM VASCULAR ACCESS DEVICES

A number of series have documented vesicant drug extravasation from vascular access devices, or VADs [62–65]. Of the two basic types of devices —implanted ports and exited catheters, or Hickman-type devices—extravasation is more commonly reported for implanted ports [62,64].

6.2.1 Extravasation from Exited Catheters

With externally accessed (exited) VADs, extravasation is truly rare [65]. The cause of VAD extravasation varies, but mechanical failure is uncommon. One report has described catheter tip erosion through the jugular vein due to a malpositioned catheter [66]. Catheter tip curling has been described in 3.6% of 500 placements of subclavian vein Hickman exited catheters. This may explain the major reason for this device failure [67]. In another case involving an exited catheter, an extravasation of 35 mg of doxorubicin into the chest wall caused immediate severe pain, swelling, and a classic burning sensation over the entire left chest wall [68]. This set of symptoms was treated with intravenous methylprednisolone and topical ice to the chest wall, along with removal of the catheter. While the site remained indurated, the underlying soft tissues did not ulcerate. Five other cases of drug extravasation from Hickman-type catheters following the use of a split-sheath introducer needle were described [69]. One of these caused an extravasation of doxorubicin into the subcutaneous chest wall tissues, ultimately necessitating a mastectomy to resolve extensive chest wall ulceration and necrosis. Despite these two severe cases of doxorubicin extravasation, Hickman-type catheters have the best overall safety record for preventing extravasations and resultant injuries.

6.2.2 Extravasation from Implanted VADs

Extravasations are more common from implanted VADs than with Hickman catheters primarily because of the difficulty of properly accessing the port septum [62–64,70]. The major problem, namely, incomplete or partial needle insertion through the septum, is compounded if the port is implanted (deeply) if the patient is obese [70], if the patient remains active, and especially when long-term infusions are attempted. The nonsecure access of the port is a consistent design problem of these popular devices, wherein superficial taping is the usual means of securing the needle in place after insertion through the port septum. Other rare complications that may also cause extravasation for implanted VADs include fracture or disconnection of the outflow catheter [71]. Laceration of the outflow catheter has also been documented as a rare complication leading to extravasation [72].

Overall, it has been estimated that the incidence of extravasation from implanted ports approaches 5%, although severe local irritation has occurred in only 1.2% of these cases [63,73]. In an early series, Reed et al. described extravasation of inotropic drugs or chemotherapy agents in five patients [62]; skin necrosis immediately above the port septum was observed in three of these patients (two receiving dobutamine and one receiving fluorouracil). In each case, the implanted device was removed and further therapy was delivered via a newly inserted Hickman-type catheter. Partial displacement of the needle outside the port septum was felt to be the primary contributing factor in these extravasations.

Drug extravasation was reported in 1 of 25 patients in a Scandinavian trial wherein the median functional survival time of port implantation was 16 months. The overall complication rate was only 1 every 900 days in this trial [74]. The single extravasation in this series, which involved doxorubicin, resolved uneventfully and did not require explantation of the port. In another series of 74 cancer patients receiving therapy via an implanted port, three extravasations were observed, one involving a severe doxorubicin extravasation that necessitated explantation of the port [75]. This represents an extravasation incidence of 4.1% and was the reason for port explantation in one of seven instances requiring surgical removal of the implanted device. A similar extravasation incidence of 4% was described by Greidanus et al. [76] working with the Infuse-A-Port, accessed by 90° Huber needles to deliver chemotherapy to 50 cancer patients. Neither of the two reported extravasations, which involved epirubicin and mitoxantrone, led to necrosis. Both extravasations were due to improper placement of the Huber needle in the port septum. In one case, this error was exacerbated by patient obesity, a common risk factor for such extravasations [76]. Other small series have also described rare extravasations from implanted ports, again primarily due to needle dislodgement. The reported incidence (events/total implants) was 4/40 as described by Smith [64], 1/14 as described by Soo et al. [77], 1/35 by Gyves et al. [78], 2/24 by Kerr et al. [79], and 1/32 by Winters et al. [80]. The most commonly reported risk factor in these series was obesity [76].

Other larger series have described higher incidence figures for extravasation from vascular access devices. Brothers et al. reported extravasations in 21 of 320 device placements among 300 patients, an incidence of 6.4% [72]. Most of these placements were for the delivery of cancer chemotherapy drugs, and the majority of the 21 extravasations involved vesicant chemotherapy drugs. However, necrosis occurred in only three of these patients, or 1.5% of device placements. Interestingly, this is not substantially different from the reported extravasation incidence for infusions of vesicant cancer drugs using peripheral veins [81]. Other large series have reported extravasation incidence rates of 1.5% in 128 cancer patients [71], and 4/132, or 3.3%, in a retrospective series reported by Lemmers et al. [82]. The latter series included two serious reactions, which despite local treatment, led to soft tissue necrosis immediately above the port pocket [82].

These extravasation incidence rates, as summarized in Table 2, show that Hickman-type exited catheters have a very low propensity for causing serious extravasations. In contrast, the reported aggregate extravasation incidence of about 5% for non-exited implanted devices rivals that of peripheral vein infusions. However, this may be an artifact of more diligent re-

Table 2 Incidence of Extravasation from Different Types of Vascular Access Devices

Type of VAD (no. of patients)	Number of placements	Extravasations reported		References
		Total	%	
Hickman (178)	183	1 [4.4]	2 [0.54]	Fellows 1970; Gemlo 1988; Howard 1990; Diekman 1985; Reed 1983
Totally Implanted (947)	989	48 [4.9]	12 [1.2]	Dorr [73]

porting with the newer non-exited devices. Fortunately, as with extravasations from peripheral veins, very few VAD-related extravasations result in serious toxicity (Table 2). In contrast, the recognition of extravasation may be more difficult with VADs, since (a) there is generally more tissue to absorb the extravasated fluid and (b) chest wall tissues may be less sensitive to irritant drugs than are peripheral veins, which lie closer to highly sensitive nerves. Thus, the early recognition of extravasations from VADs is an important consideration in the use of these devices.

The classic clinical manifestations of a VAD extravasation involving vesicant drug leakage from a dislodged needle include pain or burning in the port pocket, palpable swelling at the site, and/or a sensation of heat in the periport area [83]. If the extravasation is due to leakage along the catheter tunnel from a thrombus at the tip or a nicked outflow catheter, the symptoms are pain and a burning sensation along the catheter tunnel route. Sometimes this pain cannot be localized to the catheter route and is referred up the neck or through to the back. Similar symptoms of pain or swelling in the neck, back, or supraclavicular space are reported when the catheter is pinched off (e.g., by compression between the ribs and clavicle) or when the catheter has been damaged by aggressive flushing to remove a thrombus [83]. Early recognition of these signs and symptoms is important to ensure the timely cessation of any infusions and the evaluation of the patency of the device by radiographic or functional determinations.

The treatment of vesicant drug extravasations from VADs is essentially the same as for those involving peripheral veins, that is:

1. stopping the infusion at the first sign of a potential problem
2. evaluating catheter patency
3. withdrawing any remaining fluid from the device and around the port pocket area if extravasation is suspected
4. treatment with a local antidote (if known) for the specific vesicant drug extravasated

Thus, the same antidotal procedures originally developed for peripheral extravasations can be safely used for extravasations from VADs. This also includes the use of surgery to remove inoperative devices and any nonviable (and possibly drug-laden) tissues around the device. Such measures may prevent further spread of necrosis following a serious vesicant drug extravasation. In some cases, explantation surgery may involve a mastectomy and chest wall debridement, since dependent breast tissues form an effective reservoir for extravasated fluids from a VAD implanted in the chest wall. This possibility again underscores the need for close monitoring of vesicant drug infusions even through implanted VADs.

6.3 TREATMENT OF INDIVIDUAL VESICANT DRUG EXTRAVASATIONS

6.3.1 Anthracyclines and Other DNA Intercalators

DNA intercalators such as anthracyclines represent one of the largest categories of commonly used cytotoxic antitumor agents. Certainly the most frequently used agent in this group, doxorubicin and its related analogues such as idarubicin, epirubicin, daunomycin, and mitoxantrone, comprise a very large therapeutic category of agents that are known to produce extravasation ulcers in a high percentage of extravasations. For doxorubicin, extravasations have been reported to occur in up to 6% of patients when peripheral veins are used for the injection [2,3]. However, a larger review suggests that the true incidence is much lower, at 0.5% [5]. A more common local complication from doxorubicin is not extravasation, but, rather, the occurrence of the so-called venous flare reaction, representing local venous response to histamine release induced by the drug infusion [84–86]. Symptoms include a local edema, an erythematous venous streaking along the course of the vein and extending laterally from the vein, and pruritus, which is somewhat delayed in presentation. Up to 3% of doxorubicin injections may be complicated by this venous flare reaction, and although corticosteroids and antihistamines are frequently used, none has demonstrated preventive efficacy. Indeed, the complication usually does not recur even with repeated administration of the offending anthracycline drug solution. One report suggests that the incidence of localized venous flare reactions for the 4-deoxydoxorubicin esorubicin congener is even higher [18]. Thus, although common, the venous flare reaction is not a reason to permanently halt the infusion of the drug or to switch to an alternate site for administration.

On the other hand, true doxorubicin extravasations can be complex to manage because of their very slow onset for the evolution of gross ulceration. This time course may ultimately extend to several months. Thus, anthracycline extravasations involving the distal extremities, and particularly the dorsal surface of the hand, can lead to severe impairment of underlying nerves and tendons as the lesion increases over time. Several pharmacologic studies have documented significant accumulation of doxorubicin, the alcohol metabolite doxorubicinol, and in some cases the metabolized aglycone in the tissues removed from debrided extravasation sites [59–61]. These drugs have been recovered months after the extravasation, and since the known half-life of most anthracyclines ranges from 30 to 40 hours [87], this is far longer than one would anticipate from simple pharmacokinetic clearance estimates. Thus, for serious anthracycline extravasations, wherein tissue damage is impending or is already apparent, early surgical evaluation for potential debridement is very important [58].

In identifying viable tissues at surgery, two approaches may be kept in mind. First, fluorescein may adequately demarcate viable tissue margins; and second, the autofluorescence of Adriamycin under light of excitation wavelengths may be used to detect tissues that have taken up the drug and should be removed at the time of the surgical procedure [88]. It is important to note that the area of surgical excision may be somewhat wider and deeper than it appears upon gross physical inspection. Therefore, antidotes to diminish or prevent this type of toxicity have been avidly sought.

A number of anecdotal procedures have been recommended, and the usual caveats of isolated clinical case reports should be kept in mind. Specifically, since there is a 67% likelihood of a good outcome with no treatment [58], one must critically analyze all clinical anecdotes. Indeed, there are only a few prospective studies that have adequately tested the efficacy of some of the procedures in a scientifically rigorous fashion. Initial antidotes for doxorubicin included glucocorticosteroids such as hydrocortisone, given either by local injection or by topical application [3,5]. While limited activity has been suggested in a mouse model [89] and in a rabbit model [90], few of the pathological reports in rodents or in humans describe a significant inflammatory component to doxorubicin extravasations [91,92]. Therefore scientific support for the use of glucocorticosteroids has not been established. Furthermore, despite the existence of some case reports suggesting that local injection of hydrocortisone and/or topical application of corticosteroid creams may reduce Adriamycin lesions [3,5], there have been no prospective trials, and the animal data suggest that any antidotal efficacy is minimal at best [89]. Finally, the known activity of local corticosteroids to cause epidermal thinning [93] and to block normal inflammatory-based wound closure processes [94] significantly undermines the potential efficacy of glucocorticoids as antidotes to anthracycline extravasations.

Another anecdotally recommended antidote for doxorubicin is pH modification using sodium bicarbonate [95]. The rationale was to provide an alkaline environment that would cleave the glycosidic bond between the anthracycline and the amino-containing sugar portion of the molecule, rendering the inactive aglycone. While this result may be achievable in a strict chemical sense, the pH of most clinically used sodium bicarbonate solutions [8,15] is not adequate to produce cleavage of the glycosidic bond. In addition, a number of experimental studies in mice, rats, rabbits, and guinea pigs failed to demonstrate anecdotal efficacy for sodium bicarbonate as a doxorubicin antidote [96,91]. Finally, sodium bicarbonate itself has been shown to be a vesicant when inadvertently extravasated during attempts to resuscitate victims of cardiopulmonary arrest [98]. In one report, 8 out of 11 patients who experienced an extravasation of bicarbonate ultimately required a skin graft to treat large areas of soft tissue necrosis. Thus, there is no clinical rationale for the use of either hydrocortisone or sodium bicarbonate as an antidote to local extravasations of doxorubicin.

A number of antioxidant compounds have also been evaluated as doxorubicin extravasation antidotes. The rationale for using these agents is based on the known mechanism of anthracycline cardiotoxicity, which involves quinone-generated oxygen free radicals [99]. One group showed substantial anecdotal efficacy for a combination of dimethyl sulfoxide (DMSO-both an antioxidant and a topical penetration enhancer) and the vitamin E derivative antioxidant, α-tocopherol in rat skin [100]. However, the vitamin E compound alone was found to be ineffective in both mice [101] and in rats [102]. This suggests that the substantial efficacy seen in the original rodent trial was due to the DMSO component. This is reviewed in detail later.

Similarly, the antioxidant butylated hydroxytoluene (BHT) has been shown to reduce doxorubicin ulcers in mice [103]. However, this has not been tested in humans, although BHT is in a number of medications and perhaps should be evaluated in a formal clinical trial.

β-Adrenergic agents have been shown to be active in a dog model of anthracycline cardiotoxicity. They were believed to work by blocking histamine release and resultant cardiotoxicity and were subsequently evaluated in a mouse skin model of doxorubicin extravasation damage [104]. There was minimal efficacy for the β-adrenergic agonists in the mouse model, and a few anecdotal clinical reports showed no efficacy for these agents upon injection. Thus an adrenergic pharmacologic approach may not be effective in managing clinical doxorubicin extravasations.

On the other hand, a series of radical dimer compounds have shown efficacy. Koch et al. [105] used an oxymorpholinyl scaffold to synthesize these dimers and showed them to effectively inactivate quinone-containing compounds such as doxorubicin by chemical reduction [106]. Several compounds such as the radical dimer bis-(3,5-dimethyl-5-hydroxymethyl-2-oxomorphylin-3-yl), or DHM3, were shown to reduce anthracycline to the insoluble and inactive 7-deoxyaglycone metabolites [107]. DHM3 has also been shown to protect against doxorubicin lethality in animal models and is an extremely potent local antagonist to doxorubicin extravasation ulceration in an intradermal pig model. In addition to doxorubicin, the DHM3 radical dimer was shown to reduce the toxicity of other intradermally injected vesicant quinone compounds, including the anthracyclines daunorubicin, menogaril, idarubicin, epirubicin, 5-iminodaunorubicin, aclarubicin, and the quinone-containing alkylating agent mitomycin C. Unfortunately, these novel radical dimers have not been tested in the clinic, and availability even for animal testing may be limited. Clearly, though, these have one of the best chemical preclinical mechanistic profiles of any of the purported antidotes for anthracycline extravasation.

6.3.2 Topical Treatment of Doxorubicin Extravasation

One of the older controversies in managing any local venous complication entails the application of heat versus cooling. For doxorubicin extravasations, this question has been unequivocally answered in a variety of preclinical and clinical models that show the application of cold to be highly beneficial. In a controlled trial of heating and cooling in a mouse model, topical cooling dramatically reduced the peak lesion size and the duration of lesions after an intradermal injection of doxorubicin [108]. In contrast, when the same doxorubicin dose was followed by mild local heating of the skin, there was a significant increase in the area of ulceration. This follows other data indicating that heat and doxorubicin produce synergistic toxicity, even in tumor cell models in vitro [109]. The beneficial effects of cooling have been documented in the pig model, which has skin architecture similar to that of humans, and also in clinical trials [110]. Thus, there is consistent and overwhelming evidence that topical cooling of doxorubicin extravasations can dramatically reduce the size and duration of soft tissue ulceration.

The other topical antidote that is commonly used for anthracycline extravasations is dimethyl sulfoxide. DMSO has a number of beneficial characteristics, including the ability to penetrate intact skin to act as a carrying agent or penetration enhancer, antihistaminic activity, and antioxidant activity (by acting as a free radical scavenging agent) [111]. All these pharmacologic activities may be beneficial in the treatment of doxorubicin extravasation. The experimental studies again provide a convincing argument for DMSO as a topical antidote to anthracyclines [112,113]. An initial report using DMSO in Sprague-Dawley rats and Yorkshire piglets showed that a 7-day application of 100% DMSO solution completely prevented ulcers from developing both at local sites of doxorubicin injection and at distal untreated sites [112]. A second study showed that the combination of DMSO and tocopherol reduced doxorubicin skin ulcers by almost 70% and, as stated earlier, the major active component in this mixture was DMSO [102]. While there is a single negative trial in mice [101], the consistent activity in the pig model with DMSO shows that there is a good preclinical basis for the use of this agent in treating and preventing local extravasation reactions.

In addition to the preclinical models, a number of clinical anecdotal reports note the activity of DMSO. In several cases, DMSO was combined with either topical corticosteroids or ice packs and showed significant reduction of doxorubicin lesions [2,57,114]. These initial case reports were followed by a nonrandomized clinical trial of 20 consecutive patients who experienced an anthracycline extravasation and received topical DMSO treatment [116]. In this trial, 99% DMSO was applied in two applications to the involved area six times daily for 2 weeks and the lesions were fol-

Table 3 Prospective Studies of Topical DMSO and Cooling for Treating Anthracycline Extravasations

Assessable anthracycline extravasations				
Number	Drugs	99% (w/v) DMSO regimen used	Outcome (number with necrosis)	Ref.
18	Doxorubicin	Twice daily every	0	114
2	Daunorubicin	6 hours for 14 days	0	114
11	Doxorubicin	Every 8 hours for	0	115
42	Epirubicin	7 days	1	115

lowed up. Whereas the historical database suggests that at least one-third of these extravasations should result in severe ulceration [58], there were no instances of ulceration following the use of DMSO in this prospective, but nonrandomized clinical trial [114]. The treatment complications were minimal: some swelling, erythema, and a slight amount of a prickling type of sensation. With 3 months of follow-up, no symptomatology of ulceration was evident in the majority of the treated patients.

A follow-up report from the Italian Cancer Institute by Bertelli et al. [115] also used a nonrandomized prospective clinical design of treating patients who had experienced extravasation with 99% DMSO applied topically to the site every 8 hours for 7 days. Intermittent cooling for 1 hour three times daily on the first 3 days was also used, based on the pig study showing potential additive efficacy for these two anecdotal maneuvers. The results of this trial in over 140 patients experiencing a variety of vesicant reactions are shown in Table 3. Overall, the treatment was well tolerated, with mild local burning and a characteristic garlic breath odor as the only side effects of DMSO. In some cases treatment was continued for up to 6 weeks to obtain an adequate remission of the symptoms of extravasations, and toxicity was never dose limiting in any setting. These authors concluded that topical DMSO was a safe and effective local antidote that can be conveniently used with local cooling after extravasation of vesicant agents [115].

6.3.3 Daunorubicin

Daunorubicin is also a potential vesicant agent if extravasated [9–13,32]. Daunorubicin extravasation reactions are similar to those of doxorubicin in time course and symptomatology. The use of antidotes has not been as extensively evaluated, although as shown in Table 3, the use of topical DMSO appears to be equally advantageous in a small clinical series. Preclinical models have indicated a number of ineffective antidotes for daunorubicin local toxicity, including sodium bicarbonate, heparin, hyaluronidase, and isoproterenol [32]. Heating also increased ulceration (as was seen with doxorubicin) [108]. In a mouse model, cooling and DMSO were only marginally effective for daunorubicin compared to the demonstrated antidotal efficacy for doxorubicin [32]. Thus, this very similar congener of doxorubicin appears to behave similarly in terms of extravasation necrosis, and the same antidotal procedure of combining topical DMSO and cooling is recommended for treating daunorubicin extravasations.

6.3.3.1 Epirubicin

Epirubicin, the 4-hydroxyl epimer of doxorubicin, has been shown to be more potent on a molar basis than the parent compound and potentially to possess less cardiotoxicity. Experimental antidotes for epirubicin include the DHM3 radical dimer and, from the clinical literature, topical DMSO, which was shown to be highly effective as an extravasation antidote [115]. Thus for epirubicin the same antidotal procedure is recommended, consisting of the combination of topical DMSO and topical cooling based on the clinical and preclinical data.

6.3.3.2 Idarubicin

Idarubicin is the 4-demethoxy derivative of daunorubicin, which similarly exceeds the parent compound in antitumor potency. Overall, it has a similar toxicity profile, although metabolically idarubicin should be considered a prodrug for the more active 13-dihydro (alcohol) metabolite. Little extravasation antidote information is available for idarubicin, and only a few clinical case reports describe moderately severe idarubicin skin extravasations. Most of these did not require surgical intervention [116,117]. Based on the similarity of cytotoxic mechanisms, however, topical DMSO and cooling are recommended to treat serious idarubicin extravasations.

6.3.4 Liposomal Anthracyclines

Liposomal doxorubicin has been put into a number of liposomal formulations and is commercially available in the United States in a pegilated liposome with a trade name of Doxil. Experimental studies in rodent models have shown that when injected intradermally, this agent is relatively nontoxic [51,52], and clinical reports in the Kaposi sarcoma population confirm that in a large number of extravasation reactions no local toxicity is produced [118].

Lipsomal daunorubicin (DaunoXome) has also been shown to be a nonvesicant in both preclinical models [53] and clinical extravasation anecdotes [54]. Thus, it appears that the liposomal encapsulation of the anthracyclines doxorubicin and daunorubicin results in markedly less local toxicity potential than is found with the parent compounds. At this time no antidotal maneuvers are recommended for treating inadvertent extravasations of the liposomal anthracyclines.

6.3.4.1 Mitoxantrone

Mitoxantrone (Novantrone) is an anthracene-containing antitumor agent that shares some mechanistic effects with doxorubicin, principally intercalation into DNA and inhibition of topoisomerase II. However, mitoxantrone does not produce oxygen free radicals, a striking difference from the anthracyclines. There are a number of anecdotal case reports of mitoxantrone extravasation in humans [33,37], but only two of these cases required surgical intervention to remove lesions [35,119]. The larger clinical experience describes no extravasation reactions with mitoxantrone, suggesting that this agent is a very weak vesicant. Indeed, most extravasations simply discolor the subcutaneous tissues, only rarely causing significant local toxicity. In an animal model, the drug was markedly nontoxic even following the intradermal injection of doses that produce systemic lethality [36]. Because of the lack of a predictive animal model, and the paucity of clinical reports showing severe toxicity, we have no data on potential antidote treatment other than surgical excision of lesions that appear to be of moderate to severe intensity. Furthermore, since mitoxantrone lacks some mechanisms common to the other anthracyclines such as oxygen free radical production [120], it is not clear whether the same types of antidote could be effective for this compound.

6.3.4.2 Amsacrine

Amsacrine is an investigational, acridine-based, anthracycline-containing antitumor agent that has been shown to be active in refractory acute myelogenous leukemia. In an animal model it does produce dose-dependent skin ulcers at clinically relevant doses [32]. In this model, topical DMSO significantly reduced amsacrine-induced skin ulcerations in contrast to other experimental antidotes, which were ineffective. The ineffective procedures included administration of sodium bicarbonate and corticosteroids. Topical heating significantly enhanced skin ulceration [32]. Thus, for any clinical extravasations of amsacrine, topical DMSO is highly recommended. The inclusion of cold for this agent is not established, since it was not shown to be effective in the animal model [32], and there are no clinical anecdotes to guide dosing. Clearly, heat is contraindicated for treating amsacrine extravasations.

6.3.4.3 Dactinomycin

Dactinomycin (or actinomycin D) was the prototype for the entire DNA intercalating series of agents. It was also shown to produce severe skin ulcers if extravasated in humans [16]. In a quantitative skin ulceration trial in mice, dactinomycin produced dose-dependent skin lesions. It has also been shown to be locally toxic in a guinea pig and rat paw local inflammatory model [14,15]. The histologic pattern of skin damage from dactinomycin in guinea pigs was shown to involve coagulative necrosis, with an acute inflammatory component noted after low dose injections of the drug. Like other anthracycline extravasations, regranulation or repair of damaged tissues was markedly retarded. This suggests that either surgical excision or local antidotal procedures are vitally needed to manage extravasations occurring in the clinic. However, in a mouse model of intradermal dactinomycin toxicity, neither topical cooling nor topical DMSO was effective [32]. Thus, overall, it is unclear what antidotal procedures should be used for an extravasation of dactinomycin in the clinic. Heat is clearly contraindicated, since it causes significant synergistic skin toxicity in the mouse model [32]. The possibility that DMSO would be effective cannot be ruled out, since the mouse model did not accurately predict the substantial clinical efficacy for topical DMSO with doxorubicin [101].

6.3.5 DNA Alkylating Agents

A number of alkylating agents have been listed as potential or confirmed vesicants in humans. The list of confirmed vesicants includes the prototype alkylator mechlorethamine or nitrogen mustard [16,22] and the aziridine-based alkylating agent mitomycin C [23–25]. Several other alkylating agents, such as carboplatin and ifosfamide, have been shown to have experimental vesicant activity, but only in preclinical models using very high doses [121]. Several other DNA-binding drugs, such as the nitrosurea carmustine (BCNU) [55] and the triazine-based agent dacarbazine (DTIC), appear to be irritants, but not vesicants. Finally, the platinum-containing agent cisplatin appears to be relatively nonvesicant in humans, despite a few reports of toxicity in clinical anecdotes [38–40]. In animal models, the drug was also relatively nontoxic [15,36]. Thus, overall among the DNA-binding drugs, only two agents consistently cause extravasation toxicity in humans: mechlorethamine and mitomycin C.

6.3.5.1 Mechlorethamine

Mechlorethamine, the prototype for bifunctional alkylating agents, is administered intravenously in the treatment of Hodgkins disease and occasionally topically for the cutaneous T-cell lymphoma mycosis fungoides. This agent has been unequivocally shown to have vesicant activity and in humans, serious extravasations can produce severe and prolonged ulceration of skin and underlying soft tissues [22]. In one case of nitrogen mustard extravasation, the dorsum of the hand required over 5 months to heal. In another patient in this series, skin grafting did not provide effective wound closure [16]. The hallmarks of nitrogen mustard extravasations are immediate pain, swelling, and thrombophlebitis. Indeed, the latter complication may be seen even in the absence of a frank extravasation [22]. Reportedly, this toxicity can be reduced by diluting the drug during the injection, by administering the drug through the tubing of a freely flowing intravenous setup [22]. Clearly, nitrogen mustard can be quite toxic to veins even if no extravasation occurs, and treated patients may show severe paravenous hyperpigmentation requiring months for resolution even in the absence of extravasation.

In terms of systemic antidotes, the inorganic sulfur compound sodium thiosulfate has been comprehensively evaluated as an antidote to nitrogen mustard [122,123]. Original studies in mice and dogs showed that intravenous sodium thiosulfate can neutralize nitrogen mustard systemically. The maximal protective benefit was gained when thiol administration preceded nitrogen mustard by 15 minutes, but simultaneous administration was also effective [123]. In the case of systemic administration, thiosulfate was inactive when given at any time after nitrogen mustard. The effective dose ratio for the systemic use of 10% sodium thiosulfate was 120:1 (thiosulfate/nitrogen mustard, mg/mg) [122]. Interestingly, the intravenous injection of thiosulfate did not protect the mice in this study from soft tissue ulceration due to subcutaneous mechlorethamine injection [123]. There are also case reports of the use of thiosulfate to treat inadvertent mechlorethamine extravasations in patients. In one severe case, a dose of 30 mg was inadvertently injected intramuscularly into the buttock of a 55-year-old psoriasis patient. This error was not recognized for 5 hours, but then a regimen of 5 mL of isotonic (0.166 M) sodium thiosulfate was given intramuscularly for five doses. This treatment completely prevented skin and soft tissue ulceration [124]. In addition, the peripheral white blood count in the patient remained stable, suggesting that the intramuscular injections of thiosulfate provided antidotal activity both locally and systemically.

Experimental studies in the BALB/c mouse model have confirmed that thiosulfate provides significant protection against nitrogen mustard skin ulceration. At doses relevant to human clinical doses of mechlorethamine, thiosulfate was shown to provide dose-dependent inhibition of nitrogen mustard–induced skin ulcerations when injected immediately after nitrogen mustard. The treatment was ineffective in the mouse model when the thiosulfate injection was delayed and when a dose ratio of less than 200:1 (thiosulfate:nitrogen mustard, mg/mg) was used [125]. Ineffective antidotes evaluated in this mouse model included sodium chloride, hyaluronidase, dimethyl sulfoxide, hydrocortisone, and both topical heat and cooling. And DMSO and the spreading factor enzyme hyaluronidase actually increased the severity of nitrogen mustard skin ulcerations in the mouse model [125].

In this mouse model, thiosulfate was the only effective nitrogen mustard antidote. The recommended treatment for clinical extravasations of mechlorethamine involves the isotonic, 0.166 M solution. This thiosulfate solution can be simply prepared from a 10% (w/v) solution by adding 6 mL of sterile water to 4 mL of the 10% sodium thiosulfate, yielding a 0.166 M isotonic sodium thiosulfate solution. Because this agent inactivates nitrogen mustard on contact, it is important during the antidotal procedure to inject the sodium thiosulfate solution into all areas that might have been exposed to the nitrogen mustard solution. Since sodium thiosulfate is extremely well tolerated, repeat injections of the antidotal agent several times following the extravasation are probably helpful in preventing toxicity.

6.3.5.2 Mitomycin C

Mitomycin C is an aziridine-containing alkylating agent derived from a *Streptomyces* species. This drug is known to produce significant extravasation reactions, with some unusual attributes [23–25]. While most mitomycin C extravasation reactions are noted by immediate symptomatology, such as pain and local swelling, a substantial minority may be clinically silent for several months after the injection [23,126]. In one nursing series, the average time for the onset of such delayed extravasation symptomatology was 13 weeks [23]. Because of the slow onset of these lesions, immediate diagnosis and treatment may not be possible. Another unusual complication of some mitomycin extravasations is a distal presentation of the lesion [127]. This anomaly is marked by apparent extravasation or soft tissue deposition of drug and subsequent ulceration occurring at sites quite removed from the original injection site. Thus, mitomycin C can be a very problematic extravasation vesicant. There are several series of anecdotal reports of patients experiencing mitomycin C extravasations [23–25]. In one series of three patients, severe pain and swelling were noted during the intravenous infusion through peripheral veins on the hand, wrist, and forearm [24]. In these cases, corticosteroids were administered by means of the injection of hydrocortisone and by the use of topical 0.1% triamcinolone cream. However, all these cases progressed to painful ulcerations within 2 weeks of the extravasation. Subsequently each of the patients required surgical debridement for both wound and local pain control. Recall types of reaction have also been reported for mitomycin C [128]. In one report, a recall extravasation response apparently occurred 75 days after the first mitomycin C injection. This is reminiscent of the delayed radiation recall phenomenon seen with combinations of anthracyclines and ionizing radiation and occasionally with repeated injections of anthracyclines. Sunlight also appears to synergize with mitomycin C–induced skin necrosis [129].

Most other clinical series with mitomycin C have noted a similar pattern of delayed development of necrosis in some patients. In the cases of delayed onset of symptoms, only surgical procedures are thought to provide any effective treatment. For acute presentations, initial animal studies have shown that corticosteroids do not offer effective experimental treatments for soft tissue damage due to mitomycin C as examined in a rabbit model [130] and in a mouse model [131]. In the latter study, a large group of potential antidotes were evaluated and surprisingly, topical dimethyl sulfoxide was shown to be highly effective [131]. Inactive antidotes in this mouse trial included hyaluronidase, diphenhydramine, hydrocortisone, vitamin E, and the sulfhydryl *N*-acetylcysteine (Table 4). The single application of topical DMSO in the mouse model was shown to provide nearly complete protection against subsequent ulceration following an intradermal injection of mitomycin C. Sodium thiosulfate also had marginal activity when injected intradermally. However, it was clearly not as effective as topical DMSO [131]. The application of topical DMSO on the mouse provided complete

Table 4 Mitomycin C Extravasation Antidotes

Ineffective in mice [131]	Effective in Trials	
	Experimental	Clinical
Diphenhydramine	DMSO [131]	DMSO [132,133]
Fumaric acid	Radical dimer	
Heparin	Sodium thiosulfate [145]	
Hyaluronidase		
Hydrocortisone		
Isoproterenol		
Lidocaine		
N-Acetylcysteine		
Topical cooling or heating		
Vitamin E		

protection against mitomycin C skin toxicity, although there was no apparent effect on enhanced uptake of the drug out of the skin site [131]. Finally, the radical dimer DMH3 has been shown to be active both in the pig model [107] and in a murine model of mitomycin C skin toxicity [R. Dorr, unpublished data]. Because of its experimental nature and lack of clinical availability, however, DMH3 cannot be considered to be a front-line antidote for mitomycin C.

At least two case reports have described clinical benefits of using mitomycin C as a local antidote in cancer patients. Ludwig et al., who treated several patients with topical DMSO and showed that there was effective prevention of necrosis following a mitomycin C extravasation into the forearm [132]. In this case, topical DMSO was combined with 10% vitamin E and applied as dressings to the site every 12 hours for 2 days. Another case report by Alberts and Dorr showed that DMSO can be effective for both delayed and acute presentations of mitomycin C extravasations [133]. In these two cases, topical 99% DMSO was applied on the same schedule used in the anthracycline series: every 6 hours for several weeks following the event. There was excellent pain control in this small mitomycin C series and near complete prevention of moderate to severe soft tissue injury following documented extravasation of significant amounts of mitomycin C. One patient in this trial discontinued the DMSO treatment and experienced immediate recurrence of pain and swelling, which then was diminished by reapplications of the DMSO. Thus, while there are no prospective clinical trials of topical DMSO, this agent appears to be highly effective in both animal studies and anecdotal case reports, and therefore should be considered to be a front-line antidote for serious mitomycin C extravasations.

6.3.6 Platinum-Containing Agents

Two platinum-containing agents are currently widely used in the clinic: cisplatin and the related agent carboplatin. Both agents produce DNA damage and antitumor efficacy by binding to a single DNA strand in a process distinct from that of the classic alkylating agents. There are a few clinical case reports describing severe cisplatin extravasation injury [38–40,134]. However, several of these cases represent very special situations. In one case, mild fibrosis and a moderate degree of cellulitis were noted on a forearm of a patient treated with a concentrated (0.42 mg/mL) solution of cisplatin [39]. The lesion that developed was initially treated with warm soaks and peaked in its intensity 2 weeks after the extravasation. Resolution proceeded over the next 2 months. There were no subsequent skin ulcers or limitation of motion, and cisplatin was readministered later to this patient without incident. The second case also involved the use of a highly concentrated cisplatin infusion (0.75 mg/mL) in a patient who was restrained [38]. A large amount of this solution extravasated into the dorsum of the hand before the condition was recognized. There was no local pharmacologic treatment given and over the next 2 weeks pain, swelling, and inflammation developed, followed by a large necrotic lesion. This ultimately involved the extensor tendons and subcutaneous fat requiring a surgical debridement and split-thickness skin graft [38].

Another case involved a serious extravasation of a 1 mg/mL solution into the right humoral artery of a 48-year-old fibrosarcoma patient [40]. While only a small volume (1.5 mL) was felt to have been extravasated, local corticosteroids were injected multiple times into the site around the extravasation area. Despite this treatment, erythema and edema were followed by vesicular eruption over a 6-day period. Topical corticosteroids and antibiotics were then prescribed but did not prevent the development of a 3-cm blackened scar over the area on the forearm. This peaked in intensity approximately 1 month after the event. A final case involved cisplatin extravasation into the forearm resulting in severe cellulitis [134].

Many of these cases are similar in that the solutions of cisplatin that extravasated were highly concentrated (>0.4 mg/mL) and had been infused over a short time period in small dilution volumes. Animal models have not been able to demonstrate dose-dependent cisplatin lesions. The agent does not appear to produce significant soft tissue ulceration in rodents even following the injection of systemically lethal concentrations into the skin [36]. However, the same antidote used for nitrogen mustard, sodium thiosulfate, is known to be an effective antidote for cisplatin [135]. Thus, for serious extravasations involving large amounts of highly concentrated solutions of cisplatin, the local injection of the isotonic (0.16 M) thiosulfate solution is recommended for cisplatin extravasations. Again, however, the treatment of typical extravasations involving small amounts of more dilute solutions is probably not necessary due to the very concentration-dependent propensity of causing extravasation necrosis with this agent.

Carboplatin has also been implicated in an animal model as a potential vesicant [121]. However, there are no confirmatory clinical series or case reports and, therefore, antidote studies have not been performed. The slower activation of carboplatin to its active DNA binding moiety, and its better water solubility and tolerance compared to cisplatin, argue that clinical extravasations of carboplatin be conservatively followed, and that no antidotal procedures are required.

6.3.7 Other DNA-Binding Agents

Several compounds also bind to DNA in mechanisms that are somewhat similar to that of the classical alkylating agents. The nitrosurea carmustine or bis-chloroethylnitrosurea, BCNU, is a highly lipophilic agent which is known to cross-link DNA and also has protein carbamoylating activity in vivo [136]. However, there are virtually no reports of serious extravasation reactions for carmustine and in animal models that dose-dependent skin lesions could not be produced (R. Dorr, unpublished studies). Thus, while carmustine does produce significant thrombophlebitis and occasional superficial venous irritation, it does not appear to be associated with extravasation necrosis and no antidotal procedures are recommended.

6.3.8 Dacarbazine (DTIC)

DTIC is a triazine-containing anticancer agent that produces highly reactive methylene groups thought to induce monoalkylation of DNA [137]. The drug has been shown to cause phlebitis, and it has been suggested that this condition is worsened by exposure of the solution to light [138]. However, not all authors have found this to be the case, and the drug is typically well tolerated even though phlebitis is rarely reported. Mouse studies using intradermal DTIC showed that the agent was primarily an irritant but not a vesicant. In a dose-dependent model using intradermal injections in mouse skin, no consistent skin lesions could be created [56]. Thus, even extremely high doses given intradermally produced only very small ulcers, which healed very briskly. Using this high-dose intradermal model, a number of local adjuvants were evaluated including heat, cooling, topical DMSO, hyaluronidase, saline injected, and topical hydrocortisone. The one procedure that reduced DTIC lesions significantly involved the injection of sodium thiosulfate at a twice-isotonic concentration of 0.33 M. However, the paucity of clinical data documenting DTIC's potential as a vesicant drug suggests that DTIC extravasation reactions should be managed conservatively and that no local antidotes should be given. In the event of an extremely severe extravasation of a large amount of drug with apparent local toxicity, the injection of 0.166 M sodium thiosulfate might be used as an experimental antidotal procedure.

6.3.9 Vinca Alkaloid Extravasation

Vinca alkaloids used in the treatment of cancer include vincristine (Oncovin), vinblastine (Velban), vindesine (Eldisine), and vinorelbine (Navelbine). Each of these agents has been shown to be a potential vesicant, and extravasations can produce both neurologic and soft tissue ulcerogenic activities [26–31]. With vincristine, many of the reported extravasations have occurred in children, causing significant lesions in pediatric patients with solid tumors [139] or leukemias [26,28]. As with other vesicants, most vincristine extravasations produce initial marked pain, erythema, and localized swelling within minutes. Skin blisters can form after several days, and resolution may not be complete for several weeks. As is the case with anthracycline extravasations, however, most vinca alkaloid extravasations do not produce frank soft tissue ulceration [58].

An unusual aspect of vinca alkaloid extravasations is an occasional delayed presentation of symptoms. In one case, an 8-hour infusion of vinblastine in a peripheral vein was initially unremarkable but resulted in a severe extravasation reaction on the dorsum of the hand several weeks after drug administration [27]. This particular patient had an arterial venous fistula on the same arm used for the vinblastine infusion, and a partial obstruction of the fistula may have produced a retrograde flow of blood in the vein used for the infusion. Although skin necrosis occurred in this patient, it resolved slowly over a 6-month period and local surgery was not required for closure.

Another series of patients receiving the vinblastine derivative vindesine, by peripheral vein, experienced a number of delayed-onset reactions [31]. In these cases the symptoms of pain and swelling at the extravasation site were delayed for periods of several hours up to a day after drug administration. Most of these delayed vindesine extravasations occurred in veins on the dorsum of the hand, and several resulted in severe painful skin ulcers 3 weeks after the extravasation. As with the prior vinblastine case, these vindesine-induced lesions healed slowly over a 6-month period without requiring surgery. However, in many of these cases, localized tingling paresthesias and residual sensory deficits remained even after the superficial skin lesions over the extravasation sites had healed. This clearly suggests that for both the more typical immediate onset and for the delayed extravasation reactions, antidotal treatments would be very beneficial to reduce this morbidity.

Longer infusions of vinca alkaloids have been utilized in an attempt to enhance antitumor activity based on the cell cycle dependence of this class of agents. As with the short-term infusions, extravasation reactions have occurred from prolonged infusions of vincristine [140,141] as well as vinblastine [142]. These extravasations produced swelling and phlebitis, although skin necrosis was not described in any of the patients. Most of the reactions resolved after 1–2 weeks, possibly because the drug extravasated had been present in lower concentration.

A number of putative antidotes to vinca alkaloid extravasation have been tested, including folinic acid [143], glutamic acid [144], sodium bicarbonate [130], and hyaluronidase and glucocorticosteroids [145,145]. However, there are relatively few controlled studies available to support efficacy claims of any particular antidote. For example, in two case reports involving subcutaneous hydrocortisone, there was a beneficial outcome

[146,162]. Even so, since most vesicant extravasations do not cause ulceration, statistically this is the most likely event with any of the vesicant agents.

In preclinical models of vinca alkaloid skin toxicity, several studies have suggested important differences from other classes of vesicant drugs. In a guinea pig model, subcutaneous vincristine and vinblastine were shown to be nontoxic [90]. In contrast, intradermally injected vinca alkaloids produced substantial soft tissue ulceration at all concentrations tested, including those equivalent to 1% of the human vincristine or vinblastine therapeutic dose [90]. In this guinea pig study, the skin toxicity was not due to an immunologic or prior sensitization reaction, but instead occurred as a direct and immediate consequence of drug injection into the skin. Histologically, the vinca alkaloid lesions in the guinea pigs were associated with an acute hemorrhagic inflammation. Preservation of granulation was noted from both capillary and fibroblast cell proliferation. This is another contrast with the anthracyclines, for which inflammatory healing reactions in the immediate extravasation site, tend to be retarded or absent. This may also explain why relatively few vinca alkaloid lesions result in long-term soft tissue damage and impairment. Clearly these findings separate the vinca class of vesicants from the anthracyclines.

In rodent models, there have also been important differences from the anthracyclines. In one study, skin lesions in mice were produced only after repeated intradermal vinca alkaloid administrations using a 7-day dosing interval [5]. In this case a pattern of diffuse inflammatory lesions was produced that suggested a local hypersensitivity etiology. No antidotes were tested in this study. In a subsequent rabbit model study, intradermal vincristine injections produced inconsistent skin ulcers, which developed slowly over 7 days and had resolved completely by 17 days after intradermal injection [147]. Histopathologic examination of this lesion showed extensive neutrophil infiltration, with dermal separation occurring within days of the intradermal injection. Despite the evidence of inflammatory response, locally administered corticosteroids such as dexamethasone did not reduce or prevent these skin ulcers. There was also no reduction in the consistent occurrence of induration with dexamethasone given after intradermal viscristine in the rabbit model [136].

In a more quantitative trial of intradermal vinca alkaloid injections in the mouse model, vinblastine or vincristine was tested against a variety of experimental antidotes (Table 5). Since a number of antidotes have been suggested from the prior anecdotal case report literature, all these were tested using the intradermal injection of vincristine or vinblastine followed by treatment with each adjuvant. Of this large list of agents, only three procedures were shown to be consistently effective and they have a consistent theme:

Table 5 Extravasation Antidotes to Vinca Alkaloids

	Effective in	
Ineffective in animal models	Animal models [26]	Clinical cases [154]
Calcium Leucovorin	0.9% Sodium chloride	Hyaluronidase
Diphenhydramine	Topical heating	
Hydrocortisone[a]	Hyaluronidase	
Isoproterenol		
Sodium bicarbonate		
Topical cooling[a]		
Vitamin A cream[a]		

[a]Significantly increased skin ulceration [26].

significant dilution of the locally injected vinca alkaloid. As indicated in Table 5, these are the injection of normal saline, the application of topical heating, and the intradermal injection of hyaluronidase, a spreading factor enzyme. All these treatments could be acting to dilute the drug to a less toxic local concentration. Of these procedures, injection of hyaluronidase was most effective at reducing the amount of drug in the tissues, as noted in radiolabeled vinblastine uptake studies in the mouse [26]. Similar effects were also shown to follow the application of mild skin warming, in an effort to produce local vasodilation and promote systemic uptake of the intradermal drug.

The enzyme hyaluronidase is well established for this type of local dilution activity. It is known to act as an enzymatic spreading factor and works by temporarily dissolving the hyaluronic acid bonds that hold tissue planes together [148–150]. Hyaluronidase had formerly seen clinical use as an adjuvant to increase subcutaneous fluid absorption and as an aid in promoting drug resorption from subcutaneous spaces [149]. The typical dose in the latter setting for the subcutaneous administration of large amounts of fluid has been 150 units of enzymatic activity added to the subcutaneously injected infusate. This dose can effectively promote the systemic absorption of up to a liter of subcutaneously administered fluids [148].

Other experiments have shown that hyaluronidase can promote the absorption of inadvertently extravasated antibiotics such as nafcillin in neonates [150], and experimental extravasations of hyperosmolar hyperalimentation solutions [149] or radiopaque contrast media [151]. Hyaluronidase has also been shown to be effective for all the commercially used vincas, including vinorelbine [26,154].

6.3.10 Vinorelbine (Navelbine)

Vinorelbine (Navelbine) is a newer semisynthetic vinca alkaloid structurally related to vinblastine. Local site reactions have been reported in 10% of patients receiving weekly short intravenous infusions [152]. Most often, venous irritation is reported, a toxicity that may be worsened if the infusion time is increased from 6–10 minutes to 20–30 minutes [153]. Most venous irritation from vinorelbine is mild, however, and local venous toxicity of grade 3 or higher is rarely reported. Thus, while a 15% venous irritation incidence was described in one breast cancer series, only 1 of 115 patients in this trial experienced grade 3 pain and/or irritation. However, because the drug is often given by weekly infusions, cumulative venous toxicities can ensue, leading to more troublesome degrees of toxicity.

While no serious extravasation injuries have been clinically reported, the close chemical similarity of vinorelbine to other vinca alkaloids with established vesicant potential suggests that vinorelbine may also have vesicant activity if inadvertently extravasated. Indeed, the drug has been shown to produce dose-dependent skin ulcers in a mouse skin toxicity model [29].

Antidotes to vinorelbine extravasations have been studied in a mouse model. Intradermal vinorelbine doses of 0.01–0.5 mg produced skin lesions that healed slowly over 2–3 weeks, depending on the dose [29]. Antidote studies showed that only one adjuvant, intradermal hyaluronidase at a murine dose of 15 units, effectively reduced vinorelbine-induced skin toxicity. Other maneuvers, including topical heating or cooling, were not effective. Thus, vinorelbine is a probable vesicant and extravasations should be treated with subcutaneous hyaluronidase at the human-equivalent dose of 150–300 units in 2–3 mL of normal saline.

The clinical use of hyaluronidase as an antidote to the extravasation of vinca alkaloids was studied in a pilot trial by Bertelli et al. [154]. In this trial patients who experienced an extravasation of vincristine, vinblastine, or vinorelbine were treated with 250 units of hyaluronidase diluted in 6 mL of normal saline, administered through the indwelling needle if still in place. If the needle had been removed after the extravasation, a separate series of six subcutaneous injections was given around the extravasation site, using a 25-gauge needle. Steroids were not used. Cold packs and pressure dressings were also avoided in this trial. None of the seven patients in this small series developed skin necrosis [154]. The treatment was also very well tolerated. This provides presumptive confirmation of the antidotal efficacy of locally injected hyaluronidase as a treatment for extravasations of all the vinca alkaloids. In addition, there are unreported cases involving the delayed-onset type of vinca extravasation reactions wherein hyaluronidase has also been shown to be effective, albeit to a lesser degree than when given immediately after an extravasation. Thus, hyaluronidase should be considered as the local antidote of choice for treating all classes of vinca alkaloid extravasations.

6.3.11 Taxanes

The taxanes, paclitaxel (Taxol, Bristol-Myers Squibb) and docetaxel (Taxotere, Rhône-Poulenc Rorer), represent a unique class of tubulin-binding anticancer agents. These drugs induce abnormal, excessive tubulin polymerization [155] and are highly active in several solid tumors including ovarian, lung, and breast cancers. While the dose-limiting clinical toxicities are myelosuppression and/or peripheral neuropathy, local venous and perivenous toxicities have been observed, particularly with the most commonly used taxane, paclitaxel [156]. While extravasations of paclitaxel occurred throughout its phase I/II testing period, none of these initial events caused severe local toxicity [157,158]. A review of this literature reveals an extravasation incidence of 2.8%, all of grade 2 (mild to moderate) severity according to the criteria of the National Cancer Institute [45]. Indeed, the usual sequelae of an extravasation of paclitaxel from a peripheral venipuncture site involve only erythema, slight swelling, and (rarely) pain or residual inflammation [157,158].

Two more recent reports, however, have described more serious toxicities [45,46]. In the first report, skin toxicity of at least grade 1 was observed in three patients among a series of 69 infusions in 24 patients [45]. In this retrospective report, Ajani et al. described three serious extravasations following the first, second, or third course of therapy in one patient, each [45]. One patient developed a painful erythematous nodule at an infusion site on the left forearm 5 days after starting a 24-hour infusion of 250 mg/m^2. The 2 cm (diameter) nodule was tender but did not ulcerate and was rated as grade 2. However, a biopsy of this nodule showed extensive coagulative necrosis of soft tissue adjacent to the site. Fortunately, this lesion healed without specific intervention. Another grade 2 lesion of 2 cm size occurred on a second patient on day 7 of the second course of paclitaxel. Some peeling of the skin was noted over this time period. In the third patient, pain and swelling occurred on day 2 of the first course of paclitaxel therapy, given through a vein on the wrist. The widest diameter of this grade 2 lesion was 5 cm, and although the swelling and pain subsided without ulceration, superficial damage and skin peeling remained present 73 days after the extravasation [46].

A second report from this institution described more severe lesions among 17 patients who experienced an extravasation of paclitaxel [46]. There were 19 instances of extravasation of paclitaxel from a peripheral vein among 955 courses, or approximately 2%. Clinical signs of extravasation consisted of mild discomfort, erythema, and edema. These occurred during the infusion in only 8 of 19 (42%) of extravasations. In other words, delayed signs and symptoms occurred in the majority of patients experiencing local toxicity. Typical lesions were darkly discolored, raised, rounded, and indurated, with moderate pain present. Approximately two-thirds of the lesions were only grade 2 in severity, but lesions in four patients (21%) were of grade 3 severity with central ulcerations present. This translates to a severe extravasation incidence of only 4 in 955 or 0.4%. Four of these lesions manifested cellulitis requiring antibiotic therapy, and in one patient ulceration persisted for 6 months (up to the time of death from advancing disease). Importantly, only one patient in this series required surgical excision of a lesion, which had persisted for 12 months.

Soft tissue recall injuries have also been described following paclitaxel extravasation from peripheral veins [47,48,156,157]. In one case, recurrent pain, swelling, and erythema occurred at the hand site of an extravasation that had occurred a month earlier. Symptoms were noted 8 hours after a repeated paclitaxel infusion in a lower extremity vein. This gradually resolved over one week [47]. Another recall reaction was characterized by severe local site irritation 6 weeks after a paclitaxel infusion involving a sizable extravasation [156]. The symptoms of pain, sensory loss, and functional deficit occurred 3 weeks after an uncomplicated infusion of paclitaxel. In the initial infusion, extravasation of approximately one-fifth of the 175 mg/m^2 dose occurred into the tissues around the right antecubital vein. The initial and subsequent localization and escalation of the pain and swelling at the antecubital extravasation site suggest that neuropathic toxicities can be both prolonged and additive at local sites of paclitaxel extravasation.

In another paclitaxel extravasation recall reaction, a patient experienced an initial large extravasation of drug solution. The extravasated area of the forearm, measuring 8 cm × 12 cm, was painful and displayed erythema and induration. This was followed by superficial skin peeling but no ulceration. At the time of the next infusion 21 days later, the site had healed almost completely and paclitaxel was given uneventfully through an implanted central venous catheter. Two days later a painful, erythematous, and swollen nodule reappeared at the prior extravasation site on the forearm. This resolved after 8 days [48]. Another unusual recall reaction occurred following 15 subcutaneous injections of ''homeopathic'' doses of paclitaxel into the abdominal wall of a patient with ovarian cancer. The reaction ensued when several therapeutic paclitaxel doses of 175 mg/m^2 each were administered intravenously. Red nodules appeared at three abdominal sites of prior subcutaneous paclitaxel administration after one intravenous dose, and these progressed to frank ulcerations after two more intravenous doses had been administered. Histologic examination showed necrosis of skin and a mixed inflammatory infiltration. The most severe nodules were excised, and although 10 more courses of intravenous paclitaxel were administered, there was no further worsening of the remaining abdominal sites [157].

In addition to peripheral vein extravasations of paclitaxel, there is at least one case of severe injury following paclitaxel extravasation from a vascular access device implanted in the chest wall of an adult female patient with adenocarcinoma. It is estimated that nearly 100 mg/m^2 of the 175 mg/m^2 dose extravasated into a 10 cm × 15 cm area of the chest wall, creating extensive necrosis over a 5 cm × 11 cm area. Port explantation and surgical excision down to the pectoralis major fascia were required. This case shows that large extravasations of paclitaxel can cause severe toxicity regardless of whether the attempted administration is via peripheral or central veins.

Several local antidotes to paclitaxel extravasations have been proposed from these various anecdotal case reports. In the second report from the M. D. Anderson clinic, 16 of 19 local extravasations were treated initially with warm compresses and two with ice compresses. Only one patient received no local therapy [46]. Another case report, from Birmingham, England, described a complex pharmacologic treatment of three paclitaxel extravasations [158]. Initially, the extravasation sites were aspirated and dexamethasone and chlorpheniramine were injected subcutaneously, followed in 30 minutes by hyaluronidase, 1500 U/2 mL, again given by subcutaneous injection. None of these lesions resulted in local necrosis [158].

A quantitative paclitaxel skin toxicity study in a mouse skin model evaluated a number of putative antidotes to paclitaxel extravasation [159]. These included injected saline, albumin, hyaluronidase or hydrocortisone, and topical dimethyl sulfoxide, as well as heating and cooling. None of the topical treatments were effective. Similarly, most of the injected agents did not reduce or prevent skin lesions caused by an intradermal injection of paclitaxel. The only injected agent that showed efficacy as a local antidote was hyaluronidase. This treatment did not totally eliminate toxicity, but it significantly reduced the size and duration of paclitaxel skin lesions. At the lower intradermal paclitaxel dose of 0.6 mg, a single hyaluronidase injection of 15 units reduced the mean skin ulcer size by 95%. At the higher paclitaxel dose of 1.2 mg, hyaluronidase reduced skin ulcer sizes by over 50% [159]. This study also showed that the commercial paclitaxel solvent system, containing Cremophor EL and ethanol, produced small skin lesions. Thus, the diluent may be a minor contributor to the drug's local toxicity potential.

Finally, a pilot clinical experience with hyaluronidase as a paclitaxel extravasation antidote has been reported by Bertelli et al. of the Italian National Cancer Institute [160]. Five patients experiencing paclitaxel extravasation were treated with hyaluronidase (250 units in 6 mL) injected into and around the extravasation site. Local symptoms, consisting of pain, swelling, and erythema, subsided in all five patients, and no further therapy was required. Two other patients experiencing a docetaxel (Taxotere) extravasation were similarly treated with hyaluronidase. In one patient, all local symptoms disappeared rapidly and in the other, an intense local inflammatory reaction at the forearm extravasation site subsided slowly over a period of several days. Necrosis was not evident in either patient. Although this is not a controlled study, the preliminary clinical findings suggest that hyaluronidase is a useful local antidote for taxane extravasations.

Overall the taxanes comprise a class of weak vesicants. The question then of when to treat taxane extravasations is difficult, since paclitaxel-induced necrosis is a very rare event, even when extravasation is documented. Also, whether hyaluronidase would be effective for delayed or "recall" reactions to paclitaxel extravasation is unknown. However, it is clear that some extravasations of taxanes, and especially paclitaxel, can cause severe local toxicity if untreated. Therefore, a prudent but empirical recommendation would be to treat any extravasation wherein a relatively sizable percent of the dose ($\geq$10%) is estimated to have extravasated. This is consistent with the reported cases of severe local toxicity following large taxane extravasations. The high safety margin of subcutaneous hyaluronidase also argues for its routine use in treating any potentially serious taxane extravasation. Dosing of hyaluronidase for adult patients should be in the range of 250–300 units (in a small volume of 2–5 mL), injected once, into and around the extravasation site. Other local maneuvers, such as cold, heat, corticosteroids, and DMSO, are not recommended for treating paclitaxel extravasations because of their lack of efficacy in animal models, and because no corroborating clinical case reports are available.

6.3.12 Epipodophyllotoxins

The semisynthetic epipodophyllotoxins include the agents etoposide (VP-16) and teniposide (VM-26). Both drugs inhibit topoisomerase II, but they occasionally produce phlebitis and local swelling at injection sites. There is one description of severe skin ulceration following the extravasation of etoposide in humans [8]. However, the relative paucity of other cases suggests that etoposide is usually a nonvesicant agent. Similar case reports for VM-26 are not available, and given the widespread use of these agents in the clinic, as well as numerous extravasations that have occurred without incident, we must consider that these have a relatively low vesicant potential.

In one animal trial looking at the podophyllotoxins, the solvent system used for the commercial etoposide formulation, which contains polysorbate

80 and Cremophor EL, was shown to produce a measurable degree of skin toxicity on its own [161]. This suggests that lipophilic detergents like Cremophor EL and polysorbate 80 (Tween 80) can produce local skin toxicities that may be greater than that of the drug they are used to solubilize. Antidote studies performed with both epipodophyllotoxins in the intradermal mouse model suggest that hyaluronidase is an effective antidote and that for any severe extravasations of either VP-16 or VM-26, the use of hyaluronidase might be considered in humans. However, it is unlikely that either epipodophyllotoxin comprises a major extravasation risk, since both have a low propensity to cause serious extravasation reactions. Moreover, they are most commonly given in dilute solutions, which would preclude the subcutaneous delivery of a large amount of concentrated drug.

6.4 CONCLUSIONS AND SUMMARY RECOMMENDATIONS

As this chapter has shown, there are three distinct mechanistic categories of vesicant antitumor agents:

- DNA intercalators, primarily the anthracyclines
- DNA-binding agents (e.g., the alkylating agents nitrogen mustard and mitomycin C)
- the vinca alkaloids

Agents that have elicited sporadic reports of severe ulceration include the taxanes and, very rarely, cisplatin. These two agents should really be considered to be weak potential vesicants, since extremely large extravasated amounts of concentrated solution are needed to produce a serious reaction.

The chapter has also shown that a very large number of antidotes have been proposed for these various vesicant drugs, although relatively few have demonstrated consistent efficacy in either preclinical or clinical settings. The recognized effective antidotes are summarized in Table 6. This shows that practicing oncologists need to have readily available only a small number of antidotes. These include a means of topical cooling and a source of topical DMSO for the anthracyclines. A commercial source of medical-grade DMSO is available in the United States under the trade name Cryoserve, from Research Industries Corporation, Salt Lake City, Utah. Although officially indicated for cryopreservation of human bone marrow cells in vitro, this sterile, pyrogen-free material is supplied as a 99% (w/v) concentration in a 70 mL pour-top bottle that is suitable for use as a topical anthracycline antidote. In addition to extravasations of the anthracyclines such as doxorubicin and other DNA-binding agents, DMSO has investigational utility as a topical

Table 6 Recommended Extravasation Antidotes for Vesicant Chemotherapy Drugs

	Recommended antidotes	
Vesicant drug	Agents	Specific regimen
DNA intercalators		
Doxorubicin, daunorubicin, epirubicin	Topical cooling	Apply ice packs on/off site 15 minutes each hour for first day
	99% w/v DMSO	Apply to site four to six times daily for 2 weeks; use no occlusive dressing
DNA-binding agents		
Mechlorethamine, cisplatin (large extravasations only)	0.166 M sodium thiosulfate	Inject 2–3 mL into site; repeat up to four times
Mitomycin C	99% DMSO	Apply to site four to six times daily for 2 weeks; use no occlusive dressing
Tubulin-binding agents		
Vincristine, vinblastine, vindesine, vinorelbine paclitaxel (large extravasations only)	Hyaluronidase	Inject 150–300 units (in 1.5–3.0 mL) into site

treatment for the severe skin lesions associated with chronic dosing of (non-extravasated) liposomal doxorubicin, and extravasations of mitomycin C. For the alkylating agent nitrogen mustard, which is infrequently used, sodium thiosulfate is a very effective antidote. This agent, at its isotonic 0.166 M concentration, could also comprise a useful antidote for cisplatin extravasations, but only when a very large amount of a concentrated solution has extravasated and requires treatment.

Of all the extravasation antidotes, hyaluronidase perhaps has the best-defined rationale and efficacy as an antidote for extravasations of vinca alkaloids and paclitaxel. It is available in a sterile lyophilized form as well as a ready-to-use solution and is highly effective and nontoxic as a local antidote. It should be considered to be the antidote of choice and used in all situations involving extravasations of the standard vinca alkaloids. In this setting it may even be useful for those rare cases of delayed presentations of symptoms. For taxane extravasations it may also be considered to be the antidote of choice, but should be used only in when a large amount of the solution has extravasated.

As this chapter has shown, the use of vascular access devices has reduced, but not completely eliminated, the risk of extravasation injury. Indeed, there are an increasing number of case reports of severe extravasation involving totally vascular access devices. These numbers probably will be reduced with the advent of better devices to "lock" the drug delivery needle into the septum of the implanted device. This simple improvement could prevent the most common cause of extravasation from an implanted vascular access device. Extravasation injury remains a consistent problem in oncology practice, and the rapid use of appropriate antidotes should be considered for all vesicant extravasations. Such measures will help to mitigate, but not always prevent, severe ulceration injury. Since some injuries will not be sufficiently reduced or prevented by antidotes, close monitoring of all vesicant infusions and early consultation with surgical experts will continue to be necessary to adequately manage serious extravasation reactions.

REFERENCES

1. Rudolph R, Stein RS, Pattillo RA. Skin ulcers due to Adriamycin. Cancer 1976:38:1087–1094.
2. Reilly JJ, Neifeld JP, Rosenberg SA. Clinical course and management of accidental Adriamycin extravasation. Cancer 1977:40:2053–2056.
3. Barlock AL, Howser DM, Hubbard SM. Nursing management of Adriamycin extravasation. Am J Nurs 1979:137:94–96.
4. Mehta P, Najar N. Skin ulceration due to faulty Adriamycin administration. Clin Pediatr 1978:17:663–664.
5. Laughlin RA, Landeen JM, Habal MB. The management of inadvertent subcutaneous Adriamycin infiltration. Am J Surg 1979:137:408–412.
6. Linder RM, Upton J, Osteen R. Management of extensive doxorubicin hydrochloride extravasation injuries. J Hand Surg 1983:8:32–38.
7. Bowers DG Jr, Lynch JB. Adriamycin extravasation. Plast Reconstr Surg 1978:61:86–92.
8. Preuss P, Partoft S. Cytostatic extravasations. Ann Plast Surg 1987:19:323–329.
9. Lippman M, Zager R, Jenderson ES. High dose daunorubicin (NSC-83142) in the treatment of advanced acute myelogenous leukemia. Cancer Chemother Rep 1972:56:755–760.
10. Greene W, Huffman D, Wiernik PH, Schimpff S, Benjamin R, Bachur N. High-dose daunorubicin therapy for acute nonlymphocytic leukemia: Correlation of response and toxicity with pharmacokinetics and intracellular daunorubicin reductase activity. Cancer 1972:30:1419–1427.
11. Dragon LH, Braine HG. Necrosis of the hand after daunorubicin infusion distal to an arteriovenous fistula. Ann Intern Med 1979:91:58–59.

12. Barr RD, Benton SG, Belbeck LW. Soft tissue necrosis induced by extravasated cancer chemotherapeutic agents. J Natl Cancer Inst 1981:66:1129–1136.
13. Wiernik PH, Serpick AA. A randomized clinical trial of daunorubicin and a combination of prednisone, vincristine, 6-mercaptopurine and methotrexate in adult acute nonlymphocytic leukemia. Cancer Res 1972:32:2023–2026.
14. Gin SN, Rice S, Bacchetti P. Characteristic features of actinomycin D–induced paw inflammation of the rat. Exp Mol Pathol 1975:23:367–378.
15. Buchanan GR, Buchsbaum HJ, O'Banion K, Gojer B. Extravasation of dactinomycin, vincristine, and cisplatin: Studies in an animal model. Med Pediatr Oncol 1985:13:375–380.
16. Chait LA, Dinner MI. Ulceration caused by cytotoxic drugs. S Afr Med J 1975:49:1935–1936.
17. Ganzina F. 4′-Epi-doxorubicin, a new analogue of doxorubicin: A preliminary overview of preclinical and clinical data. Cancer Treat Rev 1983:10:1–22.
18. Lee KM, Dorr RT, Robertone A. High incidence of local venous reactions to esorubicin. Invest New Drugs 1987:5:31–35.
19. Stanton GF, Raymond V, Wittes RE, Schulman P, Budman D, Baratz R, Williams L, Petroni GR, Geller NL, Hancock C. Phase I and clinical pharmacological evaluation of 4′-deoxydoxorubicin in patients with advanced cancer. Cancer Res 1985:45:1862–1868.
20. Kreis W, Rottach C, Budman DR, Chan K, Schulman P, Allen SL, Weiselberg L, Vinciguerra V. Pharmacokinetic and phase I evaluation of esorubicin (4′-deoxydoxorubicin) by continuous infusion over forty-eight hours in patients with leukemia. Cancer Res 1988:48:5580–5584.
21. Ferrari L, Rossi, A, Brambilla C, Bonfante V, Villani F, Crippa F, Bonadonna G. Phase I study with 4′-deoxydoxorubicin. Invest New Drugs 1984:2:287–295.
22. Goodman LS, Wintrobe MM, Dameshek W, Goodman MJ, Gilman A, McLennan MT. Nitrogen mustard therapy. Use of methyl-bis(beta-chloroethyl)amine hydrochloride and tris(beta-chloroethyl)amine hydrochloride for Hodgkin's disease, lymphosarcoma, leukemia and certain allied and miscellaneous disorders. JAMA 1984:251(17):2255–2261.
23. Wood HA, Ellerhorst-Ryan JM. Delayed adverse skin reactions associated with mitomycin-C administration. Oncol Nurs Forum 1984:11:14–18.
24. Argenta LC, Manders EK. Mitomycin C extravasation injuries. Cancer 1983: 51:1080–1082.
25. Khanna AK, Khanna A, Asthana AK, Misra MK. Mitomycin C extravasation ulcers. J Surg Oncol 1985:28:108–110.
26. Dorr RT, Alberts DS. Vinca alkaloid skin toxicity: Antidote and drug disposition studies in the mouse. J Natl Cancer Inst 1985:74:113–120.
27. Gill DP, Eakin DL, Weiss GB. Cutaneous necrosis from chemotherapy in a patient with an arteriovenous fistula. Cancer Treat Rep 1981:65:352–353.
28. James DH, George P. Vincristine in children with malignant solid tumors. J Pediatr 1964:64:534–541.

29. Dorr RT, Bool KL. Antidote studies of vinorelbine-induced skin ulceration in the mouse. Cancer Chemother Pharmacol 1995:36:290–292.
30. Jones S, Winer E, Vogel C, Laufman L, Hutchins L, O'Rourke M, Lembersky B, Budman D, Bigley J, Hohneker J. Randomized comparison of vinorelbine and melphalan in anthracycline-refractory advanced breast cancer. J Clin Oncol 1995:13(10):2567–2574.
31. Dorr RT, Jones SE. Inapparent infiltrations associated with vindesine administration. Med Pediatr Oncol 1979:6:285–288.
32. Soble MJ, Dorr RT, Plezia P, Breckenridge S. Dose-dependent skin ulcers in mice treated with DNA binding antitumor antibiotics. Cancer Chemother Pharmacol 1987:20:33–36.
33. Alberts DS, Griffiths KS, Goodman GE, Herman TS, Murray E. Phase I clinical trial of mitoxantrone: A new anthracenedione anticancer drug. Cancer Chemother Pharmacol 1980:5:11–15.
34. Anderson KC, Cohen GI, Garnick MB. Phase II trial of mitoxantrone. Cancer Treat Rep 1982:65:1929–1931.
35. Peters FTM, Beijnen JH, ten Bokkel-Huinink WT. Mitoxantrone extravasation injury. Cancer Treat Rep 1987:71:992–993.
36. Dorr RT, Alberts DS, Soble MJ. Lack of experimental vesicant activity for the anticancer agents cisplatin, melphalan, and mitoxantrone. Cancer Chemother Pharmacol 1986:16:91–94.
37. Von Hoff DD, Pollard E, Kuhn J. Phase I clinical investigation of 1,4-dihydroxy-5,8-bis(2[2-dihydrocloride]) (NSC 301739), a new anthracenedione. Cancer Res 1980:1516:1518.
38. Leyden M, Sullivan J. Full thickness skin necrosis due to inadvertent interstitial infusion of cisplatin. Cancer Treat Rep 1983:67(2):199.
39. Lewis KP, Medina WD. Cellulitis and fibrosis due to *cis*-diamminedichloroplatinum(II) (platinol) infiltration. Cancer Treat Rep 1980:64:1162–1163.
40. Algarra SM, Dy C, Bilbao I, Aparicio LA. Cutaneous necrosis after intraarterial treatment with cisplatin. Cancer Treat Rep 1986:70:687–688.
41. Teta JB, O'Connor L. Local tissue damage from 5-fluorouracil extravasation. Oncol Nurs Forum 1984:11:77.
42. Reed WP, Newman KA, Applefeld MM, Sutton FJ. Drug extravasation as a complication of venous access ports. Ann Intern Med 1985:102:788–790.
43. Seyfer AE, Solimando DA Jr. Toxic lesions of the hand associated with chemotherapy. J Hand Surg 1983:8:39–42.
44. Bicher A, Levenback C, Burke TW, Morris M, Warner D, DeJesus Y, Gershenson DM. Infusion site soft-tissue injury after paclitaxel administration. Cancer 1995:76(1):116–120.
45. Ajani JA, Dodd LG, Daugherty K, Warkentin D, Ilson DH. Taxol-induced soft-tissue injury secondary to extravasation: Characterization by histopathology and clinical course. J Natl Cancer Inst 1994:86(1):51–53.
46. Bicher A, Levenback C, Burke TW, Morris M, Warner D, DeJesus Y, Gershenson DM. Infusion site soft-tissue injury after paclitaxel administration. Cancer 1995:76:116–120.

47. Shapiro J, Richardson GE. Paclitaxel-induced "recall" soft tissue injury occurring at the site of previous extravasation with subsequent intravenous treatment in a different limb. J Clin Oncol 1994:12(10):2237–2238.
48. Meehan JL, Sporn JR. Case report of Taxol administration via central vein producing a recall reaction at a site of prior Taxol extravasation. J Natl Cancer Inst 1994:86(16):1250–1251.
49. Ravdin PM, Burris HA III, Cook G, Eisenberg P, Kane M, Bierman WA, Mortimer J, Genevois E, Bellet RE. Phase II trial of docetaxel in advanced anthracycline-resistant or anthracenedione-resistant breast cancer. J Clin Oncol 1995:13:2879–2885.
50. ten Bokkel Huinink WW, Prove AM, Piccart M, Steward W, Tursz T, Wanders J, Franklin H, Clavel M, Verweij J, Alakl M, Bayssas M, Kaye SB. A phase II trial with docetaxel (Taxotere®) in second line treatment with chemotherapy for advanced breast cancer. Ann Oncol 1994:5:527–532.
51. Forssen EA, Tokes ZA. Attenuation of dermal toxicity of doxorubicin by liposome encapsulation. Cancer Treat Rep 1983:67:481–484.
52. Balazsovits JAE, Mayer LD, Bally MB, Cullis PR, McDonell M, Ginsberg RS, Falk RE. Analysis of the effect of liposome encapsulation on the vesicant properties, acute and cardiac toxicities, and antitumor efficacy of doxorubicin. Cancer Chemother Pharmacol 1989:23:81–86.
53. Forssen EA, Ross ME. DaunoXome® treatment of solid tumors: Preclinical and clinical investigations. J Liposome Res 1994:4:481–512.
54. Guaglianone P, Chan K, DelaFlor-Weiss E, Hanisch R, Jeffers S, Sharma D, Muggia F. Phase I and pharmacologic study of liposomal daunorubicin (DaunoXome). Invest New Drugs 1994:12:103–110.
55. Dorr RT. Antidotes to vesicant chemotherapy extravasations. Blood Rev 1990: 4:41–60.
56. Dorr RT, Alberts DS, Einspahr J, Mason-Liddil N, Soble M. Experimental dacarbazine antitumor activity and skin toxicity in relation to light exposure and pharmacologic antidotes. Cancer Treat Rep 1987:71:267–272.
57. Armand JP. CPT-11: Clinical experience in phase I studies. Semin Oncol 1996:23(1 supple 3):27–33.
58. Larson DL. Treatment of tissue extravasation by antitumor agents. Cancer 1982:49:1796–1799.
59. Garnick M, Israel M, Knetarpal IV, Luce J. Persistence of anthracycline levels following dermal and subcutaneous Adriamycin extravasation (abstr). Proc Am Soc Clin Oncol 1981:22:173.
60. Sonneveld P, Wassenaar HA, Nooter K. Long persistence of doxorubicin in human skin after extravasation. Cancer Treat Rep 1984:68:895–896.
61. Dorr RT, Dordal MS, Koenig LM, Taylor CW, McCloskey TM. High doxorubicin tissue levels in a patient experiencing extravasation during a four-day infusion. Cancer 1989:64:2462–2464.
62. Reed WP, Newman KA, Applefeld MM, Sutton FJ. Drug extravasation as a complication of venous access ports. Ann Intern Med 1985:102:788–790.
63. Schulmeister L. Needle dislodgement from implanted venous access devices: Inpatient and outpatient experiences. J Intravenous Nurs 1989:12:90–92.

64. Smith RE. A practical subcutaneous infusion port system for cancer patients. A Southeastern Ohio Cancer Center study. Ohio State Med J 1985:81:743–746.
65. Pessa M, Howard R. Complications of Hickman–Broviac catheters. Surg Gynecol Obstet 1985:161:256–260.
66. Fellows KE. Radiographic observation of the indwelling venous catheter. Postgrad Med 1970:47:61–62.
67. Conces DJ, Holden RW. Aberrant locations and complications in initial placement of subclavian vein catheters. Arch Surg 1984:119:293–295.
68. Diekmann J, Ransom J. Extravasation of doxorubicin from a Hickman™ catheter: A case presentation. Oncol Nurs Forum 1985:12:50–52.
69. Gemlo BT, Rayner AA, Swanson RJ, Young JA, Hormann JF, Hohn DC. A serious complication of the split-sheath introducer technique for venous access. Arch Surg 1988:123:490–492.
70. Kerr IG, Iscoe N, Sone M, Hanna S. Venous access ports. Ann Intern Med 1985:103:637–638.
71. Freytes CO, Reid P, Smith KL. Long-term experience with a totally implanted catheter system in cancer patients. J Surg Oncol 1990:45:99–102.
72. Brothers TE, von Moll LK, Niederhuber JE, Roberts JA, Walker-Andrews S, Ensminger WD. Experience with subcutaneous infusion ports in three hundred patients. Surg Gynecol Obstet 1988:4:295–301.
73. Dorr RT. Extravasation from vascular access devices. In: B Hickman, S Herbst, eds. Vascular Access and Other Related Devices.
74. Brincker H, Saeter G. Fifty-five patient years' experience with a totally implanted system for intravenous chemotherapy. Cancer 1986:57:1124–1129.
75. Bothe A Jr, Piccione W, Ambrosino JJ, Benotti PN, Lokich JJ. Implantable central venous access system. Am J Surg 1984:147:565–569.
76. Greidanus J, DeVries EGE, Nieweg MB, De Langen ZJ, Willemse PHB. Evaluation of a totally implanted venous access port and portable pump in a continuous chemotherapy infusion schedule on an outpatient basis. Eur J Cancer Clin Oncol 1987:23(11):1653–1657.
77. Soo KC, Davidson TI, Selby P, Westbury G. Long-term venous access using a subcutaneous implantable drug delivery system. Ann R Coll Surg Eng 1985:67:263–265.
78. Gyves J, Ensminger W, Niederhuber J, Liepman M, Cozzi E, Doan K, Dakhil S, Wheeler R. Totally implanted system for intravenous chemotherapy in patients with cancer. Am J Med 1982:73:841–845.
79. Kerr IG, Deangelis C, Assaad DM, Hanna SS. Drug extravasation along the route of a peritoneal catheter during intraperitoneal chemotherapy. Cancer 1987:60:1731–1733.
80. Winters V, Peters B, Coila S, Jones L. A trial with a new peripheral implanted vascular access device. Oncol Nurs Forum 1990:17:891–896.
81. Upton J, Mulliken JB, Murray JE. Major intravenous extravasation injuries. Am J Surg 1979:137:497–506.
82. Lemmers NWM, Gels ME, Sleijfer DT, Plukker J, van der Graaf WTA, de Langen ZJ, Droste JHJ, Schraffordt Koops H, Hoekstra HJ. Complications of

venous access ports in 132 patients with disseminated testicular cancer treated with polychemotherapy. J Clin Oncol 1996:14:2916–2922.

83. Wickham RS. Advances in venous access devices and nursing management strategies. Nurs Clin North Am 1990:25:345–364.
84. Etcubanas E, Wilbur JR. Uncommon side effects of Adriamycin (NSC-123127). Cancer Chemother Rep 1974:58(part 1):757–758.
85. Souhami L Jr, Feld R. Urticaria following intravenous doxorubicin administration. JAMA 1987:240:1624–1626.
86. Vogelzang NJ. "Adriamycin flare:" A skin reaction resembling extravasation. Cancer Treat Rep 1979:63:2067–2069.
87. Piscitelli SC, Rodvold KA, Rushing DA, Tewksbury DA. Pharmacokinetics and pharmacodynamics of doxorubicin in patients with small cell lung cancer. Clin Pharmacol Ther 1993:53:555–561.
88. Cohen FJ, Manganaro J, Bezozo RC. Identification of involved tissue during surgical treatment of doxorubicin-induced extravasation necrosis. J Hand Surg 1983:8:43–45.
89. Dorr T, Alberts DS, Chen HSG. The limited role of corticosteroids in ameliorating experimental doxorubicin skin toxicity in the mouse. Cancer Chemother Pharmacol 1980:5:17–20.
90. Barr RD, Sertic J. Soft-tissue necrosis induced by extravasated cancer chemotherapeutic agents: A study of active intervention. Br J Cancer 1981:44:267–269.
91. Luedke DW, Kennedy PS, Rietschel RL. Histopathogenesis of skin and subcutaneous injury induced by Adriamycin. Plast Reconstr Surg 1979:63:463–465.
92. Rudolph R, Larson DL. Etiology and treatment of chemotherapeutic agent extravasation injuries: A review. J Clin Oncol 1987:5(7):1116–1126.
93. Gottlieb NL, Penneys NS. Spontaneous skin tearing during systemic corticosteroid treatment. JAMA 1980:243(12):1260–1261.
94. Ehrlich HP, Hunt TK. Effects of cortisone and vitamin A on wound healing. Ann Surg 1968:167(3):324–328.
95. Zweig J, Kabakow B. An apparently effective countermeasure for doxorubicin extravasation (letter). JAMA 1978:239:2116.
96. Kappel B, Hindenburg AA, Taub RN. Treatment of anthracycline extravasation—A warning against the use of sodium bicarbonate. J Clin Oncol 1987:5:825–826.
97. Bartkowski-Dodds L, Daniels JR. Use of sodium bicarbonate as a means of ameliorating doxorubicin-induced dermal necrosis in rats. Cancer Chemother Pharmacol 1980:4:179–181.
98. Jackson IT, Robinson DW. Severe tissue damage following accidental subcutaneous infusion of bicarbonate solution. Scott Med J 1976:21:200–201.
99. Bachur NR, Gee MV, Friedman RD. Nuclear catalyzed antibiotic free radical formation. Cancer Res 1982:42:1078–1081.
100. Svingen BA, Powis G, Appel PL, Scott M. Protection against Adriamycin-induced skin necrosis in the rat by dimethyl sulfoxide and α-tocopheral. Cancer Res 1981:41:3395–3399.

101. Dorr RT, Alberts DS. Failure of DMSO and vitamin E to prevent doxorubicin skin ulceration in the mouse. Cancer Treat Rep 1983:67:499–501.
102. Coleman JJ III, Walker AP, Didolkar MS. Treatment of Adriamycin-induced skin ulcers: A prospective controlled study. J Surg Oncol 1983:22:129–135.
103. Daugherty JP, Khurana A. Amelioration of doxorubicin-induced skin necrosis in mice by butylated hydroxytoluene. Cancer Chemother Pharmacol 1985:14: 243–246.
104. Dorr RT, Alberts DS. Pharmacologic antidotes to experimental doxorubicin skin toxicity: A suggested role for beta-adrenergic compounds. Cancer Treat Rep 1981:65:1001–1006.
105. Barone AD, Atkinson RF, Wharry DL, Koch TH. In vitro reactivity of the meso and DL dimers of the 3,5,5-trimethyl-2-oxomorpholin-3-ylradical with Adriamycin and daunomycin. J Am Chem Soc 1981:103:1606–1607.
106. Averbuch SD, Boldt M, Gaudiano G, Stern JB, Koch TH, Bachur NR. Experimental chemotherapy-induced skin necrosis in swine: Mechanistic studies of anthracycline antibiotic toxicity and protection with a radical dimer compound. J Clin Invest 1988:81:142–148.
107. Averbuch SD, Gaudiano G, Koch TH, Bachur NR. Doxorubicin-induced skin necrosis in the swine model: Protection with a novel radical dimer. J Clin Oncol 1986:4:88–94.
108. Dorr RT, Alberts DS, Stone A. Cold protection and heat enhancement of doxorubicin skin toxicity in the mouse. Cancer Treat Rep 1985:69:431–437.
109. Ohnoshi T, Ohnuma T, Beranek JT, Holland JF. Combined cytoxicity effect of hyperthermia and anthracycline antibiotics on human tumor cells. J Natl Cancer Inst 1985:74:275–281.
110. Harwood KV, Bachur N. Evaluation of dimethyl sulfoxide and local cooling as antidotes for doxorubicin extravasation in a pig model. Oncol Nurs Forum 1987:14(1):39–44.
111. David NA. The pharmacology of dimethyl sulphoxide 6544. Annu Rev Pharmacol 1972:12:353–374.
112. Desai MH, Teres D. Prevention of doxorubicin-induced skin ulcers in the rat and pig with dimethyl sulfoxide (DMSO). Cancer Treat Rep 1982:66:1371–1374.
113. Nobbs P, Barr RD. Soft-tissue injury caused by antineoplastic drugs is inhibited by topical dimethyl sulphoxide and alpha tocopherol. Br J Cancer 1983: 48:873–876.
114. Olver IN, Aisner J, Hament A, Buchanon L, Bishop JF, Kaplan RS. A prospective study of topical dimethylsulfoxide for treatment anthracycline extravasation. J Clin Oncol 1988:6(11):1732–1735.
115. Bertelli G, Gozza A, Farno GB, Vidili MG, Silvestro S, Venturini M, Del Mastro L, Garrone O, Rosso R, Dini D. Topical dimethylsulfoxide for the prevention of soft tissue injury after extravasation of vesicant cytotoxic drugs: A prospective clinical study. J Clin Oncol 1995:13(11):2851–2855.
116. Daghestani AN, Arlin ZA, Leyland-Jones B, Gee TS, Kempin SJ, Mertelsmann R, Budman D, Schulman P, Baratz R, Williams L. Phase I and II clinical

and pharmacological study of 4-demethoxydaunorubicin (idarubicin) in adult patients with acute leukemia. Cancer Res 1985:45:1408–1412.

117. Harousseau JL, Hurteloup P, Reiffers J, Rigal-Huguet F, Hayat M, Dufour P, Le Prise PY, Monconduit M, Jaubert J, Carcassonne Y. Idarubicin in the treatment of relapsed or refractory acute myeloid leukemia (letter). Cancer Treat Rep 1987:71:991–992.
118. Madhavan S, Northfelt DW. Lack of vesicant injury following extravasation of liposomal doxorubicin. J Natl Cancer Inst 1995:87(20):1556–1557.
119. Khoury GG. Local tissue damage as a result of extravasation of mitoxantrone. Br Med J 1986:292:802.
120. Kharasch ED, Novak RF. Inhibition of microsomal oxidative drug metabolism by 1,4-bis{2-[(2-hydroxyethyl)amino]-ethylamino}-9,10-anthracenedione diacetate, a new antineoplastic agent. Mol Pharmacol 1982:22:471–478.
121. Mutch Marnocha RS, Hutson PR. Intradermal carboplatin and ifosfamide extravasation in the mouse. Cancer 1992:70:850–853.
122. Hatiboglu I, Mihich E, Moore GE, Nichol CA. Use of sodium thiosulfate as a neutralizing agent during regional administration of nitrogen mustard: An experimental study. Ann Surg 1962:156:994–1001.
123. Bonadonna G, Karnofsky DA. Protection studies with sodium thiosulfate against methyl bis(β-chloroethyl)amine hydrochloride (HN_2) and its ethyleimmonium derivative. Clin Pharmacol Ther 1965:6:50–64.
124. Owen OE, Dellatorre DL, Van Scott EJ, Cohen MR. Accidental intramuscular injection of mechlorethamine. Cancer 1980:45:2225–2226.
125. Dorr RT, Soble M, Alberts DS. Efficacy of sodium thiosulfate as a local antidote to mechlorethamine skin toxicity in the mouse. Cancer Chemother Pharmacol 1988:22:299–302.
126. Aizawa H, Tagami H. Delayed tissue necrosis due to mitomycin C. Acta Dermatol Venereol Suppl (Stockholm) 1987:67:364–366.
127. Johnston-Early A, Cohen M. Mitomycin-C-induced skin ulceration remote from infusion site. Cancer Treat Rep 1981:65:5–6.
128. Bartkowski-Dodds L, Reville B. Extensive tissue ulceration due to apparent sensitivity reactions to mitomycin. Cancer Treat Rep 1985:69:925–927.
129. Fuller B, Lind M, Bonomi P. Mitomycin C extravasation exacerbated by sunlight. Ann Intern Med 1981:94:542.
130. Ignoffo RJ, Tomlin W, Rubinstein E, Friedman MA. A model for skin toxicity of antineoplastic drugs: Doxorubicin (DOX), mitomycin-C (MMC), and vincristine (VCR). Clin Res 1981:29:437A.
131. Dorr RT, Soble M, Liddil JD, Keller JH. Mitomycin C skin toxicity studies in mice: Reduced ulceration and altered pharmacokinetics with topical dimethyl sulfoxide. J Clin Oncol 1986:4:1399–1404.
132. Ludwig CV, Stoll H, Obrist R. Prevention of ocytotoxic drug-induced skin ulcers with dimethylsulfoxide (DMSO) and alpha-tocopherol. Eur J Clin Oncol 1987:23:327–329.
133. Alberts DS, Dorr RT. Case report: Topical DMSO for mitomycin C–induced skin ulceration. Oncol Nurs Forum 1991:18(4):693–695.

134. Fields S, Koeller J, Topper RL, Guritz G, Von Hoff DD. Local soft tissue toxicity following cisplatin extravasation. J Natl Cancer Inst 1990:82:1689–1650.
135. Howell SB, Taetle R. Effect of sodium thiosulfate on *cis*-dichlorodiammin-platinum(II) toxicity and antitumor activity in L1210 leukemia. Cancer Treat Rep 1980:64:611–616.
136. Hill DL, Kirk MC, Struck RF. Microsomal metabolism of nitrosoureas. Cancer Res 1975:35:296–301.
137. Carter SK, Friedman MA. 5-(3,3-Dimethyl-1-triazeno)-imidazole-4-carboxamide (DTIC, DIC, NSC-45388)—A new antitumor agent with activity against malignant melanoma. Eur J Cancer 1972:8:85–92.
138. Baird GM, Willoughby MLN. Photodegradation of dacarbazine (letter). Lancet 1978:ii:681.
139. Carbone PP, Bono V, Frei E III, Brindley CO. Clinical studies of vincristine. Blood 1963:640–647.
140. Costa G, Hreshchyshyn MM, Holland JF. Initial clinical studies with vincristine. Cancer Chemother Rep 1963:27:91–96.
141. Jackson DV, Sethi VS, Spurr CL, Willard V, White DR, Richards F, Stuart JJ, Muss HB, Cooper MR, Homesley HD, Jobson VW, Castle MC. Intravenous vincristine infusion: Phase I trial. Cancer 1981:48:2559–2564.
142. Yap HY, Blumenschein GR, Keating MJ. Vinblastine given as a continuous five day infusion in the treatment of refractory advanced breast cancer. Cancer Treat Rep 1980:64:279–283.
143. Grush OC, Morgan SK. Folinic acid rescue for vincristine toxicity. Clin Toxicol 1979:14:71–78.
144. Jackson DV, Wells HB, Atkins JN, Zekan PJ, White DR, Richards F II, Cruz JM, Muss HB. Amelioration of vincristine neurotoxicity by glutamic acid. Am J Med 1988:84:1016–1022.
145. Johnson IS, Armstrong JG, Gorman M, Burnett JP. The vinca alkaloids: A new class of oncolytic agents. Cancer Res 1963:23:1390–1427.
146. Choy DS. Effective treatment of inadvertent intramuscular administration of vincristine (letter). JAMA 1979:241:695.
147. Harrison B, Godefroid R, SunWoo Y, Luedke D, Luedke S. Histopathological evolution of vincristine (VCR) skin toxicity and treatment with local dexamethasone (DXM) (abstr). Proc Am Soc Clin Oncol 1983:2:86.
148. Britton RC, Habif DV. Clinical uses of hyaluronidase: A current review. Surgery 1953:33:917–940.
149. Laurie SWS, Wilson KL, Kernahan DA, Bauer BS, Vistnes LM. Intravenous extravasation injuries: The effectiveness of hyaluronidase in their treatment. Ann Plast Surg 1984:13(3):191–194.
150. Zenk KE, Dungy CI, Greene GR. Nafcillin extravasation injury. Am J Dis Child 1981:135:1113–1114.
151. Elam EA, Dorr RT, Lagel KE, Pond GD. Cutaneous ulceration due to contrast extravasation: Assessment of injury and potential antidotes. Invest Radiol 1990:26:13–16.

152. Le Chevalier T, Brisgand D, Douillard J-Y, Pujol J-L, Alberola V, Monnier A, Rivière A, Lianes P, Chomy P, Cigolari S, Gottfried M, Ruffie P, Panizo A, Gaspard M-H, Ravaioli A, Besenval M, Besson F, Martinez A, Berthaud P, Tursz T. Randomized study of vinorelbine and cisplatin versus vindesine and cisplatin versus vinorelbine alone in advanced non-small-cell lung cancer: Results of a European multicenter trial including 612 patients. J Clin Oncol 1994:12:360–367.
153. Rittenberg CN, Gralla RJ, Rehmeyer TA. Assessing and managing venous irritation associated with vinorelbine tartrate (Navelbine®). Oncol Nurs Forum 1995:22(4):707–710.
154. Bertelli G, Dini D, Forno GB, Gozza FS, Silvestro S, Venturini M, Rosso R, Pronzato P. Hyaluronidase as an antidote to extravasation of vinca alkaloids: Clinical results. J Cancer Res Clin Oncol 1994:120:505–506.
155. Link CJ Jr, Sarosy GA, Kohn EC, Christian MC, Davis P. Cutaneous manifestations of Taxol® therapy. Invest New Drugs 1995:13:261–263.
156. Hidalgo M, Benito J, Colomer R, Paz-Ares L. Recall reaction of a severe local peripheral neuropathy after paclitaxel extravasation. J Natl Cancer Inst 1996:88(18):1320.
157. Du Bois A, Kommoss FGM, Pfisterer J, Luck HJ, Meerpohl HG. Paclitaxel-induced "recall" soft tissue ulcerations occurring at the site of previous subcutaneous administration of paclitaxel in low doses. Gynecol Oncol 1996:60: 94–96.
158. Stanley A, Marsh S. The management of paclitaxel (Taxol®) extravasation. J Oncol Pharm Pract 1995:1:24.
159. Dorr RT, Snead K, Liddil JD. Skin ulceration potential of paclitaxel in a mouse skin model in vivo. Cancer 1996:78:152–156.
160. Bertelli G, Cafferata MA, Ardizzoni A, Gozza A, Rosso R. Skin ulceration potential of paclitaxel in a mouse skin model in vivo. Cancer 1997:79(11): 2266–2268.
161. Dorr RT, Alberts DS. Skin ulceration potential without therapeutic anticancer activity for epipodophyllotoxin commercial diluents. Invest New Drugs 1983: 1:151–159.
162. Bellone JD. Treatment of vincristine extravasation (letter). J Amer Med Assoc 1981:245:343.

IV

ORGAN TOXICITY INDUCED BY CYTOSTATIC AGENTS

7

Nephrotoxicity and Urotoxicity of Chemotherapeutic Agents

RODERICK SKINNER
Sir James Spence Institute of Child Health, University of Newcastle upon Tyne, Newcastle upon Tyne, England

This chapter describes the toxic effects of cytotoxic drugs on the kidneys, and on the urinary tract, especially the bladder. Although many cytotoxic drugs may damage the kidneys, ifosfamide and cisplatin cause most episodes of clinically important nephrotoxicity [1]. Likewise, urinary tract toxicity is usually due to cyclophosphamide or ifosfamide [2].

7.1 NEPHROTOXICITY

Impairment of renal function is an important complication of cancer with many potential causes, including the malignant process itself and consequences of its treatment (e.g., chemotherapy, radiotherapy, immunotherapy, surgery, or supportive treatment) [3]. In many clinical situations renal damage may be multifactorial—for example, after bone marrow transplantation (BMT), where chemotherapy, radiotherapy, and supportive treatment may all contribute [4]. Chemotherapy may lead to acute or chronic nephrotoxicity, or both (Table 1). Acute renal damage may limit further treatment or even threaten life, while chronic toxicity may cause considerable morbidity. The renal tubules are especially vulnerable to toxicity because of their generous blood supply and metabolic capacity. Proximal tubular toxicity is particularly common but often overlooked, while glomerular and distal tubular damage may also cause clinically significant problems. The most important cytotoxic drugs likely to cause renal toxicity are cisplatin and ifosfamide, both of

Table 1 Nephrotoxic Chemotherapy Agents

Cytotoxic agents with potentially severe and frequent nephrotoxicity
Cisplatin
Ifosfamide
Cytotoxic agents with clinically important but less frequent nephrotoxicity
Carboplatin
Methotrexate (especially high-dose)
Nitrosoureas (especially semustine)
Cytotoxic agents with less well-documented nephrotoxicity
Anthracyclines (daunorubicin, doxorubicin)
5-Azacytidine
Cyclophosphamide
Cytosine arabinoside
Melphalan
Mithramycin
Mitomycin C
Streptozotocin
6-Thioguanine

which are used extensively because of their efficacy in many solid tumors. Up to 30% of children treated with ifosfamide may develop severe tubular toxicity [5], and 30–60% suffer substantial renal damage after cisplatin [6]. Nephrotoxicity due to other cytotoxic drugs is less frequent, but carboplatin, methotrexate, and nitrosoureas may cause serious damage [3,7]. Rarely, significant renal damage may occur after cytotoxic drugs not usually regarded as major nephrotoxins.

By the year 2000, about 0.1% of young adults will be survivors of a childhood malignancy, and up to 50% of these may have received a platinum agent, ifosfamide, or high-dose methotrexate. Even if some suffer subclinical toxicity only, the potential for chronic morbidity in later life is very worrying, especially in children and young adults. Therefore, attempts to reduce the frequency and severity of nephrotoxicity are very important.

7.1.1 Assessment of Chemotherapy-Associated Nephrotoxicity

Informed evaluation of renal toxicity requires an understanding of the mechanisms by which the kidney regulates fluid and electrolyte balance and excretes metabolic and toxic waste products. Each human kidney is composed of about a million nephrons, each comprising a glomerulus, a proximal tubule, a loop of Henle, and a distal tubule, draining into a collecting duct. Separate evaluation of glomerular, proximal, and distal tubular function is necessary because of their distinct roles. Glomerular filtration leads to the formation of an "ultrafiltrate," which then enters the proximal nephron, where it is progressively modified by tubular reabsorption and secretion. Tubular secretion eliminates endogenous and exogenous toxic substances. Finally, acidification and concentration of the ultrafiltrate occur in the distal nephron, with the formation of urine. In functional terms, the proximal nephron can be considered to include both the proximal convoluted tubule and the loop of Henle, and the distal nephron to comprise the distal convoluted tubule, the collecting tubule and collecting duct.

Nevertheless, it is possible to undertake a detailed evaluation of renal toxicity, for example, by using a standardized investigation protocol (Table

Table 2 Protocol for Investigation of Nephrotoxicity in Children

Function	Investigation
Glomerular function	
	Serum creatinine concentration
	Glomerular filtration rate (GFR, measured by $[^{51}Cr]$EDTA plasma clearance)
Proximal tubular function	
	Blood and urine concentrations of sodium, potassium, chloride, bicarbonate, creatinine, calcium, magnesium, phosphate, glucose, urate, with calculation of fractional excretion (FE) of sodium, calcium, magnesium, phosphate, glucose, urate; and of renal tubular threshold of phosphate (T_{m_p}/GFR)
	Urine excretion of low molecular weight (LMW) proteins (e.g., retinol-binding protein, RBP) and amino acids
Distal tubular function	
	Early morning urine pH and osmolality
	Assessment of renal control of acid–base balance
	I-deamino-8-D-arginine vasopressin (DDAVP) test (in patients with low urine osmolalities)
Bone chemistry	
	Blood alkaline phosphatase activity
	Radiological assessment (in patients with hypophosphatemic rickets)
General aspects of renal function	
	Urine excretion of renal tubular enzymes (RTEs) (e.g., N-acetylglucosaminidase, NAG)
	Blood concentrations and urine excretion of albumin, protein
	Urine analysis and microscopy
	Blood pressure
	Height and weight

Source: Ref. 9.

2) that has been validated in a large number of children [8,9]. Investigations with varying levels of sensitivity are included to allow assessment of both clinical problems and subtle degrees of subclinical renal dysfunction.

7.1.2 Ifosfamide Nephrotoxicity

Early clinical studies in adults described glomerular toxicity after high bolus doses of ifosfamide without mesna [10]. Subsequent reports revealed that ifosfamide may cause any combination of glomerular, proximal, or distal tubular toxicities (Table 3), with a very wide range of severity [5]. There is relatively little clear information concerning the incidence of acute renal toxicity, but Stuart-Harris et al. [11] described chronic renal damage in 9.5% of adults, while in children the incidence of severe chronic toxicity has ranged from 1.4% [12] to about 30% [13,14], depending on the measures of toxicity used. In adults, glomerular toxicity may be manifest as a reversible reduction in glomerular filtration rate (GFR), potentially fatal acute renal failure (ARF), or chronic renal failure (CRF) [11,15–18]. Features of proximal tubular toxicity range from glycosuria [19] to a Fanconi syndrome, also including phosphaturia and bicarbonaturia [15,20]. Clinically relevant consequences include hypophosphatemia and/or proximal renal tubular acidosis (RTA) [15]. Distal tubular damage may lead to impaired urine acidification or concentration, causing RTA or nephrogenic diabetes insipidus (NDI), respectively [15].

In children, early studies failed to reveal any evidence of nephrotoxicity. However, since the late 1980s, there have been many reports of severe nephrotoxicity persisting after treatment with ifosfamide, causing any combination of glomerular and tubular impairments, although proximal tubular damage is usually predominant. There is much interindividual variability in the onset, nature, and severity of nephrotoxicity, but some children are severely affected. Initially transient acute tubular damage often becomes more persistent and severe with further treatment, and may then be accompanied by glomerular impairment. Both acute and chronic deterioration in glomerular function may occur [21,22], and the latter may be irreversible or even progress long after cessation of treatment [23]. Acute and chronic subclinical proximal tubular toxicity may lead to glycosuria and/or aminoaciduria, increased urine excretion of low molecular weight (LMW) proteins, including retinol-binding protein (RBP), α_1-microglobulin (α_1-M) and β_2-microglobulin (β_2-M), or of the proximal tubular antigen adenosine deaminase–binding protein (ADBP) [24–28]. More severe damage leads to phosphaturia, kaluria, and bicarbonaturia, and, more rarely, to calciuria and magnesuria, amounting to a Fanconi syndrome [13,14,28–30], often with gradual onset but only partial recovery. Distal tubular toxicity appears to be much rarer,

Table 3 Ifosfamide Nephrotoxicity: Clinical Features and Risk Factors[a]

Glomerular toxicity
Elevated blood creatinine concentration
Reduced GFR
Acute renal failure
Chronic renal failure
Proximal tubular toxicity
Aminoaciduria
Glycosuria
Increased urinary excretion of
LMW proteins (e.g., RBP)
Proximal tubular antigens (e.g., adenosine deaminase-binding protein, ADBP)
Fanconi syndrome (as above, plus phosphaturia, bicarbonaturia, kaluria), leading to
Hypophosphatemia and hypophosphatemic rickets (HR)
Proximal renal tubular acidosis (RTA)
Hypokalemia
Calciuria, magnesuria, natriuria (rarely)
Distal tubular toxicity
Subclinical impairment of urinary acidification
Subclinical impairment of urinary concentration
Distal RTA
Nephrogenic diabetes insipidus (NDI)
Tubular toxicity (proximal or distal localization uncertain)
Increased urinary excretion of RTEs (e.g., NAG)
Renal toxicity (glomerular or tubular localization uncertain)
Proteinuria
Urinary granular cast excretion
Hypertension
Growth failure (related to chronic HR and/or RTA)
Potential risk factors
Cumulative ifosfamide dose
Age at treatment
Previous or concurrent cisplatin (or other potential nephrotoxins)
Preexisting renal impairment or tumor invasion
Interindividual variability in ifosfamide pharmacokinetics
Ifosfamide administration method (no evidence at present)

[a]Boldface indicates clinically relevant feature of toxicity.

but chronic NDI has been described [13,29]. Raised urinary excretion of renal tubular enzymes (RTEs) [31] reflects tubular damage in general.

The clinical consequences of ifosfamide-induced nephrotoxicity in children include hypophosphatemic rickets (HR), RTA, and NDI [13,29,32]. Rarely, hypertension may occur [33]. CRF, HR, and RTA are likely to cause growth impairment in children [34]. Clinical management includes the prevention or treatment of manifestations of tubular toxicity, especially HR and RTA in growing children. This may necessitate frequent ($\geq$ 3 times daily) high-dose supplementation with oral or intravenous (IV) phosphate or bicarbonate, or less commonly other electrolytes. Although 1α-hydroxy vitamin D_3 may be necessary occasionally, vitamin D preparations are best avoided in normocalcemic patients in view of the risk of metastatic calcification and nephrocalcinosis. The degree of reversibility of ifosfamide nephrotoxicity remains uncertain. Many reports describe partial or complete recovery between courses or after ifosfamide discontinuation [20], but both glomerular [11,23] and tubular function [35] may deteriorate after the end of treatment. Partial recovery from severe renal damage may occur [36], but complete resolution appears to be very rare [37].

Risk factors suggested for the development of nephrotoxicity after ifosfamide include age, cumulative ifosfamide dose, administration method, previous or concurrent cisplatin (or other potential nephrotoxins), and preexisting renal impairment or tumor invasion. Most published reports of severe toxicity have been in infants and young children, who may be more susceptible both to proximal tubular toxicity, and to its consequences, especially growth failure [38,39]. However, ifosfamide may cause severe renal damage at any age. Children receiving higher total doses of ifosfamide (> 60–100 g/m^2) appear to be at greater risk [13,38], but extensive damage has occurred after much lower doses [29]. There is no convincing evidence that the method of IV administration of ifosfamide (bolus, short or continuous infusion) influences the risk of nephrotoxicity. The incidence and severity of ifosfamide nephrotoxicity appears to be increased by prior cisplatin therapy [12,40], while combination with very-high-dose carboplatin may cause severe toxicity [41]. Severe renal damage has been reported in patients with prior unilateral nephrectomy, renal impairment, or tumor infiltration [22,30], but it is unknown whether the incidence of such damage is increased. The factors above, especially age, dose, and cisplatin, may influence the frequency of nephrotoxicity in groups of patients, but they are of little predictive value in individual patients, possibly because the interindividual variability in ifosfamide metabolism is large.

The few reported histopathological examinations of renal biopsy samples have described focal proximal tubular changes with relatively little or no glomerular damage [42]. The balance of evidence suggests a toxic, rather than immunopathological, lesion. However, the pathogenesis of ifosfamide nephrotoxicity is still poorly understood. Initial reports predated the introduction of mesna [10,15], and recent studies in rats and in vitro proximal renal tubular cell cultures have demonstrated cellular toxicity due to the drug or a metabolite [43,44]. Although ifosfamide and cyclophosphamide are qualitatively similar in their pharmacology and metabolism, quantitative differences provide important clues [5]. Ifosfamide is activated by ring hydroxylation to 4-hydroxyifosfamide/aldoifosfamide, which may either decompose to isophosphoramide mustard (the active alkylating metabolite) and acrolein, or undergo oxidation to inactive carboxyifosfamide via aldehyde dehydrogenase (ALDH). In addition, side chain dechlorethylation to chloroacetaldehyde (CAA) may account for up to 50% of metabolism in some patients. Unchanged ifosfamide and its metabolites are excreted in urine. In contrast, cyclophosphamide metabolism yields very little CAA. After IV injection, mesna (a synthetic thiol capable of detoxification of reactive ifosfamide metabolites, including CAA and acrolein) is rapidly oxidized in plasma to dimesna. Both mesna and dimesna are cleared by glomerular filtration and excreted, or taken up by renal tubular cells. Evidence from studies in rats suggests that administration schedules of mesna may influence its pharmacokinetics, but the clinical importance of this observation is unclear [5].

There is much interindividual variability in the nature and extent of ifosfamide metabolism, as well as dose and schedule dependence. Although CAA is generated in large amounts from ifosfamide, the factors above lead to considerable variability in its production and urinary excretion. CAA is highly toxic to epithelial cells and may induce an experimental Fanconi syndrome in the $LLCPK_1$ cell line (a proximal tubular model) and in the isolated perfused rat kidney, possibly by inhibiting active transport and increasing tubular cell membrane permeability [45,46]. Therefore, CAA may account for the occurrence of renal toxicity after ifosfamide but not cyclosphosphamide, as well as its variable severity. Although mesna should be capable of detoxifying CAA, it may be relatively difficult to prevent tubular damage due to the short tubular "transit time" of mesna. However, at least in theory, alternative mesna administration protocols may be more efficacious [5].

Until its pathogenesis is understood more completely, efforts to prevent ifosfamide nephrotoxicity in patients rely on minimizing known risk factors. Cumulative doses exceeding 100 g/m^2 (perhaps > 60 g/m^2) should be avoided, and the drug must be used carefully in children 5 years of age or less, in patients previously given cisplatin, and in those with poor renal function. Other potentially nephrotoxic drugs should be used sparingly. Vigorous IV hydration and mesna regimens to aid dilution, inactivation, and excretion of toxic ifosfamide metabolites are likely to reduce nephrotoxicity to some degree, but there is no rationale or published evidence to support the use of alkalinization. Even these precautions will not prevent all episodes of serious nephrotoxicity, and it may be very difficult to balance the risk–benefit ratio of ifosfamide against that of cyclophosphamide in these clinical situations [5]. Recently published work in a rat model suggests that oral glycine supplementation may ameliorate ifosfamide nephrotoxicity [43], but the efficacy of this approach in humans has yet to be confirmed in a clinical trial.

7.1.3 Cisplatin Nephrotoxicity

Preclinical studies in several animal species predicted that renal damage would be a major adverse effect of cisplatin in humans (Table 4) [47,48]. In adults, acute glomerular impairment may range from mild biochemical changes to potentially fatal ARF [49,50], while CRF may develop insidiously [47,48]. Plasma creatinine concentration and endogenous creatinine clearance are insensitive indicators of glomerular toxicity due to cisplatin [51], suggesting that such damage may be commoner than is generally appreciated. Transient or chronic magnesuria and resultant hypomagnesemia are the commonest manifestations of proximal tubular toxicity [52,53]. Hypocalcemia and hypokalemia occur commonly in adults, although the mechanism is unclear [52,54]. Dissociation of tubular calcium and magnesium handling, with chronic hypocalciuria, magnesuria, and hypomagnesemia, may be due to a distal convoluted tubule lesion [55]. Alternatively, it has been suggested that hypocalcemia may be due to hypomagnesemia-induced impairment of parathyroid hormone [56]. Similarly, kaluria and hypomagnesemia may both contribute to hypokalemia, while natriuria may lead to hyponatremia [54,56–58]. Acute and generally reversible aminoaciduria, glycosuria, and increased urine excretion of RBP, β_2-M, *N*-acetylglucosaminidase (NAG), alanine aminopeptidase (AAP), and β-galactosidase have been described [58,59]. Persistent hypertension may occur [60] owing to renovascular mechanisms in some cases [61].

In children, the reported incidence of glomerular toxicity has varied from about 20% [62] to more than 80% [63], while that of hypomagnesemia has varied from about 30% [6] to 100% [64], depending on the nature and timing of investigation. Glomerular impairment may cause an acute or chronic fall in GFR or rise in plasma creatinine concentration [6,63,65,66], or occasionally, ARF [67]. Proximal nephron damage may cause transient or permanent magnesuria and hypomagnesemia [6,66,68]. Occasionally hypokalemia, hypocalcemia, natriuria with hyponatremia, glycosuria, phosphaturia, and elevated urine β_2-M excretion may occur [64,69]. There have been

Table 4 Cisplatin Nephrotoxicity: Clinical Features and Risk Factors[a]

Glomerular toxicity
Elevated blood creatinine concentration
Reduced GFR
Acute renal failure
Chronic renal failure
Proximal tubular toxicity
Increased urinary excretion of
Magnesium, potassium, sodium, glucose, ?calcium
Amino acids
LMW proteins (e.g., RBP)
The consequences of proximal tubular toxicity include
Hypomagnesemia
Hypocalcemia
Hypokalemia
Hyponatremia
Distal tubular toxicity
Impairment of water and sodium reabsorption
Syndrome of hypomagnesemia—hypokalemia with hypocalciuria
Tubular toxicity (proximal or distal localization uncertain)
Increased urinary excretion of RTEs (e.g., NAG)
Renal toxicity (glomerular or tubular localization uncertain)
Albuminuria, proteinuria
Urinary tubular cell cast excretion
Hypertension
Potential risk factors
Age at treatment
Cumulative cisplatin dose, or dose/course, or cisplatin dose rate/course
Cisplatin administration method
Other potential nephrotoxins
Interindividual variability in cisplatin pharmacokinetics

[a]Boldface indicates clinically relevant feature of toxicity.

no specific investigations of distal tubular function after cisplatin treatment in children. However, chronic magnesuria, hypomagnesemia, hypocalciuria, with normocalcemia or mild hypercalcemia, and mild hypokalemic metabolic alkalosis may result from dissociation of magnesium and calcium handling at a distal convoluted tubular lesion [68]. Transient rises in urine AAP and NAG excretion reflect generalized tubular damage [70]. Occasionally, hypertension may occur [71].

The clinical consequences of cisplatin nephrotoxicity include ARF or CRF, and hypomagnesemia, which may cause paresthesias, tremors, tetany, and convulsions [56,65]. Many reports have emphasized the apparent irreversibility of cisplatin nephrotoxicity. Two studies in children have suggested that glomerular impairment, but not hypomagnesemia, may improve somewhat with time [6,72]. There is little clear information about the importance of patient- and treatment-related risk factors for cisplatin nephrotoxicity. These may include age, dose and administration schedule, other potentially concurrent nephrotoxic treatment, and interindividual differences in cisplatin pharmacokinetics. Older age may be a risk factor in adults [73], but in children there is no clear relationship between age and GFR or hypomagnesemia [6,72]. Daugaard found less glomerular and tubular toxicity in adults after low-dose (i.e., 20 $mg/m^2/d$) than after high-dose cisplatin (i.e., 40 $mg/m^2/d$) treatments [51,58], and the rate of cisplatin administration may also be important in children [72]. Some studies in adults and children have suggested a relationship between cumulative dose and nephrotoxicity [52,74], but others have not [6,72]. It is generally accepted that prolonged continuous infusion of cisplatin with saline hyperhydration, with or without mannitol osmotic diuresis, reduces nephrotoxicity [75]. Administration of other potential nephrotoxins, including ifosfamide and methotrexate, may increase renal toxicity [76]. Interindividual variability in cisplatin pharmacokinetics may be important. A significant correlation between the peak plasma concentration of free platinum after the first course of cisplatin and glomerular toxicity after four courses has been described in adults [77]. It is possible but unproven that monitoring of pharmacokinetic parameters may allow subsequent treatment modification to reduce the risk of renal damage. The management of cisplatin nephrotoxicity involves correction of hypomagnesemia, which may also correct concomitant hypocalcemia [56]. However, it is not clear whether routine long-term replacement treatment is necessary, and there has been no detailed study of the clinical consequences of chronic cisplatin-induced hypomagnesemia in long-term survivors.

Most studies of autopsy and renal biopsy histopathological samples in adults have shown variable tubular changes but no glomerular abnormalities [49]. The chronicity of cisplatin nephrotoxicity may be related to long-term retention of platinum in human tissues, including the kidney [78]. The pathogenesis of cisplatin nephrotoxicity remains unclear, and it is even uncertain whether a proximal or distal tubular lesion, or indeed both, is primarily responsible. The pharmacology of cisplatin in humans is complex [79]. After rapid distribution, substantial protein binding occurs, mainly to plasma proteins but also to cellular proteins, with both reversible and irreversible elements [80]. The terminal half-life of total platinum is long (20–80 h), probably because protein-bound platinum is removed only slowly. Net tubular secretion of cisplatin occurs; the details of tubular handling are poorly understood, but both reabsorption and secretion may be involved. In plasma, with a relatively high chloride concentration, the neutral dichlorocisplatin complex predominates, whereas the more reactive aquated species will prevail in the low-chloride intracellular environment, possibly leading to formation of nephrotoxic metabolites [81]. This is the rationale for the use of hypertonic saline hydration with cisplatin. There has been considerable interest in the possibility that cisplatin nephrotoxicity may be mediated by tubular transport and accumulation of the drug or a (so far, unidentified) toxic metabolite [82,83]. There is conflicting evidence concerning whether cisplatin nephrotoxicity might be initiated by renal arteriolar vasoconstriction [54,84], possibly via mechanisms involving adenosine, platelet-activating factor (PAF), or thromboxane A_2 [85–87]. There is similar uncertainty about the subcellular basis of cisplatin nephrotoxicity, although a variety of events may be involved, including binding to biological nucleophiles and proteins such as glutathione, inhibition of enzymes including ATPase, reduction in cellular and nuclear synthetic activity, especially of DNA and RNA, and damage to mitochondrial DNA and enzymes [79,88,89]. However, the relevance of these processes to nephrotoxicity remains unclear.

Since cisplatin is likely to remain in frequent use until improved analogues are introduced, much research has been performed in attempts to prevent or mitigate its nephrotoxicity [75,90]. The addition of prophylactic IV magnesium supplements to hydration fluid reduces the frequency and severity of hypomagnesemia [91]. Prolonged cisplatin infusions with hypertonic saline hydration regimens, with or without mannitol or frusemide diuresis, are used widely, although their efficacy has been difficult to evaluate [75], and nephroprotection is incomplete [54]. A multitude of pharmacological methods of modifying cisplatin nephrotoxicity have been investigated, but none has found widespread acceptance yet because of the uncertainty about the mechanism of toxicity and the lack of clear evidence to demonstrate improvements in the therapeutic index of cisplatin [90]. Among many other substances, the drugs studied for their protective effect have included a variety of sulfur-containing compounds such as sodium thiosulfate, WR-2721, DDTC (sodium diethyldithiocarbamate), mesna, biotin, cephalexin, and sulfathiazole, all of which probably react with nephrotoxic cisplatin metabolites to form less toxic products [90,92].

A second pharmacological approach has involved inhibition of tubular cisplatin transport—for example, by probenecid (organic anion transport) or cimetidine (organic cation transport) [93,94]. Another method has used drugs to counteract possible mediators of renal vasoconstriction, including aminophylline (to block adenosine) and BN 52063 (to antagonize PAF) [85,86]. Numerous cisplatin analogues (e.g., ormaplatin, oxaliplatin, zeniplatin) and complexes (e.g., with alginates, methionine, procaine hydrochloride) have been investigated in the hope of achieving pharmacokinetic and pharmacodynamic properties that lead to reduced nephrotoxicity without loss of cytotoxic efficacy. Novel pharmaceutical approaches under evaluation include liposomal and microsphere preparations.

7.1.4 Carboplatin-Induced Nephrotoxicity

Carboplatin is gaining wider acceptance as an adjunct or alternative to cisplatin therapy in view of its activity in several adult and pediatric tumors, and its distinct toxicity profile (Table 5) [95]. Preclinical animal studies suggested that carboplatin causes considerably less biochemical and histopathological evidence of nephrotoxicity than cisplatin [96]. An early study in adults supported this impression, reporting that only 3 of 60 patients suffered a significant fall in GFR [97]. Subsequent reports have described renal toxicity similar to, but usually milder than, that seen after cisplatin. Mild degrees of glomerular impairment may occur [97–99]. There have been very few reports of ARF, which may be reversible [100–102]. Hypomagnesemia, usually reversible and presumably due to magnesuria, may occur [103]. Transient natriuria and symptomatic hyponatremia have been

Table 5 Carboplatin Nephrotoxicity: Clinical Features and Risk Factors[a]

Glomerular toxicity
Elevated blood creatinine concentration
Reduced GFR
Acute renal failure (very rare)
Proximal tubular toxicity
Hypomagnesemia (magnesuria not yet demonstrated)
Natriuria and **hyponatremia**
Increased urinary excretion of LMW proteins (e.g., β_2-microglobulin, β_2-M)
Tubular toxicity (proximal or distal localization uncertain)
Increased urinary excretion of RTEs (e.g., NAG)
Renal toxicity (glomerular or tubular localization uncertain)
Albuminuria, proteinuria
Potential risk factors
Other potentially nephrotoxic treatment (including cisplatin)
Preexisting renal impairment (limited evidence)

[a]Boldface indicates clinically relevant feature of toxicity.

reported [104]. Acute increases in urinary excretion of β_2-M reflect subclinical proximal tubular toxicity, while those in NAG and β-glucuronidase are due to subclinical tubular toxicity in general [96,97].

The few reports of carboplatin nephrotoxicity in children describe reversible and generally mild toxicity. The incidence of glomerular impairment has ranged from 0% [105] to about 25% [106], and that of hypomagnesemia from 0% [107] to 10% [108]. Glomerular impairment is generally absent [105] or mild, with a small reduction in GFR [106]. Interpretation of the only report of serious glomerular damage, describing ARF in four children treated with high-dose carboplatin, is complicated by the concomitant administration of melphalan [109]. Transient hypomagnesemia has been described occasionally [96]. Clinical sequelae of carboplatin nephrotoxicity are rare, and usually fully reversible, except for rare cases of ARF [101] and hypomagnesemia [103].

The small amount of information about risk factors for carboplatin nephrotoxicity originates from adult studies and fails to reveal clear relationships between individual or cumulative carboplatin doses, age or sex, and nephrotoxicity [100,102]. It has been suggested that hydration reduces the risk of nephrotoxicity with high-dose carboplatin [110], but it appears unnecessary with conventional doses of 400–600 mg/m^2. Although one study found that previous cisplatin was not a risk factor for glomerular damage after carboplatin [102], ARF has been reported in patients given prior cisplatin [100,101]. Renal excretion is the major route of carboplatin clearance, and patients with preexisting renal impairment may be more susceptible to nephrotoxicity [96,100].

A report of histopathological findings in carboplatin nephrotoxicity describes interstitial nephritis in two women; one also had "toxic" tubular changes, revealed on electron microscopy [101], but since both patients received the drug intraperitoneally, these findings may not be representative of carboplatin nephrotoxicity. It is usually assumed that cisplatin and carboplatin nephrotoxicity share the same mechanism, but that the greater frequency and severity of cisplatin toxicity may be due to an increased ability to form one or more putative nephrotoxic metabolites, perhaps as a result of the increased lability of its chloride ligands compared to the cyclobutane dicarboxylate group of carboplatin [111].

7.1.5 Nephrotoxicity Due to Other Cytotoxic Drugs Used in Both Adults and Children

Initial studies of low-dose IV methotrexate administration revealed glomerular impairment and tubular cell necrosis. Renal toxicity, although sometimes reversible, contributed to severe systemic toxicity due to reduced methotrexate excretion [112]. High-dose IV methotrexate (HD-MTX) regimens (> 1 g/m^2) can cause renal damage which, although potentially reversible, may be severe or even fatal [113]. Subclinical acute nephrotoxicity may occur in children after HD-MTX administration, with considerable reductions in GFR [114], and increases in urinary excretion of RTEs and ADBP [25]. In addition to altering glomerular hemodynamics and causing direct tubular toxicity, methotrexate or a metabolite precipitates inside the distal nephron, causing intrarenal obstruction and ARF, usually nonoliguric [3]. Methotrexate nephrotoxicity is prevented or ameliorated greatly by prophylactic IV fluid regimens to prevent tubular precipitation by urinary dilution, alkalinization to increase solubility, and folinic acid rescue to avert systemic toxicity [113,115].

Melphalan may be associated with nephrotoxicity, usually when given in high doses prior to BMT, but it is often difficult to separate its effects from those of other concurrent nephrotoxic insults. Two of eight adults developed transiently elevated blood urea concentrations, but IV hydration ameliorated renal toxicity [116]. A later report of melphalan and total body irradiation (TBI) described glomerular toxicity in a third of patients. However, high-dose cyclophosphamide and TBI caused similar toxicity, and cyclosporin A may have contributed to renal damage, which was again reduced by hydration [117]. ARF and proximal tubular damage occurred after very-high-dose melphalan in an adolescent [118].

Chronic glomerular impairment occurred after doxorubicin treatment in an elderly man, with gradual recovery [119]. Renal biopsy showed ultrastructural changes similar to those seen after daunorubicin in rats and doxorubicin in rabbits [120,121]. In contrast to ifosfamide, its structural isomer, there is very little evidence that cyclophosphamide causes renal toxicity. Reversible proteinuria and hematuria have been reported in a patient given IV and intraperitoneal cyclophosphamide [122]. An antidiuretic effect, due to direct distal nephron damage, facilitates water reabsorption, which may lead to inappropriate urinary concentration and potentially fatal dilutional hyponatremia [123,124]. Cytosine arabinoside was associated with glomerular toxicity in 55–85% of a series of adults, with some deaths from multifactorial ARF [125].

The structurally similar nitrosourea compounds, carmustine (BCNU), lomustine (CCNU), and semustine (methyl-CCNU), share a capacity to cause chronic irreversible glomerular impairment, often developing after completion of treatment. Semustine appears to be the most nephrotoxic. In six children receiving more than 1500 mg/m^2, end-stage renal failure (ESRF) developed in four and CRF in one. Renal histology revealed glomerulosclerosis, tubular loss, and interstitial fibrosis [126]. A dose limit of 1200 mg/m^2 has been recommended [127]. Nephrotoxicity due to the other nitrosoureas is rarer. Of 89 patients given carmustine, 4 adults developed mild glomerular impairment with an insidious onset [128]. Slowly progressive ESRF may follow lomustine treatment [129]. The pathogenesis of nitrosourea nephrotoxicity is unclear, but a toxic electrophilic metabolite may be responsible [127].

Nephrotoxicity has not been reported after oral 6-thioguanine despite much use in children, but acute glomerular impairment occurred in 12 of 66 adults, with severe toxicity in 4 who were given IV boluses. However, renal function recovered in most patients [130]. Direct renal toxicity has not been described, but it has been suggested that actinomycin D may sensitize the kidney to damage from radiation doses that do not normally cause nephropathy [131], and impair compensatory renal hypertrophy in children with Wilms tumor [132]. Rarely, vincristine may cause hyponatremia due to inappropriate vasopressin secretion [133].

7.1.6 Nephrotoxicity due to Cytotoxic Drugs Used Predominantly in Adults

Although usually reversible, tubular toxicity caused aminoaciduria, glycosuria, phosphaturia, hypophosphatemia, bicarbonaturia, RTA, natriuria, polyuria, hypocalcemia, hypomagnesemia, and mild glomerular damage, and may have contributed to death in 4 of 22 patients given 5-azacytidine [134]. Mithramycin may cause acute or chronic glomerular impairment, as well as transient falls in the plasma calcium and phosphate concentrations, albeit without calciuria or phosphaturia, probably due to inhibition of RNA synthesis [135].

There are many reports of nephrotoxicity occurring in adults receiving mitomycin C, with two clinically distinct patterns of renal damage [7,136]. Acute, progressive glomerular impairment with hypertension, proteinuria, hematuria, and microangiopathic hemolytic anemia, is frequently rapidly fatal (cancer-associated hemolytic uraemic syndrome, C-HUS), while slowly progressive damage without microangiopathic hemolysis also often leads to renal failure and death. Histology shows vascular damage in both types. C-HUS usually occurs only after repeated courses of mitomycin C and may be delayed. Streptozotocin is a rarely used nitrosourea compound that may cause mild glomerular impairment or ARF, while tubular toxicity may range from aminoaciduria and glycosuria to a Fanconi syndrome [137]. Although usually mild and reversible, nephrotoxicity may contribute to death [138]. Streptozotocin nephrotoxicity is clearly distinct from that of other nitrosoureas and may be due to an active methyl metabolite [138].

7.2 UROTOXICITY

Urinary tract toxicity mainly affects the bladder, presumably owing to the presence of urinary stasis, while the ureters and urethra are rarely damaged. Hemorrhagic cystitis (HC) may follow treatment with the oxazaphosphorine drugs cyclophosphamide and ifosfamide, pelvic radiotherapy, or occasionally, intravesical installation of other drugs [2]. HC is particularly common in patients undergoing BMT, when the potential causes include high-dose cyclophosphamide, TBI, and primary infection with or reactivation of papovavirus BK, adenovirus, and cytomegalovirus occurring as a result of profound immunosuppression; other potential precipitating factors include bacterial urinary tract infections (UTIs) and episodes of graft-versus-host disease (GVHD) requiring further immunosuppressive treatment [139]. Papovavirus BK is commonly found in the urine (and blood) of patients with HC after BMT, although it is unclear how important it is in the pathogenesis of HC, since it may also be found in patients who do not have HC [140].

HC after cyclophosphamide was first reported in 1959 [141] and its reported incidence has ranged from about 5% to 60%, depending mainly on the patient group studied (e.g., 8–27% in BMT patients), and whether prophylactic mesna was given [2,139]. The incidence may be relatively higher after ifosfamide because higher doses may be given (compared to cyclophosphamide), but mesna ameliorates this toxicity in most patients [142]. The onset of HC may occur during oxazaphosphorine therapy, or days or even months after its completion. Severity may range from asymptomatic microscopic to major hematuria with severe bladder and urethral spasms and pain, passage of clots, and sometimes acute urinary retention due to bladder outlet or urethral obstruction by clot [2]. Severe HC may cause life-threatening hemorrhage, bladder perforation, or renal failure due to urinary tract obstruction by clot, and may occasionally contribute to death [2]. Ultrasound examination may reveal a thickened bladder wall, intravesical clots, and hydronephrosis. Even severe HC is usually (but not invariably) self-limiting, albeit only after several months in some patients [139,143]. However, recurrences weeks after apparent resolution of HC may be associated with viral reactivation, or with episodes of GVHD or bacterial UTI [139]. Although many patients recover completely from HC, some suffer persistent urinary symptoms, including frequency, dysuria, urgency, and incontinence due to bladder fibrosis and dysfunction; furthermore, transitional cell carcinoma of the bladder has been reported in 5% of patients with HC, occurring 1–12 years after the start of cyclophosphamide treatment [143].

The clinical management of established HC is very difficult, especially in severe cases. Supportive care is of paramount importance, comprising discontinuation of any ongoing precipitating treatments (e.g., oxazaphosphorine drug or radiotherapy), vigorous hydration to achieve high urine flow rates and minimize intravesical clot retention, aggressive platelet support to reduce bleeding, and symptomatic treatment with antispasmodics (e.g., oxybutynin) and analgesics (e.g., opiates) to control the distressing pain. Urinary alkalinization is no longer recommended, since it may exacerbate HC [144]. These measures may be sufficient to control mild cases, but they will fail to prevent deterioration in severe cases. Surgical intervention is frequently employed, including urethral catheterization, continuous bladder irrigation (via either a urethral or a suprapubic catheter), urinary diversion procedures, or rarely in life-threatening bleeding, embolization or ligation of the internal iliac artery, or even cystectomy [2]. Several pharmacological strategies have been used in patients with severe and refractory HC, including intravesical installation of prostacyclins (PGE_2, PGE_1, or $PGF_{2\alpha}$), alum, formalin, phenol or silver nitrate, intravenous vasopressin, intravenous or oral antifibrinolytic agents (tranexamic acid, aminocaproic acid), and oral conjugated estrogen [2]. However, it has been difficult to evaluate the efficacy of these treatments, not only because of the lack of controlled trials and the tendency of HC to improve with time, but because the side effects of treatment may be considerable (e.g., severe bladder pain with intravesical installations, clot retention with antifibrinolytics). Vidarabine has been used occasionally in patients with HC associated with urine excretion of papovavirus or adenovirus, but the evidence for its efficacy remains preliminary [145].

The histopathological findings in oxazaphosphorine-induced HC include mucosal edema, ulceration, subendothelial telangiectasia, and submucosal fibrosis [143], and the pathogenesis is thought to involve direct toxic damage by acrolein [144]. Prevention is clearly preferable to treatment of severe HC, and the use of IV hyperhydration and mesna with ifosfamide or high-dose cyclophosphamide (≥ 1 g/m^2/course) to inactivate acrolein and other potentially urotoxic metabolites [146] achieves this aim in the majority of patients, although the details of the mesna administration schedule may be important in determining its efficacy [147].

REFERENCES

1. Skinner R. Strategies to prevent nephrotoxicity of anticancer drugs. Curr Opin Oncol 1995:7:310–315.
2. West NJ. Prevention and treatment of hemorrhagic cystitis. Pharmacotherapy 1997:17:696–706.
3. Rieselbach RE, Garnick MB. Renal diseases induced by antineoplastic agents. In: RW Schrier, CW Gottschalk, eds. Diseases of the Kidney, 4th ed. Boston: Little, Brown, 1988, pp 1275–1299.
4. Berg U, Bolme P. Renal function in children following bone marrow transplantation. Transplant Proc 1989:21:3092–3094.

5. Skinner R, Sharkey IM, Pearson ADJ, Craft AW. Ifosfamide, mesna and nephrotoxicity in children. J Clin Oncol 1993:11:173–190.
6. Brock PR, Koliouskas DE, Barratt TM, Yeomans E, Pritchard J. Partial reversibility of cisplatin nephrotoxicity in children. J Pediatr 1991:118:531–534.
7. Fillastre JP, Viotte G, Morin JP, Moulin B. Nephrotoxicity of antitumoral agents. Adv Nephrol 1988:17:175–218.
8. Skinner R. A study of the nephrotoxicity caused by cytotoxic drugs in children with cancer. Ph.D. dissertation, University of Newcastle upon Tyne, 1995.
9. Skinner R, Pearson ADJ, Coulthard MG, Skillen AW, Hodson AW, Goldfinch ME, Gibb I, Craft AW. Assessment of chemotherapy-associated nephrotoxicity in children with cancer. Cancer Chemother Pharmacol 1991:28:81–92.
10. van Dyk JJ, Falkson HC, van der Merwe AM, Falkson G. Unexpected toxicity in patients treated with iphosphamide. Cancer Res 1972:32:921–924.
11. Stuart-Harris RC, Harper PG, Parsons CA, Kaye SB, Mooney CA, Gowing NF, Wiltshaw E. High-dose alkylation therapy using ifosfamide infusion with mesna in the treatment of adult advanced soft-tissue sarcoma. Cancer Chemother Pharmacol 1983:11:69–72.
12. Pratt CB, Meyer WH, Jenkins JJ, Avery L, McKay CP, Wyatt RJ, Hancock ML. Ifosfamide, Fanconi's syndrome, and rickets. J Clin Oncol 1991:9:1495–1499.
13. Skinner R, Pearson ADJ, English MW, Price L, Wyllie RA, Coulthard MG, Craft AW. Risk factors for ifosfamide nephrotoxicity in children. Lancet 1996:348:578–580.
14. Ashraf MS, Brady J, Breatnach F, Deasy PF, O'Meara A. Ifosfamide nephrotoxicity in paediatric cancer patients. Eur J Paediatr 1994:153:90–94.
15. DeFronzo RA, Abeloff M, Braine H, Humphrey RL, Davis PJ. Renal dysfunction after treatment with isophosphamide (NSC-109724). Cancer Chemother Rep 1974:58:375–382.
16. Sangster G, Kaye SB, Calman KC, Dalton JF. Failure of 2-mercaptoethane sulphonate sodium (mesna) to protect against ifosfamide nephrotoxicity. Eur J Cancer Clin Oncol 1984:20:435–436.
17. Loehrer PJ, Lauer R, Roth BJ, Williams SD, Kalasinski LA, Einhorn LH. Salvage therapy in recurrent germ cell cancer: Ifosfamide and cisplatin plus either vinblastine or etoposide. Ann Intern Med 1988:109:540–546.
18. Sutton GP, Blessing JA, Homesley HD, Berman ML, Malfetano J. Phase II trial of ifosfamide and mesna in advanced ovarian carcinoma: A Gynecologic Oncology Group study. J Clin Oncol 1989:7:1672–1676.
19. Bremner DN, McCormick JS, Thomson JWW. Clinical trial of isophosphamide (NSC-109724)—Results and side effects. Cancer Chemother Rep 1974:58:889–893.
20. Patterson WP, Khojasteh A. Ifosfamide-induced renal tubular defects. Cancer 1989:63:649–651.
21. Jurgens H, Exner U, Kuhl J, Ritter J, Treuner J, Weiner P, Winkler K, Gobel U. High-dose ifosfamide with mesna uroprotection in Ewing's sarcoma. Cancer Chemother Pharmacol 1989:24(suppl):S40–S44.

22. Burk CD, Restaino I, Kaplan BS, Meadows AT. Ifosfamide-induced renal tubular dysfunction and rickets in children with Wilms tumor. J Pediatr 1990: 117:331–335.
23. Prasad VK, Lewis IJ, Aparicio SR, Heney D, Hale JP, Bailey CC, Kinsey SE. Progressive glomerular toxicity of ifosfamide in children. Med Pediatr Oncol 1996:27:149–155.
24. Rossi R, Kist C, Wurster U, Kulpmann W-R, Ehrich JHH. Estimation of ifosfamide/cisplatinum-induced renal toxicity by urinary protein analysis. Pediatr Nephrol 1994:8:151–156.
25. Goren MP, Wright RK, Horowitz ME, Pratt CB. Cancer chemotherapy-induced tubular nephrotoxicity evaluated by immunochemical determination of urinary adenosine deaminase binding protein. Am J Clin Pathol 1986:86:780–783.
26. Al Sheyyab M, Worthington D, Beetham R, Stevens M. The assessment of subclinical ifosfamide-induced renal tubular toxicity using urinary excretion of retinol-binding protein. Pediatr Hematol Oncol 1993:10:119–128.
27. Heney D, Wheeldon J, Rushworth P, Chapman C, Lewis IJ, Bailey CC. Progressive renal toxicity due to ifosfamide. Arch Dis Child 1991:66:966–970.
28. De Schepper J, Hachimi-Idrissi S, Verboven M, Piepsz A, Otten J. Renal function abnormalities after ifosfamide treatment in children. Acta Paediatr 1993:82:373–376.
29. Smeitink J, Verreussel M, Schroder C, Lippens R. Nephrotoxicity associated with ifosfamide. Eur J Pediatr 1988:148:164–166.
30. Rossi R, Ehrich JHH. Partial and complete de Toni–Debre–Fanconi syndrome after ifosfamide chemotherapy for childhood malignancy. Eur J Clin Pharmacol 1993:44 (suppl 1):S43–S45.
31. Goren MP, Pratt CB, Viar MJ. Tubular nephrotoxicity during long-term ifosfamide and mesna therapy. Cancer Chemother Pharmacol 1989:25:70–72.
32. Sweeney LE. Hypophosphataemic rickets after ifosfamide treatment in children. Clin Radiol 1993:47:345–347.
33. Schwartzman E, Scopinaro M, Angueyra N. Phase II study of ifosfamide as a single drug for relapsed paediatric patients. Cancer Chemother Pharmacol 1989:24(suppl):S11–S12.
34. De Schepper J, Stevens G, Verboven M, Baeta C, Otten J. Ifosfamide-induced Fanconi's syndrome with growth failure in a 2-year-old child. Am J Pediatr Hematol Oncol 1991:13:39–41.
35. Caron HN, Abeling N, van Gennip A, de Kraker J, Voute PA. Hyperaminoaciduria identifies patients at risk of developing renal tubular toxicity associated with ifosfamide and platinate containing regimens. Med Pediatr Oncol 1992:20:42–47.
36. Van Gool S, Brock P, Wijndaele G, Van de Casseye W, Kruger M, Proesmans W, Casteels-Van Daele M. Reversible hypophosphatemic rickets following ifosfamide treatment. Med Pediatr Oncol 1992:20:254–257.
37. Ashraf MS, Skinner R, English MW, Craft AW, Pearson ADJ. Late reversibility of chronic ifosfamide-associated nephrotoxicity in a child. Med Pediatr Oncol 1997:28:62–64.

38. Raney B, Ensign LG, Foreman J, Khan F, Newton W, Ortega J, Ragab A, Wharam M, Wiener E, Maurer H. Renal toxicity of ifosfamide in pilot regimens of the Intergroup Rhabdomyosarcoma Study for patients with gross residual disease. Am J Pediatr Hematol Oncol 1994:16:286–295.
39. Shore R, Greenberg M, Geary D, Koren G. Iphosphamide-induced nephrotoxicity in children. Pediatr Nephrol 1992:6:162–165.
40. Rossi R, Danzebrink S, Hillebrand D, Linnenberger K, Ullrich K, Jurgens H. Ifosfamide-induced subclinical nephrotoxicity and its potentiation by cisplatinum. Med Pediatr Oncol 1994:22:27–32.
41. Elias AD, Ayash LJ, Eder JP, Wheeler C, Deary J, Weissman L, Schryber S, Hunt M, Critchlow J, Schnipper L, Frei E, Antman KH. A phase I study of high-dose ifosfamide and escalating doses of carboplatin with autologous bone marrow support. J Clin Oncol 1991:9:320–327.
42. Morland BJ, Mann JR, Milford DV, Raafat F, Stevens MCG. Ifosfamide nephrotoxicity in children: Histopathological features in two cases. Med Pediatr Oncol 1996:27:57–61.
43. Nissim I, Weinberg JM. Glycine attenuates Fanconi syndrome induced by maleate or ifosfamide in rats. Kidney Int 1996:49:684–695.
44. Mohrmann M, Ansorge S, Schmich U, Schonfeld B, Brandis M. Toxicity of ifosfamide, cyclophosphamide and their metabolites in renal tubular cells in culture. Pediatr Nephrol 1994:8:157–163.
45. Mohrmann M, Pauli A, Walkenhorst H, Schonfeld B, Brandis M. Effect of ifosfamide metabolites on sodium-dependent phosphate transport in a model of proximal tubular cells ($LLC-PK_1$) in culture. Renal Physiol Biochem 1993: 16:285–298.
46. Zamlauski-Tucker MJ, Morris ME, Springate JE. Ifosfamide metabolite chloroacetaldehyde causes Fanconi syndrome in the perfused rat kidney. Toxicol Appl Pharmacol 1994:129:170–175.
47. Lippman AJ, Helsen C, Helson L, Krakoff IH. Clinical trials of *cis*-diamminedichloroplatinum (NSC-119875). Cancer Chemother Rep 1973:57:191–200.
48. Madias NE, Harrington JT. Platinum nephrotoxicity. Am J Med 1978:65:307–314.
49. Gonzalez-Vitale JC, Hayes DM, Cvitkovic E, Sternberg SS. The renal pathology in clinical trials of *cis*-platinum(II) diamminedichloride. Cancer 1977: 39:1362–1371.
50. Hayes DM, Cvitkovic E, Golley RB, Scheiner E, Helson L, Krakoff IH. High dose *cis*-platinum diamminedichloride. Amelioration of renal toxicity by mannitol diuresis. Cancer 1977:39:1372–1381.
51. Daugaard G, Rossing N, Rorth M. Effects of cisplatin on different measures of glomerular function in the human kidney with special emphasis on high-dose. Cancer Chemother Pharmacol 1988:21:163–167.
52. Lam M, Adelstein DJ. Hypomagnesemia and renal magnesium wasting in patients treated with cisplatin. Am J Kidney Dis 1986:8:164–169.
53. Schilsky RL, Barbock A, Ozols RF. Persistent hypomagnesemia following cisplatin chemotherapy for testicular cancer. Cancer Treatment Rep 1982:66: 1767–1769.

54. Daugaard G, Abildgaard U. Cisplatin nephrotoxicity. Cancer Chemother Pharmacol 1989:25:1–9.
55. Mavichak V, Coppin CML, Wong NLM, Dirks JH, Walker V, Sutton RAL. Renal magnesium wasting and hypocalciuria in chronic *cis*-platinum nephropathy in man. Clin Sci 1988:75:203–207.
56. Bellin SL, Selim M. Cisplatin-induced hypomagnesemia with seizures: A case report and review of the literature. Gynecol Oncol 1988:30:104–113.
57. Kurtzberg J, Dennis VW, Kinney TR. Cisplatinum-induced renal salt wasting. Med Pediatr Oncol 1984:12:150–154.
58. Daugaard G, Abildgaard U, Holsten-Rathlou NH, Bruunshuus I, Bucher D, Leyssac PP. Renal tubular function in patients treated with high-dose cisplatin. Clin Pharmacol Ther 1988:44:164–172.
59. Verplanke AJW, Herber RFM, de Wit R, Veenhof CHN. Comparison of renal function parameters in the assessment of cis-platin induced nephrotoxicity. Nephron 1994:66:267–272.
60. Stoter G, Koopman A, Vendrik CPJ, Struyvenberg A, Sleijfer DT, Willemse PHB, Koops HS, van Oosterom AT, ten Bokhel Huinink WW, Pinedo HM. Ten-year survival and late sequelae in testicular cancer patients treated with cisplatin, vinblastine and bleomycin. J Clin Oncol 1989:7:1009–1104.
61. Harrell RM, Sibley R, Vogelzang NJ. Renal vascular lesions after chemotherapy with vinblastine, bleomycin and cisplatin. Am J Med 1982:23:429–433.
62. Kamalaker P, Freeman AI, Higby DJ, Wallace HJ Jr, Sinks LF. Clinical response and toxicity with *cis*-dichlorodiammine-platinum(II) in children. Cancer Treatment Rep 1977:61:835–839.
63. Womer RB, Pritchard J, Barratt TM. Renal toxicity of cisplatin in children. J Pediatr 1985:106:659–663.
64. Hayes FA, Green AA, Casper J, Cornet J, Evans WE. Clinical evaluation of sequentially scheduled cisplatin and VM26 in neuroblastoma: Response and toxicity. Cancer 1981:48:1715–1718.
65. Pratt CB, Hayes A, Green AA, Evans WE, Senzer N, Howarth CB, Ransom JL, Crom W. Pharmacokinetic evaluation of cisplatin in children with malignant solid tumors: A phase II study. Cancer Treatment Rep 1981:65:1021–1026.
66. Hartmann O, Pinkerton CR, Philip T, Zucker JM, Breatnach F. Very-high-dose cisplatin and etoposide in children with untreated advanced neuroblastoma. J Clin Oncol 1988:6:44–50.
67. Gomez Campdera FJ, Gonzalez P, Carrillo A, Estelles MC, Rengel M. Cisplatin nephrotoxicity: Symptomatic hypomagnesemia and renal failure. Int J Pediatr Nephrol 1986:7:151–152.
68. Bianchetti MG, Kanaka C, Ridolfi-Luthy A, Wagner HP, Hirt A, Paunier L, Peheim E, Oetliker OH. Chronic renal magnesium loss, hypocalciuria and mild hypokalaemic metabolic alkalosis after cisplatin. Pediatr Nephrol 1990:4:219–222.
69. Vassal G, Rubie H, Kalifa C, Hartmann O, Lemerle J. Hyponatremia and renal sodium wasting in patients receiving cisplatinum. Pediatr Hematol Oncol 1987:4:337–344.

70. Goren MP, Wright RK, Horowitz ME. Cumulative renal tubular damage associated with cisplatin nephrotoxicity. Cancer Chemother Pharmacol 1986:18: 69–73.
71. Ettinger LJ, Douglass HO, Higby DJ, Mindell ER, Nime F, Ghoorah J, Freeman AI. Adjuvant adriamycin and *cis*-diamminedichloroplatinum (*cis*-platinum) in primary osteosarcoma. Cancer 1981:47:248–254.
72. Skinner R, Pearson ADJ, English MW, Price L, Wyllie RA, Coulthard MG, Craft AW. Cisplatin dose rate as a risk factor for nephrotoxicity in children. Br J Cancer 1998:77:1677–1682.
73. Blom JHM, Kurth KH, Splinter TAW. Renal function, serum calcium and magnesium during treatment of advanced bladder carcinoma with *cis*-dichlorodiamineplatinum: Impact of tumour site, patient age and magnesium suppletion. Int Urol Nephrol 1985:17:331–339.
74. Bianchetti MG, Kanaka C, Oetliker OH. Bartter-like syndrome, hypomagnesemia associated with hypocalciuria, and isolated hypocalciuria: Late sequelae after treatment with cisplatin, Pediatr Nephrol 1990:4:C33 (Abstr).
75. Finley RS, Fortner CL, Grove WR. Cisplatin nephrotoxicity: A summary of preventive interventions. Drug Intell Clin Pharm 1985:19:362–367.
76. Preiss R, Brovtsyn VK, Perevodchikova NI, Bychkor MB, Huller H, Belova LA, Michailov P. Effect of methotrexate on the pharmacokinetics and renal excretion of cisplatin. Eur J Clin Pharmacol 1988:34:139–144.
77. Reece PA, Stafford I, Russell J, Khan M, Gill PG. Creatinine clearance as a predictor of ultrafilterable platinum disposition in cancer patients treated with cisplatin: Relationship between peak ultrafilterable platinum plasma levels and nephrotoxicity. J Clin Oncol 1987:5:304–309.
78. Tothill P, Klys HS, Matheson LM, McKay K, Smyth JF. The long-term retention of platinum in human tissues following the administration of cisplatin or carboplatin for cancer chemotherapy. Eur J Cancer 1992:28:1358–1361.
79. Borch RF. The platinum anti-tumor drugs. In: G Powis, RA Prough, eds. Metabolism and Action of Anti-cancer Drugs. London: Taylor & Francis, 1987, pp 163–193.
80. Daley-Yates PT, McBrien DCH. The renal fractional clearance of platinum antitumour compounds in relation to nephrotoxicity. Biochem Pharmacol 1985:34:1423–1428.
81. Daley-Yates PT, McBrien DCH. Cisplatin (*cis*-dichlorodiammineplatinum II) nephrotoxicity. In: PH Bach, FW Bonner, JW Bridges, EA Lock, eds. Nephrotoxicity—Assessment and Pathogenesis. Chichester: Wiley, 1981, pp 356–370.
82. Caterson R, Etheredge S, Snitch P, Duggin G. Mechanisms of renal excretion of *cis*-dichlorodiammine platinum. Res Commun Chem Pathol Pharmacol 1983:41:255–264.
83. Williams PD, Hottendorf GH. Effect of cisplatin on organic ion transport in membrane vesicles from rat kidney cortex. Cancer Treatment Rep 1985:69: 875–880.
84. Barros EJG, Boim MA, Santos OFP, Schor N. Effect of cisplatin on glomerular haemodynamics. Braz J Med Biol Res 1989:22:1295–1301.

85. Heidemann HT, Muller S, Mertins L, Stepan G, Hoffmann K, Ohnhaus EE. Effect of aminophylline on cisplatin nephrotoxicity in the rat. Br J Pharmacol 1989:97:313–318.
86. Dos Santos OFP, Boim MA, Barros EJG, Pirotsky E, Braquet P, Schor N. Effect of platelet-activating factor antagonist BN 52063 on the nephrotoxicity of cisplatin. Lipids 1991:26:1324–1328.
87. Blochl-Daum B, Pehamberger H, Kurz C, Kyrle P-A, Wagner O, Muller M, Monitzer B, Eichler H-G. Effects of cisplatin on urinary thromboxane B_2 excretion. Clin Pharmacol Ther 1995:58:418–424.
88. Singh G. A possible cellular mechanism of cisplatin-induced nephrotoxicity. Toxicology 1989:58:71–80.
89. Yasumasu T, Ueda T, Uozumi J, Mihara Y, Kumazawu J. Comparative study of cisplatin and carboplatin on pharmacokinetics, nephrotoxicity and effect on renal nuclear DNA synthesis in rats. Pharmacol Toxicol 1992:70:143–147.
90. Gandara DR, Perez EA, Wiebe V, de Gregorio MW. Cisplatin chemoprotection and rescue: Pharmacologic modulation of toxicity. Semin Oncol 1991: 18(suppl 3):49–55.
91. Kibirige MS, Morris Jones PH, Addison GM. Prevention of cisplatin-induced hypomagnesemia. Pediatr Hematol Oncol 1988:5:1–6.
92. Jones MM, Basinger MA, Holscher MA. Control of the nephrotoxicity of cisplatin by clinically used sulfur-containing compounds. Fundam Appl Toxicol 1992:18:181–188.
93. Jacobs C, Kaubisch S, Halsey J, Lum BL, Gosland M, Coleman CN, Sikic BI. The use of probenecid as a chemoprotector against cisplatin nephrotoxicity. Cancer 1991:67:1518–1524.
94. Sleijfer DT, Offerman JJG, Mulder NH, Verweij M, Van Der Hem GK, Schraffordt Koops H, Meijer S. The protective potential of the combination of verapamil and cimetidine on cisplatin-induced nephrotoxicity in man. Cancer 1987:60:2823–2828.
95. Doz F, Pinkerton R. What is the place of carboplatin in paediatric oncology? Eur J Cancer 1994:30A:194–201.
96. Foster BJ, Clagett-Carr K, Leyland-Jones B, Hoth D. Results of NCI-sponsored phase I trials with carboplatin. Cancer Treatment Rev 1985:12(suppl A):43–49.
97. Calvert AH, Harland SJ, Newell DR, Siddik ZH, Jones AC, McElwain TJ, Raju S, Wiltshaw E, Smith IE, Baker JM, Harrap KR. Early clinical studies with *cis*-diammine-1,1-cyclobutane dicarboxylate platinumII. Cancer Chemother Pharmacol 1982:9:140–147.
98. Mason MD, Nicholls J, Horwich A. The effect of carboplatin on renal function in patients with metastatic germ cell tumours. Br J Cancer 1991:63:630–633.
99. Sleijfer DT, Smit EF, Meijer S, Mulder NH, Postmus PE. Acute and cumulative effects of carboplatin on renal function. Br J Cancer 1989:60:116–120.
100. Curt GA, Grygiel JJ, Corden BJ, Ozols RF, Weiss RB, Tell DT, Myers CE, Collins JM. A phase I and pharmacokinetic study of diamminecyclobutane-dicarboxylato-platinum (NSC 241240). Cancer Res 1983:43:4470–4473.

101. McDonald BR, Kirmani S, Vasquez M, Mehta RL. Acute renal failure associated with the use of intraperitoneal carboplatin: A report of two cases and review of the literature. Am J Med 1991:90:386–391.
102. Shea TC, Flaherty M, Elias A, Eder JP, Antman K, Begg C, Schnipper L, Frei E III, Henner WD. A phase I clinical and pharmacokinetic study of carboplatin and autologous bone marrow support. J Clin Oncol 1989:7:651–661.
103. Leyvraz S, Ohnuma T, Lassus M, Holland JF. Phase I study of carboplatin in patients with advanced cancer, intermittent intravenous bolus, and 24-hour infusion. J Clin Oncol 1985:3:1385–1392.
104. Welborn J, Meyers FJ, O'Grady LF. Renal salt wasting and carboplatinum [letter]. Ann Intern Med 1988:108:640.
105. Brandt LJ, Broadbent V. Nephrotoxicity following carboplatin use in children: Is routine monitoring of renal function necessary? Med Pediatr Oncol 1993: 21:31–35.
106. Pinkerton CR, Broadbent V, Horwich A, Levitt J, McElwain TJ, Meller ST, Mott M, Oakhill A, Pritchard J. JEB—A carboplatin-based regimen for malignant germ cell tumours in children. Br J Cancer 1990:62:257–262.
107. Lewis IJ, Stevens MCG, Pearson ADJ, Pinkerton CR, Barnes JM. Carboplatin activity in cisplatin treated neuroblastoma. Adv Neuroblastoma Res 1991:3: 553–559.
108. Ettinger LJ, Siegel SE, Baum ES, Moel DI, Gaynon PS. Phase I pediatric trial of *cis*-diammine-1,1-cyclobutane dicarboxylate platinumII (NSC 241240, CBDCA). Am Soc Clin Oncol Abstr 1984:1:44.
109. Gordon SJ, Pearson ADJ, Reid MM, Craft AW. Toxicity of single-day high-dose vincristine, melphalan, etoposide, and carboplatin consolidation with autologous bone marrow rescue in advanced neuroblastoma. Eur J Cancer 1992: 28A:1319–1323.
110. Reed E, Jacob J. Carboplatin and renal dysfunction [letter]. Ann Intern Med 1989:110:409.
111. Siddik ZH, Dible SE, Boxall FE, Harrap KR. Renal pharmacokinetics and toxicity of cisplatin and carboplatin in animals. In: DCH McBrien, TF Slater, eds. Biochemical Mechanisms of Platinum Antitumour Drugs. Oxford: IRL Press, 1986, pp 171–198.
112. Condit PT, Chanes RE, Joel W. Renal toxicity of methotrexate. Cancer 1969: 23:126–131.
113. Von Hoff DD, Penta JS, Helman LJ, Slavik M. Incidence of drug-related deaths secondary to high-dose methotrexate and citrovorum factor administration. Cancer Treatment Rep 1977:61:745–748.
114. Abelson HT, Fosburg MT, Beardsley GP, Goorin AM, Gorka C, Link M, Link D. Methotrexate-induced renal impairment: Clinical studies and rescue from systemic toxicity with high-dose Leucovorin and thymidine. J Clin Oncol 1983:1:208–216.
115. Pitman SW, Frei EI. Weekly methotrexate–calcium Leucovorin rescue: Effect of alkalinization; pharmacokinetics in the CNS; and use in CNS non-Hodgkin's lymphoma. Cancer Treatment Rep 1977:61:695–701.

116. McElwain TJ, Hedley DW, Burton G, Clink HM, Gordon MY, Jarman M, Juttner CA, Millar JL, Milsted RAV, Prentice G, Smith IE, Spence D, Woods M. Marrow autotransplantation accelerates haematological recovery in patients with malignant melanoma treated with high-dose melphalan. Br J Cancer 1979:40:72–80.
117. Helenglass G, Powles RL, McElwain TJ, Lakhani A, Milan S, Gore M, Nandi A, Zuiable A, Perren T, Forgensen G, Treleaven J, Hamilton C, Millar J. Melphalan and total body irradiation (TBI) versus cyclophosphamide and TBI as conditioning for allogeneic matched sibling bone marrow transplants for acute myeloblastic leukaemia in first remission. Bone Marrow Transplant 1988:3:21–29.
118. Alix JL, Swiercz P, Schaerer R, Mousseau M, Cordonnier D, Couderc P, Michallet M. Nephrotoxicité du melphalan utilisé à haute dose. La Presse Med 1983:12:575–576.
119. Burke JF, Laucius JF, Brodovsky HS, Soriano RZ. Doxorubicin hydrochloride–associated renal failure. Arch Intern Med 1977:137:385–388.
120. Fajardo LF, Eltringham JR, Stewart JR, Klauher MR. Adriamycin nephrotoxicity. Lab Invest 1980:43:242–253.
121. Sternberg SS. Cross-striated fibrils and other ultrastructural alterations in glomeruli of rats with daunomycin nephrosis. Lab Invest 1970:23:39–51.
122. Lopes VM. Cyclophosphamide nephrotoxicity in man [letter]. Lancet 1967:i:1060.
123. DeFronzo RA, Colvin OM, Braine H, Robertson GL, Davis PJ. Cyclophosphamide and the kidney. Cancer 1974:33:483–491.
124. Harlow PJ, DeClerck YA, Shore NA, Ortega JA, Carranza A, Heuser E. A fatal case of inappropriate ADH secretion induced by cyclophosphamide therapy. Cancer 1979:44:896–898.
125. Slavin RE, Dias MA, Saral R. Cytosine arabinoside induced gastrointestinal toxic alterations in sequential chemotherapeutic protocols. A clinico-pathologic study of 33 patients. Cancer 1978:42:1747–1759.
126. Harman WE, Cohen HJ, Schneeberger EE, Grupe WE. Chronic renal failure in children treated with methyl CCNU. N Engl J Med 1979:300:1200–1203.
127. Weiss RB, Posada JG, Jr., Kramer RA, Boyd MR. Nephrotoxicity of semustine. Cancer Treatment Rep 1983:67:1105–1112.
128. Schacht RG, Feiner HD, Gallo GR, Lieberman A, Baldwin DS. Nephrotoxicity of nitrosoureas. Cancer 1981:48:1328–1334.
129. Silver HKB, Morton DL. CCNU nephrotoxicity following sustained remission in oat cell carcinoma. Cancer Treatment Rep 1979:63:226–227.
130. Presant CA, Denes AE, Klein L, Garrett S, Metter GE. Phase I and preliminary phase II observations of high-dose intermittent 6-thioguanine. Cancer Treatment Rep 1980:64:1109–1113.
131. Arneil GC, Emmanuel IG, Flatman GE, Harris F, Young DG, Zachary RB. Nephritis in two children after irradiation and chemotherapy for nephroblastoma. Lancet 1974:i:960–963.
132. Makipernaa A, Koskimies O, Jaaskelainen J, Teppo A-M, Siimes MA. Renal growth and function 11–28 years after treatment of Wilms' tumour. Eur J Pediatr 1991:150:444–447.

133. Robertson GL, Bhoopalam N, Zelkowitz LJ. Vincristine neurotoxicity and abnormal secretion of antidiuretic hormone. Arch Intern Med 1973:132: 717–720.
134. Peterson BA, Collins AJ, Vogelzang NJ, Bloomfield CD. 5-Azacytidine and renal tubular dysfunction. Blood 1981:57:182–185.
135. Kennedy BJ. Metabolic and toxic effects of mithramycin during tumor therapy. Am J Med 1970:49:494–503.
136. Hanna WT, Krauss S, Regester RF, Murphy WM. Renal disease after mitomycin C therapy. Cancer 1981:48:2583–2588.
137. Sadoff L. Nephrotoxicity of streptozotocin (NSC-85998). Cancer Chemother Rep 1970:54:457–459.
138. Schein PS, O'Connell MJ, Blom J, Hubbard S, Magrath IT, Bergevin P, Wiernik PH, Ziegler JL, DeVita VT. Clinical antitumor activity and toxicity of streptozotocin (NSC-85998). Cancer 1974:34:993–1000.
139. Russell SJ, Vowels MR, Vale T. Haemorrhagic cystitis in paediatric bone marrow transplant patients: An association with infective agents, GVHD and prior cyclophosphamide. Bone Marrow Transplant 1994:13:533–539.
140. Bogdanovic G, Ljungman P, Wang F, Dalianis T: Presence of human polyomavirus DNA in the peripheral circulation of bone marrow transplant patients with and without hemorrhagic cystitis. Bone Marrow Transplant 1996: 17:573–576.
141. Coggins PR, Ravdin RG, Eisman SH. Clinical pharmacology and preliminary evaluation of Cytoxan (cyclophosphamide). Cancer Chemother Rep 1959:3: 9–11.
142. Zalupski M, Baker LH. Ifosfamide. J Natl Cancer Inst 1988:80:556–566.
143. Stillwell TJ, Benson RC. Cyclophosphamide-induced hemorrhagic cystitis. Cancer 1988:61:451–457.
144. Brock N, Pohl J, Stekar J. Studies on the urotoxicity of oxazaphosphorine cytostatics and its prevention—I: experimental studies on the urotoxicity of alkylating compounds. Eur J Cancer 1981:17:595–607.
145. Kawakami M, Ueda S, Maeda T, Karasuno T, Teshima H, Hiraoko A, Nakamura H, Tanaka K, Masaoka T. Vidarabine therapy for virus-associated cystitis after allogeneic bone marrow transplantation. Bone Marrow Transplant 1997:20:485–490.
146. Brock N, Pohl J, Stekar J, Scheef W. Studies on the urotoxicity of oxazaphosphorine cytostatics and its prevention—III: profile of action of sodium 2-mercaptoethane sulfonate (mesna). Eur J Cancer Clin Oncol 1982:18: 1377–1387.
147. Fleming RA, Cruz JM, Webb CD, Kucera GL, Perry JJ, Hurd DD. Urinary elimination of cyclophosphamide alkylating metabolites and free thiols following two administration schedules of high-dose cyclophosphamide and mesna. Bone Marrow Transplant 1996:17:497–501.

8

Hepatotoxicity Induced by Cytostatic Drugs

HANS-PETER LIPP, JOACHIM BOOS, EUGEN J. VERSPOHL, EUGENE Y. KRYNETSKI, and WILLIAM E. EVANS

8.1 OVERVIEW

HANS-PETER LIPP
University of Tübingen, Tübingen, Germany

8.1.1 INTRODUCTION

High concentrations of cytotoxic drugs reach the liver either via the hepatic artery after IV administration or via the portal vein if administered orally. However, hepatotoxicity is of comparatively low incidence regarding treatment protocols with antineoplastic agents (Table 1) [1–3].

It has been suggested that the constitutive slow proliferation of hepatocytes and the high detoxification capacity of the liver may be of particular importance in this regard. Even a prodrug like cyclophosphamide induces severe hepatic side effects only rarely, though it may be given in very high doses [4]. The chemotherapy-induced hepatic changes range from hepatocellular necrosis, fatty changes, cholestasis, fibrosis, even cirrhosis, veno-occlusive diseases (VOD), and most often, an elevation of liver enzymes [1].

8.1.2 Assessment of Hepatobiliary Disease and Liver Dysfunction

Hepatobiliary disease is routinely deduced from abnormal results of standard biochemical liver tests, including aspartate aminotransferase (AST), alkaline phosphatase, bilirubin, and albumin (Table 2 and 3). However, these tests do not measure true liver function because they lack specificity in predicting disease severity. Thus, it appears that dynamic liver function based on the disposition of a test drug may be a more attractive approach to the assessment of hepatic dysfunction regarding metabolic clearance [5].

Possibly the use of the "MEGX assay" will be established as a more reliable and sensitive indicator of hepatic dysfunction. This test is based on the conversion, in the liver, of the drug lidocaine to MEGX (monoethylglycine xylide) by cytochrome-P450-mediated oxidative N-deethylation (Fig. 1). It has been demonstrated that normal subjects and patients with liver cirrhosis can be clearly differentiated from each other with respect to liver function by the MEGX assay [6]. A change in hepatic blood flow or a decrease in constitutive cytochrome P450 activity will result in an impairment of lidocaine metabolism and MEGX formation, whereas renal dysfunction does not have any influence on lidocaine or MEGX clearance.

Table 1 Cytostatics That Commonly Cause Hepatotoxic Side Effects

Drug	Clinical signs of liver dysfunction
Asparaginase	Fatty changes in the liver; increase of AST (SGOT), ALT (SGPT), serum alkaline phosphatase, direct and indirect bilirubin and ammonia; decrease in clotting factors; pancreatitis [decreased insulin synthesis, hyperglycemia].
High-dose busulfan	Hepatic veno-occlusive disease.
Carmustine	Generally mild and reversible hepatotoxicity (increase in liver enzymes).
Streptozocin	Minimal transient increase in serum concentrations of AST (SGOT), ALT (SGPT), LDH, and/or alkaline phosphatase.
Mercaptopurine and azathioprine	Rapid onset of jaundice, cholestasis, ascites, hepatic encephalopathy, and/or elevated hepatic enzyme concentrations, hepatic fibrosis (incidence increases from 0–6% to about 40% when dosage exceeds 2.5 mg/kg/d).
Methotrexate	Acute (transient elevation of liver enzymes) and chronic hepatotoxicity (hepatic fibrosis or cirrhosis). The latter has generally been associated with prolonged MTX therapy and cumulative doses of more than 1.5 g.
Paclitaxel	Abnormalities in liver function tests (increase in serum ALT as well as serum AST; increase in serum bilirubin may occur in 8% of patients).

Table 2 Criteria for Hepatic Function

Hepatic function	Thrombotest (%)	Asp-AT[a] (U/L)	Albumin (g/L)	Bilirubin (μM)
Good	>40	<51	>34	<36
Fair	25–39	51–200	28–34	36–68
Poor	<25	>200	>28	>68

[a]Asp-AT, aspartate aminotransferase.
Source: Ref. 3.

Table 3 Normal Range of Laboratory Tests Regarding Liver Function

Constituent	Traditional	SI	Conversion factor
Alanine aminotransferase (ALT, SGPT) in serum	0–35 U/L	0–0.58 μkat/L	0.01667
Albumine in serum	4–6 g/dL	40–60 g/L	10
Alkaline phosphatase (AP) in serum	30–120 U/L	0.5–2.0 μkat/L	0.01667
Ammonia in plasma			
As ammonia (NH_3)	10–80 μg/dL	5–50 μmol/L	0.5872
As ammonium (NH_4^+)	10–85 μg/dL	5–50 μmol/L	0.5543
As nitrogen (N)	10–65 μg/dL	5–50 μmol/L	0.7139
Aspartate aminotransferase (AST, SGOT) in serum	0–35 U/L	0–0.58 μkat/L	0.01667
Bilirubin in serum			
Total	0,1–1,0 mg/dL	2–18 μmol/L	17.1
Conjugated (direct form)	0–0,2 mg/dL	0–4 μmol/L	17.1
γ-Glutamyl transferase (GGT) in serum	0–30 U/L	0–0.5 μkat/L	0.01667

Source: Adapted from SI unit conversion guide, N Engl J Med 1992:56–107.

It seems to be a major advantage that the MEGX assay is rapid and easy to perform. The recommended low dose of 1 mg/kg lidocaine (injected over 1–2 min) appears to be safe. In contrast to the indocyanine green (ICG) test, several blood collections can be circumvented by the MEGX-assay. In summary, the MEGX assay appears to be a promising approach for the assessment of individual hepatic function in cancer patients (Fig. 1).

8.1.3 Interpretation of Abnormal Liver Function Tests

In normal subjects the total bilirubin level should not exceed 1.0 mg/dL (Table 2). Around 70% is indirect (unconjugated) bilirubin, whereas about 30% is direct bilirubin, primarily as glucuronidated bilirubin. In cases of "unconjugated hyperbilirubinemia," more than 80% may be indirect bilirubin, which indicates hemolysis or Gilbert syndrome. In the former situation, the total bilirubin levels rarely exceed 6.0 mg/dL total bilirubin in serum.

If more than 50% of the total bilirubin is conjugated ("conjugated hyperbilirubinemia"), hepatocellular dysfunction, cholestasis, and bile duct obstruction cannot be excluded.

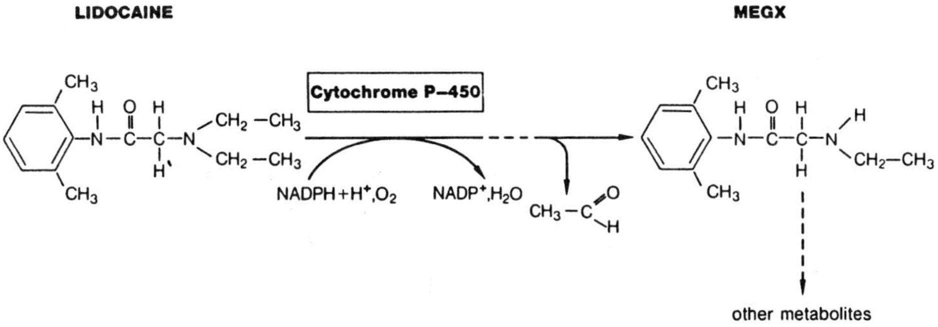

LIDOCAINE

MEGX

Cytochrome P-450

NADPH+H⁺,O₂ NADP⁺,H₂O

CH_3-CHO

other metabolites

Fig. 1 Principles of the MGEX liver function test.

If the bilirubin level exceeds 25–30 mg/dL, bile duct obstruction by gallstones seems to be unlikely because conjugated bilirubin can be excreted by the kidney in cases of extrahepatic cholestasis.

The transaminases are enzymes that catalyze the transfer of amino groups from aspartate and alanine to ketoglutaric acid. The aspartate aminotransferase (AST: formerly designated serum glutamic-oxaloacetic transaminase [SGOT]) is not restricted to the liver, whereas the alanine aminotransferase (ALT, SGPT) is predominantly expressed in the hepatic tissue. Thus, an increase of the latter seems to be a better indicator of liver cell injury, whereas an isolated increase of AST without concomitant ALT elevation may primarily indicate a cardiac or muscle disease.

The alkaline phosphatase (AP) is primarily expressed in the liver and the bone. Its synthesis by the bile duct epithelial cells is frequently increased if bile ducts are obstructed. Levels of AP are also increased in cases of hyperthyroidism, cardiac failure, lymphoma, and hypernephroma. However, if γ-glutamyltransferase (GGT) is elevated simultaneously, an underlying liver dysfunction is very probable. If bilirubin levels are in the normal range in spite of high AP levels, granulomatous or infiltrative diseases of the liver are very likely.

A hypoalbuminemia may indicate a progressive liver disease because the circulating half-life of albumin averages 3 weeks. Sometimes, the serum albumin concentrations decline more rapidly in cases of severe liver disease.

In conclusion, liver function tests based on transaminase, bilirubin, and albumin levels in serum must be interpreted very carefully. An AST increase must be confirmed by ALT elevation, an AP-increase should be confirmed by GGT elevation, if hepatic dysfunction is to be diagnosed. An exemplary clinical approach to the interpretation of abnormal liver function test results was presented by Kamath [5].

8.1.4 Hepatotoxicity of Cytostatics

In general, cytostatics are rarely associated with the development of hepatic disease (Table 3). Especially high-dose busulfan, dacarbazine, the nitrosoureas, several antimetabolites, and L-asparaginase have been reported to induce hepatotoxic side effects [1–3].

8.1.4.1 Asparaginase Preparations (see also Section 8.2)

Liver function abnormalities are evident in most patients treated with asparaginase preparations. AST (SGOT), ALT (SGPT), and serum alkaline phosphatase, direct as well as indirect bilirubin levels, and plasma ammonia concentrations can be severely increased [7,8].

Treatment with L-asparaginase results in a rapid reduction of plasma asparagine and glutamine levels, which in turn leads to inhibition of hepatic protein biosynthesis. As a consequence, besides other side effects, thromboembolic complications (incidence ranges from 1 to 17%, dependent on dose) and hemorrhage are serious complications induced by L-asparaginase therapy [9–12].

Impairment of pancreatic function occus rather frequently, too, after L-asparaginase administration. Thus, a hypoinsulinemia with concomitant hyperglycemia may develop, amylase levels in plasma may be increased, and a sometimes fulminant pancreatitis may develop. Although hyperglycemia is usually transient and resolves after discontinuation of the drug, some patients have died of diabetic ketoacidosis [13–15]. In common, other asparaginase preparations, like erwinase or pegaspargase, are also associated with an increased risk of hepatotoxicity [9,15–17].

8.1.4.2 Alkylating Agents

High-Dose Busulfan (HD-Busulfan)

The dose-limiting organ toxicity of high-dose busulfan (HD-busulfan) is hepatic veno-occlusive disease (HVOD) [18,19]. This severe side effect occurs in approximately 15–20% of patients after bone marrow transplantation. The syndrome consists of liver damage manifested by the occlusion of hepatic venules via fibrin thrombi and sinusoidal congestion. Risk factors include prior intensive chemotherapy (particularly based on alkylating agents) and radiation, prior hepatitis, and persistent fever during posttransplant period [18,19].

A higher incidence of HVOD occurred in patients receiving the combination of HD-busulfan/HD-cyclophosphamide than those who were treated with HD-busulfan/HD-cytarabine or HD-busulfan/HD-etoposide [20].

Levels of circulating antithrombin III and protein C are usually decreased in patients with HVOD. The lower concentrations of these substances may significantly contribute to the progressive hepatic disease, even resulting in hemorrhagic complications [21].

It is not fully understood which regimen would most successfully counteract busulfan-induced HVOD. Recently a combination of plasminogen activator (bolus administration) and antithrombin III (continuous infusion) was demonstrated to be useful in reversing the course of HVOD without increased risk of bleeding in contrast to unfractionated heparin [21].

The pathogenesis of busulfan-induced HVOD remains obscure. However, there appears to be a correlation between high AUC values of unchanged busulfan and the occurrence of HVOD. In this context one must keep in mind the extraordinarily high interindividual variability of busulfan disposition in cancer patients [22,23].

Based on their pharmacokinetic studies, Dix and colleagues recently suggested that an initial AUC of more than 1500 μmol × min/L may be a very critical risk factor for the development of HVOD. As a consequence, it may be reasonable to use a busulfan test dose to calculate the individual pharmacokinetic course before HD-busulfan is started [22,24].

Dacarbazine

Single-agent dacarbazine (DTIC) reportedly has induced hepatic vein thrombosis and potentially fatal hepatocellular necrosis (incidence about 0.01%). However, the complicated clinical situation (e.g., concomitant administration of other antineoplastic agents) often does not allow a clear correlation between the use of dacarbazine and the onset of symptoms. Concomitant eosinophilic infiltrates indicate that hepatotoxicity may be partially based on allergic reactions [25–27].

Nitrosoureas

Generally mild and reversible hepatotoxicity related to the use of carmustine has been reported in up to 26% of patients. Serum transaminase, alkaline phosphatase, and bilirubin concentrations may be increased, whereas the incidence of jaundice is rather rare.

A mild transient increase of AST (SGOT), ALT (SGPT), and lactate dehydrogenase (LDH) levels was recorded in about 25% of patients after the IV administration of streptozocin. An elevation of serum bilirubin concentrations and hypoalbuminemia has also been recorded. The incidence of severe and fatal hepatic effects, however, is rare in conventional therapy, in contrast to high-dose therapy [28,29].

8.1.4.3 Antimetabolites

Mercaptopurine and Azathioprine (see also Section 8.3)

Hepatotoxic side effects induced by mercaptopurine (6-MP) are manifested in rapid onset of jaundice, intrahepatic cholestasis, ascites, hepatic encephalopathy, and/or increased liver enzymes. As a consequence, liver function must be closely monitored during 6-MP therapy [30–32].

The incidence of hepatic dysfunction appears to be increased if the daily dosage exceeds 2.5 mg/kg. The biochemical pathogenesis of 6-MP-induced hepatotoxicity is not yet fully understood. It is likely that liver dysfunction and jaundice resolve after discontinuation of therapy [31].

The nitroimidazole derivative of 6-MP, azathioprine, is also able to induce hepatotoxic side effects [33–37]. It has been speculated that patients who convert azathioprine rather rapidly to 6-MP may be at higher risk of developing increased serum bilirubin and alkaline phosphatase levels [32].

Only very rarely has 6-thioguanine, which is structurally related to 6-mercaptopurine, been associated with the onset of HVOD and other hepatotoxic symptoms [38,39].

Methotrexate

Conventional as well as high doses of methotrexate (MTX) have been associated with the onset of acute as well as chronic hepatotoxic side effects [40–43]. Serum transaminases are frequently elevated 24–72 hours after administration of MTX, but in most cases the increase of liver enzymes is transient and asymptomatic [41].

During long-term therapy (e.g., > 2 years or longer with frequent small doses daily and a cumulative dose of more than 1500 mg), however, severe irreversible hepatotoxicity, including hepatic fibrosis and liver cirrhosis requiring hepatic allotransplantation, may develop. Conditions like alcoholism, obesity, or diabetes may predispose patients to develop progressive hepatic changes. Thus far, the greatest problem appears to be the lack of a specific pathologic indicator capable of leading to timely diagnoses. The potential reversibility of such lesions following discontinuation of therapy is currently unknown [44–47].

5-Fluorouracil

After receiving hepatic arterial infusions of 5-fluorouracil or the structurally related floxuridine, some patients may develop biliary sclerosis. This hepatotoxic side effect is an event associated primarily with the use of hepatic arterial infusion rather than IV administration of these drugs. Jaundice and elevation of several liver enzymes may develop between 3 and 21 months after the initiation of therapy; clinically, cholangiographic changes that resemble signs of primary sclerotic cholangitis may be diagnosed [48–50].

The biochemical background of this toxicity is not yet fully understood; however, high levels of a conjugate consisting of chenodeoxycholic acid and α-fluoro-β-alanine have been isolated from bile. This unphysiological bile acid conjugate probably differs in its detergent effect from the natural occurring chenodeoxycholic acid and may lead to progressive solubilization of biliary membrane components [48].

Cytarabine

Cytarabine (Ara-C) is rarely associated with the onset of hepatic dysfunction (e.g., jaundice; increases in serum bilirubin concentrations, transaminases, and alkaline phosphatase). Veno-occlusive hepatic disease also is a very rare event associated with the use of Ara-C [51,52].

8.1.4.4 Other Potentially Hepatotoxic Cytostatics

Paclitaxel

Abnormalities in liver function tests can be observed in patients after IV administration of paclitaxel. However, the incidence of increased serum ALT concentrations, increased serum alkaline phosphatase, and increased serum AST (SGOT) levels is low. Elevated bilirubin concentrations were recorded in about 8% of cancer patients.

Paclitaxel should be administered with caution in patients with hepatic dysfunction, however, because the liver plays an important role in paclitaxel metabolism [53,54].

High-Dose Etoposide

The use of high-dose etoposide has been associated with the onset of hepatotoxic symptoms, particularly an increase of serum bilirubin (sometimes leading to jaundice) and liver enzymes (e.g., AST and alkaline phosphatase). However, these effects are generally transient [55,56].

Dactinomycin

Dactinomycin should be administered with extreme caution in the first 2 months after radiation therapy in patients treated for right-sided Wilms tumor, because hepatomegaly, elevated liver enzymes, and ascites have been reported [57,58].

REFERENCES TO SECTION 8.1

1. Perry MC. Chemotherapeutic agents and hepatotoxicity. Semin Oncol 1992: 19:551–565.
2. Menard DB, Gisselbrecht C, Marly M, et al. Antineoplastic agents and the liver. Gastroenterology 1980:78:142–164.
3. Koren G, Beatty K, Steo A, et al. The effects of impaired liver function on the elimination of antineoplastic agents. Ann Pharmacother 1992:26:363–371.
4. Goldberg JW, Lidsky MD. Cyclophosphamide-associated hepatotoxicity. South Med J 1985:78:222–223.
5. Kamath PS. Clinical approach to the patient with abnormal liver test results. Mayo Clin Proc 1996:71:1089–1095.
6. Oellerich M, Burdelski M, Lautz H-U, et al. Lidocain metabolite formation as a measure of liver function in patients with cirrhosis. Ther Drug Monit 1990: 12:219–226.
7. Haskell CM, Canellos GP, Leventhal BG, et al. L-Asparaginase: Therapeutic and toxic effects in patients with neoplastic disease. N Engl J Med 1969:281: 1028–1034.
8. Durden DL, Salazar AM, Distasio JA. Kinetic analysis of hepatotoxicity associated with antineoplastic asparaginase. Cancer Res 1983:43:1602–1605.
9. Boos J, Werber G, Ahlke E, et al. Monitoring of asparaginase activity and asparagine levels in children on different asparaginase preparations. Eur J Cancer 1996:32A:1544–1550.
10. Asselin BL, Whitin JC, Cappola DJ, et al. Comparative pharmacokinetic studies of three asparaginase preparations. J Clin Oncol 1993:11:1780–1786.
11. Glasmacher A, Kleinschmidt R, Unkrig C, Metzger J, Scharf RE. Coagulation disorders induced by L-asparaginase: Correction with and without fresh-frozen plasma. Infusionsther Transfusionsmed 1997:24:138–143.
12. Rodeghiero F, Mannucci PM, Vigano S, et al. Liver dysfunction rather than intravascular coagulation as the main cause of low protein C and antithrombin III in acute leukemia. Blood 1984:63:965–969.
13. MacEwan E, Rosenthal R, Matus R, et al. A preliminary study on the evaluation of asparaginase. Cancer 1987:59:2011–2015.
14. Haskell CM, Canellos GP, Leventhal BG, et al. L-Asparaginase: Therapeutic and toxic effects in patients with neoplastic disease. N Engl J Med 1969:281: 1028–1034.
15. Holle LM. Pegaspargase: An alternative? Ann Pharmacother 1997:31:616–624.
16. Koerholz D, Brueck M, Nuernberger W, et al. Chemical and immunological characteristics of four different L-asparaginase preparations. Eur J Hematol 1989:42:417–424.
17. Ettinger LJ, Kurtzberg J, Voute PA, et al. An open-label multicenter study of polyethylene glycol-L-asparaginase for the treatment of acute lymphoblastic leukemia. Cancer 1995:75:1176–1181.
18. Morris LE, Guthrie TH. Busulfan-induced hepatitis. Am J Gastroenterol 1988: 83:682–683.

19. Buggia I, Locatelli F, Regazzi MB, Zecca M. Busulfan. Ann Pharmacother 1994:28:1055–1062.
20. Morgan M, Dodds A, Atkinson K, Szer J, et al. The toxicity of busulphan and cyclophosphamide as the preparative regimen for bone marrow transplantation. Br J Haematol 1991:77:529–534.
21. Patton DF, Harper JL, Wooldridge TN, et al. Treatment of veno-occlusive disease of the liver with bolus tissue plasminogen activator and continuous infusion antithrombin III concentrate. Bone Marrow Transplant 1996:14:443–447.
22. Dix SP, Wingard JR, Mullins RE, et al. Association of busulfan area under the curve with veno-occlusive disease following BMT. Bone Marrow Transplant 1996:17:225–230.
23. Vassal G, Koscielny S, Challine D, Valteau-Couanet D, et al. Busulfan disposition and hepatic veno-occlusive disease in children undergoing bone-marrow transplantation. Cancer Chemother Pharmacol 1996:37:247–253.
24. Grochow LB. Busulfan disposition: The role of therapeutic drug monitoring in bone marrow transplantation induction regimes. Semin Oncol 1993:20(suppl 4):18–25.
25. Sutherland CM, Krementz ET. Hepatic toxicity of DTIC. Cancer Treatment Rep 1981:65:321–322.
26. Ceci G, Bella M, Mellisari M, et al. Fatal hepatic vascular toxicity of DTIC. Cancer 1988:61:1988–1991.
27. Erichsen C, Jonsson R. Veno-occlusive liver disease after dacarbazine therapy (DTIC) for melanoma. J Surg Oncol 1984:27:268–270.
28. De Vita VT, Carbone PP, Owens AH, et al. Clinical trials with 1,3-bis(2-chloroethyl)-1-nitrosourea, NSC-409962. Cancer Res 1965:25:1876–1881.
29. Wolff SN. High-dose carmustine and high-dose etoposide: A treatment regimen resulting in enhanced hepatic toxicity. Cancer Treatment Rep 1986:70:1464–1465.
30. McIlvanie SK, MacCarthy JD. Hepatitis in association with prolonged 6-mercaptopurine therapy. Blood 1959:14:80–90.
31. Gross R. Hepatotoxicity of 6-mercaptopurine and azathioprine [letter]. Mayo Clin Proc 1994:69:498.
32. Shorey J, Schenker S, Suki WN, et al. Hepatotoxicity of mercaptopurine. Arch Intern Med 1968:122:54–58.
33. Jeurissen MEC, Boerbooms AMT, van de Putte LBA, et al. Azathioprine induced fever, chills, rash and hepatotoxicity in rheumatoid arthritis. Ann Rheum Dis 1990:49:25–27.
34. Aguilar HI, Burgart LJ, Geller A, Rakela J. Azathioprine-induced lymphoma manifesting as fulminant hepatic failure. Mayo Clin Proc 1997:72:643–645.
35. Stetter M, Schmidl M, Krapf R. Azathioprine hypersensitivity mimicking Goodpasture's syndrome. Am J Kidney Dis 1994:23(6):874–877.
36. Small P, Lichter M. Probable azathioprine hepatotoxicity. A case report. Ann Allergy 1989:62:518–520.
37. Read AE, Wiesner RH, LaBrecque DR, et al. Hepatic veno-occlusive disease associated with renal transplantation and azathioprine therapy. Ann Intern Med 1986:104:651–655.

38. Gill RA, Onstad GR, Cardamone JM, et al. Hepatic veno-occlusive disease caused by 6-thioguanine. Ann Intern Med 1982:96:58–60.
39. Satti MB, Weinbren K, Gordon-Smith EC. 6-Thioguanine as a cause of toxic veno-occlusive disease of the liver. J Clin Pathol 1982:35:1086–1091.
40. McIntosh S, Davidson DL, O'Brien RT, et al. Methotrexate hepatotoxicity in children with leukemia. J Pediatr 1977:90:1019–1021.
41. Tolman KG, Clegg DO, Lee RG, et al. Methotrexate and the liver. J Rheumatol 1985:12:29–34.
42. Weber BL, Tanyer G, Poplack DG, et al. Transient acute hepatotoxicity of high-dose methotrexate therapy during childhood. Natl Cancer Inst Monogr 1987:5:207–212.
43. Willkens RF, Leonard PA, Clegg DO, et al. Liver histology in patients receiving low dose pulse methotrexate for the treatment of rheumatoid arthritis. Ann Rheum Dis 1990:49:591–593.
44. MacKenzie AH. Hepatotoxicity of prolonged methotrexate therapy for rheumatoid arthritis. Clevel and Clin Q 1985:52:129–135.
45. Podurgiel BJ, McGill DB, Ludwig J, et al. Liver injury associated with methotrexate therapy for psoriasis. Mayo Clin Proc 1973:48:787–792.
46. Lanse SB, Arnold GL, Gowans JDC, et al. Low incidence of hepatotoxicity associated with long-term, low dose oral methotrexate in treatment of refractory psoriasis, psoriatic arthritis and rheumatoid arthritis: An acceptable risk/benefit ratio. Dig Dis Sci 1985:30:104–109.
47. Lewis JH, Schiff E. Methotrexate-induced chronic liver injury: Guidelines for detection and prevention. Am J Gastroenterol 1988:88:1337–1345.
48. Sweeny DJ, Martin M, Diasio RB. *N*-Chenodeoxycholyl-2-fluoro-β-alanine: A biliary metabolite of 5-fluorouracil in humans. Drug Metab Dispos 1988:16: 892–894.
49. Hohn D, Melnick J, Stagg R, et al. Biliary sclerosis in patients receiving hepatic arterial infusion of floxuridine. J Clin Oncol 1985:3:98–102.
50. Pettavel J, Gardiol D, Bergier N, et al. Fatal liver cirrhosis associated with long-term arterial infusion of floxuridine. Lancet 1986:2:1162–1163.
51. Pizzuto J, Aviles A, Ramosi E, et al. Cytosine arabinoside induced liver damage. Histopathologic demonstration. Med Pediatr Oncol 1983:11:287–290.
52. George CB, Mansour RP, Redmond J, et al. Hepatic dysfunction and jaundice following high-dose cytosine arabinoside. Cancer 1984:54:2360–2362.
53. Pazdur R, Kudelka AP, Kavanagh JJ, et al. The taxoids: Paclitaxel (Taxol) and docetaxel (Taxotere). Cancer Treatment Rev 1993:19:351–386.
54. Tamura T, Sasaki Y, Eguchi K, et al. Phase I and pharmacokinetic study of paclitaxel by 24-hour intravenous infusion. Jpn J Cancer Res 1994:85(10): 1057–1062.
55. Tran A, Housset C, Boboc B, et al. Etoposide (VP16-213) induced hepatitis. Report of three cases following standard dose treatments. J Hepatol 1991:2: 36–39.
56. Johnson DH, Greco FA, Wolff SN. Etoposide-induced hepatic injury: A potential complication of high-dose therapy. Cancer Treatment Rep 1983:2:36–39.

57. Pritchard J, Raine J, Wallendszus K. Hepatotoxicity of actinomycin D. Lancet 1989:1:168.
58. Raine J, Bowman A, Wallendszus K, et al. Hepatopathy–thrombocytopenia syndrome—A complication of dactinomycin therapy of Wilm's tumor: A report from the United Kingdom Children's Cancer Study Group. J Clin Oncol 1991: 9:268–273.

8.2 LIVER, PANCREAS, AND COAGULATION DISORDERS

JOACHIM BOOS and EUGEN J. VERSPOHL
University of Münster, Münster, Germany

8.2.1 Introduction

L-Asparaginase is an antineoplastic agent [1]. Kidd observed that guinea pig serum inhibited growth of transplanted lymphomas in mice [2], an effect that was later demonstrated to be due to the L-asparaginase activity of the serum [3]. Old et al. were the first to show its effectiveness in cancer treatment (animal trials) [4]. It is also effective in inducing remission of acute lymphoblastic leukemia (ALL) in up to 60% of human patients [5–7]. Approximately 90–95% of children with newly diagnosed ALL reach complete remission when treated with L-asparaginase in combination with other compounds [8]. This chapter extensively reviews liver, pancreas, and coagulation disorders with respect to L-asparaginase therapy.

8.2.2 Mechanism of Action

L-Asparaginase has a unique mechanism of action: it induces the specific depletion of L-asparagine, which results in the death of tumor cells (e.g., lymphoblastic leukemia cells) lacking an endogenous synthetic capacity for L-asparagine from aspartic acid [9]. L-Asparagine is not an essential amino acid in general, but it is essential for lymphoblasts. Asparaginase hydrolyzes L-asparagine into aspartic acid and ammonia and thus deprives tumor cells of a necessary substrate for their protein synthesis (Fig. 2).

8.2.3 Asparaginase Preparations

A couple of different biological sources of asparaginase have been used in clinical practice [10]. While the anaerobic bacterium *Vibrio succinogenes* was applied only in single early trials [11], products based on *Escherichia coli* [12] and *Erwinia chrysanthemi* [13] are marketed for widespread clinical use.

Early on, significant differences in pharmacokinetics were encountered with batches from different commercial sources even if only preparations derived from *E. coli* were employed, and half-lives of about 11 and 22 hours were seen with two different batches [14]. Still, even today different prep-

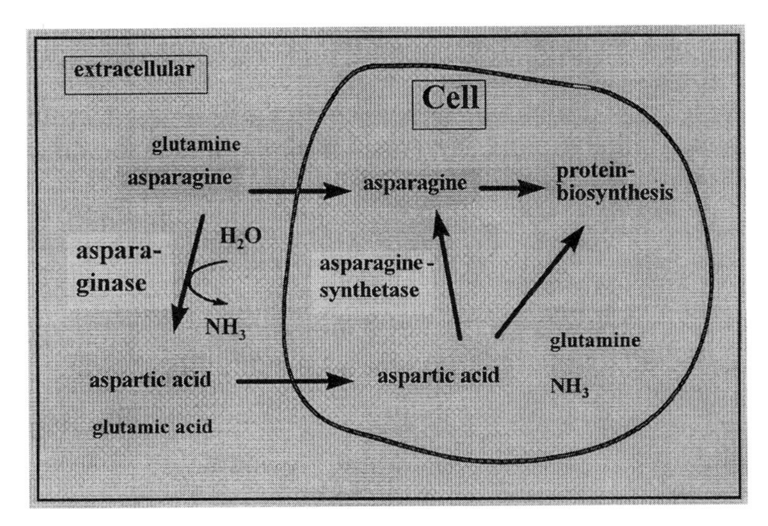

Fig. 2 Mechanism of action for L-asparaginase.

arations are being used in the same treatment schedule, and significant variations of treatment intensity show up in monitoring [15]. The main benefit of *Erwinia* asparaginase, which has a significantly shorter half-life [16], was the lack of cross-resistance with *E. coli* asparaginase after allergic reactions [17] and the long-lasting impression of a reduced risk of severe side effects with this drug [18]. A recent randomized clinical trial, however, clearly indicated that the reduced toxicity and lower pharmacokinetic treatment intensity of the *Erwinia* preparation translates into a significantly higher relapse rate in acute lymphoblastic leukemia [19] and lymphoma [20].

Another preparation has recently been developed and placed on the market. In this product, PEG-asparaginase, *E. coli* asparaginase is conjugated to polyethylene glycol, aiming at a prolonged half-life and reduced immunogenicity and toxicity [16,21].

8.2.4 Analytical Problems

Asparaginase differs from all other clinically used anticancer drugs in that it is an active enzyme. The enzymatic activity can be stopped if relatively high amounts of chemical inhibitors are added directly at the time of withdrawal [22]. In the clinical routine, however, such inhibitors are difficult to handle and normally not available. It must be realized that in the case of asparaginase many of the observed changes in laboratory parameters may be highly influenced by enzymatic activity after withdrawal and, therefore, may be partly artificial. Dependent on temperature and time, the desaminating activity results in a decrease of asparagine and glutamine and an increase of aspartic and glutamic acids and, most significantly, ammonia. The glutaminase activity is lower than the asparaginase activity, but this is of minor importance in most samples because in the absence of asparagine, glutamine becomes the favorite substrate. In addition, moderate direct interactions with most of the proteins mentioned have been demonstrated in blood in vitro [23].

Laboratory findings in children on asparaginase therapy, therefore, must be very cautiously interpreted, keeping in mind the possibility of preanalytical errors. This is especially true for high analytical ammonia levels when clinical correlates are lacking.

It is not unusual for fibrinogen to become undetectable during repeated applications of asparaginase. Although this surely represents a decrease in fibrinogen (see below), low concentrations of this hypofibrinogenemia may be detected. Fibrin(ogen) degradation products, which often are present as a consequence of hypercoagulability and fibrinolysis, interfere negatively because they inhibit fibrin polymerization if the fibrometer assay is used for the analysis of clotting time [24,25].

8.2.5 Toxicity (Side Effects) in General

The toxicity of asparaginase is well known [26–28]. Side effects are obvious in 30–90% of the patients [29]. The toxicity of asparaginase preparations is often difficult to evaluate, since they usually are combined with other chemotherapeutics such as vincristine, cyclophosphamide, methotrexate, and corticoids.

Asparaginase toxicity reports include fever, neurologic dysfunctions, tremor, drowsiness, lethargy, confusion, granulocytopenia, lymphopenia, thrombocytopenia, parotitis (a rare case), weight loss, nausea, vomiting, gastrointestinal toxicity with abdominal distension and pain, diarrhea, malabsorption, anorexia, elevated blood ammonia, renal disturbances, diabetes (nonketotic hyperglycemia) and hypersensitivity reactions, severe sepsis, and other specific abnormalities as discussed later [9,30–35]. Regression in spleen size was observed in one dog [36]. In contrast to other cytostatics, asparaginase only rarely causes myelosuppression, mucositis, and alopecia.

Hypersensitivity symptoms may vary from urticaria to hypotension, bronchospasm, and cardiac arrest [37,38]. Limiting hypersensitivity reactions were cumulatively present in more than 70% of patients using *E. coli* asparaginase [39] and could be considerably decreased or abolished when therapy was switched to PEG-L-asparaginase [39]. PEG-asparaginase does not show hypersensitivity reactions, as was emphasized by some authors [40–42]. Antiasparaginase antibodies may accelerate enzyme clearance [16] and consequently reduce therapeutic effectiveness [43].

Toxicity in several animals, including mice, rats, rabbits, dogs, and monkeys, has been reviewed [44]. Data of animals are difficult to extrapolate, since the plasma half-life is 2.5 hours in mice and in earlier literature approximately 18 hours in man [44,45]; the exact activity half-lives were 1.24 ± 0.17 days (*E. coli* asparaginase), 0.65 ± 0.13 day (*Erwinia chrysanthemi* asparaginase), and 5.73 ± 3.24 days (PEG-asparaginase) [16].

8.2.6 Liver

8.2.6.1 General Comments

Hepatotoxicity is a property of many antineoplastic agents, including doxorubicin, bleomycin, cyclophosphamide, 5-fluorouracil, hydroxyurea, paclitaxel, and mitoxantrone (for review, see Ref. 46). Their slow division rate compared with blood stem cells and mucosa makes hepatocytes less sensitive to toxic compounds than at least some other tissues. The liver dysfunction induced by *E. coli* asparaginase is well documented in both human and animal systems [27,47–53]. It can lead to extremely severe, sometimes fatal dysfunction of the liver. Steatosis is one result of such damage.

In general, compounds can reach the liver either by way of the hepatic artery (when intravenously applied) or the portal vein (when perorally applied). The liver is an important metabolizing organ for antineoplastic compounds. However, it is not absolutely clear whether asparaginase is hepatically metabolized or whether there is a biliary excretion. It is known that L-asparaginase is not cleaved by proteases in humans [54].

8.2.6.2 Frequency of Liver Damage

It was reported that liver dysfunction due to asparaginase occurred in 33 out of 35 patients, though increments in liver function tests [bilirubin, aspartate aminotransferase (AST: formerly SGOT), and alkaline phosphatase (AP)] were mild—probably because single doses were relatively low (200 IU/kg/day) [26]. In other trials an incidence of 75% was observed [49]. Others estimated a decrease in albumin to occur in 71 and 82% of children and adults, respectively [27]; retention of bromsulfalein (BSP) at 45 minutes (up to 40%) was observed in 57 and 84%, aspartate aminotransferase (AST) elevation in 46 and 63%, rise in total serum bilirubin in 29 and 51%, elevation of alkaline phosphatase in 31 and 47%, elevated 5′-nucleotidase in 15 and 26% of children and adults, respectively, in each case [27].

Frequency of L-asparaginase (from *E. coli*) hepatotoxicity is far above of that of other compounds with high incidence such as streptozotocin and mithramycin (used in earlier times). Hepatic toxicity does not appear to be increased by combinations with, for example, Ara-C [55].

Types of Hepatotoxicity

The phenotypes of hepatotoxicity of antineoplastic agents are as follows:

hepatocellular necrosis [increase in AST and alanine aminotransferase (ALT: formerly SGPT]
fatty degeneration (steatosis) including cirrhosis and/or fibrosis
intrahepatic cholestasis (increase in AP, γ-glutamyltransferase, and bilirubin)
liver fibrosis
veno-occlusive diseases

The first three phenotypes are most typical but not exclusive for asparaginase.

The hepatic dysfunction induced by asparaginase can be differentiated into two types.

1. Reversible: an acute, non-dose-dependent decrease of the synthesis of albumin and clotting factors which is apparent shortly after the start of therapy with a high frequency.
2. Irreversible: dose-dependent fatty degenerative changes of livers, appearing subacutely.

In a case report (the first with respect to liver toxicity) the liver was greatly enlarged [53]. Indicators of abnormal liver function are raised bilirubin, raised liver enzymes, and/or prolonged prothrombin time [18]. In addition, delayed bromsulfalein clearance; increased levels of AST and increased levels of alkaline phosphatases have been observed [49].

The same outcome is demonstrated using a murine model, namely, quantitation of extractable lipid from livers of asparaginase-treated BALB/c mice (a model for diffuse microfatty changes within hepatocytes as seen in human pathology) [56]: the hepatotoxicity of *E. coli* asparaginase in this model parallels the toxicity in humans; a rapid increase in liver lipid levels is observed [56]. Morphologically, asparaginase-induced liver damage results in diffuse fatty metamorphosis. Dependent on the study such changes vary from 42 to 87% [27,28,57,58]. Marked steatosis can even be observed without evidence for biochemical abnormalities [47].

A clear statement, however, is difficult, since other clinically important factors cannot be ruled out, and these in turn may induce hepatotoxic symptoms such as metastases, viral hepatitis, sepsis, and drug interactions. Induced effects due to drugs given simultaneously also may be present.

Such secondary effects due to liver dysfunction as a higher risk of thrombosis of therapy and a higher risk of hemorrhagia later on may develop and are discussed later. The liver dysfunction induced by asparaginase causes a decrease in the hepatic clearance of vincristine, which is often included in the therapy regimen; additionally, administration of vincristine 12–24 hours prior to asparaginase is recommended, to minimize direct drug–drug interaction.

The control of hepatic function is mandatory during asparaginase therapy. Interactions with other compounds with established hepatotoxicity must be kept in mind.

8.2.7 Liver Damage Dependent on the Source of Asparaginase?

While in the above-mentioned murine model *E. coli* asparaginase is clearly hepatotoxic, this outcome was not observed with *V. succinogenes* asparaginase [56], and the damage was much less pronounced when *Erwinia chrysanthemi* asparaginase was used [56]. A hypothetical mechanism that may account for these differences is discussed later.

When *Erwinia* asparaginase and *E. coli* asparaginase were compared, the latter appeared to result in more side effects, including hepatotoxicity in children (besides increased overt bleeding during sepsis, hypofibrinogenemia) [18]; the odds ratio is 0.47 (with 0.08 and 2.68 as 95% confidence intervals) for hepatomegaly and 0.42 (0.11 and 1.54) for abnormal liver function test [18] possibly indicating a slight disadvantage of *E. coli* asparaginase. In this study, only *E. coli* asparaginase decreased plasma antithrombin III, a sensitive indicator of hepatocellular function, and decreased albumin [18].

The *Erwinia* preparations in some clinical trials did not sufficiently deplete serum from asparagine [59,60]. Additionally, the half-life of *Erwinia* asparaginase is shorter than that of *E. coli* asparaginase [61]. Both these results may contribute to the lesser toxicity. In the above-mentioned investigation, however, the toxicity of *Erwinia* asparaginase was less pronounced and the antileukemic efficacy was nevertheless similar [18]. It cannot be excluded that variations in results (effects and side effects including hepatotoxicity) are due to the different asparaginase dose schedules used and are influenced by antibodies to asparaginase [62], thereby changing the biological effect and the kinetics in different investigations.

In the older literature, *Vibrio succinogenes* asparaginase appeared to be less hepatotoxic in an experiment with mice [56,63].

Toxicity features of other sources of L-asparaginase were summarized by Ho et al. [45].

8.2.8 Modified Asparaginases and Liver Function

Asparaginase was covalently coupled to PEG as outlined earlier. Within 14 days PEG-asparaginase showed increases in AST, with approximately 14–

24% (toxicity grades I and II) and increases in serum glutamic oxaloacetic transaminase with approx. 10% (toxicity grades III and IV) [21]. Other grade III and IV toxicities include transaminase elevation by 21% [64] and hypoalbuminemia by 7% [64]. Additionally, serum albumin was decreased and bilirubin levels increased, but there was no hepatic failure [21]. Thus the lack of a huge difference in toxicity was not unexpected, since both compounds should act the same way (see Section 8.2.9). There is a tendency for hepatotoxicity to be slightly increased when the PEG-coupled asparaginase is used instead of the native asparaginase (incidence of 71–59%) [21]; the number of patients, however, probably was too small to substantiate this view. The Pediatric Oncology Group and the reviewing of the regimen protocols by the Clinical Trials Evaluation Program nevertheless came to the statement in 1993 that the protocols must be reviewed with respect to toxicities (e.g., liver toxicities when combinations of PEG-asparaginase with IV methotrexate, 6-mercaptopurine, or cytosine arabinoside are used with the possible result of modifying the protocols). Additionally in preliminary reports other authors show an increase in toxicity by PEG-asparaginase compared with the native asparaginase [65].

Polymeric conjugates of L-asparaginase with homologous albumin were compared with free L-asparaginase for antitumor activity using a mouse model. Though its higher effectiveness is known to be due to less biodegradation, no data are available on the frequency of side effects [66].

Some experiments were done in dogs: malignant lymphomas in dogs are a good experimental–therapeutic model for non-Hodgkin lymphoma in man [67]. PEG-asparaginase (*E. coli* derived) had a tendency to improve survival time that was not, however, statistically relevant [68]. The use of PEG-asparaginase in dogs produced much less toxicity compared with uncoupled original asparaginase [68], whereas efficacy was as good (see above). The advantages and disadvantages of pegaspargase were recently reviewed [69].

8.2.9 Mechanism Leading to Liver Toxicity

The biosynthesis of asparagine in mammalian systems is primarily mediated through a glutamine-dependent transamidation reaction catalyzed by asparagine synthetase [70,71]. This is why glutamine deprivation can be expected to block the biosynthetic pathway by which normal cells escape the toxic effects of asparagine depletion. It was speculated that the toxic effect may be the result of the capability of commercial asparaginases to hydrolyze both asparagine and glutamine (glutaminase activity) [72,73]. It was clearly shown that the degree of glutaminase activity varies between different sources [74]: in one investigation it accounted for 2% in *E. coli* preparations and 10% in an *Erwinia chrysanthemi* preparation [73]. The K_m values of various asparaginases for glutamine are in the range of $1-6 \times 10^{-3}$ M (reviewed in Ref. 10). Thus the present inherent glutaminase activity is not the most important factor; rather, it is the ability of asparaginases primarily to convert glutamine in the absence of asparagine. In fact, patients show both a decrease of serum asparagine and glutamine [75]. Probably protein synthesis in the liver is impaired as a result of the decrease in asparagine and glutamine: the changes in plasma glutamine and asparagine resemble changes in protein concentration observed in plasma [76,77]. Additionally, a rise of glutamic acid occurs [15,78].

Primary cultures of rat hepatocytes were used to show that L-asparaginase was able to inhibit protein synthesis only when levels of glutamine were reduced to a critical level of below 10 nmol per milligram of cell protein [71]. Therefore, it appears reasonable to assume that glutaminase-free asparaginase from, say, *Vibrio succinogenes*, is not hepatotoxic. In fact it was shown that hepatocellular dysfunction does not occur when a glutaminase-free asparaginase from *V. succinogenes* was used in animal studies [56], even when used for a longer period; it does not induce fatty infiltration of the liver, as was observed with *E. coli* asparaginase [56,79]. There are, however, no confirmatory data for patients (and in a clinical monitoring program steady-state concentrations of glutamine were shown to stay within normal ranges, thus not supporting the hypothesis of glutamine depletion as primary trigger of hepatotoxicity in man [15]).

In another publication, a threshold was defined for glutamine depletion that led to diminished protein synthesis in rat hepatocytes [73]. Even when a glutaminase-free enzyme preparation was used, there was still an effect (reduction) on plasma cholesterol, but this was the only effect [56].

The decrease in protein synthesis is again reflected in results obtained with BALB/c mice 2 and 3 weeks after starting *E. coli* asparaginase treatment: body weight was reduced by 19 and 15%, respectively [56]; however, liver weight was reduced much more by 31 and 15%, respectively [56]. Again, this effect was much less pronounced when *Erwinia chrysanthemi* asparaginase was used, corroborating the toxicity data [56].

Other possible mechanisms that may be involved in causing liver toxicity include the following:

1. L-Asparaginase is a sensitizing agent with high molecular weight (anaphylactic reactions are described); however, there is no clear proof yet that such a mechanism is involved in liver toxicity.
2. A role of contamination with bacterial endotoxins was suggested [26]. This possible mechanism was ruled out by some authors [80]. It has been postulated that the toxic hepatitis (as well as pancre-

atitis, hypoalbuminemia, and coagulation abnormalities) are secondary to contamination not only with glutaminase but also with endotoxin.
3. Asparaginase inhibits early mitosis in regenerating rat liver [81].
4. The most attractive theory implicates the inhibition of protein synthesis inhibition, as is evidenced by diffuse protein depression including clotting factors. Even hypocholesterolemia can be related to this mechanism, since a decreased synthesis of proteins transporting cholesterol was observed [48].

It is hard to say to what extent the one mechanism or another is additionally involved in hepatic toxicity.

Interestingly *V. succinogenes* asparaginase shows less hepatotoxicity as was outlined earlier [56] and additionally does not show immunosuppression [56]. It is far from clear whether impurities in the preparations (e.g., bacterial endotoxins) are responsible for hepatotoxic effects.

8.2.9.1 Hyperlipidemia (Liver)

Asparaginase can cause abnormal lipid metabolism [27]. Hyperlipidemia is rare after asparaginase and—even severe hyperlipidemia is random, transient, and benign [82]. The underlying mechanism is not clear.

Serum cholesterol was decreased in some studies by 80% [14]. Other patients were asymptomatic: cholesterol peaked to up to 1750 mg/dL [83].

Possible causes of hyperlipidemia could include the impaired metabolism of dietary fat, modulation of protein components of lipoproteins and increased production of lipoproteins by the liver. Maybe a decrease in synthesis by hepatocytes of apoprotein-E receptors is involved; these receptors, which are known to be inhibited by either asparaginase or glucocorticoids, are needed for the elimination of chylomicrons from serum. Hyperlipidemia was not interpreted as a reason to modify the therapy doses [82].

Whereas lipids from livers of *E. coli*–treated mice rose quickly, they did not differ from controls when *V. succinogenes* asparaginase was used [56].

8.2.10 Dose Dependency of Liver Damage

The type of hepatic damage depends on the application form and the dose. Reducing the *E. coli* asparaginase dose to thrice 6000 IU/m^2, served to lower the hepatic complications [56]. Reducing dosages of *E. coli* asparaginase results in limited hepatotoxic complications without compromising therapeutic efficacy [83–86]. Nevertheless, very sensitive indicators of hepatic damage stay elevated even after the dose has been reduced.

In cultured rat hepatocytes a clear dose dependency of hepatotoxic effects (decreased protein synthesis) was demonstrated for *E. coli* asparaginase [73] but in vivo, there is only one study indicating a dependency between hepatic parameter changes and dose [28], and it is questioned by others.

8.2.11 Time-Dependence of Liver Damage

In one study the reduction in liver weight in BALB/c mice after *E. coli* asparaginase treatment was not observed until the second week [56]. After the fourth week the weight had returned to normal [56]. Even during the first and second weeks of asparaginase treatment there was a major increase in lipid concentration in the liver of the mice [56]. Hepatic dysfunction became biochemically evident as early as 2 weeks after start of treatment [56]. After at least 4 weeks liver function normalized in most cases [56]. In cultured rat hepatocytes a clear time dependency of hepatoxic effects (decreased protein synthesis) was demonstrated for *E. coli* asparaginase [73].

Maximum disturbances were increase of bilirubin after 12 days [53], alkaline phosphatase after 38 days, AST after 29 days, and cholesterol after 39 days [53]; since data were not gathered at all time points, the exact peaks are not clear.

Hepatic lipoidosis may persist for up to 261 days after the last dose of L-asparaginase [28]. Other indicators (e.g., liver function test disturbances) normally regress rapidly, mostly within 2 weeks after completion of the therapy [28].

8.2.12 Age Dependency of Liver Toxicity

From the data obtained by Oettgen et al. it is clear that adults are more susceptible to liver damage than children are [27]; this was outlined earlier (see Section 8.2.6.2). Others as well pointed out that damage was more often seen in adults [26]. The development of liver function after cessation of therapy has been described [87]: the authors suggest carefully monitoring various parameters such as serum ALT and bile secretion (various cholic acid ratios).

8.2.13 Secondary Effects Due to Liver Damage

E. coli asparaginase induced a decrease in plasma levels of albumin, antithrombin, cholesterol, phospholipids, and triglycerides [56]; however, in most cases an increase in triglycerides is observed [88]. Coagulation and fibrinolytic disturbances are directly related to hepatic toxicity (outlined below in Section 8.2.16). The time-dependent decrease in plasma triglycerides and cholesterol rather parallels the increase in total extractable liver lipid due to *E. coli* asparaginase [56]. Again, there were no secondary effects in response to *Erwinia chrysanthemi* enzyme with respect to plasma cholesterol and triglycerides [56], which parallels its less hepatotoxic effects.

8.2.14 Pancreas

8.2.14.1 General Comments

L-Asparaginase can lead to extremely severe and in some cases fatal dysfunction of the pancreas [89–96], although this complication is uncommon. Acute pancreatonecrosis was recorded [97], and a hemorrhagic pancreatitis and fat necrosis over the pancreas were described [98]. Asparaginase-induced hemorrhagic pancreatitis is rare: serious damage occurs in less than 0.5% of patients treated with this drug. Altogether pancreatitis sums to 2–16% [99]. Ninety-three publications on pancreatitis have been reviewed [100].

In addition to asparaginase, the following drugs seem to cause pancreatitis: azathioprine, thiazides, sulfonamides, furosemide, estrogens, valproic acid, and tetracycline (reviewed in Ref. 100). Originally in the 1980s, the evidence for asparaginase inducing pancreatitis was less convincing [101]. Also the combination of the agents prednisone and L-asparaginase has been demonstrated to produce pancreatic injury.

An early diagnosis of pancreatitis in many cases is not possible because symptoms are vague, physical findings may be minimal, and laboratory studies are frequently inconclusive until the injury is severe. Abdominal sonography as a monitor of pancreatic size and structure has proven to be helpful in the diagnosis of subclinical and early pancreatic injury [102]. Sonograms were useful only in confirming clinical and/or laboratory evidence of pancreatitis, but were of no value in making the early or preclinical diagnosis of drug-induced pancreatitis in the context of asparaginase treatment [103].

In addition to humans, acute pancreatitis was observed in animals (dogs) [104]. When *E. coli* asparaginase and *Erwinia* asparaginase were compared, acute pancreatitis was more often observed with *E. coli* asparaginase (odds ratio of 0.05 with 95% confidence intervals of 0.01 and 0.31) [18]. Thus *Erwinia* asparaginase has a lower frequency of producing pancreatitis (as well as other side effects such as neurological effects and sepsis).

When PEG-asparaginase was used in one trial no pancreatitis (increase in amylase) was seen; the trial covered a very small number of patients, however, [21,105]. In another trial clinical and biochemical pancreatitis was seen in 7% with PEG-asparaginase [64,104,105]. Others state that toxic pancreatitis was moderate and disappeared after 10–20 days of discontinuation of the drug [106]. Pancreatitis seemed to be reduced when PEG-asparaginase instead of *E. coli* asparaginase was used (from 8.8% to 5.7%) [65]. Pancreatitis is increased from virtually 0 to 10 or 15% by switching from PEG-asparaginase to a combination of PEG-asparaginase with methotrexate, 6-mercaptopurine, or cytosine arabinoside—therapeutic regimes that were tried but later discarded. We actually observed two cases of severe pancreatitis in the context of the Berlin-Frank-first-Münster study (BFM) reinduction therapy, indicating that the use of the pegylated compound definitively does not overcome this clinical problem.

8.2.14.2 Mechanism of Disturbance

Little is known in general about the pathogenesis of drug-induced pancreatitis [101]. It was suggested that like other side effects (toxic hepatitis, hypoalbuminemia, coagulation abnormalities), the pancreatitis may also be a secondary effect to contamination with glutaminase or endotoxin. This possibility was intensively discussed in Section 8.2.9. In general, the mechanisms suggested for drug-induced pancreatitis include pancreatic duct constriction, immunosuppression, cytotoxic, osmotic, pressure, or metabolic effects, arteriolar thrombosis, direct cellular toxicity, and hepatic involvement.

Clinical and laboratory improvements were evident after treatment with somatostatin, with no complications of pancreatitis [107].

8.2.14.3 Pseudocyst Formation

The progression of pancreatitis to pseudocyst formation in some patients has been reported repeatedly [108] but is less well addressed. The subsequent development of a pseudocyst, with progressive increase in size and development of obstructive symptoms, requires surgical decompression [109]. Transgastric cytogastrostomy was successfully carried out [109]. The pseudocyst is managed in some cases with intravenous hyperalimentation and antibiotics [110], but nonsurgical management over protracted periods of time was less effective in another investigation [111]. Surgical drainage (internal or external) was in some cases successful in eradicating the pseudocyst; in these cases there was no further evidence for a subsequent pancreatic disease to occur [111]. The pseudocyst, on the other hand, may resolve spontaneously in one month without complication [110] and surgical intervention, therefore, will be the exception. One adolescent male developed acute pancreatitis and pseudocyst of the pancreas 16 weeks after cessation (a huge delay) of intramuscular L-asparaginase [112].

8.2.14.4 Endocrine Function

Sometimes after a pancreatitis hyperglycemia additionally occurs [113]; an epigastrial tumor is palpable and gradually grows in size. A CT scan and abdominal ultrasonography may reveal a pancreatic pseudocyst [113]. Hyperglycemia is observed, sometimes with accompanying ketoacidosis. Insulin treatment was necessary and effective in at least two reports [114,115]. Pancreatitis may add to this situation [116]. Hyperglycemia may also occur as a complication in patients when L-asparaginase is combined with (diabetogenic) steroids [117]; the reported incidence is about 10% [117].

Independently a direct impairment of endocrine pancreas function may develop [30,33,118–120]: asparaginase therapy induced a significant reduction in basal and peak blood glucose by an unknown mechanism, with resulting decreased insulin and C-peptide levels, while glucagon was not modified. The conserved C-peptide–insulin molar ratio suggests the interference of L-asparaginase with proinsulin synthesis and not granular processing. This indicates a decreased insulin reserve with a preserved, although reduced, β-cell function [119].

In rat or human islets of Langerhans in vitro, both the accumulation of insulin in the medium and the content of insulin and glucagon in the islets were significantly reduced in the presence of 100 mU/mL L-asparaginase [121]. In contrast to data of other researchers [119], 0.1 U/mL asparaginase caused roughly a 50% reduction in insulin biosynthesis [121]. Following L-asparaginase, there was a fall in both plasma insulin and gastrin [122].

Pancreatic Carcinoma Treatment

An attempt was made to cure a pancreatic carcinoma with asparaginase; this approach is of no therapeutic value. Patients with advanced nonresectable pancreatic carcinoma had been chosen because the tumor had demonstrated in vitro sensitivity to the drug [123]. However, with respect to islet cell carcinoma of the pancreas, L-asparaginase (140,000 units) infused into the hepatic artery resulted in a remission from disabling hypoglycemia for 9 months in a man [122].

The therapies attempted stem from in vitro investigations: the effects of *E. coli* L-asparaginase on cultured human pancreatic carcinoma (MIA PaCa-2) have been studied [124,125]. The enzyme (1 U/mL) inhibited growth and protein synthesis in both MIA PaCa-2 and PANC-1, another pancreatic carcinoma cell line. The effect of L-asparaginase on cultured pancreatic carcinoma cells was believed to be exerted at least partly through its L-glutaminase activity. However, asparaginase derived from *Vibrio succinogenes*, which is virtually free of L-glutaminase activity, is equally inhibitory to MIA PaCa-2 cell growth but does not affect protein synthesis [124]. It is, therefore, possible that the inhibition of growth of cultured pancreatic carcinoma cells by *E. coli* asparaginase is a combined function of both its L-asparaginase and L-glutaminase activity [124].

8.2.15 Blood

The side effects of L-asparaginase on the blood system include slight to moderate depression of all strains of cellular elements and significant changes in the composition of soluble components including glucose, calcium and electrolytes, hepatic enzyme levels, bilirubin in some cases, cholesterol and triglyceride levels, ammonia, urea, nitrogen in many patients, and amino acid pattern and decrease of many protein components in almost all patients [27].

Leukopenia, anemia, and thrombocytopenia have repeatedly been reported in the context of asparaginase therapy and have been included in the side effects lists of handbooks and databases [126]. While some studies reported a lack of L-asparaginase-related myelosuppression without going into details [57,127], other publications, including reports of patients treated with asparaginase alone, showed very moderate bone marrow suppression. In children on single-drug asparaginase in remission, Mathe et al. [128] observed a minimal decrease in thrombocyte counts and a reduction of white blood cells down to about 50% and in neutrophils to about 30% of start levels. Children with active leukemia treated in this trial did not show any additional decrease of their neutrophil counts. Since only a few studies focused on toxicity with single-drug therapy and clear-cut phase I trials, the dose-limiting toxicity and schedule remain undefined; most observations are deduced from combined treatment modalities, most commonly with prednisolone, vincristine, or anthracyclines. Land et al. reported severe leukopenia in 2 of 105 children treated for ALL both with additional vincristine and corticoids; no severe bone marrow toxicity was observed in a subgroup receiving asparaginase monotherapy [58]. A comparison of the induction therapy of the phase I and II trials showed that the addition of *E. coli* asparaginase to vincristine and prednisone was paralleled by a slightly more intense leukopenia and significantly better blast cell regression after 3 weeks of treatment [129].

During the last decade, the development of PEG-asparaginase again raised additional studies focusing on the pattern of side effects [130]. Relevant myelotoxicity, however, was not observed in these trials, even after prolonged duration of treatment and asparagine depletion up to 12 months [131].

In summary, although leukopenia and thrombocytopenia have been reported repeatedly, severe cytopenia seems to be a rare event, and compared with the effects of other cytostatic drugs the bone marrow suppression induced by L-asparaginase is of minor importance.

8.2.16 The Coagulation System

Inhibition of protein synthesis can be observed in roughly 100% of patients on asparaginase therapy and includes decreased levels of albumin, α-globulin, β-globulin, insulin, thyroxin-binding protein, lipoproteins, and, most important, many proteins involved in the homeostasis of blood coagulation.

8.2.16.1 Bleeding and Thrombosis

Hemorrhage, disseminated intravascular coagulation (DIC), and thromboembolic events all have been reported repeatedly. The physiological basis of these clinical events includes effects of the prevalent leukemia, thrombocytopenia induced by different additionally administered anticancer drugs, and a significant decrease in plasma proteins, and especially in essential proteins for coagulation and fibrinolysis primarily induced by asparaginase (for review see Ref. 132). The decrease in plasma proteins offers a stringent rationale for those clinical observations, which were strictly related to asparaginase treatment.

In the first comprehensive report on asparaginase toxicity, approximately 6% of patients on asparaginase treatment reportedly experienced bleeding symptoms [27]. The majority of these patients, however, were in terminal-stage leukemia with severe thrombocytopenia or were bleeding from their tumors.

In a group of 238 children and adults treated with asparaginase, the incidence of minor bleeding was 2.1% and a single case of hemaphtoe as lethal complication occurred [133]. In addition, the incidence of thromboembolic complications was 4.2% in this group. In a questionnaire to all centers involved in the German ALL/NHL-BFM trials, 13 of 471 children were identified who suffered from severe hemorrhages or thrombosis, again more than 50% in the central nervous system [134]. While earlier publications reported 1–2% thrombosis [85], in studies focusing especially on L-asparaginase toxicity, 10–15% of the children developed vascular accidents [135,136].

In summary, bleeding seems to be a rare event and thrombosis a more common and much more dramatic complication.

8.2.16.2 Pathophysiological Changes

Subclinical disturbances in the highly sensitive and regulated system of activating and inhibiting protein cascades (see Fig. 3) seem to be a constant

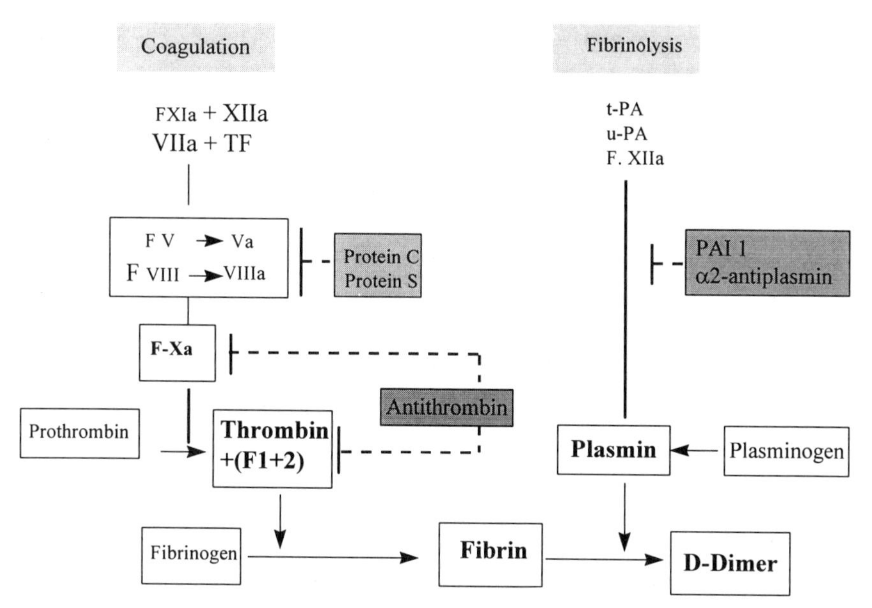

Fig. 3 PA and u-PA, tissue and unbound plasminogen activator, respectively. Proteins in activation and inhibition of coagulation and fibrinolysis schematically (Scheme according to Nowak-Göttl et al. [136]).

circumstance in asparaginase treatment. In general they can split into three different categories [57,134–140] (for reviews Refs. 132, 141):

a significant decrease of factors of the activating downstream cascade of coagulation proteins including II, V, VIII, IX–XIII, fibrinogen, and others indicating a risk of bleeding

a significant reduction of proteins inhibiting coagulation activation [e.g., protein C, protein S, and antithrombin (AT)] or counterregulating the clotting process (e.g., plasminogen)

an increase in the activity of other factors indicating a state of hypercoagulobility [e.g., von Willebrand factor (vWf), prothrombin fragments 1 + 2, and plasminogen activator inhibitor 1 (PAI-1)]

The pathophysiological impact of these changes and their interrelations are not completely understood, but the published data fit together to establish a model that could explain most of the analytical and clinical observations (Fig. 4). The overall decrease in protein synthesis due to reduced availability of asparagine and in some circumstances glutamine probably is one of the major occurrences. The mentioned proteins all contain about 5% asparagine

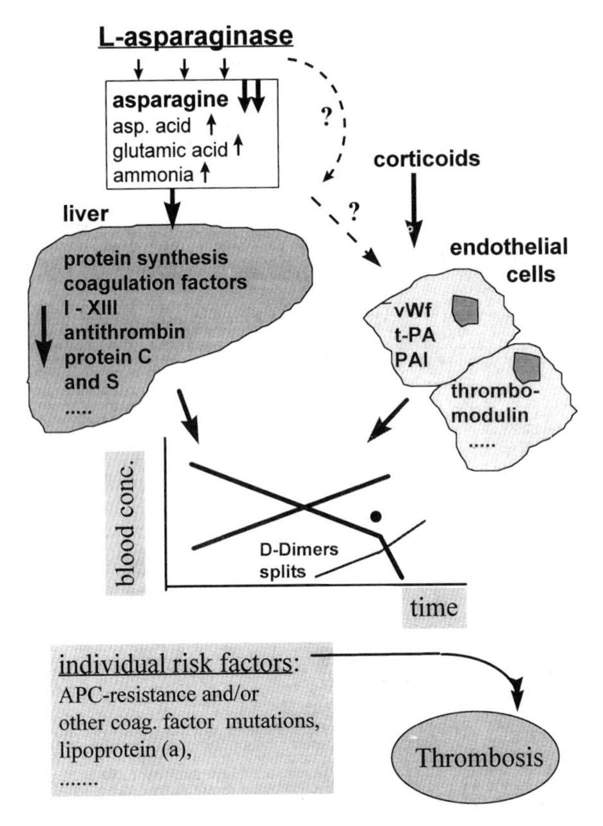

Fig. 4 Model of the development of thrombosis on L-asparaginase treatment: APC (activated protein C).

(summarized in Ref. 141) and their synthesis, therefore, is related to the availability of this amino acid or to its synthesis. Although besides other tissues, pancreas and the liver express the highest amounts of asparagine synthetase in man [142,143], the capacity or the distribution within these organs does not allow sufficient protein synthesis and function. As a function of time, the concentration then drops and the hypoproteinemia, therefore, reaches the maximum roughly a week after onset of asparaginase treatment [133,134].

The timing of the vascular events fits this dynamic of protein reduction in most of the reported cases and studies (reviewed in Refs. 132, 141) and the onset of pancreatic toxicity as well.

In contrast to the general protein decrease, an increase in von Willebrand factor, thrombomodulin, and fibrin degradation products can be observed in many children [136]. The most plausible explanation for this phenomenon is a release from endothelial cells and thrombocytes. Activation of endothelial factors like vWf and tissue plasminogen activator (t-PA) have been shown in vitro with asparaginase and to a much higher extent with corticoids [144]. It is still a matter of speculation whether the enzyme asparaginase directly interferes with membranes, receptors, or (coagulation) proteins or whether the continuing release of unphysiological amounts of aspartic and glutamic acid contributes to endothelial toxicity.

The combination of an endothelial factor release with a general state of hypercoagulability on the reduced fibrinolytic potential then may result in thrombosis rather than bleeding. The formation of fibrin and the subsequent fibrinolysis, as well as the ongoing depletion of counterregulating factors, increase the velocity of the general consumption of the coagulation system in asparaginase treatment. The analytical determination of fibrin degradation products indicates in this situation that fibrinolysis happens to a higher extent. The parallel decrease of inhibitory factors like AT then is an additional indicator of an increased risk of a clinical prothrombotic state event.

Since despite changes in the pattern of pro- and anticoagulatory proteolytic proteins, this complex system nevertheless remains stable without clinical relevant symptoms, the major questions involve the individual degree of disturbances in the protein pattern and whether the regulatory systems of fibrin formation and fibrinolysis become unbalanced, resulting in bleeding or thrombosis. Why is the labile system influenced by asparaginase effects, and why is the influence of the corticoids normally applied in parallel compensated in most patients, with only a subgroup experiencing severe imbalances?

8.2.16.3 Additional Risk Factors

In such a highly regulated system, which is stressed by treatment with corticoids and asparaginase and borderline compensated, additional individual risk factors become important. At the time of the observed thromboembolic events, patients normally are in remission, which normally rules out persisting leukemia as a cause. A familial history of thrombotic events and the existence of molecular mutations predisposing to thromboembolic accidents, however, contribute significantly to the risk of decompensation of the coagulation system during asparaginase treatment.

All the following conditions were highly overrepresented in children with thromboembolic events:

the mutation of factor V R506Q [145], resulting in resistance to the inhibitory effect of protein C
elevated lipoprotein (a) [146], which is closely homologous to plasminogen [147] and complementary, inhibiting its functional binding
genetic variation in the prothrombin gene, resulting in inadequate function [148]
mutations in antithrombin, protein C, or protein S

Therefore, these conditions are now known to increase the risk of such events significantly [149,150]. About 80% of the children with one or more of these predisposing factors present suffered from thrombosis. In addition to the familial predisposition, the use of central lines clearly correlated with the risk of thrombosis in this prospective analysis.

In summary, reduction of protein synthesis induced by asparaginase and endothelial toxicity by corticoids and to a still not well-defined extent by asparaginase itself add up to an inborn risk of thrombophilia and then induce thromboembolic events. Central lines contribute to this overall risk, and the same should be expected for any other circumstances (e.g., dehydration, septicemia, immobilization) that increases the general tendency of vascular events.

8.2.16.4 Influence of Treatment Schedule and Dose Intensity

Inasmuch as it is not the enzyme itself but the disappearance of substrates and possibly of metabolic products that provide the basis of toxicity, it may be easily understood that even the highest individual single dosages do not result in enhanced toxicity. Phase I trials escalating single doses of L-asparaginase are lacking, but single infusions of 90,000 U/m^2 [151] did not result in unusual toxicity in a multicenter trial. The correlation of the asparaginase dose schedule with the observed toxicity is difficult because the complete pattern of side effects may occur without any asparaginase during antileukemic induction therapy with vincristine and prednisolone. The early systematic summary of side effects accounted for the impression that dosages higher than 5000 U/m^2 applied daily increased the unintentional effects [27]. With increasing experience with the currently used schedules of 6000 U/m^2 three times a week of 10,000 U/m^2 every third day, differences of toxic potential between the various marketed preparations (see above) became evident; in particular, a reduced toxicity of *Erwinia* asparaginase in comparison to *E. coli* preparations has been reported [18,152]. The same drug, however, shows a much more rapid elimination [16], a significantly lower treatment intensity, defined as degree and time of asparagine depletion [15], and in treatment protocols with repetitive applications, a continuous loss of activity with increasing numbers of applications [60,153]. In parallel, others reported an insufficient depletion of asparagine in the cerebrospinal fluid with this drug if applied at the same dose schedule as *E. coli* preparations [154].

From today's point of view, this phenomenon of silent inactivation in many patients in combination with the short half-life correlates to an impression of reduced toxicity of *Erwinia* asparaginase and, unfortunately, to a significant higher relapse rate for children with leukemia and lymphoma [19,20]. In the clinical trials, however, *Erwinia* and *E. coli* asparaginase have been used on identical dose schedules, and in this respect the actual dose intensity differs significantly. Nevertheless, an investigation on 11 patients treated with 15,000 U/m^2 erwinase daily again indicated reduced toxicity in the coagulation system in this small group [155]. On the other hand, pharmacokinetic data were not reported with this dose schedule.

Even different preparations based on *E. coli* today show significantly different pharmacokinetics, trough levels, and pharmacodynamics [15], including differences in the degree and pattern of coagulation disturbances [156] and the changes in fibrinolytic proteins correlated with the asparaginase plasma activities [157]. Because of its longer half-life, a more bioactive preparation based on an *E. coli* source produced by Kyowa Hakko, in Japan, induced in parallel significantly more changes in the analytical coagulation pattern. In a subsequent dose reduction trial with this drug, the decrease of these effects on coagulation and fibrinolysis could be reduced but not avoided [158,159], and even with individual drug monitoring and targeting to trough levels of roughly 100 U/L, thrombosis has been observed. Under these stricter conditions, however, thrombotic events were restricted to children with a predisposition to familial thrombophilia (see Fig. 4).

In summary, toxic side effects, especially on coagulation and fibrinolysis, depend on the time of effective asparaginase treatment and successful asparagine depletion. Schedules not successfully depleting the organism from this amino acid over time are less toxic but, unfortunately, less effective, too. A significant increase of asparaginase activities, to levels much higher than necessary for asparagine depletion, is expected to increase side effects again.

Whether *Erwinia* asparaginase has a broader therapeutic gain and induces fewer problems is still an open question, and the answer requires clinical trials applying the different preparations on dosages adapted to their own pharmacokinetic characteristics.

The major factor for the development of vascular events, however, is the individual predisposition of the patients and eventually additional risk factors like central lines or others.

8.2.16.5 Supportive Treatment of Coagulation Disturbances

Given the complex changes in the counterbalanced systems of coagulation and fibrinolysis, with a tendency toward hypercoagulability, the substitution of single coagulation factors like fibrinogen has no rationale and may increase the risk of thrombosis. The substitution of fresh frozen plasma as a preparation including more or less all factors involved might theoretically be beneficial, but the prophylactic application in the case of significant fibrinogen reduction, did not significantly improve the coagulatory situation [160,161]. Possibly this was due to the limitations in the applicable volume in these trials to 10–20 mL/kg. Extensive substitution of fresh frozen plasma (FFP) three times daily in combination with antithrombin was shown to increase most of the parameters analyzed on those days [162]. Substitution of FFP, therefore, requires consequent application of significant volumes and should be restricted to patients in special individual situations.

The supplementation of antithrombin has been intensively investigated, and substitution schedules have been reported [163,164] because this protein most likely can be expected to act as a break in the asparaginase-induced situation (Figs. 3 and 4). In fact, AT supplementation is able to achieve high levels of this protein during the time of asparaginase treatment and to reduce or prevent the markers of activation of the hemostatic system in adults [165] and children [166]. A dynamic increase in D-dimer formation paralleled with a decrease of AT concentration, therefore, is an easily measurable indicator of enhanced thrombin formation and fibrinolysis indicating hypercoagulation and the threat of thrombotic events. Again, however, studies are required to test the hypothesis that prophylactic AT administration really reduces the risk and incidence of thrombosis in asparaginase-treated patients.

The same is true for the question whether the administration of normal or low molecular weight heparins will reduce asparaginase side effects on the coagulation system.

In situations with noncoagulatory side effects, very few patients have been supplemented with intravenous application of asparagine, and positive effects are reported [38]. From the practical point of view, the toxic changes normally disappear rapidly after the end of asparagine treatment. The supplementation of asparagine theoretically is a two-side coin. On one side, the basis of protein synthesis reduction, the asparagine depletion can be overcome and the liver might immediately synthesize lacking proteins. On the other side, the asparaginase is still circulating and is expected to deplete the supplemented amounts of asparagine rapidly, resulting in a significant increase in aspartic acid and ammonia, both with an unknown contribution to the imbalanced systems.

The idea of routine asparagine supplementation, therefore, cannot be recommended as a causal treatment. Thus far it has not been investigated systematically, but it can be kept in mind for an experimental indication when supportive treatment modalities cannot stabilize the situation.

REFERENCES TO SECTION 8.2

1. Broome JD. L-Asparaginase: Discovery and development as a tumor-inhibitory agent. Cancer Treatment Rep 1981:65:111–114.
2. Kidd JG. Regression of transplanted lymphomas induced in vivo by means of normal guinea pig serum. J Exp Med 1953:98:565–582.
3. Broome JD. Evidence that the L-asparaginase activity of guinea pig serum is responsible for its antilymphoma effects. Nature (London) 1961:191:1114–1115.
4. Old LJ, Boyse EA, Campbell HA, Brodey RS, Ridler J, Teller JD. Treatment of lymphosarcoma in the dog with L-asparaginase. Cancer 1967:20:1066–1070.
5. Hill JM, Roberts J, Loeb E, Khan A, MacLellan A, Hill RW. L-asparaginase therapy for leukemia and other malignant neoplasms. JAMA 1967:202:882–888.
6. Tallai L, Tan CC, Oettgen HF, Wollner N, McCarthy M, Helson L, Burchenal J, Karnofsky DA, Murphy ML. L-Asparaginase in 111 children with leukemia and solid tumors. Proc Am Assoc Cancer Res 1969:10:92 (Abstr).
7. Jaffe N, Traggis D, Das L, Frauenberger G, Hann HW, Kim BS, Bishop Y. Favorable remission induction rate with twice weekly doses of L-asparaginase. Cancer Res 1973:33:1–4.
8. Ortega JA, Nesbit ME Jr, Donaldson MH, Hittle RE, Weiner J, Karon M, Hammond D. L-Asparaginase, vincristine, and prednisone for induction of first remission in acute lymphocytic leukemia. Cancer Res 1977:37:535–540.
9. Capizzi RL, Bertino JR, Skeel RT, Creasey WA, Zanes R, Peterson RG, Handschumacher RE. L-Asparaginase: Clinical, biochemical, pharmacological and immunological studies. Ann Intern Med 1971:74:893–901.
10. Wriston JC, Yellin TO: L-Asparaginase: A review. Adv Enzymol Relat Areas Mol Biol 1973:39:195–248.
11. Kafkewitz D, Goodman D. L-Asparaginase production by the rumen anaerobe *Vibrio succinogenes*. Appl Microbiol 1974:27:206–209.
12. Mashburn LT, Wriston JC Jr. Tumor inhibition effect of L-Asparaginase from *Escherichia coli*. Arch Biochem Biophys 1964:105:450–452.
13. Wade HE, Elswoth R, Herbert D, Keppie J, Sargeant K. A new L-asparaginase with antitumour activity? Lancet 1968:2:776–777.
14. Schwartz MK, Lash ED, Oettgen HF, Tomao FA. L-Asparaginase activity in plasma and other biological fluids. Cancer 1970:25:244–252.
15. Boos J, Werber G, Ahlke E, Schulze-Westhoff P, Nowak-Göttl U, Würthwein G, Verspohl EJ, Ritter J, Jürgens H. Monitoring of asparaginase activity and

asparagine levels in children on different asparaginase preparations. Eur J Cancer 1996:32A:1544–1550.
16. Asselin BL, Within JC, Coppola DJ, Rupp IP, Sallan SE, Cohen HJ. Comparative pharmacokinetic studies of three asparaginase preparations. J Clin Oncol 1993:11:1780–1786.
17. Ohnuma T, Holland JF, Meyer P. *Erwinia caratovora* asparaginase in patients with prior anaphylaxis to asparaginase from *E. coli*. Cancer 1972:30:376–381.
18. Eden OB, Shaw MP, Lilleyman JS, Richards S. Nonrandomized study comparing toxicity of *Escherichia coli* and *Erwinia* asparaginase in children with leukemia. Med Pediatr Oncol 1990:18:497–502.
19. Otten J, Suciu S, Lutz P, Benoit Y, Robert A, Thyss A, Plouvier E, Ferster A, Méchinaud F, Mazingue F, Brock P, Villmer E, Solbu G, Waterkeyn C, Philippe N. The importance of L-asparaginase (A'ase) in the treatment of acute lymphoblastic leukemia (ALL) in children: Results of the EORTC 58881 randomized phase III trial showing greater efficiency of *Escherichia coli (E. coli)* as compared to *Erwinia (Erw)* A'ase. Blood 1996:88 (suppl 1/1):669.
20. Paquement H, Philippe N, Méchinaud F, Robert A, Vilmer E, Francotte N, Millot F, Waterkeyn C, Solbu G, Suciu S, Otten J. EORTC Children's Leukemia Study Group: Importance of L-asparaginase (ASP), detrimental effects of additional cytosine-arabinosine (Ara-C), and of IV 6-mercaptopurine (6-MP) in the treatment of lymphoblastic non-Hodgkin lymphoma (LB-NHL): Results of the EORTC 58881 randomized trial. Med Pediatr Oncol 1997:29: 429-P-160.
21. Ettinger LJ, Kurtzberg J, Voute PA, Jürgens H, Halpern SL. An open-label, multicenter study of polyethylene glycol–L-asparaginase for the treatment of acute lymphoblastic leukemia. Cancer 1995:75:1176–1181.
22. Asselin BL, Lorenson MY, Whitin JC, Coppola DJ, Kende AS, Blakeley RL, Chohen HJ. Measurement of serum L-asparagine in the presence of L-asparaginase requires the presence of an L-asparaginase inhibitor. Cancer Res 1991: 51:6568–6573.
23. Nowak-Göttl U, Boos J, Wolff JEA, Lill H, Veltmann H, Werber G, Ahlke E, Jürgens H. Asparaginase decreases clotting factors in vitro: A possible pitfall? Int J Clin Lab Res 1995:25:146–148.
24. Hoffmann M, Greenberg CS. The effect of fibrin polymerization inhibitors on quantitative measurements of plasma fibrinogen. Am J Clin Pathol 1987: 8:490–493.
25. Alving B, Bell WR. Methods for correcting inhibitory effects of fibrinogen degradation products in fibrinogen determinations. Thromb Res 1976:9:1–8.
26. Haskell CM, Canellos GP, Leventhal BG, Carbone PP, Block JB, Serpick AA, Selawry OS. L-Asparaginase—Effects in patients with neoplastic disease. N Engl J Med 1969:281:1028–1034.
27. Oettgen HF, Stephenson PA, Schwartz MK, Leeper RD, Tallal L, Tan CC, Clarkson BD, Goldberg RD, Kiakoff IA, Karnofsky DA, Murphy ML, Burchenal JH. Toxicity of *E. coli* L-asparaginase in man. Cancer 1970:253–278.

28. Pratt CM, Johnson WW. Duration and severity of fatty metamorphosis of liver following L-asparaginase therapy. Cancer 1971:28:361–364.
29. Chabner B. Enzyme therapy: L-Asparaginase. In: B Chabner, ed. Pharmacologic Principles of Cancer Chemotherapy. Philadelphia: Saunders, 1982, pp 435–443.
30. Winick NJ, Bowman WP, Kamen BA, Roach ES, Rollins N, Jacaruso D, Buchanan GR. Unexpected acute neurologic toxicity in the treatment of children with acute lymphoblastic leukemia. J Natl Cancer Inst 1992:84:252–256.
31. Pui CH, Burghen GA, Bowman WP, Aur RJA. Risk factors for hyperglycemia in children with leukemia receiving L-asparaginase and prednisone. J Pediatr 1981:99:(1)46–50.
32. Ertel IJ, Nesbit ME, Hammond D, Weiner J, Sather H. Effective dose of L-asparaginase for induction of remission in previously treated children with acute lymphocytic leukemia: A report from Children's Cancer Study Group. Cancer Res 1979:39:3893–3896.
33. Charan VD, Desai N, Singh AP, Choudhry VP. Diabetes mellitus and pancreatitis as a complication of L-asparaginase therapy. Indian Pediatr 1993:30: 809–810.
34. Haskell CM. L-Asparaginase: Human toxicology and single agent activity in nonleukemic neoplasms. Cancer Treatment Rep 1981:65(suppl 4):57–59.
35. Sica S, Pagano L, Salutari P, Di-Mario A, Rutella S, Leone G. Acute parotitis during induction therapy including L-asparaginase in acute lymphoblastic leukemia. Ann Hematol 1994:68(2):91–92.
36. MacEwen EG, Rosenthal R, Matus R, Viau AT, Abuchowski A. A preliminary study on the evaluation of asparaginase. Cancer 1987:59:2011–2015.
37. Tallai L, Tan CC, Oettgen HF, Wollner N, McCarthy M, Helson L, Burchenal J, Karnofsky D, Murphy ML. *E. coli* L-asparaginase in the treatment of leukemia and solid tumours in 131 children. Cancer 1970:25:306–320.
38. Ohnuma T, Holland JF, Sinks LF. Biochemical and pharmacological studies with L-asparaginase in man. Cancer Res 1970:30:2297–2305.
39. Kurtzberg J. A new look at PEG-L-asparaginase and other asparaginases in hematological malignancies. Cancer Invest 1994:12(suppl 1):59–60.
40. Bendich A, Kafkewitz D, Abuchowski A, Davis FF. Immunological effects of native and polyethylene glycol-modified asparaginase from *Vibrio succinogenes* and *Escherichia coli* in normal and tumor-bearing mice. Clin Exp Immunol 1982:48:273–278.
41. Distasio JA, Niederman RA, Kafkewitz D. Antilymphoma activity of a glutaminase-free L-asparaginase of microbial origin. Proc Soc Exp Biol Med 1977:155:528–531.
42. Koerholz D, Brueck M, Nuernberger W, Juergens H, Goebel U, Wahn V. Chemical and immunological characteristics of four different L-asparaginase preparations. Eur J Haematol 1989:42:417–424.
43. Goldberg AI, Cooney DA, Glynn JP, Homan ER, Gaston MR, Milman HA. The effects of immunization to L-asparaginase on antitumor and enzymatic activity. Cancer Res 1973:33:256–261.

44. Charles LM, Bono VH Jr. A review of the preclinical antitumor activity and toxicity of L-asparaginase derived from *E. coli.* Cancer Treatment Rep 1981: 65:39–46.
45. Ho DHW, Thetford BS, Carter CJK. Clinical pharmacologic studies of L-asparaginase. Pharmacol Ther 1979:11:408–417.
46. Ménard DB, Gisselbrecht C, Marty M, Reyes F, Dhumeaux D. Antineoplastic agents and the liver. Gastroenterology 1980:78:142–164.
47. Woods WG, O'Leary M, Nesbit ME. Life-threatening neuropathy and hepatotoxicity in infants during induction therapy for acute lymphoblastic leukemia. J Pediatr 1981:98:642–645.
48. Canellos GP, Haskell CM, Arseneau J, Carbone PP. Hypoalbuminemic and hypocholesterolemic effect of L-asparaginase (NSC-109,229) treatment in man. A preliminary report. Cancer Chemother Rep 1969:53:67–69.
49. Capizzi RL, Bertino JR, Handschumacher RE. L-Asparaginase. Annu Rev Med 1970:21:431–444.
50. Schein PS, Rakieten N, Gordon BM, Davis RD, Rau DP. The toxicity of *Escherichia coli* L-asparaginase. Cancer Res 1969:29:426–434.
51. Cairo MS. Adverse reactions of L-asparaginase. Am J Pediatr Hematol Oncol 1982:4(3):335–339.
52. Woods WG, O'Leary M, Nesbit ME. Life-threatening neuropathy and hepatotoxicity in infants during induction therapy for acute lymphoblastic leukemia. J Pediatr 1981:98(4):642–645.
53. Jenkins R, Perlin E. Severe hepatotoxicity from *Escherichia coli* L-asparaginase. J Natl Med Assoc 1987:79(7):775–779.
54. Brueck M, Koerholz D, Nuernbeerger W, Juergens H, Goebel U, Wahn V. Elimination of L-asparaginase in children treated for acute lymphoblastic leukemia. Dev Pharmacol Ther 1989:12:200–204.
55. Amadori S, Papa G, Avvisati G, Petti MC, Motta M, Salvagnini M, Meloni G, Martelli M, Monarca B, Mandelli F. Sequential combination of systemic high-dose Ara-C and asparaginase for the treatment of central nervous system leukemia and lymphoma. J Clin Oncol 1984:2(2):98–101.
56. Durden DL, Salazar AM, Distasio JA. Kinetic analysis of hepatotoxicity associated with antineoplastic asparaginases. Cancer Res 1983:43(4):1602–1605.
57. Whitecar JP Jr, Bodey GP, Harris JE, Freireich EJ. L-Asparaginase. N Engl J Med 1970:282:732–734.
58. Land VJ, Sutow WW, Fernbach DJ, Lane DM, Williams TE. Toxicity of L-asparaginase in children with advanced leukemia. Cancer 1972:30:339–347.
59. Rizzari C, Gentili D, D'Incalci M, Orlandoni D, Zucchetti M, Tschuemperlin B, Conter V, Maser G. Inadequate L-asparagine (L-ASN) depletion after repeated courses of *Erwinia* L-asparaginase (L-ASP) administration in children with acute lymphoblastic leukemia (ALL). Med Pediatr Oncol 25(4):282 Abstr. P-13, 1995.
60. Boos J, Nowak-Göttl U, Jürgens H, Fleischhack G, Bode U. Loss of activity of *Erwinia* asparaginase on repeat applications. J Clin Oncol 1995:13:2474–2475.

61. Asselin BL, Cohen HJ. Clearance of L-asparaginase (ASNase) in patients with acute lymphoblastic leukemia (ALL). Pediatr Res 1988:23(4):336A.
62. Grebanier A, Chen R, Franklin A, Scudiery D, Fisherman JD, Kurtzberg J, Asselin B, Poplack D. Antibodies to asparaginase after pharmacokinetics and decrease enzyme activity in patients on asparaginase therapy. Proc Am Assoc Cancer Res 1993:34:304.
63. Distasio JA, Salazar AM, Nadji M, Durden DI. Glutaminase-free asparaginase from *Vibrio succinogenes*: An antilymphoma enzyme lacking hepatotoxicity. Int J Cancer 1982:30:343–347.
64. Ettinger LJ, Lerner ED, Johnson RW. A toxicity study of Oncaspar® (PEG-asparaginase) in children with acute lymphoblastic leukemia (ALL). Med Pediatr Oncol 1994:23:278.
65. Asselin B, Gelber R, Sallan S. Relative toxicity of *E. coli* L-asparaginase and pegaspargase (peg) in newly diagnosed childhood acute lymphoblastic leukemia (ALL). Med Pediatr Oncol 1993:21:556.
66. Poznansky MJ, Shandling M, Salkie MA, Elliott J, Lau E. Advantages in the use of L-asparaginase–albumin polymer as an antitumor agent. Cancer Res 1982:42(3):1020–1025.
67. Strandstrom HV, Bowen JM. Canine leukemia–lymphoma complex: A model for human hematopoietic malignancies. In: DS Yohn, and JR Blakerslee, eds. Advances in Comparative Leukemia Research. New York, Elsevier/North-Holland, 1982, pp 447–450.
68. Teske E, Ruttemann GR, van Heerde P, Misdorp W. Polyethylene glycol-L-asparaginase versus native L-asparaginase in canine non-Hodgkin's lymphoma. Eur J Cancer 1990:26(8):891–895.
69. Holle LM. Pegaspargase: An alternative? Ann Pharmacother 1997:31:616–623.
70. Woods JS, Handschumacher RE. Hepatic homeostasis of plasma L-asparagine. 1971:221:1785–1790.
71. Villa P, Corada M, Bartosek I. L-Asparaginase-effects on inhibition of protein synthesis and lowering of the glutamine content in cultured rat hepatocytes. Toxicol Lett 1986:32:235–241.
72. Benezra D, Pitaro R, Birkenfeld U, Hochman A. Reversal of the immunosuppressive effect of L-asparaginase by L-glutamine. Nature New Biol 1972: 236:80–82.
73. Urten JR, Handschumacher RE. Enzyme therapy. In: FF Becker, ed. Cancer: A Comprehensive Treatise, vol 5. New York: Plenum Press, 1977, pp 457–487.
74. Wade HE, Phillips AP. Automated determination of bacterial asparaginase and glutaminase. Anal Biochem 1971:44:189–199.
75. Miller HK, Salser JS, Balis ME. Amino acid levels following L-asparagine amidohydrolase (EC 3.5.1.1) therapy. Cancer Res 1969:29:183–187.
76. Ollenschläger G, Roth E, Linkesch W, Jansen S, Simmel A, Mödder B. Asparaginase-induced derangements of glutamine metabolism: The pathogenetic basis for some drug-related side-effects. Eur J Clin Invest 1988:18:512–516.

77. Woodward CN, Sur P, Capizzi RL, Modest JE. Serum amino acid levels in leukemic mice after L-asparaginase treatment. Biochem Med Metab Biol 1988:39:199–207.
78. Korinthenberg R, Ullrich K, Ritter J, Stephani U. Electrolytes, amino acids and proteins in lumbar CSF during the treatment of acute leukemia in childhood. Acta Paediatr Scand 1990:79:334–342.
79. Distasio JA, Salazar AM, Nadji M, Durden DL. Glutaminase-free asparaginase from *Vibrio succinogenes*: An anti-lymphoma enzyme lacking hepatotoxicity. Int J Cancer 1982:30:343–347.
80. Rutter DA. Toxicity of asparaginases. Lancet 1975:1:1293–1294.
81. Becker FF, Broome JD. L-Asparaginase: Inhibition of early mitosis in regenerating rat liver. Science 1967:156:1602–1603.
82. Konya H, Tamura S, Miyazaki E, Inque N, Okamoto T, Takemoto Y, Kohsaki M, Kanemaru A, Kakishita E. L-Asparaginase-induced hyperlipidemia in a case of acute lymphoblastic leukemia. Jpn J Clin Hematol 1991:32(3):250–254.
83. Buchanan GR, Holtkamp CA. Reduced antithrombin III levels during L-asparaginase therapy. Med Pediatr Oncol 1980:8:7–14.
84. Cairo MS, Lazarus K, Gilmore RL, Baelner RL. Intracranial hemorrhage and focal seizures secondary to use of L-asparaginase during induction therapy of acute lymphocytic leukemia. J Pediatr 1980:97:829–833.
85. Priest JR, Ramsay NKC, Bennett AJ, Krivit W, Edson JR. The effect of L-asparaginase on antithrombin, plasminogen and plasma coagulation during therapy for acute lymphoblastic leukemia. J Pediatr 1982:100:990–995.
86. Priest JR, Ramsay NKC, Steinherz PG, Tubergen DG, Cairo MS, Sitzr AL, Bishop AJ, White L, Trigg MD, Levitt CJ, Cich JA, Coccia PF. A syndrome of thrombosis and hemorrhage complicating L-asparaginase therapy for childhood acute lymphoblastic leukemia. J Pediatr 1982:100:984–989.
87. Bessho F, Kinumaki H, Yokota S, Hayashi Y, Kobayashi M, Kamoshita S. Liver function studies in children with acute lymphocytic leukemia after cessation of therapy. Med Pediatr Oncol 1994:23:111–115.
88. Tozuka M, Yamauchi K, Hidaka H, Nakabayashi T, Okumura NS, Katsuyama T. Characterization of hypertriglyceridemia induced by L-asparaginase therapy for acute lymphoblastic leukemia and malignant lymphoma. Ann Clin Lab Sci 1997:27:351–357.
89. McLean R, Martin S, Lam Po Tang PR. Fatal case of L-asparaginase induced pancreatitis. Lancet 1982:2:1401–1402.
90. Yang CM, Hsieh YL, Hwang B. Acute pancreatitis in association with L-asparaginase therapy: Report of one case. Chung-Hua I Hsueh Tsa Chih, Taipei 1993:51(1):74–77.
91. Frick TW, Speiser DE, Bimmler D, Largiader F. Drug-induced acute pancreatitis: Further criticism. Dig Dis 1993:11(2):113–132.
92. Nakashima Y, Howard JM. Drug-induced acute pancreatitis. Surg Gynecol Obstet 1977:145(1):105–109.
93. Tan CL, Chiang SP, Wee KP. Acute haemorrhagic pancreatitis following L-asparaginase therapy in acute lymphoblastic leukaemia—A case report. Singapore Med J 1974:15(4):278–282.

94. Weetman RM, Baehner RL. Latent onset of clinical pancreatitis in children receiving L-asparaginase therapy. Cancer 1974:34(3):780–785.
95. Shaw MT, Barnes CC, Madden FJ, Bagshawe KD. L-Asparaginase and pancreatitis. Lancet 1970:2(675):721.
96. Underwood TW, Frye CB. Drug-induced pancreatitis. Clin Pharm 1993:12(6): 440–448.
97. Kondrat'eva NA, Kruglova GV, Lorie IuI, Koshel' IV, Kurmashov VI. [L-asparaginase study results (phase II of the clinical trials)] (in Russian). Antibiotiki 1980:25(9):686–689.
98. Jain R, Ramanan SV. Iatrogenic pancreatitis. A fatal complication in the induction therapy for acute lymphocytic leukemia. Arch Intern Med 1978: 138(11):1726.
99. Sadoff J, Hwang S, Rosenfeld D, Ettinger L, Spigland N. Surgical pancreatic complications induced by L-asparaginase. J Pediatr Surg 1997:32(6):860–863.
100. Dobrilla G, Felder M, Chilovi F. Acute drug-induced pancreatitis (in German). Schweiz Med Wochenschr 1985:115(25):850–858.
101. Mallory A, Kern F Jr. Drug-induced pancreatitis: A critical review. Gastroenterology 1980:78(4):813–820.
102. Samuels BI, Culbert SJ, Okamura J, Sullivan MP. Early detection of chemotherapy-related pancreatic enlargement in children using abdominal sonography: A preliminary report. Cancer 1976:38(4):1515–1523.
103. Nguyen DL, Wilson DA, Engelman ED, Sexauer CL, Nitschke R. Serial sonograms to detect pancreatitis in children receiving L-asparaginase. South Med J 1987:80(9):1133–1136.
104. Hanson JF, Carpenter RH. Fatal acute systemic anaphylaxis and hemorrhagic pancreatitis following asparaginase treatment in a dog. J Am Anim Assoc 1983:19:977–980.
105. Park YK, Abuchowski A, Davis S, Davis F. Pharmacology of *Escherichia coli* L-asparaginase polyethylene glycol adduct. Anticancer Res 1981:1:373–376.
106. Volkova MA, Maiakova SA, Kaletin GI, Kurdiukov BV, Frenkel MA, Protasova AK, Tupitsyn NN, Fleishman BV. Use of long-acting L-asparaginase (PEG-asparaginase) in acute lymphoblastic leukemia. Gematol Transfusiol 1994:39:3–6.
107. Cheung YF, Lee CW, Chan CF, Chan KL, Lau YL, Yeung CY. Somatostatin therapy in L-asparaginase-induced pancreatitis. Med Pediatr Oncol 1994: 22(6):421–424.
108. Koniver GA, Scott JE. Pancreatitis with pseudocyst: A complication of L-asparaginase therapy for leukemia. Del Med J 1978:50(6):330–332.
109. Greenstein R, Nogeire C, Ohnuma T, Greenstein A. Management of asparaginase induced hemorrhagic pancreatitis complicated by pseudocyst. Cancer 1979:43(2):718–722.
110. Yu CH, Lin KH, Lin DT, Chen RL, Horng YC, Chang MH. L-Asparaginase-related pancreatic pseudocyst: Report of a case. J Formosan Med Assoc 1994: 93(5):441–444.

111. Caniano DA, Browne AF, Boles ET Jr. Pancreatic pseudocyst complicating treatment of acute lymphoblastic leukemia. J Pediatr Surg 1985:20(4):452–455.
112. Bertolone SJ, Fuenfer MM, Groff DB, Patel CC. A delayed pancreatic pseudocyst formations belongs to the long-term complication of L-asparaginase treatment. Cancer 1982:50(12):2964–2966.
113. Yasui I, Shimokawa T, Kasai M, Yamada H, Watanabe E, Takeyama H, Satake T. A case of ALL complicated with acute pancreatitis and pancreatic pseudocyst caused by L-asparaginase (in Japanese). Gan To Kagaku Ryoho 1993: 20(1):149–152.
114. Uysal K, Uguz A, Olgun N, Sarialiglu F, Buyukgebiz A. Hyperglycemia and acute parotitis related to L-asparaginase therapy. J Pediatr Endocrinol Metab 1966:9:627–629.
115. Brodkiewicz A, Kamienska E, Urasinski T, Peregud-Pogorzelski J. Hyperglycemia as a side effect of using L-asparaginase in children with acute lymphoblastic leukemia. Acta Haematol Pol 1995:26:99–101.
116. Cetin M, Yetgin S, Kara A, Tuncer AM, Gunay M, Gumruk F, Gurgey A. Hyperglycemia, ketoacidosis and other complications of L-asparaginase in children with acute lymphoblastic leukemia. J Med 1994:25:219–229.
117. Wang YJ, Chu HY, Shu SG, Chi CS. Hyperglycemia induced by chemotherapeutic agents used in acute lymphoblastic leukemia: Report of three cases. Chung-Hua I Hsueh Tsa Chih, Taipei 1993:51(6):457–461.
118. Capizzi RL. Asparaginase revisited. Leuk Lymphoma 1993:10:147–150.
119. Meschi F, di Natale B, Rondanini GF, Uderzo C, Jankovic M, Masera G, Chiumello G. Pancreatic endocrine function in leukemic children treated with L-asparaginase. Horm Res 1981:15(4):237–241.
120. Package insert. Oncaspar (pegaspargase). Collegeville, PA: Rhône-Poulenc Rorer, November 1994.
121. Clausen N, Nielsen JH. Direct long-term effects of L-asparaginase on rat and human pancreatic islets. Pediatr Res 1989:26(2):158–161.
122. Warne G, Adie R, Hansky J, Martin FI, Varigos G. Prolonged control of hypoglycaemia by L-asparaginase in islet cell carcinoma producing insulin and gastrin. Aust NZ J Med 1975:5(5):466–468.
123. Lessner HE, Valenstein S, Kaplan R, DeSimone P, Yunis A. Phase II study of L-asparaginase in the treatment of pancreatic carcinoma. Cancer Treatment Rep 1980:64(12):1359–1361.
124. Wu MC, Arimura GK, Yunis AA. Mechanism of sensitivity of cultured pancreatic carcinoma to asparaginase. Int J Cancer 1978:22(6):728–733.
125. Yunis AA, Arimura GK, Russin DJ. Human pancreatic carcinoma (MIA PaCa-2) in continuous culture: Sensitivity to asparaginase. Int J Cancer 1977:19(1): 218–235.
126. Gleman CR, Rumack BH, Sayre ND, eds. Drugdex System. Englewood, CO: Micromedex, Inc. December 1997.
127. Jaffe N, Traggis D, Das L, Moloney WC, Hann HW, Kim BS, Mair R. L-Asparaginase in the treatment of neoplastic diseases in children. Cancer Res 1971:31:942–949.

128. Mathe G, Amiel JL, Clarysse A, Hayat M, Schwarzenberg L, Schneider M. La L-asparaginase dans le traitement des leucémies aigues. Sem Hop Paris 1970:46:1135–1140.
129. Johnston PGB, Hardisty RM, Kay HEM, Smith PG. Myelosuppressive effect of Colaspase (L-asparaginase) in initial treatment of acute lymphoblastic leukemia. Br Med J 1974:3:81–83.
130. Patel SS, Benfield P. Pegaspargase (polyethylene glycol-L-asparaginase). Clin Immunother 1996:5:492–496.
131. Kawashima K, Takeshima H, Higashi Y, Hamaguchi M, Sugie H, Imamura I, Wada H. High efficacy of monomethoxapolyethyleneglycol-conjugated L-asparaginase (PEG2-ASP) in two patients with hematological malignancies. Leuk Res 1991:15:525–530.
132. Mitchel LG, Sutor AH, Andrew M. Hemostasis in childhood acute lymphoblastic leukemia: Coagulopathy induced by disease and treatment. Sem Thromb Hemostasis 1995:21:390–401.
133. Gugliotta L, Mazzucconi MG, Leone G, Belmonte MM, Defazio D, Annino L, Mandeli F. L-Asparaginase and haemostasis: A Gimema retrospective study on the incidence of thrombosis and haemorrhage in ALL patients. Thromb Haemostasis 1991:65:1021.
134. Sutor AH, Niemeyer C, Sauter S, Witt I, Kaufmehl K, Rombach A, Brandis M, Riehm H. Gerinnungsveränderungen bei Behandlung mit den Protokollen ALL-BFM-90 und NHL-BFM-90. Klin Paediatr 1992:204:264–273.
135. Mitchel L, Hoogendoorn H, Giles AR, Vegh P, Andrew M. Increased endogenous thrombin generation in children with acute lymphoblastic leukemia: Risk of thrombotic complications in L-asparaginase-induced antithrombin III deficiency. Blood 1994:83:386–391.
136. Nowak-Göttl U, Wolff JEA, Kuhn N, Boos J, Kehrel B, Lilienweiss V, Schwabe D, Jürgens H. Enhanced thrombin generation, P-von Willebrand factor, P-fibrin D-dimer and P-plasminogen activator inhibitor 1: Predictive for venous thrombosis in asparaginase-treated children. Fibronolysis 1994: 8(suppl 2):63–65.
137. Saito M, Asakura H, Jokaji H, Uotani C, Kumabashiri I, Ito K, Matsuda T. Changes in hemostatic and fibrinolytic proteins in patients receiving L-asparaginase therapy. Am J Hematol 1989:32:20–23.
138. Bauer K, Teitel JM, Rosenberg RD: L-Asparaginase induced antithrombin III deficiency: Evidence against the production of a hypercoagulable state. Thromb Res 1983:29:437–442.
139. Pui CH, Chesney CM, Weed J, Jackson CW. Altered von Willebrand factor molecule in children with thrombosis following asparaginase–prednisone–vincristine therapy for leukemia. J Clin Oncol 1985:3:1266–1272.
140. Gralnik HR, Henry PH. L-Asparaginase induced coagulopathy. Proc Am Assoc Cancer Res 1969:10:32.
141. Andrew M, Brooker L, Mitchell L. Acquired antithrombin II deficiency secondary to asparaginase therapy in childhood acute lymphoblastic leukemia. Blood Coagulation Fibrinol 1994:5:524–536.

142. Prager MD, Bachynski N. Asparagine synthetase in normal and malignant tissues; Correlation with tumor sensitivity to asparaginase. Arch Biochem Biophys 1968:127:645–654.
143. Milmann HA, Cooney DA. The distribution of L-asparaginase synthetase in the principal organs of several mammalian and avian species. Biochem J 1974:142:27–35.
144. Nowak-Göttl U, Erben M, Münstermann G, Kehrel B, Boos J, Wolff JEA: Endothelial vWf and t-PA release after incubation with different concentrations of asparaginase and dexamethasone. Fibrinolyses 1996:10:55–56.
145. Dahlbäck B, Carlsson M, Svensson PJ. Familial thrombophilia due to a previously unrecognized mechanism characterized by poor anticoagulant response to activated protein C: Prediction of a cofactor to activated protein C. Proc Natl Acad Sci USA 1994:90:1004–1008.
146. Miles LA, Fless GM, Levin EG, Scanu AM, Plow EF. A potential basis for the thrombotic risk associated with lipoprotein (a). Nature 1989:339:301–303.
147. McLean JW, Tomlinson JE, Kuang WJ, Eaton DL, Chen EY, Fless GM, Scanu AM, Lawn RM. cDNA sequence of human apolipoprotein (a) is homologous to plasminogen. Nature 1987:300:132–137.
148. Poort SR, Rosendaal FR, Reitsma PH, Bertina RM. A common genetic variation in the 3′-untranslated region of the prothrombin gene is associated with elevated plasma prothrombin levels and an increase in venous thrombosis. Blood 1996:88:3698.
149. Nowak-Göttl U, Aschka I, Koch G, Boos J, Dockhorn-Dworniczak B, Deufel T, Jürgens H, Kohlhase B, Kuhn N, Laupert A, Rath B, Wolff JEA, Schneppenheim R. Resistance to activated protein C (APCR) in children with acute lymphoblastic leukemia—the need for a prospective multicentre study. Blood Coagulation Fibrinol 1995:6:761–764.
150. Nowak-Göttl U, Schneider C, Schwabe D, Schneppenheim R for the ALL-BFM Thrombophilia Study Group. Defects in the protein C anticoagulation pathway and further risks of thrombophilia—First results of the German multicentre study on thromboembolism in childhood ALL. Blood 90 (10, Suppl 1/1):72a, abstract 311, 1997.
151. Janka GE, Winkler K, Jürgens H, Göbel, U, Gutjahr P, Spaar HJ. Akute lymphoblastische Leukämie im Kindesalter: Die COALL-Studien. Klin Paediatr 1986:198:171–177.
152. Kauze A, Jelenska M, Palester-Chlebowczyk M, Ochocka M. Influence of L-asparaginase *Escherichia coli* and *Erwinia* on antithrombin III and coagulation factors during induction therapy of acute lymphoblastic leukemia in children. In: Büchner et al., eds. Acute Leukemias, vol 6, Prognostic Factors and Treatment Strategies. Berlin: Springer-Verlag, 1997, pp 517–525.
153. Gentili D, Conter V, Rizzari C, Tschuemperlin B, Zucchetti M, Orlandomi C, Dincalci M, Masera G. L-Asparagine depletion in plasma and cerebrospinal fluid of children with acute lymphoblastic leukemia during subsequent exposures to *Erwinia* L-asparaginase. Ann Oncol 1996:7:725–730.
154. Dibenedetto SP, Di Cataldo A, Ragusa A, Meli C, Lo Nigro L. Levels of L-

asparaginase in CSF after intramuscular administration of asparaginase from *Erwinia* in children with acute lymphoblastic leukemia. J Clin Oncol 1995: 13:339–344.

155. Carlsson H, Stockelberg D, Tengborn L, Braide I, Carneskog J, Kutti J. Effects of *Erwinia*-asparaginase on the coagulation system. Eur J Haematol 1995:55:289–293.
156. Nowak-Göttl U, Boos J, Wolff JEA, Werber G, Ahlke E, Pollmann H, Jürgens H. Influence of two different *E. coli* asparaginase preparations on coagulation and fibrolysis: A randomized trial. Fibrinolysis 1994:8(suppl 2):66–68.
157. Nowak-Göttl U, Werber G, Ziemann D, Ahlke E, Boos J. Influence of two different *Escherichia coli* asparaginase preparations on fibrinolytic proteins in childhood ALL. Haematologica 1996:81:127–131.
158. Ahlke E, Nowak-Göttl U, Schulze-Westhoff P, Werber G, Börste H, Würthwein G, Jürgens H, Boos J. Dose reduction of asparaginase under pharmacokinetic and pharmakodynamic control during induction therapy in children with acute lymphoblastic leukemia. Br J Haematol 1997:96:657–681.
159. Nowak-Göttl U, Ahlke E, Schulze-Westhoff P, Boos J. Changes in coagulation and fibrinolysis in childhood ALL: A two-step dose reduction of one *E. coli* asparaginase preparation. Br J Haematol 1996:95:123–126.
160. Nowak-Göttl U, Rath B, Binder M, Hasel JU, Wolff JEA, Husemann S, Ritter J. Inefficacy of fresh frozen plasma in the treatment of L-asparaginase-induced coagulation factor deficiencies during ALL induction therapy. Haematologica 1995:80:451–453.
161. Halton JM, Mitchell L, Vegh P, Eves M, Andrew ME. Fresh frozen plasma has no beneficial effect on the hemostatic system in children receiving *L*-asparaginase. Am J Hematol 1994:47:157–161.
162. Zaunschirm A, Muntean W. Correction of hemostatic imbalances induced by L-asparaginase therapy in children with acute lymphoblastic leukemia. Pediatr Hematol Oncol 1986:3:19–25.
163. Gugliotta L, D'Angelo A, Mattiolo Belmone M, Vigano-D'Angelo S, Colombo G, Catani L, Gianni L, Lauria F, Tura S. Hypercoagulobility during L-asparaginase treatment: The effect of antithrombin III supplementation in vivo. Br J Haematol 1990:74:465–470.
164. Belmonte MM, Gugliotta L, Delvos U, Catani L, Vianelli N, Cascione ML, Belardinelli AR, Mottola L, Tura S. A regimen for antithrombin III substitution in patients with acute lymphoblastic leukemia under treatment with L-asparaginase. Haematologica 1991:76:209–214.
165. Mazzucconi MG, Gugliotta L, Leone G, Dragoni F, Belmonte MM, DeStefano V, Chistolini A, Tura S, Mandelli F. Antithrombin III infusion suppresses the hypercoagulable state in adult acute lymphoblastic leukaemia patients treated with low dose of *Escherichia coli* L-asparaginase. A Gimema study. Blood Coagulation Fibrinol 1994:5:23–28.
166. Nowak-Göttl U, Kuhn N, Wolff JEA, Boos J, Kehrel B, Rath B, Jürgens H. Inhibition of hypercoagulation by antithrombin substitution in *E. coli* L-asparaginase-treated children. Eur J Haematol 1996:56:35–38.

8.3 MERCAPTOPURINE AND RELATED COMPOUNDS

EUGENE Y. KRYNETSKI and WILLIAM E. EVANS
St. Jude Children's Research Hospital, Memphis, Tennessee

List of Abbreviations

DNPS	*de novo* purine synthesis
HPRT	hypoxanthine phosphoribosyltransferase (IMP: pyrophosphate phosphoribosyltransferase, EC 2.4.2.8)
IDP	inosine 5′-diphosphate
IMP	inosine 5′-monophosphate
meMP	*S*-methylmercaptopurine
meMPR	*S*-methylmercaptopurine riboside
meTGN	*S*-methylthioguanosine phosphates
MP	6-mercaptopurine
MPR	6-mercaptopurine riboside
PRPP-AT	Ribosylamine 5-phosphate: pyrophosphate phosphoribosyltransferase (glutamate amidating), EC 2.4.2.14
SAM	*S*-adneosylmethionine
TG	6-thioguanine
TGN	6-thioguanosine nucleotides (mono-, di-, and triphosphates: 6thio GMP, 6thio GDP, and 6thio GTP, respectively)
TIMP	Thioinosine 5′-monophosphate
TPMT	Thiopurine *S*-methyltransferase
TXMP	Thioxanthosine 5′-monophosphate

8.3.1 Introduction

Despite extensive studies during the last 40 years, the mechanism of action of thiopurines remains obscure. Similar to other cytotoxic drugs, there are multiple potential targets for thiopurines, and their therapeutic or toxic effects may reflect several complementary mechanisms. This may be why determinants of the cytotoxic effects of thiopurines have been so elusive. Traditionally, two processes are considered to be the key events in exerting thiopurine toxicity: (a) inhibition of enzymes involved in de novo purine biosynthesis and (b) incorporation of thiopurine nucleotides into nucleic acids. By interacting with enzymes along biosynthetic pathways, thiopurines inhibit their activity and cause a misbalance of important cellular components—nucleotides. By incorporating into DNA, thiopurines interrupt the normal replication, storage, and processing of genetic information.

Considering cell death (apoptosis) as an active process triggered by various signals, one can hypothesize that the cytotoxic effect of mercaptopurine (MP) and thioguanine (TG) generates this signal either in a direct (DNA modification) or indirect (misbalance of nucleotides) way [1]. Thus, cell sensitivity and resistance to thiopurine treatment may be determined in large part by the nature of these signals and their transduction.

8.3.2 Thiopurines: Metabolism and Mechanism of Action

8.3.2.1 Thiopurine Metabolites Interfere with Purine Biosynthesis

Historically, the initial studies of MP and TG action were focused on interactions of these drugs and their metabolites with major nucleotide metabolic pathways. MP and TG are inactive prodrugs, requiring metabolism to thiopurine nucleotides to exert cytotoxicity (Fig. 5). Incorporation of thiopurines into biosynthetic pathways is achieved via the "salvage pathway" normally exploited by cells to reutilize nucleobases after breakdown of nucleosides. As depicted in Fig. 5, TG is metabolized directly to TGMP by HPRT (route B), while MP must first be metabolized to TIMP, then TXMP, before metabolism to TGMP (route A). In this way, a number of thiopurine nucleotides are formed that are structural analogues of natural nucleotides and therefore are able to interact with cellular components. Alternatively, these two drugs can undergo S-methylation catalyzed by thiopurine *S*-methyltransferase (TPMT), or oxidation to thiouric acid (TU) by xanthine oxidase (TG must be deaminated to thioxanthine before being oxidized by xanthine oxidase). However, hematopoietic tissues do not have measurable xanthine oxidase activity [2], leaving S-methylation as the major competing metabolic pathway in these cells. TPMT-catalyzed methylation of MP and TG yields the corresponding S-methylated thiopurine bases (Fig. 5), both of which are inactive metabolites. The effectiveness of MP/TG in inhibiting cell growth is primarily dependent on their transformation to ribonucleotides, the initial step being catalyzed by hypoxanthine phosphoribosyltransferase (IMP: pyrophosphate phosphoribosyltransferase, EC 2.4.2.8). The reaction of phosphoribosylation (a transfer of a phosphoribosyl moiety) of guanine, hypoxanthine, MP, and TG is catalyzed by the same enzyme, resulting in the corresponding nucleotide [3]. Both MP and TG are relatively good substrates for HPRT: Michaelis constants for hypoxanthine, guanine, MP, and TG are 4.0, 2.7, 10, and 10 μM, respectively. These numbers do not differ greatly

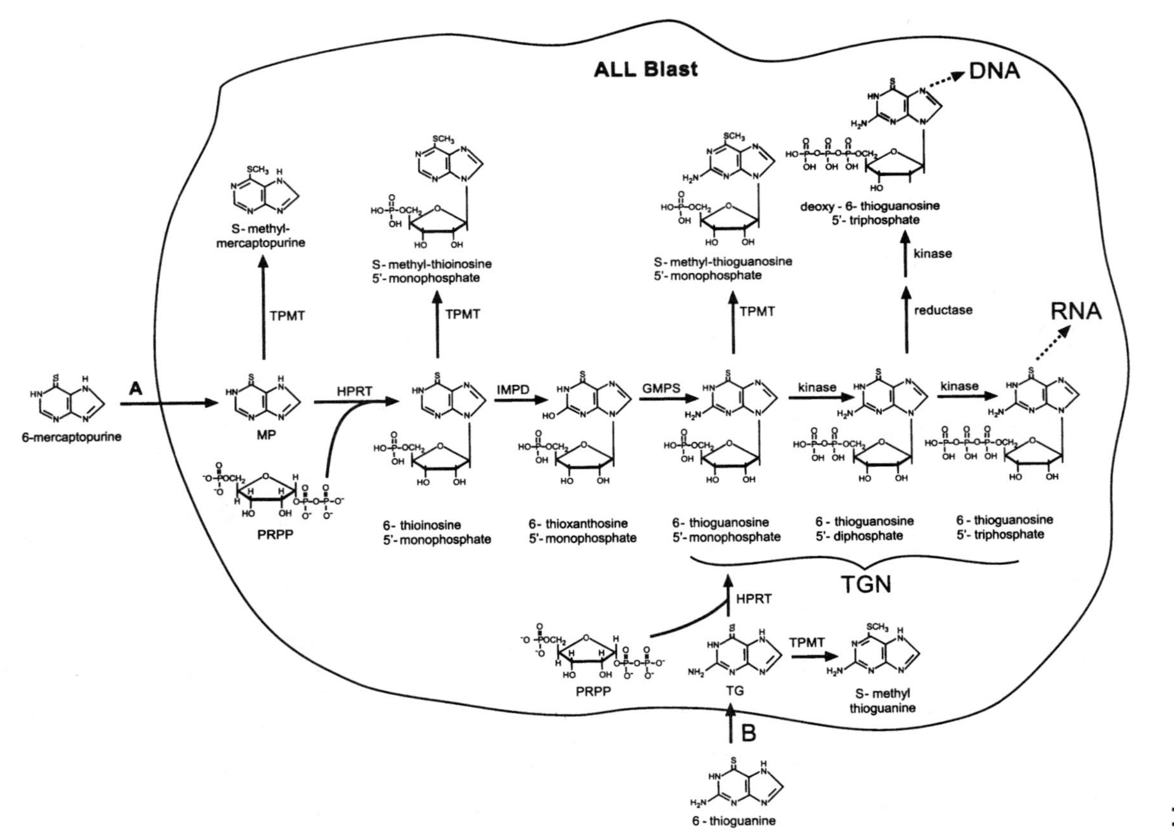

Fig. 5 Metabolism of MP (A) and TG (B) in human leukemia cells: HPRT, hypoxanthine phosphoribosyltransferase; IMPD, inosine monophosphate dehydrogenase; GMPS, guanosine monophosphate synthetase; TPMT, thiopurine *S*-methyltransferase; PRPP, phosphoribosylpyrophosphate. (Modified and reproduced with publisher's permission, from Krynetski et al, Mol Pharmacol 1995:47:1141–1147.)

from those for Ehrlich ascites tumor cells, yeast, and human erythrocytes [3]. The corresponding nucleotides formed in this reaction (IMPGMP, dGMP, TIMP, and TGMP) are inhibitors of HPRT activity by a feedback mechanism [4].

Resulting thiopurine nucleotides TIMP and TGMP inhibit certain enzymes involved into purine metabolism: PPRP-amidotransferase [ribosylamine 5-phosphate: pyrophosphate phosphoribosyltransferase (glutamate amidating), EC 2.4.2.14], IMP dehydrogenase (IMP:NAD and oxidoreductase, EC 1.2.1.14), and TGMP inhibits GMP kinase. The last reaction is of notable interest because TGMP can also serve as a substrate for ATP:GMP phosphotransferase, but the reaction rate is less than 1% of the rate obtained with GMP [5]. This is a critical step in thiopurine activation, since incorporation into DNA becomes possible only after reduction of TGDP to the deoxy form, dTGTP and phosphorylation to dTGTP.

Strong inhibition of HPRT by thiopurine nucleotides is a notable effect, though its influence on the inhibition of cell growth is questionable, since HPRT deficiency is not a lethal cellular event and is a common mechanism by which cells acquire resistance to MP and TG.

Methylation of the S-6 in thiopurines is catalyzed by thiopurine *S*-methyltransferase, an enzyme for which biological functions and endogenous substrate(s) remain unknown. In contrast to thiopurine nucleobases, methylation of thiopurine nucleosides and nucleotides does result in active metabolites. The most abundant methylated product, *S*-methyl-6-thioinosine monophosphate (meTIMP) is a strong inhibitor of DNPS, as a result of its inhibitory effect on PRPP amidophosphoribosyltransferase.

Modification of the sulfur atom in the heterocyclic moiety of thioinosine monophosphate leads to important changes of the chemical structure and therefore alters substrate properties and stability of this molecule. Crystallographic data indicate that both MP and the corresponding nucleotide (TIMP) acquire a *thioketo* tautomeric form, with the length of the C—S bond close to the length of a double bond C═S [6]. This tautomeric form has a hydrogen atom at N-1 of the purine moiety so that the overall structure is similar to that of inosine (Fig. 6). When S-methylation occurs, the purine residue converts to a form without a hydrogen atom at the N-1 position and is therefore similar to that of the 6-aminopurines (e.g., adenine). As a consequence, substrate properties of the nucleotide (nucleoside) change. Most notably, in contrast to MPR and TGR, meMPR is not a substrate of nucleoside phosphorylases [7], and in vitro, meMPR remains intact under conditions that produce extensive cleavage of MP nucleoside to the free base. The molecular reason for this was revealed when the x-ray structures for human purine nucleoside phosphorylase were solved at 2.75 Å [8,9]. Stability of meMPR to PNP-catalyzed phosphorolysis relative to thioinosine

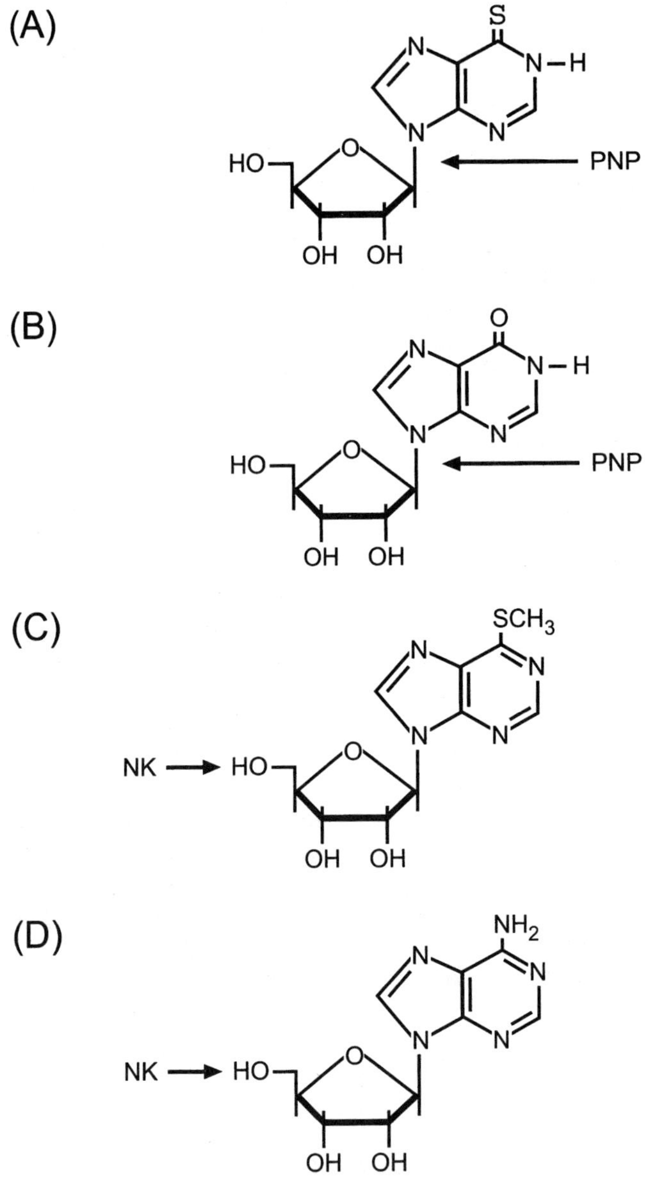

(A)

(B)

(C)

(D)

Fig. 6 Structural formulas of thioinosine (A), inosine (B), *S*-methylthioinosine (C), and adenosine (D). Arrows indicate sites of action of purine nucleoside phosphorylase (PNP) and nucleoside kinase (NK).

can best be explained from the hydrogen bond pattern entailing hydrogen bonds in the enzyme–substrate complex [10]. Evidently, N-1 and S-6 in thioinosine fit this pattern of the noncovalent bonding, whereas meMPR does not. Stability of meMPR to the action of PNP is one reason for substantial accumulation of meTIMP in the cells. The extensive conversion of meMPR to the nucleotide in cells that fail to convert MPR to the nucleotide indicates that meMPR is a substrate for adenosine kinase (ATP: adenosine 5′-phosphotransferase, EC 2.7.1.20) that does not act on MPR [11]. The structural reason for the phosphorylation of meMPR but not MPR by adenosine kinase is also explained by the same difference in the chemical structure: whereas inosine and MPR both bear a proton at N-1 (since they exist largely in lactam and thiolactam forms), adenosine and meMPR do not. The absence of a proton at N-1 of the purine ring might be more critical for activity as a substrate for the kinase than the nature of the group at the sixth position of the ring [7]. The list of enzymes sensitive to these two tautomeric forms of the purine ring is obviously not restricted to these two enzymes. For instance, meTIMP is not a substrate for 5′-monophosphate nucleotide kinases [12] and therefore cannot be converted into di- and triphosphates, which precludes its further processing and incorporation into nucleic acids. Indeed, subsequent studies revealed thioguanosine as the only triopurine derivative incorporated into DNA and RNA. Similarly, TIMP is not a substrate for guanylate kinase [12,13], and there is no significant conversion of IMP to IDP in most animal cells.

Interestingly, meMPR and its ribonucleotide are not inhibitors of HPRT [3], and meMP is not a substrate for adenine or hypoxanthine–guanine phosphoribosyltransferases [14,15]. The last observation means that the only way for cells to produce meTIMP after MP treatment is via TIMP formation and subsequent methylation catalyzed by thiopurine *S*-methyltransferase [16].

One known target of meTIMP action is the first enzyme of DNPS, namely, PRPP-amidotransferase [17]. The overall effect of inhibiting this step of DNPS may be multifactorial, since this leads to accumulation of PRPP, which may facilitate phosphoribosylation of MP and TG along the salvage pathway when PRPP is limiting [18,19]. This, in turn, leads to increased accumulation of TIMP and, correspondingly meTIMP. The higher amount of meTIMP and its much greater efficiency as an inhibitor of PRPP amidotransferase, compared to TIMP, make it likely that meTIMP is responsible for most or all of the inhibition of de novo purine synthesis produced by MP [20]. Inhibition of adenosine kinase prevented meMPR toxicity to CEM lymphoblasts, consistent with meTIMP being an active metabolite of meMPR [21,22].

It should be noted that even with the highest MP concentrations tested, the pool of purine ribonucleotide triphosphates was decreased by only 50–

60% after 24 hours of MP treatment and recovered during the next 24 hours [18,23–25]. MP depletes both ATP and GTP pools, and its antiproliferative effect on isolated peripheral blood T cells can be almost completely reversed by the addition of adenine but not guanosine. Interestingly, another thiopurine drug, azathioprine, may inhibit the proliferation of purified T cells by a completely independent mechanism, since the replenishment of both adenine and guanine ribonucleotides is not effective in reversing azathioprine inhibition of cell proliferation. It is possible that azathioprine has a generalized antiproliferative effect separable from any effect on purine metabolism [26,27].

The foregoing schematic of thiopurine metabolism implies that increased levels of TIMP formation can be achieved in several ways: (a) inhibition of DNPS, (b) induction of the "salvage pathway," and (c) inactivation of catabolic pathways; this strategy is best illustrated by simultaneous administration of the known inhibitors of DNPS. A well-known inhibitor is methotrexate (MTX), and the favorable therapeutic effect of MTX and MP is well documented. On the other hand, simultaneous addition of hypoxanthine and MP decreased the accumulation of all cellular MP metabolites, likely as a result of competitive inhibition of HPRT [28–30]. Allopurinol is an inhibitor of XO, and its coadministration can decrease the clearance of oral MP but not the systemic clearance of IV MP (which is limited more by liver blood flow and not XO activity, unlike first-pass oral clearance of MP) [31].

Based on a variety of cellular processes that involve GTP and dGTP, one may speculate that the corresponding counterparts (thioguanosine triphosphate and deoxythioguanosine triphosphate) potentially can interfere with other intra- and intercellular processes. To mention just a few hypothetical possibilities, these metabolites may affect protein biosynthesis, functioning of cytoskeleton proteins, and signal transduction.

8.3.2.2 Cytotoxic Effect of MP and TG Is Mediated Through Incorporation into DNA

The principal cytotoxic mechanism of MP and TG is generally considered to be via incorporation of thioguanine nucleotides (TGN) into DNA and RNA [32–35]. This notion is based on a relationship between delayed cytotoxicity and incorporation of thiopurines as 6-thioguanosine into nucleic acids. Inhibition of this incorporation [e.g., with mycophenolic acid, hydroxyurea, 1-β-D-arabinofuranosyl cytosine (Ara-C), or 5-fluorodeoxyuridine (FUdR)] [33,36,37] protects cells against the delayed lethal effect of MP or TG.

2′-Deoxy-6-thioguanosine 5′-triphosphate (dTGTP), a final metabolite of MP and TG is a good substrate for human DNA polymerases α, δ, and γ, with K_m values similar to those of natural substrates [38]. Cells resuspended in drug-free medium undergo lysis 1 to 2 divisions after exposure to MP or TG (delayed cytotoxic response) [33]. A number of agents other than 6-thiopurines induce delayed cytotoxic effects; a common property of these agents appears to be the ability to affect the structure of DNA [39–41]. Single-strand breaks (SSBs) were shown to accumulate in cultured Chinese hamster ovary and L1210 cells treated with thiopurines, as revealed by alkaline sucrose gradient and alkaline elution [37]. Strand breaks appeared to be related to the incorporation of TG into DNA, since the addition of cycloheximide during a 24-hour treatment with TG prevented cytotoxicity, prevented incorporation of TG into DNA, and eliminated strand breaks [42].

During the first cell division, the DNA strand incorporating TG elongates naturally [43]. However, DNA elongation is impaired in the cell cycle following TG treatment. These results indicate that because the ability to elongate the newly synthesized strand is lacking, SSBs are formed in daughter DNA synthesized from a TG-DNA template [44].

Alterations of the geometry of a thioG-containing duplex, cause DNA–protein interactions to change dramatically. For instance, some restriction endonucleases do not cleave DNA within the restriction sites containing dthioG [38,45]. dthioG incorporated at 3′ ends of DNA severely inhibits DNA ligase I–mediated ligation of DNA fragments. This implies that incorporation of dthioG at the 3′ termini of Okazaki fragments would inhibit lagging strand DNA synthesis. Moreover, since dTGTP misincorporates in place of adenine at a greater frequency than dGTP, it can have mutagenic effects [46]. Chemical reactivity of dthioG-containing DNA is also changed. For instance, dthioG-DNA is susceptible to endogenous alkylating agents such as *S*-adenosylmethionine (SAM). It has been suggested that the cytotoxicity of 6-thioguanine after incorporation into DNA depends on methylation of the thio group by *S*-adenosylmethionine to give *S*-methylthioguanine, leading to miscoding during DNA replication to give [methylthioG]*T base pairs and subsequent recognition of these base pairs by proteins of the postreplicative mismatch repair system [47,48]. On a chromosomal level, treatment with TG produces severely disrupted chromatin during phase G_2 of the cell cycle, as visualized by premature chromosome condensation [49]. The chromatid damage is a dose-related effect, appearing as sharp curling or "kinking" of chromatid at lower TG concentrations and as unilateral chromatid damage and gross chromosome disruption at higher TG concentrations [50].

Substantial evidence indicates that the principal mechanism of thiopurine cytotoxicity is triggered by thioguanine incorporation into DNA. The cytotoxic effects of MP and TG are delayed by an irreversible block of cells in the G_2 phase of the cell cycle, after TG incorporation into DNA [32,33,51]. This arrest in G_2 may be due to DNA strand breaks and the physical disruption of chromatin [42,49–51]. The time and dose relationship between the appearance of toxicity and of unilateral chromatid damage suggests that these two phenomena are related [51]. Effects of TG on RNA have also been investigated, but its role in cytotoxicity is not well defined [17,36,52,53]. One interesting mechanism found in cell culture is TG incorporation into RNA by a substitution mechanism, since it obviates the HPRT-mediated phosphoribosylation pathway [54]. Evidently, TG is directly incorporated into tRNA by queuine tRNA-phosphoribosyltransferase.

8.3.2.3 Determinants of MP/TG Cytotoxicity

A critical determinant of thiopurine toxicity is intracellular concentration of thiopurine nucleotides in the target tissues, since thiopurine bases themselves do not exert any cytotoxicity [55–57]. Consistent with the two major mechanisms of cytotoxicity discussed above, the crucial active metabolites are 2′-deoxythioguanosine triphosphate (an immediate precursor of thioguanylated DNA) and meTIMP, a potent inhibitor of the PRPP-amidotransferase. Therefore, ability to measure the content of these two thiopurine derivatives is instrumental for correlation studies aimed to support either of these hypothetical mechanisms of thiopurine activity.

Because of low concentrations of TGN in target tissues and the inability to sample tumor tissue in most patients, erythrocyte (RBC) levels of thioguanosine nucleotides (TGN) was suggested as a surrogate measure of thiopurine tissue accumulation [58]. Interpatient variability of RBC TGN concentration and its clinical importance was assessed in a study of 120 pediatric patients with acute lymphoblastic leukemia (ALL) [59]. After 49 months, of the patients who relapsed, 89% (17 of 19) had RBC TGN below the population median (275 pmol of TGN per 8×10^8 RBC). This finding suggested a minimum target thiopurine concentration in the indicator tissue (RBC), to avoid a higher risk of relapse in childhood ALL. Since most TPMT-deficient patients with severe hematopoietic toxicity have RBC TGN concentrations exceeding 2000 pmol/8×10^8 RBC, one can consider ~1500–2000 pmol/8×10^8 RBC as the upper range for TGN concentrations, to avoid severe toxicity in most patients. Because of gross interpatient variability of the observed TGN concentration as well as the distinctly different metabolism pathways and regulatory mechanisms in the indicators (RBC) and target (lymphoblast) cells, the optimal target concentrations of

TGN remains elusive, as do determinants of thiopurine resistance in leukemia cells.

In addition to measuring tissue TGN levels, it is possible to assess the activity of enzymes involved in interconversion of thiopurine. Moreover, when a correlation between the amount of messenger RNA and enzymatic activity exists, very sensitive assays [e.g., reverse transcriptase–polymerase chain reaction (RT-PCR)] can be established to estimate these activities. This approach, though indirect, makes it potentially feasible to conduct clinical studies even when the amount of patient tissue is small. Several such studies have been performed to assess correlation between corresponding enzymatic activities and the therapeutic outcome of thiopurine therapy.

Inactivation of HPRT in cell lines treated with TG or MP is considered to be a common mechanism of thiopurine resistance [34,60]. Consistent with this, decreased HPRT activity was hypothesized to be an important factor of resistance to MP therapy. Unexpectedly, no clear correlation was found between HPRT activity and in vitro sensitivity to TG in a group of patients with B-lineage ALL. Though low HPRT activities correlated with poorer prognosis in pre-B ALL, no correlation was found between HPRT activity and in vitro resistance to TG [61]. Similarly, no or only weak correlation was found between enzymatic activities of 5′-nucleotidase, alkaline phosphatase, purine nucleoside phosphorylase, and adenosine deaminase, and in vitro resistance to tiopurines [62,63]. In contrast, elevated phosphatase activity was found in human leukemia cell lines resistant to 6-thiopurines [64].

Clinical studies have established that cellular accumulation of TGN is inversely related to TPMT activity (Fig. 7) [65], presumably because high TPMT activity shunts more drug down the methylation pathway, leaving less for activation to TGNs (Fig. 5). Furthermore, several studies have documented that TPMT-deficient patients accumulate very high TGN concentrations in erythrocytes and presumably other hematopoietic tissues, leading to severe hematopoietic toxicity unless the thiopurine dosage is reduced 10- to 15-fold [66–68]. The magnitude of TGN accumulation in two TPMT-deficient patients is exemplified in Fig. 8, depicting RBC TGN concentrations 10- to 20-fold higher than the median of other patients [55]. The potential severity of thiopurine toxicity is exemplified in Fig. 9, depicting a TPMT-deficient heart transplant recipient who died of sepsis as a consequence of repeated leukopenia due to conventional doses of azathioprine, prior to the post hoc diagnosis of TPMT deficiency [69]. Thus, hematopoietic toxicity following MP and azathioprine is more likely in patients with TPMT deficiency [70,71]. Myelosuppression is the primary dose-limiting toxicity of both MP and TG. Occasional side effects of both agents include mucositis, anorexia, and mild nausea and vomiting.

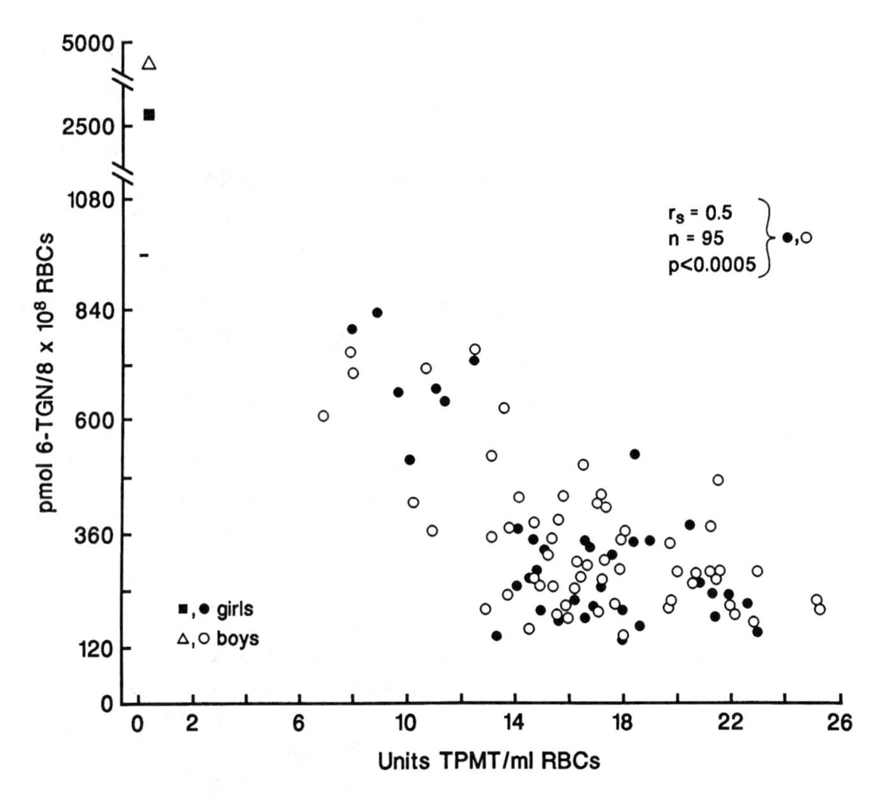

Fig. 7 Relationship between TPMT activity in erythrocytes and thioguanine nucleotide (TGN) accumulation in erythrocytes of children with acute lymphoblastic leukemia receiving uniform mercaptopurine therapy. Values depicted by circles are reproduced with publisher's permission from Lennard et al. (Lancet 1990:336:225–229), while values depicted as squares and triangles are two TPMT-deficient patients from St. Jude Children's Research Hospital (described in Refs 66 and 68).

As indicated above, meTIMP is a potent inhibitor of phosphoribosyl pyrophosphate amidotransferase (PRPP-AT), an enzyme catalyzing the first step in de novo purine synthesis [20], whereas meTGN is about 12-fold less potent as an inhibitor of PRPP-AT [72]. Moreover, meMPR was shown to be cytotoxic to human epidermoid cancer cells selected for resistance to MP, consistent with a unique mechanism of cytotoxicity for methylated metabolites of thiopurines. Thus, the total intracellular concentration of both methylated and nonmethylated thio metabolites may be important in determining the mechanism(s) by which mercaptopurine exerts its cytotoxicity [73].

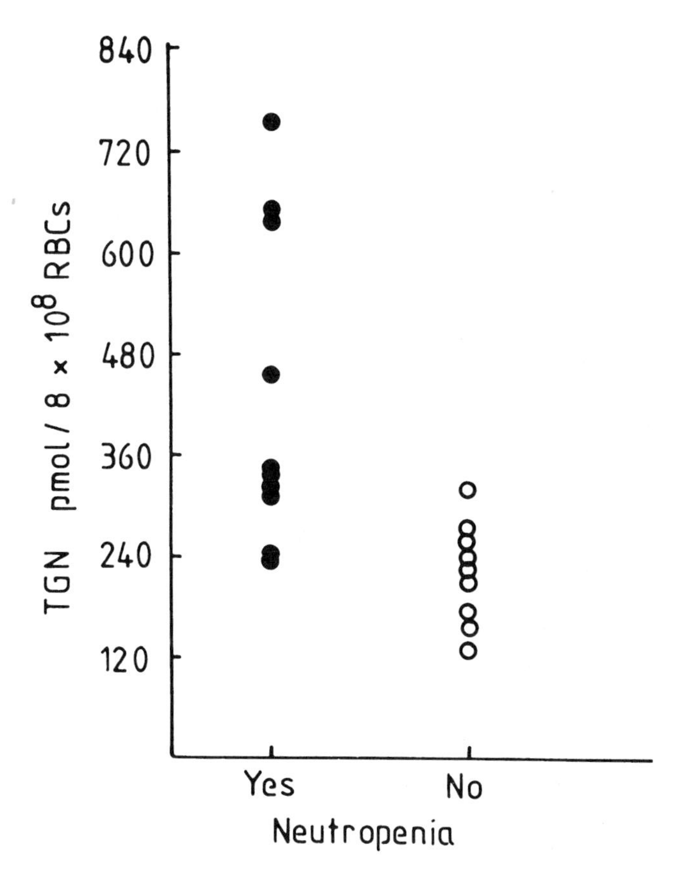

Fig. 8 Thioguanine nucleotides (TGN) measured in erythrocytes of 10 patients who developed neutropenia and nine patients who did not develop neutropenia (<1500 neutrophils/μL) during uniform therapy with mercaptopurine (75 mg m^{-2} per day PO). (Reproduced with publisher's permission from Lennard et al, Clin Pharmacol Ther 1986:40:287–292.)

8.3.3 Thiopurine *S*-Methyltransferase Is a Major Determinant of Thiopurine Toxicity

8.3.3.1 TPMT Biochemistry

Thiopurine methyltransferase (EC 2.1.1.67) is a cytoplamsic transmethylase found in humans and other mammalian species [74]. Using *S*-adenosylmethionine as a methyl donor, this enzyme catalyzes methylation of sulfur atoms in aromatic and heterocyclic compounds. Originally found in kidney and liver of rats and mice, it was shown to be present in most tissues (e.g.,

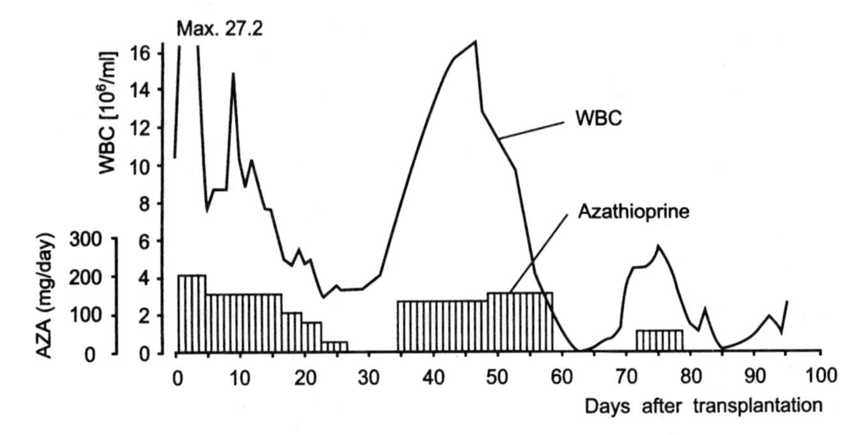

Fig. 9 White blood cell count (WBC) and azathioprine (AZA) dosage in a transplant recipient who died of sepsis during the third episode of azathioprine-induced leukopenia. There was a posthumous diagnosis of TPMT deficiency. (Reproduced with publisher's permission from Schutz et al, Lancet 1993:341:436.)

heart, blood cells, placenta, pancreas, intestine) [74–76]. Human TPMT has a molecular mass of 28 kDa, comprises 245 amino acids, and is not metal dependent. TPMT catalyzes methylation of mercaptopurine, thioguanine, thiophenols, and thiopurine nucleotides and nucleosides [77–81]. Derivatives of benzoic acid and TXMP are inhibitors of TPMT catalytic activity [80,82,83]. Human kidney TPMT has a pH optimum of 6.7 [76], whereas in erythrocytes this value is about 7.5 [84]. Ion exchange chromatography showed the presence of two isoforms of TPMT in human kidney and liver, with similar molecular weight and catalytic properties [85,86]. Given the presence of only one TPMT gene in the human genome [16] and the absence of evidence for posttranslational modification of the TPMT protein (Tai et al., unpublished), the minor peak may represent a complex of TPMT with a substrate or a cosubstrate, (e.g., *S*-adenosylmethionine), although its identity remains unknown.

No endogenous substrate is known for this enzyme, and its biological role remains obscure. The plasma of uremic patients reversibly inhibits RBC TPMT activity to a greater extent than normal plasma and contains higher concentrations of endogenous methyl acceptors than normal plasma [87]. Paradoxically, TPMT activity is higher in uremic patients, as well as in newborns who have not yet fully developed renal function [88]. The clinical and biological importance of these observations is unknown.

Using a radioincorporation assay [84] and partially purified human kidney TPMT, the K_m values for S-methylation were 383 and 557 μM for

MP and TG, respectively [79]. In contrast, an HPLC assay of the methylated product formed by erythrocyte lysates indicated that the K_m for S-methylation of MP was 83 μM [89], while a K_m of 11 μM for MP was found with heterologously expressed human TPMT [81]. Moreover, the V_{max} and K_m values for S-methylation of MP, TG, TIMP, and TGMP were comparable when assessed with recombinant human TPMT [81], while 2-hydroxy-6-mercaptopurine was not a substrate, but actually inhibited the TPMT-catalyzed reaction [79]. Thus, the polymorphism of TPMT affects the metabolism of active nucleotide metabolites of MP and TG, in addition to that of the parent drugs.

8.3.3.2 Molecular Genetics of TPMT

Partial amino acid sequence was obtained after photoaffinity labeling of TPMT [90], leading to the isolation of a human cDNA comprising 2760 nucleotides, with an open reading frame (ORF) of 735 nucleotides, encoding a protein of 245 amino acids [91]. Its identity as TPMT was confirmed by comparison of the deduced amino acid sequence with that obtained by partial amino acid sequencing of human kidney TPMT and by expressing the isolated cDNA in COS-1 cells [91]. Surprisingly, no significant homology was found with other mammalian cytosolic Ado-Met-dependent methyltransferase enzymes, nor were the hypothetical Ado-Met-binding sequences detected in this protein [91,92].

Northern analysis of total RNA extracted from different human tissues revealed three transcripts of 1.0, 1.7, and 3.2 kilobases (kb) [93] or 1.4, 2.0, and 3.6 kb [94]. Hybridization with a panel of human mRNAs isolated from different tissues demonstrated the presence of all three TPMT-homologous mRNA transcripts in all tissues tested (Fig. 10). The clinical and biological importance of tissue-specific expression to TPMT mRNA in humans has not been established, but studies have consistently revealed the highest mRNA level in kidney and liver and the lowest in brain. This observation is consistent with the level of TPMT protein in different human tissues, as revealed by Western blotting analysis using antibodies against a fusion GST-TPMT protein expressed in *E. coli* [95] (Fig. 11). Ubiquitous transcription of the TPMT gene in functionally different cells, even highly specialized tissues such as muscle and brain, may indicate an important role of TPMT in cellular metabolism.

Of interest, Southern hybridization of a human TPMT ORF fragment with a panel of DNA from various species showed the presence of homologous sequences in monkey, rat, mouse, dog, cow, and rabbit, but not chicken and yeast (Krynetski et al., unpublished). Of all the species tested, the greatest similarity in hybridization pattern was found for monkey DNA, compared to humans.

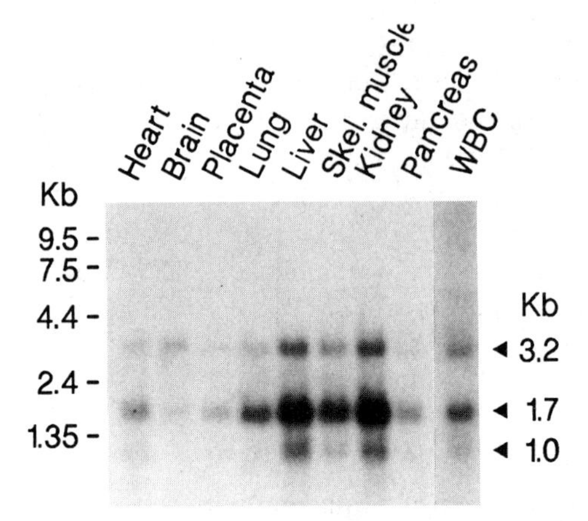

Fig. 10 Northern blot analysis of poly(A^+) RNA isolated from various human tissues and hybridized with wild-type TPMT cDNA, demonstrating the presence of multiple TPMT mRNA transcripts. Each lane contained approximately 2 μg of poly (A^+) RNA. (Reproduced with publisher's permission from Krynetski et al. Proc Natl Acad Sci USA 1995:92:949–953.)

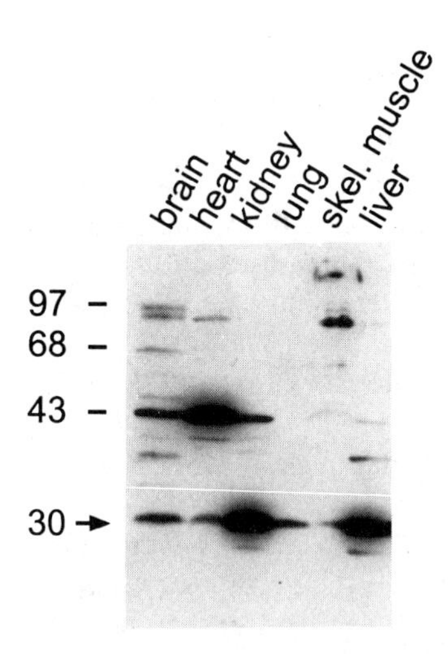

Fig. 11 Western blot analysis of human tissues (Clontech MTW) probed with polyclonal antibody raised against GST-TPMT fusion protein. Arrow indicates TPMT protein band.

Direct screening of the human lymphocyte genomic library resulted in isolation of a processed pseudogene that was mapped to chromosome 18q21.1 [94].

Two alternative approaches based on intron sequences led to isolation of the TPMT chromosomal gene [96,97]. Fluorescent in situ hybridization localized the human TPMT gene to 6p22.3 [16,96]. Though the genes isolated by the two alternative techniques are basically similar in structure (Fig. 12), substantial differences were detected in two regions. One difference is the length of intron 8, which is 1.7 kb in two clones isolated in our lab [97], compared to approximately 7 kb in that previously reported [96]. The overall distance between the 5′ end of exon 1 and the 3′ end of exon 10 in the map published by Weinshilboum and colleagues is about 30 kb, compared to 25 kb in our clones, coinciding perfectly with the 5 kb difference in intron 8 in these two clones. Southern hybridization with an intron-8-specific probe confirmed the presence of the short variant of intron 8 in genomic DNA from 18 of 18 unrelated patients [97]. The same results were obtained by "long" PCR with exon 8 and intron-8-specific primers. None of these experiments provided evidence for the longer 7 kb variant of intron 8. Failure to find the longer intron 8 for this region of the gene as reported by Szumlanski et al. [96] can be explained in two ways: (a) it exists as a rather rare allele of the TPMT gene; or (b) it represents a cloning artifact in the earlier report due to some recombination event generated in the human chromosome-6-specific Lawrist 4 cosmid library. Other differences include additional *Eco*RI sites found in intron 2 and 4, several minor nucleotide differences in intron sequences, and the longer (by 17 base pairs) promoter region [97].

8.3.4 Molecular Mechanisms of TPMT Inactivation

8.3.4.1 Variability of TPMT Activity in Humans

Activity of TPMT in humans exhibits polymorphism, which first was detected in 1980 [98]. It has been established that TPMT polymorphism is inherited as an autosomal codominant trait, with about 10% of Caucasian and African-American population having intermediate activity and 1 in 300 inheriting TPMT deficiency. TPMT deficiency results from the presence of two inactive alleles at the *TPMT* locus, and molecular mechanisms of TPMT deficiency are discussed below.

TPMT activity demonstrates significant differences among some ethnic groups. For example, racial differences in TPMT activity have been observed in the Saami population of northern Norway, where erythrocyte TPMT activity is higher compared with white subjects [99]. In a black population in Florida, TPMT activity was reported to be 33% lower than in early reports

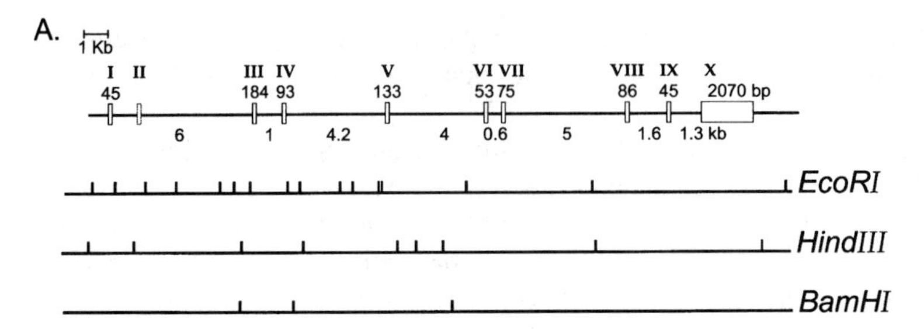

Fig. 12 Human *TPMT* gene structure and restriction maps. Boxes depict exons in the gene. TPMT exon lengths are shown in base pairs and the intron lengths are shown in kilobases. (Reproduced with publisher's permission from Krynetski et al. Pharm Res 1997:14:1672–1678.)

of white populations [100]. A smaller difference was observed in a more recent study comparing white and black Americans, with black subjects having 17% lower TPMT activity, but a similar proportion of high- and intermediate-activity phenotypes in the two populations [101]. Evidently, these differences, similar to other drug-metabolizing enzymes, stem from the relative frequencies of alleles encoding an enzyme with decreased or increased activity [102,103], but to date there have been no published studies of ethnic differences in TPMT alleles.

8.3.4.2 Genetic Polymorphism of TPMT

The initial finding of Weinshilboum and Sladek indicating the hereditary nature of TPMT deficiency in humans has been further substantiated by the recent identification of inactivating mutations in the human TPMT gene [93,95,96,104]. The "wild-type" allele is designated *TPMT*1*, and the allele with a T474C silent mutation that does not lead to any change in enzymatic activity has been designated *TPMT*1S* [105]. Currently, eight variant alleles for low levels of enzymatic activity have been reported (Fig. 13). These alleles contain point mutations leading to amino acid substitutions (*TPMT*2*, **3A*, **3B*, **3C*, **3D*, **5*, **6*), formation of a premature stop codon (*TPMT*3D*), or destruction of a splice site (*TPMT*4*). Consequences of amino acid substitutions in alleles **2*, **3A*, **3B*, and **3C* have been extensively characterized in both in vitro and in vivo experiments [95,106].

The G-to-C transversion present in the *TPMT*2* allele results in an Ala80Pro substitution [93]. Evidently, this mutation results in alteration of the three-dimensional protein structure as a result of substitution of a rigid proline for the rather flexible alanine residue. This is illustrated by the two-dimensional plot of the TPMT folding pattern calculated according to the

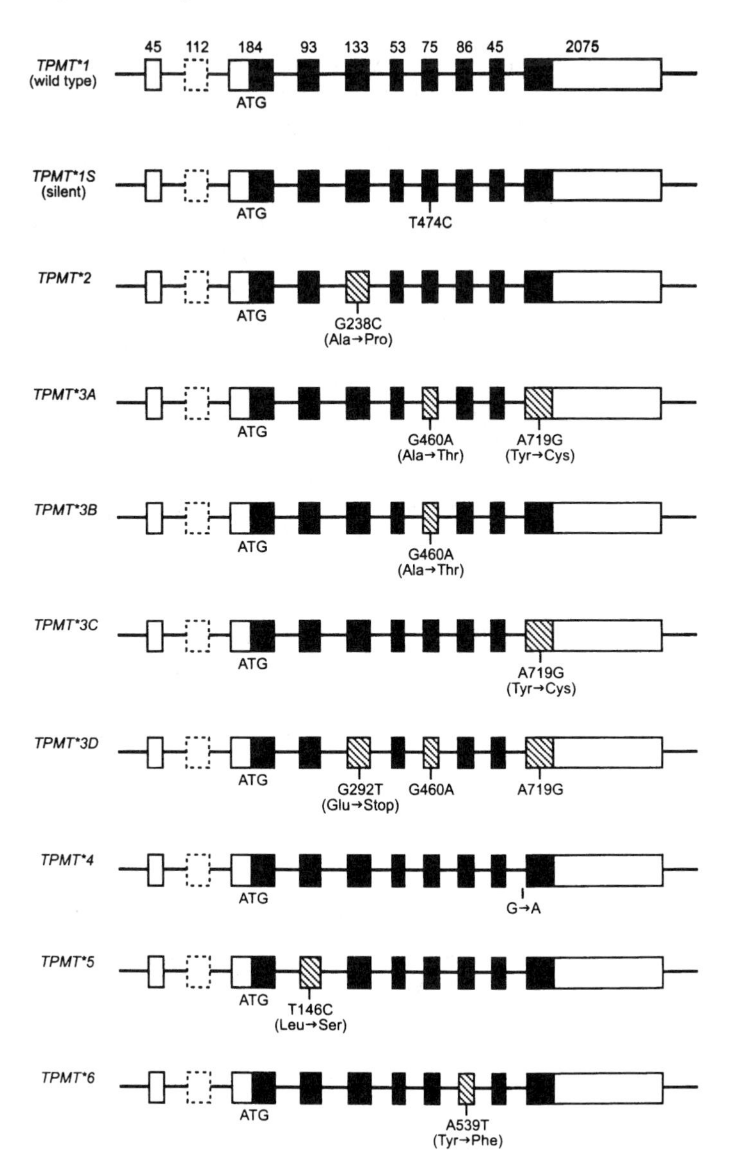

Fig. 13 Allelic variants at the human thiopurine *S*-methylotransferase (*TPMT*) locus. Boxes depict exons in the human *TPMT* gene. White boxes are untranslated regions, and black boxes represent exons in the open reading frame. Hatched boxes represent exons that contain mutations that result in changes of amino acids. The dashed box represents exon 2, which was detected in one of 16 human liver cDNAs (From Ref. 96.)

Chou–Fasman algorithm (Fig. 14). The region of the protein containing the Ala80Pro substitution has an additional turn compared to the wild-type *TPMT* structure. *TPMT*3A* mutant allele contains two nucleotide transition mutations (G460A and A719G) in the ORF, leading to the amino acid substitutions Ala154Thr and Tyr240Cys [95,96]. Heterologous expression of the *TPMT*2* and **3A* cDNA in yeast produced TPMT mRNA levels comparable to wild type, indicating that these mutations have no significant impact on transcription. However, the TPMT protein level was about 100-fold less in yeast expressing *TPMT2* and 400-fold less in yeast expressing *TPMT*3A*, compared to the wild-type cDNA, indicating a posttranscriptional mechanism for the loss of TPMT activity (see below).

A definite subpopulation of patients with heterozygous TPMT phenotype was found to have *TPMT* alleles with either the 460 or the 719 mutation [104,105], (Loennechen et al., submitted). The allele with the only mutation at position 460 was designated *TPMT*3B* and that with G719A transversion was designated *TPMT*3C*. Another inactive allele (*TPMT*3D*), found in a phenotypically heterozygous patient, contains mutations at both 460 and 719 positions, and a G292T transversion that results in a change of Glu98 to a stop codon within exon 5 [104]. Though the transcription of this allele has not been confirmed by direct sequencing of cDNA, it was assumed that this new mutation is present on the same allele as the 460 and 719 polymorphisms. Allele *TPMT*3D* and allele *TPMT*5* (T146C transition leading to

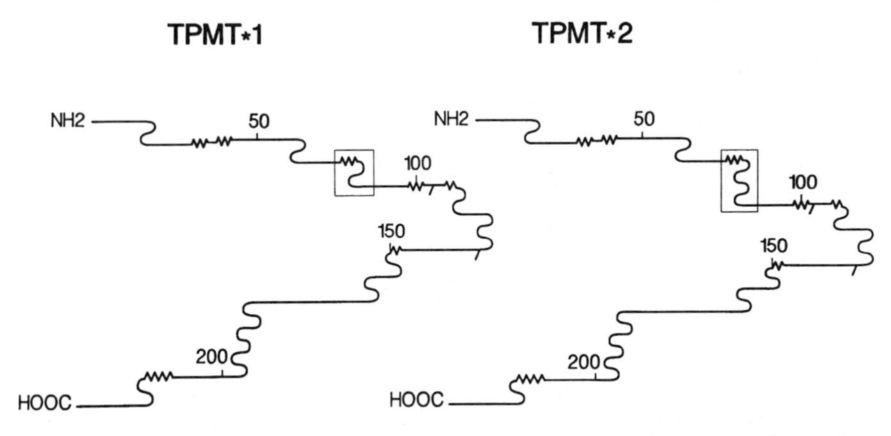

Fig. 14 Chou–Fasman prediction of the *TPMT* secondary structure. *Left panel:* wild-type *TPMT*. *Right panel: TPMT*2*, mutant *TPMT* with G238C point mutation leading to Ala80Pro change at codon 80. Additional turn due to Ala80Pro substitution is depicted in the region enclosed in the box. (Reproduced with publisher's permission, from Krynetski et al, Pharmacogenetics 1996:6:279–290.)

Leu49Ser substitution) have been found in only one person each to date, and ethnic origin was not reported in either case, thus precluding estimation of their frequency [104]. An allele *TPMT*4*, containing a mutation at the splice site for the intron 9–exon 10 junction, has also been described in a person of unreported ethnic origin [107]. If expressed, this mutation would result in an aberrantly spliced mRNA. The most common nonfunctional TPMT allele in U.S. white population is TPMR*3C [105], accounting for 68–88% of mutations, while the most prevalent mutations in other ethnic groups remain to be determined.

8.3.4.3 Catalytic Activity and Stability of the Mutant Proteins

Catalytic Activity of Mutant Proteins

Heterologous expression of wild-type and mutant forms of TPMT in yeast intrinsically devoid of TPMT activity permitted characterization of catalytic activity and protein stability. Table 4 summarizes results of kinetic experiments performed after induction of heterologous TPMT synthesis in transformed yeast cells. For all cDNAs expressed (including *TPMT*2, *3A, *3B, *3C*), the level of messenger RNA was not affected by mutations, indicative of normal synthesis of *TPMT* mRNA [93,106]. Similarly, the synthesis rate

Table 4 Kinetic Parameters of Substrate (MP) and Cosubstrate (SAM)[a] for S-Methylation of MP Catalyzed by Human TPMT cDNAs Expressed in Yeast

cDNA expressed	K_m (μM)	V_{max} (nmol/min/mg TPMT)	V_{max}/K_m (mL/min/mg TPMT)
		6MP	
Wild type	95.3 ± 5.5	260.6 ± 9.8	2.7
TPMT$_{460}$	4396 ± 1367[a]	958.5 ± 187.9[a]	.2
TPMT$_{719}$	182.5 ± 10.1	338.8 ± 13.5	1.9
*TPMT*3*	ND	ND	—
		SAM	
Wild type	6.6 ± 1.1	173.1 ± 14.1	26.2
TPMT$_{460}$	1375 ± 211[a]	704.9 ± 69.7[b]	.51
TPMT$_{719}$	9.5 ± 1.4	226.9 ± 19.1	23.9
*TPMT*3*	ND	ND	—

[a]Kinetic parameters for 6MP were estimated using 1 mM SAM; parameters for SAM were estimated at 2 mM 6MP. All values are expressed as mean SE; ND, activity not detectable.
[b]Significantly different from wild-type and *TPMT*$_{719}$ ($p < .01$).

of the TPMT protein in yeast, as well as in vitro translation in rabbit reticulocyte lysate, was not different for mutant *TPMT* cDNAs, compared to wild-type *TPMT* cDNA (106). In contrast, as discussed below (Section 8.4.3.3), the degradation rates of some mutant proteins were markedly enhanced.

The kinetic parameters for MP methylation by the mutant proteins changed substantially. Both K_m and V_{max} values for MP or SAM were significantly higher for the TPMT protein with the Ala154Thr (G460A) mutation compared to wild type, while V_{max} and K_m for the TPMT protein with only the Tyr240Cys (A719G) mutation were not significantly different from the wild type. For instance, the K_m for *TPMT*3B* was substantially greater than wild type (about 46-fold with MP, 208-fold with SAM), such that the intrinsic clearance of MP and SAM (i.e., V_{max}/K_m) for *TPMT*3B* was 13- and 51-fold lower than wild type. For comparison, the V_{max}/K_m ratio for heterologously expressed *TPMT*2* [18] was about five-fold lower than wild-type *TPMT*. These experiments clearly indicate that mutations at nucleotide positions 238 and 460 have dramatic effects on catalytic activity of TPMT. Consistent with this, the intrinsic stability of mutant *TPMT*2* and *TPMT*3* proteins was also decreased, in the absence of visible degradation of the polypeptide chain. Evidently, the dramatic effect of the mutations on TPMT activity may be explained by decreased stability of its tertiary structure, so that both catalytic activity and folding pattern are not maintained in the mutant proteins.

One interesting observation made in the course of expression experiments was notably lower level of TPMT protein in yeast cells expressing mutant cDNAs (Fig. 15) [106]. Table 5 illustrates the difference in half-lives of mutant variants compared to the wild-type TPMT. TPMT protein levels were 400-fold lower for *TPMT*3A*, and fourfold lower for *TPMT*3B* than for wild type, while *TPMT*3C* had protein levels comparable to wild type (Fig. 15). The G238C mutation (Ala80Pro) had the greatest effect on protein degradation ($t_{1/2}$ = 0.2 h), while the G460A (Ala154Tyr) mutation had a modest effect ($t_{1/2}$ = 6 h), and the A719G (Tyr240Cys) mutation alone had no effect on TPMT protein degradation in yeast. Thus, the G238C and G460A mutations may result in more disruption of the tertiary structure than the A719G mutation, consistent with more rapid degradation of *TPMT*2* and *TPMT*3B*. Moreover, when the G460A and A719G mutations are present together, as is the case for the most prevalent mutant allele in humans (*TPMT*3A*), there was a dramatic increase in the rate of protein degradation (Fig. 16A), suggesting that there is a greater effect on the tertiary structure of TPMT when both mutations are present, thus making it more susceptible to proteolysis.

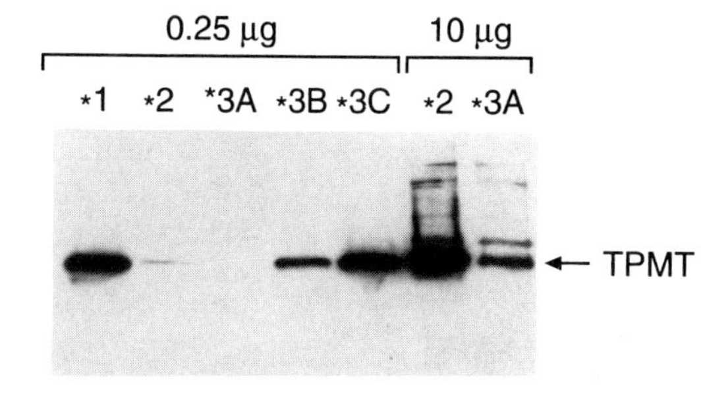

Fig. 15 Western blot of recombinant human TPMT protein in yeast cytosol expressing wild type (**1*) and mutant *TPMT* cDNAs (**2, *3A, *3B*, and **3C*) after a 24-hour culture in galactose-containing medium. The amount of total protein loaded in each lane is indicated at the top. (Reproduced with publisher's permission from Tai et al, Proc Natl Acad Sci USA 1997:94:6444–6449.)

The experiments with transgenic yeast reflect the situation in the human cells: lower TPMT protein was also observed in erythrocytes from the *TPMT*3A* propositus (Fig. 16B), indicating that the mechanism for loss of function results in lower TPMT protein levels in both yeast and humans. Furthermore, as depicted in Fig. 16C, there was a strong correlation between RBC TPMT protein levels on Western blots and RBC TPMT activity in patients with different TPMT phenotypes.

It should be recognized that the natural substrate for TPMT has not been identified, and it is not known whether mutations leading to loss of function for S-methylation of thiopurines will also affect catalytic activity

Table 5 Half-Lives and Synthesis Rates of Wild-Type and Mutant TPMT Proteins in Yeast

	Alleles[a]				
Parameter	*TPMT*1*	*TPMT*2*	*TPMT*3A*	*TPMT*3B*	*TPMT*3C*
Degradation $t_{1/2}$, h	18 (0.4)	0.2α (43), 14.8β (1)*	0.25 (6)*	6.1 (0.3)*	18 (0.3)
Formation rate, fmol/mg/h	335 (8)	409 (9)	268 (14)	349 (8)	220 (12)

*$p < 0.05$ when compared to *TPMT*1*.
[a]Data in parentheses are coefficient of variation percent.

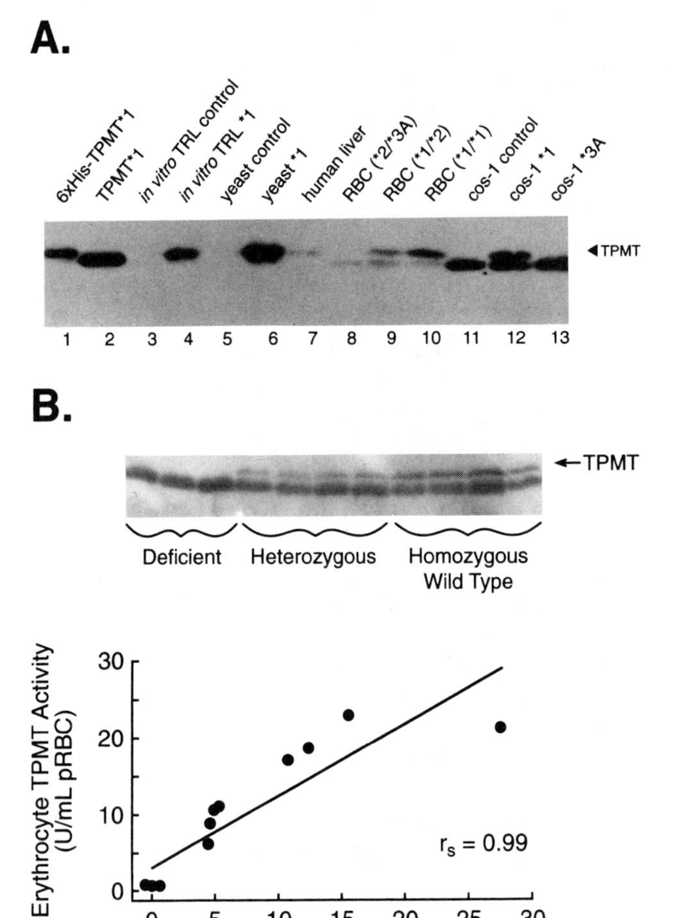

Fig. 16 (A) Western blot of purified histidine-tagged human TPMT*1 protein (0.2 ng, lane 1), TPMT*1 generated from thrombin-treated purified GST-TPMT fusion protein (2 ng, lane 2), in vitro translated control (vector alone without TPMT cDNA insert) in rabbit reticulocyte lysate (RRL) (2 μL of 1:10 dilution, lane 3), in vitro translated human TPMT*1 in RRL (2 μL of 1:10 dilution, lane 4), yeast cytosol expressing vector alone (45 ng, lane 5), yeast cytosol expressing human TPMT*1 (45 ng, lane 6), human liver cytosol (5 μg, lane 7), RBC lysates equivalent to 2 × 10^6 cells from patients with homozygous deficient (**2/*3A*)(64.3 μg, lane 8), heterozygous (**1/*2*)(87.8 μg, lane 9), or homozygous wild-type (*1/*1)(78.2 μg, lane 10) TPMT genotypes, COS-1 cells expressing vector alone (3.65 μg, lane 11), COS-1 cells expressing TPMT*1 (5.01 μg, lane 12), COS-1 cell lysate expressing

Legend continues next page

for its endogenous substrate(s). However, it is clear from the present work that enhanced protein degradation is a primary mechanism for loss of TPMT activity with *TPMT*2* and *TPMT*3A*, which represent more than 80% of mutant TPMT alleles in Caucasians [105]. Therefore, individuals inheriting these mutant alleles will have deficient metabolism of thiopurines and as yet unknown endogenous substrates.

Other Factors Affecting TPMT Activity

Although inheritance is the principal determinant of TPMT activity, other factors may also influence its in vivo activity. For example, there are data indicating that patient age [88,108] renal function [87], and thiopurine administration [65,101] alter TPMT activity in erythrocytes. Moreover, tissue-specific expression of TPMT mRNA has also been reported [93,94], with the highest expression level of TPMT mRNA in liver and kidney, and relatively low levels in brain and lung (see above, Figs. 10, 11). However, the molecular mechanisms and clinical significance of these observations remain undefined.

Mechanism of Degradation of Mutant TPMT Proteins

Western blot analysis of erythrocytes from patients with different TPMT phenotypes demonstrated strong correlation between TPMT activity and the level of TPMT protein (Fig. 16C). Moreover, the level of TPMT protein detected in yeast cells expressing wild-type and mutant forms of TPMT also revealed decreased amount of mutant proteins. Taken together with data on synthesis rates of wild-type versus mutant mRNA and TPMT protein, these data suggest that amino acid changes in the TPMT polypeptide chain result in increased proteolysis of these mutant proteins. Though it is not unusual for mutant proteins to have decreased stability within cells, mutant forms of some enzymes (e.g., p53, CFTR, steroid 21-hydroxylase) demonstrate greater stability than wild-type proteins [109–111]. Two major proteolytic pathways are responsible for the degradation of proteins in eukaryotic cells: an ATP-dependent proteasomal pathway and an ATP-independent lysosomal pathway [112,113]. Incubation of yeast cells expressing mutant forms of TPMT with chloroquine, a strong inhibitor of lysosomal metabolism, did

---

TPMT*3A (4.7 μg, lane 13). (B) Western blot of TPMT protein in RBC lysates, and correlation of erythrocyte TPMT activity and protein in 11 individuals with different TPMT phenotypes. The Spearman rank order coefficient (r_s) was 0.99 ($p < 0.001$). (Reproduced with publisher's permission from Tai et al, Proc Natl Acad Sci USA 1997:94:6444–6449.)

not decrease degradation of mutant TPMT [106]. On the other hand, proteolysis of *TPMT*2* and *TPMT*3A* was decreased in cells incubated with 2-deoxyglucose and 2,4-dinitrophenol, inhibitors of ATP synthesis. A proteasome-mediated, ATP-dependent pathway for degradation of mutant TPMT proteins was further corroborated by experiments with the *pre-1* strain of yeast with inactivated proteasomal activity [106]. Both *TPMT*2* and *TPMT*3A* were degraded more slowly in the *pre-1* strain compared with the yeast with wild-type proteasomes. One may speculate that after the initial folding pattern of the mutant protein has been disturbed, as a result of intrinsic instability, the partially denatured protein becomes vulnerable to ubiquitination and subsequent proeasome-mediated degradation.

8.3.5 Detection of TPMT Deficiency

TPMT deficiency is associated with severe hematopoietic toxicity when deficient patients are treated with standard doses of MP or azathioprine. Moreover, this toxicity can be fatal, as exemplified by the death of a TPMT-deficient heart transplant recipient treated with azathioprine (Fig. 9) (see above, [69]).

In contrast, a successful example of thiopurine therapy in a TPMT-deficient patient is exemplified by a young girl with ALL who received MP despite TPMT activity of < 1 unit/10^8 erythrocytes [66]. The level of 6-thioguanosine nucleotides in this patient's erythrocytes was seven times the population median, and the child had intolerable toxic effects during post-remission therapy with a standard dosages of MP (i.e., 50 mg/m^2/day). Subsequent therapy with 6% of this dosage yielded erythrocyte 6-thioguanosine nucleotide concentrations consistently above the population median, but avoided high concentrations with unacceptable hematopoietic toxicity. This case demonstrates that TPMT deficiency does not absolutely contraindicate MP therapy if an appropriate dosage reduction is made [66]. The ability to successfully treat TPMT-deficient patients with substantially reduced dosages of MP was subsequently corroborated by Lennard et al. [67].

Low TGN concentrations in RBC have been associated with a higher risk of relapse in children with ALL treated with an antimetabolite-based protocol [59]. Since RBC intracellular concentrations of TGN inversely correlate with TPMT activity, the possible relation of TPMT activity to relapse was studied in a group of 95 pediatric patients. Among them, a subgroup of children with decreased TGN concentrations in RBC had significantly higher TPMT activity, compared to those having TGN above the population median value [65].

It is now common to monitor RBC TGN levels in ALL patients treated with protocols containing extensive MP therapy, and it has been suggested that transplant patients be screened for TPMT deficiency or that TGN be monitored during therapy [68]. While the greatest risk of toxicity is in patients with TPMT deficiency, preliminary data indicate that the patients with heterozygous phenotypes are at intermediate risk of thiopurine toxicity [114,115]. It has also been suggested that the wide range of TPMT activity may be an important factor in determining long-term graft survival in azathioprine-treated patients; those with high activity might benefit from doses near the upper limit of those generally recommended [116].

8.3.5.1 Biochemical Assays

Originally, a method for TPMT activity determination was based on detection of the methylation products by paper chromatography, which was not practical for multiple analyses [74]. Introduction of a radiochemical extraction assay made it possible to carry out fast screening of large populations and, with some improvements, is the method currently used for monitoring TPMT activity in clinical studies [84]. This assay is based on the methylation of 6-mercaptopurine with [^{14}C-methyl]*S*-adenosylmethionine as the methyl donor. With this assay, erythrocytes are typically used as surrogate cells for drug-metabolizing tissues, and a strong correlation between TPMT activity in erythrocytes and other tissues has been confirmed [75,86,117,118]. Mercaptopurine is used in this method as an acceptor of the methyl group, and subsequent extraction of the radioactive methylated thiopurine is used to separate the reaction product from the excess of [^{14}C-methyl]SAM. Though convenient for routine clinical analyses, the extraction method can give inaccurate results with highly hydrophilic compounds that are not efficiently extracted with organic solvents.

Several variants of HPLC assays have been developed that use chromatographic determination of methylated thiopurines formed in the course of the TPMT-catalyzed reaction [81,89,119]. These methods are based on detection of 6-methylmercaptopurine or 6-methylthioguanine formed as a result of the TPMT-catalyzed reaction with nonradioactive SAM, using by UV or fluorescent detection instead of radioactive detection. A good correlation has been found between the established radiochemical assay and the newer HPLC techniques [119].

8.3.5.2 Genotyping Assays

It is anticipated, as is the case with other polymorphic drug-metabolizing enzymes, that this genetic polymorphism is caused by a limited number of inactive alleles. If so, a PCR-based diagnostic system could be developed to identify TPMT-deficient patients based on their genotype, prior to therapy with mecaptopurine, azathioprine, or thioguanine.

It should be noted that in patients who have received an RBC transfusion within 30–60 days, the TPMT activity can be significantly changed if a deficient or heterozygous patient is transfused with blood from a homozygous wild-type patient. This is illustrated by one of the TPMT-deficient patients at our hospital (genotype *TPMT*3A/*3A*), who had an activity of 9.8 U/mL pRBC 12 days after receiving 2 units of packed erythrocytes, compared to undetectable activity 4 months after the erythrocyte transfusions. Thus, this patient appeared to be TPMT heterozygotic based on her erythrocyte TPMT activity, because she had been transfused with erythrocytes from an individual with homozygous wild-type TPMT activity. To avoid similar misleading situations, we have developed molecular genetic methods that are not affected by donor erythrocytes, providing a more robust method to diagnose patients with TPMT-deficiency or heterozygosity at the *TPMT* gene locus (Fig. 17) [105]. These PCR-based methods require less than 1 μg of DNA, the amount contained in approximately 100 μL of whole blood. The reagents to determine TPMT genotype using these methods cost less than $100 and the assay can be performed in a few hours. Furthermore, "DNA chip" technology has the potential to completely automate TPMT genotype determination, once genomic DNA has been isolated from a patient.

Given the importance of MP for curative therapy of acute lymphoblastic leukemia and the expanding role of azathioprine immunosuppression in organ transplant recipients [120], a DNA-based method to prospectively diagnose TPMT deficiency offers a clinically important strategy to minimize the risk of potentially life-threatening hematopoietic toxicity in patients treated with these medications. To date, it has become possible to detect the presence of TPMT-inactivating mutations with more than 95% concordance between genotype and phenotype in American white subjects. This impressive level of concordance demonstrates the feasibility of genotyping technique in detecting genetic polymorphisms, but also indicates the existence of additional mutant alleles of TPMT yet to be found. With further studies (e.g., more broad screening of TPMT-deficient white population and studies in populations with a different genetic background), more reliable detection of deficient TPMT genotypes should soon be possible. It will also be im-

Fig. 17 Schematic of PCR-based methods to detect G238C (A), G460A (B), and A719G (C) mutations at the human *TPMT* gene locus. The bottom of each panel is an ethidium bromide stained gel depicting DNA-amplified fragments for each of the genotype and PCR conditions described. (Reproduced with publisher's permission from Yates et al, Ann Intern Med 1997:126:608–614.)

A. Detection of *TPMT* G238C

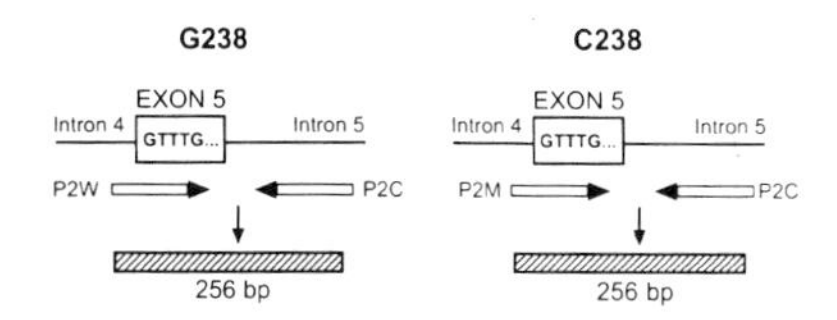

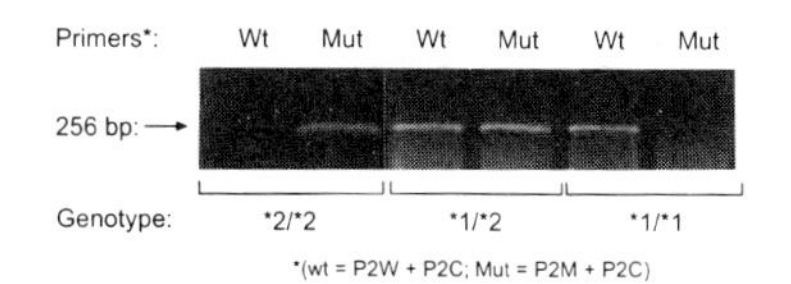

B. Detection of *TPMT* G460A

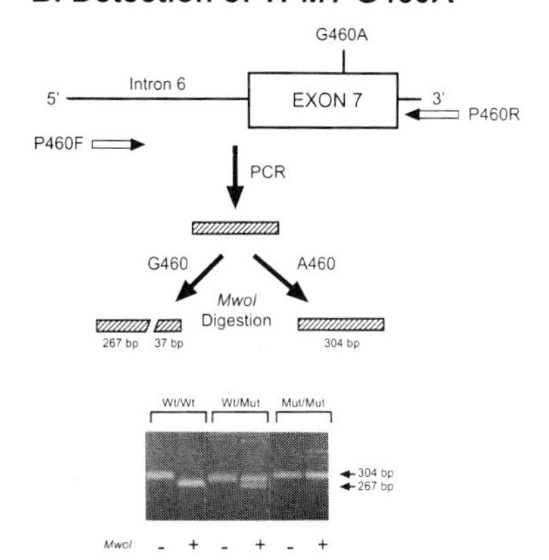

C. Detection of *TPMT* A719G

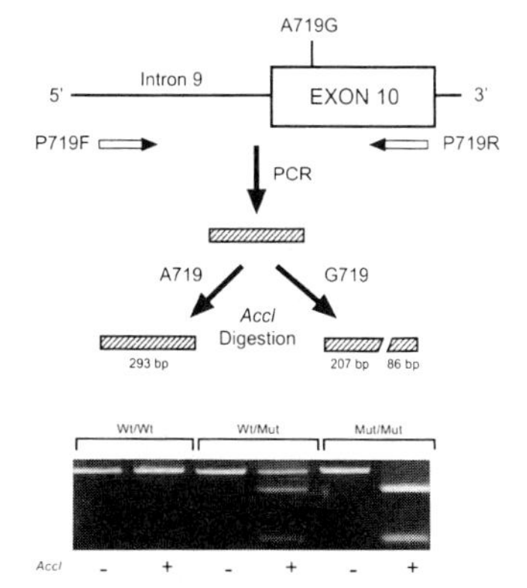

portant to determine whether these mutant alleles are the most prevalent in other racial groups, and to assess the utility of these methods in other populations. Preliminary data from a small group of African Americans (n = 9) with intermediate TPMT activity, indicates that the same TPMT mutations (i.e., G238C, G460A, and A719G) are present in the majority of heterozygotes in this ethnic group. However, the *TPMT*3C* allele was found in four of nine African Americans with heterozygous phenotypes, suggesting that this allele may be more prevalent in this ethnic group.

8.3.5.3 Immunoassays

Good correlation between enzymatic activity and TPMT protein levels has been found in different populations [88,95], providing a rationale for developing a TPMT immunoassay. The mechanisms underlying this correlation were discussed in Section 8.3.4.3. Though monoclonal antibodies for TPMT are currently unavailable, antibody raised against the partially purified protein of a recombinant fusion protein demonstrated reasonable selectivity [88,95] (Loennechen et al., submitted). The protein products of the most common mutant alleles, *TPMT*2* and *TPMT*3A*, have significantly decreased protein stability, therefore, a decreased level of protein can be detected using one of the well-developed immunoassay techniques. Spurious results with immunoassays can be produced by heterozygous RBC transfusions, as is the case for TPMT activity assays, and immunoassays could be misleading if mutations are found that produce nonfunctional but stable TPMT proteins. Nonetheless, since none of the existing methods (activity, immunoassay, genotype) are perfect, immunoassays represent a potential screening tool for identifying TPMT-deficient patients.

8.3.6 Future Prospects

Today, thiopurine *S*-methyltransferase is a classical example of a polymorphic enzyme that determines adverse effects of chemotherapy. Characterization of the molecular mechanisms of this genetically inherited trait made it possible to accurately identify patients who are at high risk of toxicity, thereby providing a rational way of choosing dosages of these important antileukemic and immunosuppressive medications. Nonetheless, certain questions remain unanswered, such as the biological role of this enzyme. In TPMT-deficient patients there is no obvious aberrant phenotype in the absence of thiopurine therapy. Given that no known TPMT substrate is an endogenous compound in mammalian species, one can only speculate as to what metabolic pathways involve TPMT. It is plausible that there are phenotype(s) connected with environmental exposures and deficiency that have not been discovered, simply because TPMT deficiency has such a low prevalence and all environmental substrates are not known. Another important point is that adjusting the dose of MP (i.e., 10- to 15-fold decrease compared to conventional doses) makes thiopurine therapy as tolerable and effective in TPMT-deficient patients as it is in those with normal TPMT activity. Thus, the same thiopurine medications can be safely and effectively used for TPMT-deficient patients, with proper dosage adjustments. Finally, elucidation of regulatory mechanisms can help to better our understanding of the metabolic pathways of MP and TG in different tissues under defined physiological conditions, which may provide important insights for decreasing toxicity in nonhematopoietic tissues.

REFERENCES TO SECTION 8.3

1. White E. Life, death, and the pursuit of apoptosis. Genes Dev 1996:10:1–15.
2. Parks DA, Granger DN. Xanthine oxidase: Biochemistry, distribution and physiology. Acta Physiol Scand 1986:548:89–99.
3. Hill DL. Hypoxanthine phosphorybosyltransferase and guanine metabolism of adenocarcinoma 755 cells. Biochem Pharmacol 1970:19:545–557.
4. Brockman RW. Biochemical aspects of mercaptopurine inhibition and resistance. Cancer Res 1963:23:1191–1201.
5. Miech RP, Parks RE, Jr., Anderson JH Jr, Sartorelli AC. An hypothesis on the mechanism of action of 6-thioguanine. Biochem Pharmacol 1967:16: 2222–2227.
6. Saenger W. Principles of Nucleic Acid Structure. New York: Springer-Verlag, 1984.
7. Bennett LL Jr, Brockman RW, Schnebli HP, Chumley, Dixon GJ, Schnabel FM Jr, Dulmadge EA, Skipper HE, Montgomery JA, Thomas HJ. Activity and mechanism of action of 6-mercaptopurine ribonucleoside in cancer cells resistant to 6-mercaptopurine. Nature 1965:205:1276–1279.
8. Ealick SE, Rule SA, Carter DC, Greenhough TJ, Babu YS, Cook WJ, Habash J, Helliwell JR, Stoeckler JD, Parks RE, Jr, Chen S-F, Bugg CE. Three-dimensional structure of human erythrocytic purine nucleoside phosphorylase at 3.2 Å resolution. J Biol Chem 1990:265:1812–1820.
9. Ealick SE, Babu YS, Bugg CE, Erion MD, Guida WC, Montgomery JA, Secrist JA III. Application of crystallographic and modelling methods in the design of purine nucleoside phosphorylase inhibitors. Proc Natl Acad Sci USA 1991:88:11540–11544.
10. Erion MD, Takabayashi K, Smith HB, Kessi J, Wagner S, Honger S, Shames SL, Ealick SE. Purine nucleoside phosphorylase. 1: Structure–function studies. Biochemistry 1997:36:11725–11734.
11. Schnebli HP, Hill DL, Bennett LL Jr. Purification and properties of adenosine kinase from human tumor cells of type H.Ep.No. 2*. J Biol Chem 1967:242: 1997–2004.

12. Miech RP, Parks RE Jr. Adenosine triphosphate:guanosine monophosphate phosphotransferase. J Biol Chem 1965:240:351–357.
13. Miech RP, Parks RE Jr, Anderson JH Jr, Sartorelli AC. An hypothesis on the mechanism of action of 6-thioguanine. Biochem Pharmacol 1967:16:2222–2227.
14. Krenitsky TA, Neil SM, Elion G, Hitchings GH. Adenine phosphoribosyltransferase from monkey liver. J Biol Chem 1969:244:4779–4784.
15. Krenitsky TA, Papaioannou R, Elion G. Human hypoxanthine phosphorybosyltransferase. J Biol Chem 1969:244:1263–1270.
16. Krynetski EY, Tai HL, Yates CR, Fessing MY, Loennechen T, Schuetz JD, Relling MV, Evans WE. Genetic polymorphism of thiopurine *S*-methyltransferase: Clinical importance and molecular mechanisms. Pharmacogenetics 1996:6:279–290.
17. LePage GA, Jones M. Purinethiols as feedback inhibitors of purine synthesis in ascites tumor cells. Cancer Res 1961:21:642–649.
18. Scholar EM, Brown PR, Parks RE Jr. Synergistic effect of 6-mercaptopurine and 6-methylmercaptopurine ribonucleoside on the level of adenine nucleotides of sarcoma 180 cells. Cancer Res 1972:32:259–269.
19. Higuchi T, Nakamura T, Wakisaka G. Metabolism of 6-mercaptopurine in human leukemic cells. Cancer Res 1976:36:3779–3783.
20. Hill DL, Bennett LL, Jr. Purification and properties of 5-phosphoribosyl pyrophosphate amidotransferase from adenocarcinoma 755 cells. Biochemistry 1969:8:122–130.
21. Bennett LL Jr, Schnebli HP, Vail MH, Allan PW, Montgomery JA. Purine ribonucleoside kinase activity and resistance to some analogs of adenosine. Mol Pharmacol 1966:2:432–443.
22. Cottam HB, Wasson DB, Shih HC, Raychaudhuri A, Di Pasquale G, Carson DA. New adenosine kinase inhibitors with oral antiinflammatory activity: Synthesis and biological evaluation. J Med Chem 1993:36:3424–3430.
23. Bokkerink JP, Stet EH, De Abreu RA, Damen FJ, Hulscher TW, Bakker MA, van Baal JA. 6-Mercaptopurine: Cytotoxicity and biochemical pharmacology in human malignant T-lymphoblasts. Biochem Pharmacol 1993:45:1455–1463.
24. Stet EH, De Abreu RA, Janssen YPG, Bokkerink JP, Trijbels FJ. A biochemical basis for synergism of 6-mercaptopurine and mycophenolic acid in Molt F4, a human malignant T-lymphoblastic cell line. Biochim Biophys Acta 1993:1180:277–282.
25. Warnick CT, Paterson ARP. Effect of methylthioinosine on nucleotide concentrations in L5178Y cells. Cancer Res 1973:33:1711–1715.
26. Dayton JS, Turka LA, Thompson CB, Mitchell BS. Comparison of the effects of mizorubine with those of azathioprine, 6-mercaptopurine, and mycophenolic acid on T lymphocyte proliferation and purine ribonucleotide metabolism. Mol Pharmacol 1992:41:671–676.
27. Crawford DJK, Maddocks JL, Jones DN, Szawlowski P. Rational design of novel immunosuppressive drugs: Analogs of azathioprine lacking the 6-mer-

captopurine substituent retain or have enhanced immunosuppressive effects. J Med Chem 1996:39:2690–2695.
28. Zimm S, Johnson GE, Poplack DG. Modulation of thiopurine cytotoxicity in the HL-60 cell line by physiological concentrations of hypoxanthine. Cancer Res 1986:46:6286–6289.
29. Hashimoto H, Kubota M, Shimizu T, Takimoto T, Kitoh T, Akiyama Y, Mikawa H. Biochemical basis of the prevention of 6-thiopurine toxicity by the nucleobases, hypoxanthine and adenine. Leuk Res 1990:14:1061–1066.
30. Liliemark J, Pettersson B, Peterson C. On the biochemical modulation of 6-mercaptopurine by methotrexate in murine WEHI-3b leukemia cells in vitro. Leuk Res 1992:16:275–280.
31. Elion GB, Callahan HN, Bieber S, Rundles RW, Hitchings GH. Potentiation by inhibition of drug degradation: 6-Substituted purines and xanthine oxidase. Biochem Pharmacol 1963:12:85–93.
32. Tidd DM, Paterson ARP. A biochemical mechanism for the delayed cytotoxic reaction of 6-mercaptopurine. Cancer Res 1974:34:738–746.
33. Tidd DM, Paterson ARP. Distinction between inhibition of purine nucleotide synthesis and the delayed cytotoxic reaction of 6-mercaptopurine. Cancer Res 1974:34:733–737.
34. Elion GB. The purine path to chemotherapy. Science 1989:24:441–447.
35. Kawahata RT, Chuang LF, Holmberg CA, Osburn BI, Chuang RY. Inhibition of human lymphoma DNA-dependent RNA polymerase activity by 6-mercaptopurine ribonucleoside triphosphate. Cancer Res 1983:43:3655–3659.
36. Tidd DM, Paterson ARP. A biochemical mechanism for the delayed cytotoxic reaction of 6-mercaptopurine. Cancer Res 1974:34:738–746.
37. Lee SH, Sartorelli AC. The effect of inhibitors of DNA biosynthesis on the cytotoxicity of 6-thioguanine. Cancer Biochem Biophys 1981:5:189–194.
38. Ling YH, Chan JY, Beattie KL, Nelson JA. Consequences of 6-thioguanine incorporation into DNA on polymerase, ligase, and endonuclease reactions. Mol Pharm 1992:42:802–807.
39. Goldenberg GJ, Alexander P. The effects of nitrogen mustard and dimethyl myleran on murine leukemia cell lines of different radiosensitivity *in vitro*. Cancer Res 1965:25:1401–1409.
40. Harrap KR, Hill BT. The selectivity of acting of alkylating agents and drug resistance. Br J Cancer 1969:23:227–234.
41. Bases RE. Some applications of tissue culture methods to radiation research. Cancer Res 1959:19:311–315.
42. Christie NT, Drake S, Meyn R, Nelson JA. 6-Thioguanine-induded DNA damage as a determinant of cytotoxicity in cultured Chinese hamster ovary cells. Cancer Res 1984:44:3665–3671.
43. Ling YH, Nelson JA, Cheng YC, Anderson RS, Beattie KL. 2′-Deoxy-6-thioguanosine 5′-triphosphate as a substrate for purified human DNA polymerases and calf thymus terminal deoxynucleotidyltransferase *in vitro*. Mol Pharmacol 1991:40:508–514.
44. Pan BF, Nelson JA. Characterizatoin of the DNA damage in 6-thioguanine-treated cells. Biochem Pharmacol 1990:40:1063–1069.

45. Iwaniec LM, Kroll JJ, Roethel WM, Maybaum J. Selective inhibition of sequence-specific protein–DNA interactions by incorporation of 6-thioguanine: Cleavage by restriction endonucleases. Mol Pharmacol 1991:39:299–306.
46. Uribe-Luna S, Quintana-Hau JD, Maldonado-Rodriguez R, Espinosa-Lara M, Beattie KL, Farquhar D, Nelson JA. Mutagenic consequences of the incorporation of 6-thioguanine into DNA. Biochem Pharmacol 1997:54:419–424.
47. Swann PF, Waters TR, Moulton DC, Xu YZ, Zheng Q, Edwards M, Mace R. Role of postreplicative DNA mismatch repair in the cytotoxic action of thioguanine. Science 1996:273:1109–1111.
48. Waters TR, Swann PF. Cytotoxic mechanism of 6-thioguanine: hMutS, the human mismatch binding heterodimer, binds to DNA containing *S*(6)-methylthioguanine. Biochemistry 1997:36:2501–2506.
49. Maybaum J, Mandel HG. Differential chromatid damage induced by 6-thioguanine in CHO cells. Exp Cell Res 1981:135:465–468.
50. Maybaum J, Mandel HG. Unilateral chromatid damage: A new basis for 6-thioguanine cytotoxicity. Cancer Res 1983:43:3852–3856.
51. Wotring LL, Roti JL. Thioguanine-induced S and G_2 blocks and their significance to the mechanism of cytotoxicity. Cancer Res 1980:40:1458–1462.
52. Nelson JA, Carpenter JW, Rose LM, Adamson DJ. Mechanisms of action of 6-thioguanine, 6-mercaptopurine, and 8-azaguanine. Cancer Res 1975:35: 2872–2878.
53. Kwan SW, Kwan SP, Mandel HG. The incorporation of 6-thioguanine into RNA fractions and its effect on RNA and protein biosynthesis in mouse sarcoma 180 ascites cells. Cancer Res 1973:33:950–955.
54. Morgan CJ, Chawdry RN, Smith AR, Siravo-Sagraves G, Trewyn RW. 6-Thioguanine-induced growth arrest in 6-mercaptopurine-resistant human leukemia cells. Cancer Res 1994:54:5387–5393.
55. Lennard L, Keen D, Lilleyman JS. Oral 6-mercaptopurine in childhood leukemia: Parent drug pharmacokinetics and active metabolite concentrations. Clin Pharmacol Ther 1986:40:287–292.
56. Lennard L, Rees CA, Lilleyman JS, Maddocks JL. Childhood leukaemia: A relationship between intracellular 6-mercaptopurine metabolites and neutropenia. Br J Clin Pharmacol 1983:16:359–363.
57. Lilleyman JS, Lennard L. Mercaptopurine metabolism and risk of relapse in childhood lymphoblastic leukaemia. Lancet 1994:343:1188–1190.
58. Lennard L, Maddocks JL. Assay of 6-thioguanine nucleotide, a major metabolite of azathioprine, 6-mercaptopurine and 6-thioguanine, in human red blood cells. J Pharm Pharmacol 1983:35:15–18.
59. Lennard L, Lilleyman JS. Variable mercaptopurine metabolism and treatment outcome in childhood lymphoblastic leukemia. J Clin Oncol 1989:7:1816–1823.
60. Albertini RJ, O'Neil JP, Nicklas JA, Heintz NH, Kelleher PC. Alterations of the *hprt* gene in human in vivo–derived 6-thioguanine-resistant T lymphocytes. Nature 1985:316:369–371.

61. Pieters R, Huismans DR, Loonen AH, Peters GJ, Hahlen K, Van Der Does-Van Den Berg A, Van Wering ER, Veerman AJ. Hypoxanthine-guanine phosphoribosyltransferase in childhood leukemia: Relation with immunophenotype, in vitro drug resistance and clinical prognosis. Int J Cancer 1992:51: 213–217.
62. Pieters R, Huismans DR, Loonen AH, Peters GJ, Hahlen K, Van Der Does-Van Den Berg A, Van Wering ER, Veerman AJ. Relation of 5′-nucleotidase and phosphatase activities with immunophenotype, drug resistance and clinical prognosis in childhood leukemia. Leuk Res 1992:16:873–880.
63. Pieters R, Huismans DR, Loonen AH, Peters GJ, Hahlen K, Van Der Does-Van Den Berg A, Van Wering ER, Veerman AJ. Adenosine deaminase and purine nucleoside phosphorylase in childhood lymphoblastic leukemia: Relation with differentiation stage, in vitro drug resistance and clinical prognosis. Leukemia 1992:6:375–380.
64. Lee MH, Hunag YM, Sartorelli AC. Alkaline phosphatase activities of 6-thiopurine-sensitive and -resistant sublines of sarcoma 180. Cancer Res 1978: 38:2413–2418.
65. Lennard L, Lilleyman JS, Van Loon J, Weinshilboum RM. Genetic variation in response to 6-mercaptopurine for childhood acute lymphoblastic leukaemia. Lancet 1990:336:225–229.
66. Evans WE, Horner M, Chu YQ, Kalwinsky D, Roberts WM. Altered mercaptopurine metabolism, toxic effects, and dosage requirement in a thiopurine methyltransferase-deficient child with acute lymphocytic leukemia. J Pediatr 1991:119:985–989.
67. Lennard L, Gibson BE, Nicole T, Lilleyman JS. Congenital thiopurine methyltransferase deficiency and 6-mercaptopurine toxicity during treatment for acute lymphoblastic leukaemia. Arch Dis Child 1993:69:577–579.
68. McLeod HL, Miller DR, Evans WE. Azathioprine-induced myelosuppression in thiopurine methyltransferase deficient heart transplant recipient [letter; comment]. Lancet 1993:341:1151.
69. Schutz E, Gummert J, Mohr F, Oellerich M. Azathioprine-induced myelosuppression in thiopurine methyltransferase deficient heart transplant recipient [letter]. Lancet 1993:341:436.
70. Lennard L, Van Loon JA, Weinshilboum RM. Pharmacogenetics of acute azathioprine toxicity: Relationship to thiopurine methyltransferase genetic polymorphism. Clin Pharmacol Ther 1989:46:149–154.
71. Leipold G, Schutz E, Oellerich M. Azathioprine-induced severe pancytopenia due to a homozygous two-point mutation of the thiopurine methyltransferase gene in a patient with juvenile HLA-B27-associated spondylarthritis. Arthritis and Rheuma 1997:40:1896–1898.
72. Allan PW, Bennett LL Jr. 6-Methylthioguanylic acid, a metabolite of 6-thioguanine. Biochem Pharmacol 1971:20:847.
73. Evans WE, Relling MV. Mercaptopurine vs. thioguanine for the treatment of acute lymphoblastic leukemia [comment]. Leuk Res 1994:18:811–814.
74. Remy CN. Metabolism of thiopyrimidines and thiopurines. J Biol Chem 1963: 238:1078–1084.

75. Woodson LC, Dunnette JH, Weinshilboum RM. Pharmacogenetics of human thiopurine methyltransferase: Kidney–erythrocyte correlation and immunotitration studies. J Pharmacol Exp Ther 1982:222:174–181.
76. Woodson LC, Weinshilboum RM. Human kidney thiopurine methyltransferase. Purification and biochemical properties. Biochem Pharmacol 1983:32: 819–826.
77. Woodson LC, Ames MM, Selassie CD, Hansch C, Weinshilboum RM. Thiopurine methyltransferase. Aromatic thio substrates and inhibition by benzoic acid derivatives. Mol Pharmacol 1983:24:471–478.
78. Ames MM, Selassie CD, Woodson LC, Van Loon JA, Hansch C, Weinshilboum RM. Thiopurine methyltransferase: Structure–activity relationships for benzoic acid inhibitors and thiophenol substrates. J Med Chem 1986:29: 354–358.
79. Deininger M, Szumlanski CL, Otterness DM, Van Loon J, Ferber W, Weinshilboum RM. Purine substrates for human thiopurine methyltransferase. Biochem Pharmacol 1994:48:2135–2138.
80. Szumlanski CL, Weinshilboum RM. Sulphasalazine inhibition of thiopurine methyltransferase: Possible mechanism for interaction with 6-mercaptopurine and azathioprine. Br J Clin Pharmacol 1995:39:456–459.
81. Krynetski EY, Krynetskaia NF, Yanishevski Y, Evans WE. Methylation of mercaptopurine, thioguanine, and their nucleotide metabolites by heterologously expressed human thiopurine *S*-methyltransferase. Mol Pharmacol 1995:47:1141–1147.
82. Lysaa R, Giverhaug T, Libaek Wold H, Aarbakke J. Inhibition of human thiopurine methyltransferase by furosemide, bendroflumethiazide, and trichlormethiazide. Eur J Clin Pharmacol 1997:49:393–396.
83. Lewis LD, Benin A, Szumlanski CL, Otterness DM, Lennard L, Weinshilboum RM, Nierenberg DW. Olsalazine and 6-mercaptopurine-related bone marrow suppression: A possible drug–drug interaction. Clin Pharmacol Ther 1997:62:464-475.
84. Weinshilboum RM, Raymond FA, Pazmino PA. Human erythrocyte thiopurine methyltransferase: Radiochemical microassay and biochemical properties. Clin Chim Acta 1978:85:323–333.
85. Van Loon JA, Weinshilboum RM. Thiopurine methyltransferase isozymes in human renal tissue. Drug Metab Dispos 1990:18:632–638.
86. Szumlanski CL, Honchel R, Scott MC, Weinshilboum RM. Human liver thiopurine methyltransferase pharmacogenetics: Biochemical properties, liver–erythrocyte correlation and presence of isozymes. Pharmacogenetics 1992:2: 148–159.
87. Pazmino PA, Sladek SL, Weinshilboum RM. Thiol S-methylation in uremia: Erythrocyte enzyme activities and plasma inhibitors. Clin Pharmacol Ther 1980:28:356–367.
88. McLeod HL, Krynetski EY, Wilimas JA, Evans WE. Higher activity of polymorphic thiopurine *S*-methyltransferase in erythrocytes from neonates compared to adults. Pharmacogenetics 1995:5:281–286.

89. Lennard L, Singleton HJ. High-performance liquid chromatographic assay of human red blood cell thiopurine methyltransferase activity. J Chromatogr B Biomed Appl 1994:661:25–33.
90. Van Loon JA, Szumlanski CL, Weinshilboum RM. Human kidney thiopurine methyltransferase. Photoaffinity labeling with *S*-adenosyl-L-methionine. Biochem Pharmacol 1992:44:775–785.
91. Honchel R, Aksoy IA, Szumlanski C, Wood TC, Otterness DM, Wieben ED, Weinshilboum RM. Human thiopurine methyltransferase: Molecular cloning and expression of T84 colon carcinoma cell cDNA. Mol Pharmacol 1993:43: 878–887.
92. Kagan RM, Clarke S. Widespread occurrence of three sequence motifs in diverse *S*-adenosylmethionine-dependent methyltransferases suggests a common structure for these enzymes. Arch Biochem Biophys 1994:310: 417–427.
93. Krynetski EY, Schuetz JD, Galpin AJ, Pui CH, Relling MV, Evans WE. A single point mutation leading to loss of catalytic activity in human thiopurine *S*-methyltransferase. Proc Natl Acad Sci USA 1995:92:949–953.
94. Lee D, Szumlanski C, Houtman J, Honchel R, Rojas K, Overhauser J. Wieben ED, Weinshilboum RM. Thiopurine methyltransferase pharmacogenetics. Cloning of human liver cDNA and a processed pseudogene on human chromosome 18q21.1. Drug Metab Dispos 1995:23:398–405.
95. Tai HL, Krynetski EY, Yates CR, Loennechen T, Fessing MY, Krynetskaia NF, Evans WE. Thiopurine *S*-methyltransferase deficiency: Two nucleotide transitions define the most prevalent mutant allele associated with loss of catalytic activity in Caucasians. Am J Hum Genet 1996:58:694–702.
96. Szumlanski C, Otterness D, Her C, Lee D, Brandriff B, Kelsell D, Spurr N, Lennard L, Wieben E, Weinshilboum R. Thiopurine methyltransferase pharmacogenetics: Human gene cloning and characterization of a common polymorphism. DNA Cell Biol 1996:15:17–30.
97. Krynetski EY, Fessing MY, Yates CR, Sun D, Schuetz JD, Evans WE. Promoter and intronic sequences of the human thiopurine *S*-methyltransferase (TPMT) gene isolated from a human *Pac1* genomic library. Pharm Res 1997: 14:1672–1678.
98. Weinshilboum RM, Sladek SL. Mercaptopurine pharmacogenetics: Monogenic inheritance of erythrocyte thiopurine methyltransferase activity. Am J Hum Genet 1980:32:651–662.
99. Klemetsdal B, Straume B, Wist E, Aarbakke J. Identification of factors regulating thiopurine methyltransferase activity in a Norwegian population. Eur J Clin Pharmacol 1993:44:147–152.
100. Jones CD, Smart C, Titus A, Blyden G, Dorvil M, Nwadike N. Thiopurine methyltransferase activity in a sample population of black subjects in Florida. Clin Pharmacol Ther 1993:53:348–353.
101. McLeod HL, Lin JS, Scott EP, Pui CH, Evans WE. Thiopurine methyltransferase activity in American white subjects and black subjects. Clin Pharmacol Ther 1994:55:15–20.

102. Evans WE, Relling MV, Rahman A, McLeod HL, Scott EP, Lin JS. Genetic basis for a lower prevalence of deficient CYP2D6 oxidative drug metabolism phenotypes in black Americans. J Clin Invest 1993:91:2150–2154.
103. Meyer UA, Zanger UM. Molecular mechanisms of genetic polymorphisms of drug metabolism. Annu Rev Pharmacol Toxicol 1997:37:269–296.
104. Otterness D, Szumlanski C, Lennard L, Klemetsdal B, Aarbakke J, Park-Hah JO, Iven H, Schmiegelow K, Branum E, O'Brien J, Weinshilboum R. Human thiopurine methyltransferase pharmacogenetics: Gene sequence polymorphisms. Clin Pharmacol Ther 1997:62:60–73.
105. Yates CR, Krynetski EY, Loennechen T, Fessing MY, Tai HL, Pui CH, Relling MV, Evans WE. Molecular diagnosis of thiopurine *S*-methyltransferase deficiency: Genetic basis for azathioprine and mercaptopurine intolerance. Ann Intern Med 1997:126:608–614.
106. Tai HL, Krynetski EY, Schuetz EG, Yanishevski Y, Evans WE. Enhanced proteolysis of thiopurine *S*-methyltransferase (TPMT) encoded by mutant alleles in humans (*TPMT*3*A, *TPMT*2*): mechanisms for the genetic polymorphism of TPMT activity. Proc Natl Acad Sci USA 1997:94:6444–6449.
107. Otterness DM, Szumlanski CL, Weinshilboum RM. Human thiopurine methyltransferase pharmacogenetics: Identification of a novel variant allele. J Invest Med 1996:44:248A (Abstr).
108. Pacifici GM, Romiti P, Giuliani L, Rane A. Thiopurine methyltransferase in humans: Development and tissue distribution. Dev Pharmacol Ther 1991:17: 16–23.
109. Welsh MJ, Smith AE. Molecular mechanisms of CFTR chloride channel dysfunction in cystic fibrosis. Cell 1993:73:1251–1254.
110. Amor M, Parker KL, Globerman H, New MI, White PC. Mutation in the CYP21B gene (Ile-172–Asn) causes steroid 21-hydroxylase deficiency. Proc Natl Acad Sci USA 1988:85:1600–1604.
111. Reich NC, Oren M, Levine AJ. Two distinct mechanisms regulate the levels of a cellular tumor antigen, p53. Mol Cell Biol 1983:3:2143–2150.
112. Ciechanover A, Schwartz AL. The ubiquitin-mediated proteolytic pathway: Mechanisms of recognition of the proteolytic substrate and involvement in the degradation of native cellular proteins. FASEB J 1994:8:182–191.
113. Olson TS, Dice JF. Regulation of protein degradation rates in eukaryotes. Curr Opin Cell Biol 1989:1:1194–1200.
114. Aarbakke J, Janka-Schaub G, Elion GB. Thiopurine biology and pharmacology. Trends Pharmacol Sci 1997:18:3–7.
115. Relling MV, Lui Q, Pui CH, Evans WE. Are patients with intermediate TPMT activity (e.g., heterozygous genotypes and phenotypes) at intermedaite risk of thiopurine hematopoietic toxicity? Second Thiopurine Symposium 1996 (Abst).
116. Chocair PR, Duley JA, Simmonds HA, Cameron JS. The importance of thiopurine methyltransferase activity for the use of azathioprine in transplant recipients. Transplantation 1992:53:1051–1056.
117. Van Loon JA, Weinshilboum RM. Thiopurine methyltransferase biochemical genetics: Human lymphocyte activity. Biochem Genet 1982:20:637–658.

118. McLeod HL, Relling MV, Liu Q, Pui CH, Evans WE. Polymorphic thiopurine methyltransferase in erythrocytes is indicative of activity in leukemic blasts from children with acute lymphoblastic leukemia. Blood 1995:85:1897–1902.
119. Jacqz-Aigrain E, Bessa E, Medard Y, Mircheva Y, Vilmer E. Thiopurine methyltransferase activity in a French population: HPLC assay conditions and effects of drugs and inhibitors. Br J Clin Pharmacol 1994:38:1–18.
120. Hollander AAM, van Saase JLCM, Kootte AMM, van Dorp WT, van Bockel HJ, van Es LA, van der Woude FJ. Beneficial effects of conversion from cyclosporin to azathioprine after kidney transplantation. Lancet 1995:345: 610–614.

9

Neurotoxicity (Including Sensory Toxicity) Induced by Cytostatics

HANS-PETER LIPP
University of Tübingen, Tübingen, Germany

9.1 INTRODUCTION

Some cytostatics provoke peripheral neuropathy or CNS toxicity regularly during or after therapy, and even more drugs may cause neurologic symptoms occasionally (Table 1) [1,2]. Sometimes the use of these drugs also is associated with sensory toxicity (e.g., hearing loss or blurred vision: Table 2) [3].

Generally, it is difficult to clearly differentiate between a drug-induced neurotoxic side effect and complications due to underlying intracerebral metastases, meningeal invasion, nervous compression by increasing tumor size, metabolic or electrolyte disorders, cerebral infections, or toxic effects induced by radiotherapy.

Although many mechanisms of drug-induced neurotoxicity remain to be clearly elucidated, in some cases correlations between special metabolic patterns and the onset of symptoms have been identified [4].

9.2 VINCA ALKALOIDS

Vinca alkaloids like vincristine and vinblastine sulfate are anticancer drugs with impressive activity against a variety of tumors, including leukemia and malignant lymphoma [5,6].

Vincristine was the first vinca alkaloid used in clinical practice. Soon after its introduction there was some evidence that neurotoxicity rather than

Table 1 Cytotoxic Drugs Causing Neurotoxicity Regularly or Occasionally

Drugs regularly causing neurotoxicity
Mitotic inhibitors: vinca alkaloids, taxanes
Antimetabolites
methotrexate, high-dose cytarabine, 5-fluorouracil, adenosine deaminase inhibitors (at higher doses)
Platinum compounds: cisplatin, oxaliplatin
Alkylating agent: ifosfamide
Drugs occasionally causing neurotoxicity
L-Asparaginase
High-dose busulfan
High-dose carmustine
Procarbazine (intravenous)
High-dose thiotepa

myelosuppression was the dose-limiting toxicity of this plant alkaloid. Because of a synergism in causing acute, reversible neurotoxicity, treatment regimens based on combined vinca alkaloids are generally not recommended [7].

Commonly, single doses of vincristine (e.g., 1.4 mg/m^2 weekly) are limited to absolute 2 mg in adult patients, to reduce the risk of severe peripheral neuropathy. This limitation is based on the observation that a full dose of vincristine (e.g. 2.8 mg) sometimes results in an unacceptably high incidence (>90%) of neurotoxicity without any proven therapeutic advantage [8]. However, very recently this rigid guideline has been questioned because the underlying interpatient pharmacokinetic variability is high and because there are large differences in susceptibility to vincristine-induced neurotoxic side effects [9].

Symptomatic vincristine-induced neuropathy can be divided into four categories, namely, peripheral neuropathy, autonomic neuropathy, cranial nerve neuropathy, and encephalopathy (Table 3) [2].

Constipation is the most prominent side effect in the autonomic nervous system, occurring as a rather early manifestation after the first vincristine dose. Some authors recommend the use of laxatives, such as lactulose, concomitantly to reduce the incidence of constipation and to diminish the risk of an accidental paralytic ileus. However, colicky abdominal pains cannot be diminished by this supportive intervention [1,2].

Symptoms of peripheral neuropathy include paresthesia in the fingers and toes, increased pinprick and impaired vibration sensations, and motor weakness, particularly of the intrinsic hand muscles and the foot as well as

Table 2 Ocular Toxicity Induced by Cancer Chemotherapy: An Overview

Drug	Symptoms and remarks
Busulfan	Posterior subcapsular cataract with a polychromatic sheen (dependent on duration of therapy and total dose)
Cisplatin	Nonspecific blurred vision, unilateral and bilateral retrobulbar neuritis, papilledema, optic neuritis, color blindness
Cyclophosphamide	Blurred vision, keratoconjunctivitis sicca, blepharoconjunctivitis, and pinpoint pupils
Deoxycoformycin	Conjunctivitis, keratitis
Cytarabine	Ocular pain, tearing, foreign body sensation, photophobia, blurred vision (induced by high-dose therapy or intrathecal administration)
Fludarabine	Decreased visual acuity, optic neuritis, photophobia
5-Fluorouracil	Blurred vision, ocular pain, photophobia, excessive lacrimation, eye irritation, irritative conjunctivitis, circumorbital edema and keratitis (incidence may range from 25 to 38%)
Methotrexate	Periorbital edema, ocular pain, blurred vision, photophobia, conjunctivitis, blepharitis and decreased reflex tear production (induced by high-dose MTX or intrathecal administration)
Mitomycin C	Blurred vision; topical use as eye drops (e.g., scleral ulcerations, necrotizing scleritis, corneal performation, cataract)
Vinca alkaloids	Ptosis, lagophthalmos, corneal hypoesthesia (onset is dependent on cumulative dose, e.g., > 18 mg vincristine)
Rare	
Anthracyclines	Lacrimation, conjunctivitis
Chlorambucil	Keratitis (after several years of long-term oral therapy)
Ifosfamide	Blurred vision and conjunctivitis
Nitrosoureas	Mild, nonspecific forms of ocular symptoms (more problems after intracarotid infusion)
Taxanes	Photopsia [flashing light across the visual field], especially after a dose of 225 mg/m^2 [and more]

Table 3 A Classification of Neurotoxic Symptoms Induced by Vinca Alkaloids

I.	Peripheral neuropathy Loss of Achilles tendon reflex and other deep tendon reflexes; paresthesia in the fingers and toes; clumsiness of the hands
II.	Injury of the autonomic system Colicky abdominal pain, constipation; paralytic ileus; urinary retention; impotence; orthostatic hypotension
III.	Cranial nerve neuropathy Reversible transient cortical blindness, bilateral ptosis, diplopia, photophobia; trigeminal nerve toxicity; facial palsy; hoarseness
IV.	Encephalopathy Seizures; syndrome of inappropriate antidiuretic hormone secretion (SIADH)

the toe dorsiflexors. The severity of peripheral neuropathy seems to be closely related to the cumulative vincristine dose (e.g., 16–20 mg) and to the duration of therapy. Sometimes, patients may experience manual clumsiness, a slapping goat, and the loss of the Achilles tendon reflex [1,2].

Cranial nerve neuropathy, which involves the optic, oculomotor, trigeminal, vagus, and facial nerves, may lead to visual disorders and diplopia [3]. Jaw pain represents a trigeminal nerve toxicity, which occurs suddenly within a few hours after the administration of vincristine and usually resolves a few days after administration [1,2].

Encephalopathy with the **s**yndrome of **i**nappropriate **a**nti**d**iuretic **h**ormone secretion (SIADH) is a rare event during vincristine therapy, since the vinca alkaloids cross the blood–brain barrier very poorly. However, after accidental intrathecal administration of vincristine a very severe and often fatal CNS toxicity develops. If the error is recognized in time, an immediate intrathecal drainage may help to remove significant amounts of the drug from the cerebrospinal fluid [10,11].

It has been suggested that drugs like folinic acid, pyridoxine, or glutamic acid might be useful as supportive agents in reducing the incidence of neurotoxic side effects induced by vinca alkaloids [12]. However, more studies are needed for further recommendations. The same is true for the corticotropin analogue Org 2766, which has been demonstrated to ameliorate the neurotoxic side effects of vincristine [13].

A comparison of the different commercially available vinca alkaloids for neurotoxic potency indicates that vincristine is the most neurotoxic one, followed by vindesine and vinblastine, whereas the novel analogue vinorelbine seems to induce neuropathy rarely. In this regard vinorelbine may represent a very interesting candidate in particular for palliative treatment of older patients [14,15]. However, if it is given to patients with preexisting sensory neuropathy or if it is combined with other potentially neurotoxic drugs, particularly the taxoids, worse neuropathy will develop [16].

The pathogenesis underlying the neurologic disorders induced by vinca alkaloids is not fully understood. An axonal degeneration and irreversible damage of the neuronal transport processes has been postulated [6]. This seems to be reasonable, because mitotic inhibitors may impair the orientation and organization of microtubules and neurofilaments within the neurons. The high neurotoxic potency of vincristine may be closely related to its extraordinarily long terminal elimination half-life, which approximates 85 hours, in comparison with 20–30 hours of the related compounds [5].

9.3 METHOTREXATE (MTX)

Regarding MTX-associated neurotoxicity we distinguish between three characteristic forms: acute, subacute, and late. The onset of neurotoxic symptoms can be primarily observed after intravenous high-dose MTX therapy and intrathecal or intraventricular administration of the drug (Table 4) [1,2,17].

9.3.1 Symptoms of Acute Neurotoxicity

Characteristic symptoms of acute neurotoxicity occurring within 24 hours of administration include nausea, emesis, headaches, somnolence, confusion, speech disorder, hemiparesis, and seizures. This strokelike encephalopathic syndrome, which is usually reversible, may also develop after moderate MTX doses. It has been postulated that an embolic-like obstruction of the small brain vessels may be responsible for the onset of this syndrome after subclinical micrometastases have been released by MTX treatment [1,2].

Table 4 Acute, Subacute, and Chronic MTX-Induced Neurotoxic Symptoms

I.	Acute strokelike encephalopathy occurring within 24 hours of administration Nausea, emesis, headaches, back pain, dizziness, somnolence, confusion, speech disorder, and hemiparesis
II.	Subacute neurotoxic symptoms occurring 7–9 days after MTX administration Affective disturbances, focal neurological deficits, transient paraparesis and pseudobulbar palsy; tremor, ataxia; visual disturbances
III.	Chronic delayed leukoencephalopathy Subtle personality changes, progressive dementia; focal seizures; spasticity and changes in consciousness; lethargy; aphasia

9.3.2 Symptoms of Subacute Neurotoxicity

Subacute neurotoxic symptoms usually occur 7–9 days after MTX administration. These symptoms can be characterized by affective disturbances, focal neurological deficits, transient paresis, and pseudobulbar palsy. Visual disturbances may also occur. Very recently, Quinn and colleagues published an interesting model to explain the mechanism of MTX-induced subacute neurotoxicity [18].

MTX reversibly inhibits the enzyme dihydrofolate reductase, which leads to an intracellular decrease of tetrahydrofolic acid and to reduced availability of the one-carbon fragments that are essential for several biochemical pathways, including the remethylation of the amino acid homocysteine to methionine. As a consequence, the use of MTX results in an increase of plasma homocysteine. Under these conditions, however, this amino acid is primarily metabolized to homocysteic acid (HCA) and cysteine sulfinic acid (CSA), which represent important excitatory amino acid neurotransmitters by binding to the *N*-methyl-D-aspartate (NMDA) receptors as endogenous agonists [18,19].

In conclusion, MTX-induced hyperhomocysteinemia appears to be responsible for the onset of vascular disease, including stroke and carotid artery stenosis, as well as neurologic deficits. From a pharmacokinetic point of view it cannot be excluded that the higher the MTX levels in the CSF and systemic circulation, the higher the amount of newly formed excitatory amino acids HCA and CSA. Quinn et al. proposed that the supportive use of betaine may overcome the MTX-induced inhibition of homocysteine remethylation, but clinical studies confirming this hypothesis are still lacking [18].

9.3.3 Symptoms of Late or Chronic Neurotoxicity

Late or chronic MTX-associated neurotoxicity is evident weeks or months following MTX administration and involves an impairment of higher cognitive functions. Persistent MTX concentrations in the CSF may favor the onset of the chronic delayed encephalopathy. This syndrome includes focal seizures, spasticity, changes in consciousness, and subtle personality changes. The neurologic disorders (including ocular toxicity) associated with high MTX concentrations in the CSF may be based on a depression of cerebral glucose metabolism as well as alterations in blood–brain barrier function [20,21].

If MTX is administered intrathecally or intraventricularly via an Omaya reservoir, acute, subacute, and chronic neurotoxic side effects may occur [22–24]. The first clinical symptoms appear within few hours after drug administration (Table 3). The incidence ranges from 5 to 40%. There is some evidence that interindividual variation of MTX peak levels and AUC values in the CSF is very high (>10-fold) after a conventional dose of 12 mg/m^2 intrathecally (Fig. 1). As a consequence, patients with high AUC values may suffer from extended neurotoxic side effects [24]. To minimize this variability, a pharmacokinetically derived MTX dosing regimen has

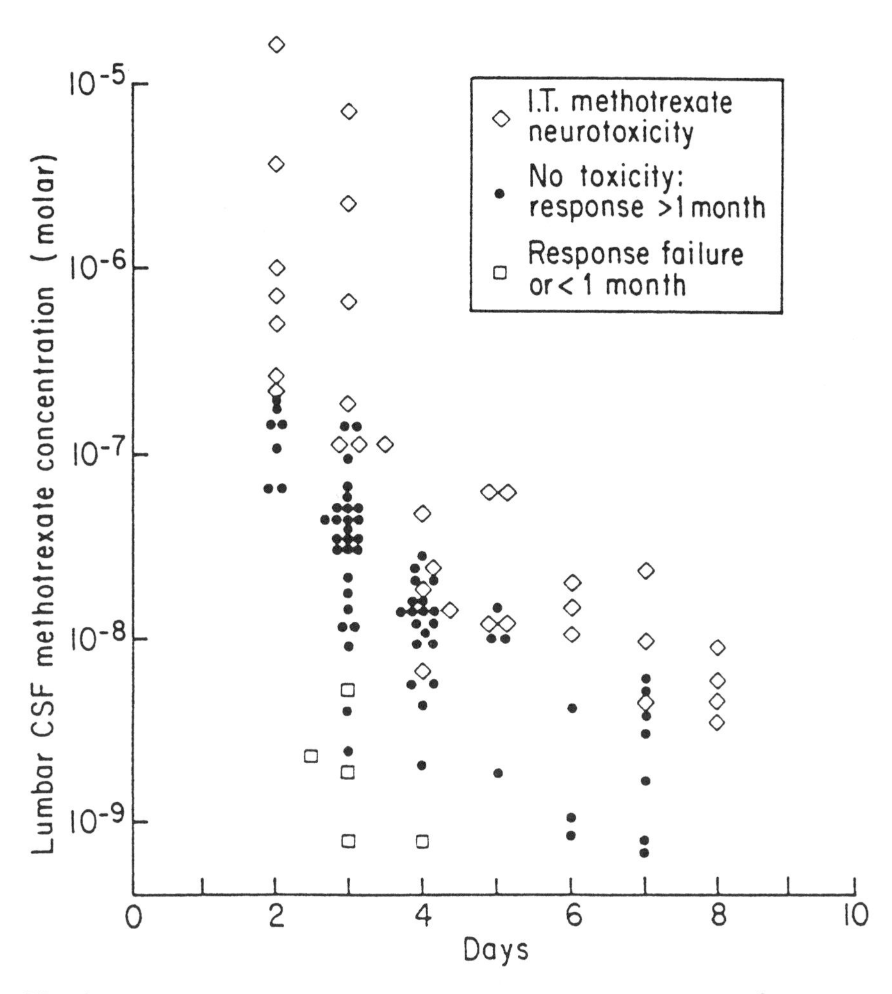

Fig. 1 CSF antifolate concentrations after intrathecal MTX (12 mg/m^2) of body surface area): rhombi, patients with neurotoxic reactions to intrathecal MTX; squares, patients who failed to achieve CNS remission or had a meningeal relapse within one month after therapy; and solid circles, patients who had neither neurotoxic reactions nor early CNS relapse. (From Ref. 21.)

been presented [25]. In cases of accidental intrathecally applied overdosage, a successful regimen consisting of ventricolumbar perfusion and intrathecal instillation of carboxypeptidase G_2 has been reported [26].

The delayed onset of leukoencephalopathic symptoms appears to be cosegregated with the concomitant use of CNS irridation, IV administration of high-dose MTX, and repeated intrathecal applications. The underlying mechanism of leukoencephalopathy is not fully understood but may be mainly based on a progressive disease including the white matter [18,27].

9.4 HIGH-DOSE CYTARABINE (HD Ara-C)

Whereas conventional therapy with cytarabine (e.g., 100–200 mg/m^2 IV, days 1–7) is rarely associated with the onset of neurotoxic symptoms, the incidence of CNS dysfunction may range from 6 to 47% when high-dose therapy (e.g., 2 × 3000 mg/m^2 for several days) is used [28]. A recent meta-analysis identified 227 cases of neurotoxicity in 2196 patients who were treated with high-dose cytarabine (HD Ara-C) [29]. The onset of symptoms, their clinical manifestation, and the proposed risk factors are briefly summarized in Table 5. Usually the symptoms resolve completely within 48 hours or several days after neurotoxic manifestation; case reports indicate, however, that the syndrome may last as long as several months [1,2]. High doses of Ara-C have been reported to induce ocular toxicity including conjunctivitis, ocular pain, tearing, photophobia, and blurred vision. In common, these symptoms last about 7 days. The use of glucocorticoid eye drops has been proven to be effective in the prevention of Ara-C-induced corneal damage [30].

There is some evidence that cumulative dose, age, sex, prior CNS disease, and renal dysfunction may be important risk factors for the development of CNS toxicity, which indicates that individual pharmacokinetic

Table 5 Clinical Characteristics of CNS Complications Induced by Cytarabine

I.	Onset of symptoms between 3 (or earlier) and 8 days after the first dose
II.	Mostly reversible symptoms Cerebellar dysfunction, seizures, altered mental status, confusion, personality changes, somnolence, cognitive dysfunction
III.	Proposed risk factors Cumulative dosages > 27 g/m^2; past history of neurological dysfunction, hepatic and renal insufficiency, age > 55 years

parameters play a substantial role in the development of CNS-toxic symptoms.

After IV administration, the drug is rapidly and extensively metabolized in hepatic and extrahepatic tissues by the enzyme cytidine deaminase, which results in the formation of the major metabolite 1-β-D-arabinofuranosyluracil (Ara-U). Ara-U is completely excreted in the urine. This metabolite, however, is able to inhibit the cytidine deaminase. If renal function is impaired, the metabolite will accumulate and impair the catabolism of cytarabine and, thus, increase particularly the CSF concentration of Ara-C and its related active triphosphate. This aspect has not yet been examined in detail, but in patients with renal dysfunction, an adjustment of the dose of high-dose cytarabine is generally recommended to reduce the risk of severe neurotoxic side effects [31,32]. If the creatinine clearance averages 60 or 45 mL/min, only 60 or 50% of the dose should be administered, respectively. If the creatinine clearance is less than 30 mL/min, high-dose Ara-C therapy is not recommended [31].

In patients with hepatic dysfunction, if the alkaline phosphatase is less than threefold above normal, no significant increase of neurotoxicity is expected during HD Ara-C. However, if total bilirubin exceeds 2.0 mg/dL, the risk of neurotoxicity may be increased during HD Ara-C [31,33–35].

CNS toxicity (paraparesis, seizures) may also occur after intrathecal or intraventricular administration of Ara-C. The acute or delayed onset of symptoms may be correlated with an interindividual low clearance of cytarabine out of the CSF [36,37].

9.5 5-FLUOROURACIL

About 5% of patients treated with 5-fluorouracil (5-FU) may develop an acute cerebellar syndrome, which is characterized by slurred speech, gross dysmetria, ataxia of the trunk and the extremities, unsteady gait, dizziness, and nystagmus. Generally these symptoms resolve within 1–6 weeks after discontinuation of the drug [1,2,38].

There has been some speculation regarding the possible pathogenesis of 5-FU-induced neurotoxicity. Because of the high neurotoxic potency of fluorocitrate in mammals (it causes cerebellar lesions that are histopathologically nearly identical to those resulting from the use of fluorouracil), it was postulated that a hitherto unknown metabolic pathway may convert the metabolite α-fluoro-β-alanine into trace amounts of fluoroacetyl–coenzyme A and fluorocitrate. This "fluorocitrate hypothesis," however, has not been confirmed by pharmacokinetic studies (Fig. 2) [39].

The validity of the "fluorocitrate hypothesis" has been further questioned based on pharmacogenetic studies. Some individuals are not able to

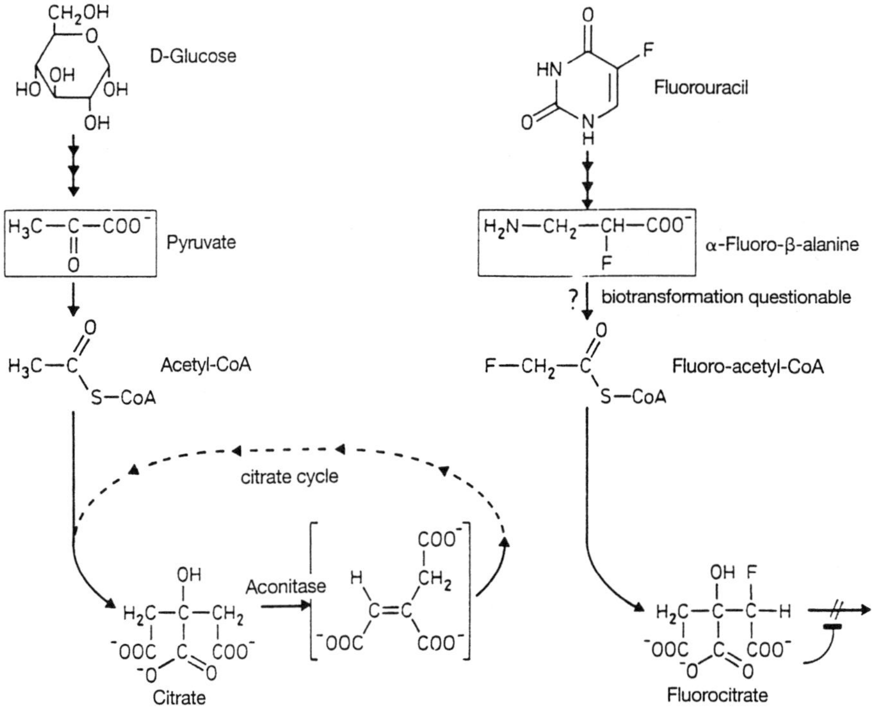

Fig. 2 The "fluorocitrate hypothesis" (for explaining 5-FU-induced neurotoxicity) is based on the theory that 5-fluoroacetyl–coenzyme A can be released during 5-FU metabolism. If this catabolite enters the citric acid cycle, 5-fluorocitrate will be formed, which is a very strong inhibitor of the enzyme aconitase and the overall citric acid cycle.

catabolize 5-fluorouracil significantly because they lack the enzyme dihydropyrimidine dehydrogenase (DPDH). Though they cannot metabolize 5-FU, they develop severe neurotoxic symptoms, indicating that particularly high concentrations of 5-FU and its related nucleotides rather than "fluorocitrate" may be responsible for the development of neurotoxicity [40,41]. There are rather high interindividual differences in DPDH expression, which may make patients more or less sensitive to the toxic side effects of 5-FU [40].

Recently, Lemaire and colleagues brought new aspects into discussion. They detected up to 1.5 mol % fluorinated impurities (e.g., fluoroacetaldehyde acetal) in a commercially available preparation of 5-fluorouracil. Furthermore, they suggested, that an adjuvant that is sometimes used, trometamol, stabilizes such impurities, which represent precursors of fluorocitrate [42,43].

9.6 IFOSFAMIDE

Ifosfamide is structurally related to cyclophosphamide, but differs from the latter in regard to its water solubility, its spectrum of activity, and its toxicity pattern. In particular, neurotoxicity is a side effect that can be observed shortly after ifosfamide rather than cyclophosphamide therapy. The incidence ranges from 10 to 20% and seems to be dose dependent. The most prominent symptoms, usually resolving within 24–72 hours of discontinuation of the drug, include confusion, somnolence, hallucinations, seizures, weakness, mutism, cranial nerve dysfunction, and extrapyramidal reactions. Individual risk factors include low serum albumine levels (<3.5 g/dL), impaired renal and hepatic function, short infusion time, decreased bicarbonate concentrations, and prior CNS disease or cranial radiation, or exposure to cisplatin [44–49].

The onset of peripheral neuropathy (e.g., extremely painful paresthesia approximately 10–14 days after the initiation of therapy) has also been associated with the use of ifosfamide but is thus far restricted to case reports. The supportive use of carbamazepine and topical capsaicin cream may be helpful in cases of peripheral neuropathy [50].

The biochemical pathogenesis of ifosfamide-induced neurotoxicity is not fully understood, however, there is some evidence that the amount of metabolically released chloroacetaldehyde plays an important role [51]. Indeed, in contrast to cyclophosphamide, which is not associated with CNS toxicity, the chloroethyl side chain of ifosfamide can be oxidized by cytochrome P450 3A4, which accounts for about 10% of the total metabolism of this oxazaphosphorine [52–55]. However, because of the underlying high interindividual variability in metabolic capacity, the amount of ifosfamide metabolized via this route may be as high as 50% [56–58].

The most important degradation product of this oxidative pathway, chloroacetaldehyde, is a well-known neurotoxic agent. According to the pharmacokinetic study of Goren and colleagues, there seems to be an obvious correlation between the incidence of neurotoxicity and the amount of chloroacetaldehyde recovered in plasma (Fig. 3) [51]. The hypothesis that chloroacetaldehyde may be the responsible neurotoxic metabolite was confirmed by the observation that the routine use of oral ifosfamide is poorly tolerated because of concomitant unacceptably high neurotoxicity, which is due to extraordinarily high levels of chloroacetaldehyde released during the first pass [44].

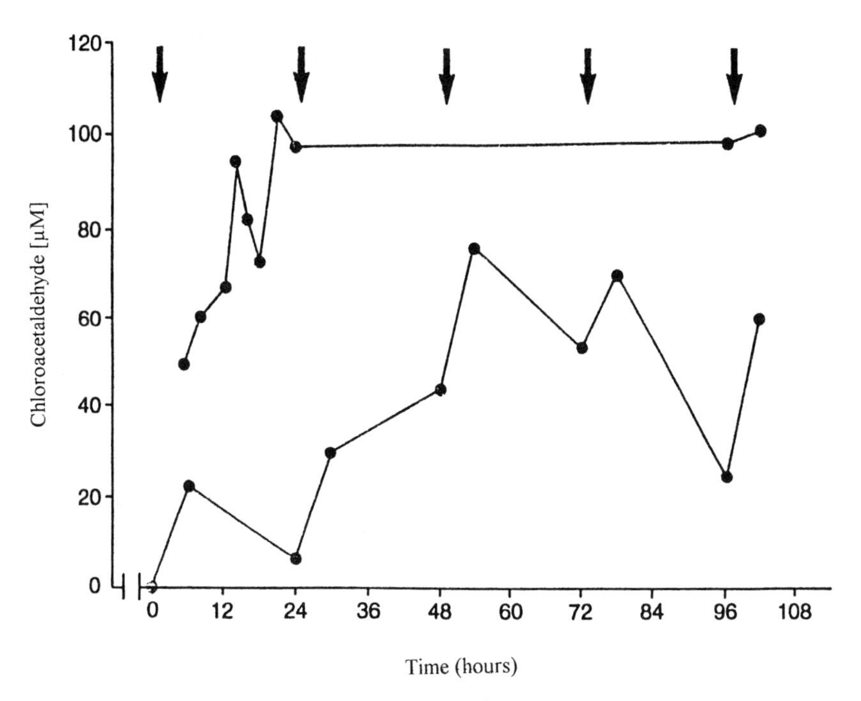

Fig. 3 Goren et al. were one of the first study groups to find a correlation between the incidence of ifosfamide-induced neurotoxicity and the plasma concentration of chloroacetaldehyde. Lower curve: patient without neurotoxicity. Dose of ifosfamide: 1.6 mg/m^2 day 1–5. (From Ref. 51).

Moreover, the possibility cannot be excluded that significant amounts of chloroacetaldehyde are additionally formed by the mitochondrial oxidation of chloroethylamine, which has been proposed to be a hydrolysis product of isophosphoramide mustard or ifosfamide [59–61].

Chloroacetaldehyde, structurally related to acetaldehyde and chloral hydrate, can be further oxidized to chloroacetic acid, which undergoes cysteine conjugation to give carboxymethylcysteine, which is further degraded into thiodiglycolic acid (Fig. 4). After decarboxylation *S*-aminoethylcysteine (thialysine), a structural analogue of lysine, is released and follows the biochemical pathway of lysine, resulting in the formation of some cyclic metabolites, including aminoethylcysteine ketimine (thialysine ketimine). This sulfur-containing cyclic imino acid appears to be a very potent inhibitor of flavoproteins, which could explain the pathogenesis of ifosfamide-induced encephalopathy [62–65].

There is some evidence that the therapeutic intravenous or prophylactic oral use of methylene blue is able to counteract the neurotoxic side effects

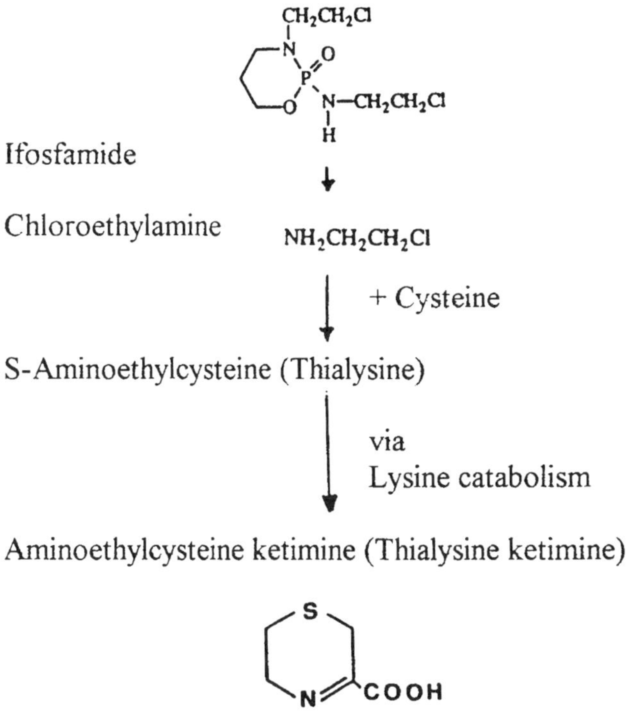

Ifosfamide

$$\downarrow$$

Chloroethylamine $NH_2CH_2CH_2Cl$

$\downarrow$ + Cysteine

S-Aminoethylcysteine (Thialysine)

$\downarrow$ via Lysine catabolism

Aminoethylcysteine ketimine (Thialysine ketimine)

Fig. 4 Metabolic pathways of ifosfamide that help to explain the neurotoxicity induced by the catabolites chloroethylamine and chloroacetaldehyde. It has been suggested that chloroacetaldehyde metabolites may enter the lysine catabolism, which would result in the formation of very neurotoxic ketimines and related compounds.

of ifosfamide. It is not fully understood whether methylene blue is able to inactivate the thialysine ketimines directly, whether it works as a temporary redox system replacement in the mitochondrial respiratory chain, or whether it inhibits the metabolic conversion of chloroethylamine to chloroacetaldehyde. According to several preliminary results, methylene blue seems to be a promising agent (e.g., 50 mg every 2–4 h, IV) in cases of ifosfamide-induced neurotoxicity [66,67].

9.7 PLATINUM ANALOGUES

The incidence of neurotoxicity associated with cisplatin therapy ranges from 30 to 100%. As a rule, cisplatin neuropathy is a cumulative, dose-related phenomenon. About 15% of patients may develop neurotoxicity at doses less than 300 mg/m^2, whereas more than 85% will suffer from neuropathy if cumulative doses exceed 300 mg/m^2. Temporary or persistent neurotoxicity reactions that may last for months remain a major dose-limiting factor with respect to the use of cisplatin in clinical oncology [68–71].

If any progradient hearing loss is not detected in time, speech may be affected and interpersonal communication rendered more difficult [72]. There is increasing evidence that the two most important ototoxic side effects, hearing loss and tinnitus, may be more dependent on the amount of the single rather than the cumulative dose [73]. As a consequence, the risk of hearing impairment, particularly at higher frequencies, may be more prominent if an absolute dose of 100 mg/m^2 rather than 50 mg/m^2 is administered in a short infusion time. Additionally, the hearing loss may progress after termination of the cisplatin therapy [72,73].

Concerning the pathogenesis of hearing loss, it is necessary to distinguish between a cisplatin-induced adverse effect and a normal consequence of aging, because hearing thresholds normally deteriorate in older patients. However, patients with preexisting hearing loss or abnormal renal function may be at a higher risk of developing severe and irreversible ototoxicity after cisplatin therapy. Additionally, since cisplatin is nephrotoxic, it may impair the renal clearance of other potentially ototoxic drugs, especially aminoglycosides [1,2,69,72,73].

Another well-known side effect of cisplatin is ocular toxicity (Table 2) [3,30]. Patients mainly suffer from nonspecific blurred vision, unilateral and bilateral retrobulbar neuritis, papilledema, optic neuritis, and color and cortical blindness. A cumulative dose of 200 mg/m^2 cisplatin appears to increase the risk of developing ophthalmological disturbances. Although blurred vision usually resolves after discontinuation of therapy, it may persist for up to 6 months [3,30,74].

Peripheral neuropathy due to cisplatin is predominantly characterized by paresthesia, numbness, and tingling. The symptoms usually begin in the extremities and may spread proximally later. All modalities of sensation may be affected, particularly the vibratory, and position appears to be most disturbed, whereas motor neuropathy usually is unaffected. Autonomic neuropathy may also occur but is generally a rare event. The same is true for the development of CNS toxicity as manifested, for example, in seizures [1,2,75].

The peripheral neuropathy induced by cisplatin shows some similarity to intoxication with heavy metals like thallium, which belongs to the same series in the periodic table. There is some evidence that the level of platinum within the dorsal root ganglia, dorsal roots, and peripheral nerves correlates with the cumulative dosage of cisplatin [30,76].

Whereas the structurally related novel compound oxaliplatin produces a dose-limiting neurotoxicity, too, the second-generation agent carboplatin offers some advantages over cisplatin with respect to nephrotoxic and neurotoxic side effects [77].

9.8 PACLITAXEL (TAXOL)

The major side effects of Taxol include myelosuppression, hypersensitivity reactions, and mucositis, but significant toxicity to the peripheral nervous system has been reported, too [78,79]. The incidence of paclitaxel-induced neurotoxicity seems to be dose dependent and appears to increase if dosages exceed 175 mg/m^2 or if dosages in this amount are infused within 1 hour rather than 3 or 24 hours [80,81]. Recently it was demonstrated that accidental extravasation of Taxol can induce delayed focal neuropathy [82].

Characteristic symptoms include glove and stocking paresthesia. Autonomic and subclinical motor nerve dysfunctions have been associated with Taxol administration, too. There is some evidence that the incidence of peripheral Taxol-induced neuropathy is increased in patients who are pretreated or concomitantly treated with other potentially neurotoxic anticancer drugs, particularly cisplatin or vinorelbine [83]. CNS toxic symptoms are rare after Taxol administration, probably because of low corresponding CNS concentrations [84]. Very probably the structurally related analogue docetaxel (Taxotere) exerts peripheral neuropathy, too, because a microtubular change in the neuron may be the underlying mechanism of taxoid-induced neurotoxicity [85].

At this point, only symptomatic interventions based on carbamazepine or amitriptyline can be recommended to decrease the symptomatology of peripheral neuropathy [82].

9.9 ADENOSINE DEAMINASE INHIBITORS

There is some evidence that the adenosine deaminase inhibitors fludarabine, cladribine, and pentostatin can induce dose-dependent symptoms of CNS toxicity [86]. Particularly after high doses, symptoms including somnolence, confusion, headache, lethargy, and seizures have been recorded. They are sometimes irreversible and may appear even after weeks and months. At the currently recommended doses, however, neurologic side effects are unusual with all three drugs [87–90].

Factors other than dose intensity that predispose to the development of neurotoxicity are less well defined. Since, however, all three drugs are excreted predominantly unchanged in the urine [87–90], the risk of accumulation and the incidence of neurotoxicity may be enhanced if the conventional dose is not adjusted to the individual underlying glomerular filtration rate [31].

The mechanism by which these purine analogues induce neurotoxicity is not fully understood. Because the human brain has rather high levels of adenosine deaminase, it may be that the higher the CSF concentrations of cladribine, pentostatin, or fludarabine, the more pronounced the levels of adenosine [91]. Adenosine itself exerts considerable neuromodulatory activity, and its accumulation in the CSF has been associated with headache, nausea, emesis, and somnolence. Theoretically, methylxanthines (e.g., aminophylline), which represent a class of adenosine receptor antagonists, should be able to ameliorate acute neurotoxicity induced by adenosine deaminase inhibitors [87].

9.10 HIGH-DOSE BUSULFAN (HD-BUSULFAN)

There is some evidence that busulfan, which can pass the blood–brain barrier to a considerable extent, is able to induce CNS toxicity (e.g., hallucinations, seizures) if the drug is given in high dosages (e.g., 4 mg/kg/d on days 1–4) [92–94]. It has been suggested that the amount of busulfan in the CSF may correlate with the severity of neurotoxicity [94].

Thus, as a rule, anticonvulsants like diazepam or phenytoin are prophylactically applied during high-dose therapy. However, phenytoin does not seem to be the ideal candidate for prophylaxis because it has been demonstrated to be a very potent inducer of busulfan metabolism, which may result in therapeutically inadequate plasma levels of busulfan [95].

9.11 HEXAMETHYLMELAMINE (HMM, ALTRETAMINE)

The use of hexamethylmelamine (HMM) is rather frequently associated with symptoms of neurotoxicity including peripheral neuropathy (e.g., paresthesia, hyporeflexia, weakness) or CNS dysfunctions (e.g., somnolence, depression, dysphagia). There is some evidence that a Parkinson-like syndrome may develop, with prominent ataxia and tremors. However, most cases of neurotoxicity are mild and reversible [96].

The biochemical pathogenesis of HMM-induced neuropathy is not fully understood. However, since in some patients neurotoxic side effects were successfully prevented by the daily oral use of 100 mg vitamin B_6

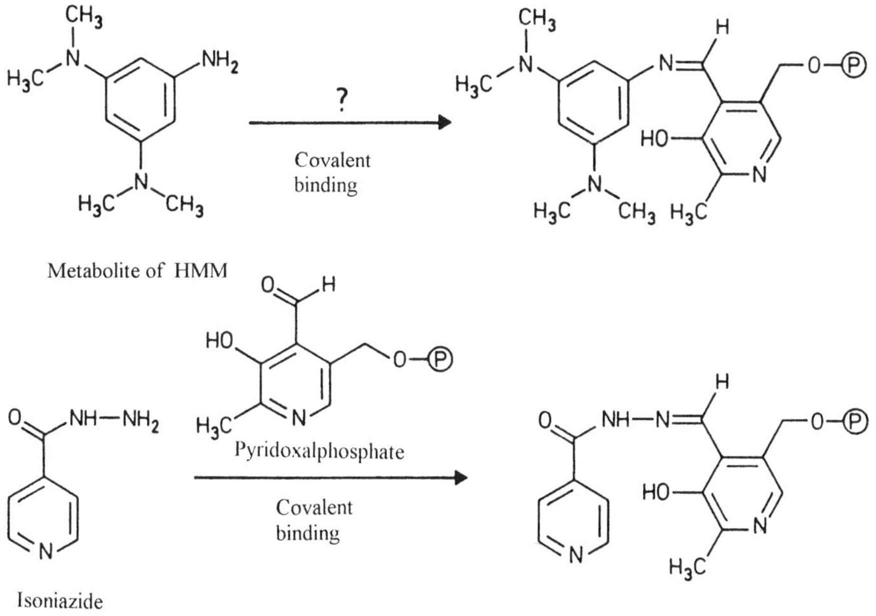

Fig. 5 Neurotoxic side effects induced by hexamethylmelamine (HMM) appear to be related to a dealkylated catabolite binding convalently to pyridoxal phosphate, which leads to a progressive systemic lack of vitamin B_6.

(pyridoxine), it can be assumed that a dealkylated metabolite of HMM is able to bind covalently to pyridoxal phosphate, leading to an inert adduct and a progressive lack of vitamin B_6 (Fig. 5). A similar mechanism has been described for the neurotoxic action of the tuberculostatic agent isoniazide [97].

9.12 CHLORAMBUCIL

Nervous system toxicity is a rather rare event during chlorambucil treatment. However, some patients may develop a chlorambucil-induced myoclonus characterized by jerking movements in the limbs and persisting stiffness [98,99]. Discontinuation of therapy, or dose reduction, results in mitigation of symptoms. The underlying mechanisms responsible for the development of neurotoxic symptoms have not yet been clearly defined. However, these side effects may be partially based on the release of the neurotoxic metabolite chloroacetaldehyde during hepatic biotransformation of chlorambucil [100].

9.13 PROCARBAZINE

Procarbazine is a hydrazine derivative with structural similarity to 1-methyl-2-benzylhydrazine, a rather cytotoxic and hepatotoxic agent. The *N*-isopropylamide side chain of procarbazine makes hepatic oxidation of the hydrazine group more difficult, hence its lower hepatotoxic potency [101].

The use of procarbazine can induce a variety of CNS reactions including paresthesia and psychosis, headache, disorientation, and seizures [102]. Since procarbazine is a monoamine oxidase inhibitor, the CNS side effects may be due to an altered metabolism of endogenous catecholamines after procarbazine has passed the blood–brain barrier [101]. As a consequence, the drug should not be taken concomitantly with tyramine-rich food (e.g., certain cheeses, red wine). Other mechanisms that may explain procarbazine-induced neurotoxicity include the formation of radicals and pyridoxal phosphate deficiency [103,104].

9.14 L-ASPARAGINASE

Adverse CNS effects of asparaginase preparations include depression (or hyperexcitability), somnolence, lethargy, and convulsions varying from mild to severe. An acute organic brain syndrome similar to acute alcoholic delirium tremens has been reported, too [105].

Because of its high molecular weight, L-asparaginase is not able to cross the blood–brain barrier. However, the elevated levels of aspartate, glutamate, and ammonia, which are released by enzymatic hydrolysis of asparagine and glutamine, may indirectly induce CNS side effects. As a consequence, cerebral protein biosynthesis may be severely impaired by the extensive systemic depletion of asparagine and glutamine [1,2].

REFERENCES

1. Kaplan RS, Wiernik PH. Neurotoxicity of antineoplastic agents. Semin Oncol 1982:9:103–130.
2. Tuxen MK, Hansen SW. Neurotoxicity secondary to antineoplastic agents. Cancer Treatment Rev 1994:20:191–214.
3. Al-Tweigeri T, Nabholtz J-M, Mackey JR. Ocular toxicity and cancer chemotherapy. Cancer 1996:78:1359–1373.
4. Lipp H-P. Prevention and management of anticancer drug toxicity—The significance of clinical pharmacokinetics. Jena: Universität Jena, 1995.
5. Zhou XJ, Rahmani R. Preclinical and clinical pharmacology of vinca alkaloids. Drugs 1992:44(suppl 4):1–16.
6. Hacker MP. The toxicity of vinca alkaloids. In: G Powis, MP Hacker, eds. The Toxicity of Anticancer Drugs. New York: Pergamon Press, 1991, pp 151–160.

7. Stewart DJ, Maroun JA, Lefebvre B, Heringer R. Neurotoxicity and efficacy of combined vinca alkaloids in breast cancer. Cancer Treatment Rep 1986:70:571–573.
8. Haim N, Epelbaum R, Ben-Shahar M, et al. Full dose vincristine (without 2-mg dose limit) in the treatment of lymphomas. Cancer 1994:73:2515–2519.
9. McCune JS, Lindley C. Appropriateness of maximum-dose guidelines for vincristine. Am J Health-Syst Pharm 1997:54:1755–1758.
10. Shepherd DA, Steuber CP, Starling KA, Fernbach DJ. Accidental intrathecal administration of vincristine. Med Pediatr Oncol 1978:5:85–88.
11. Slyter H, Liwnicz B, Herrick MK, Mason R. Fatal myeloencephalopathy caused by intrathecal vincristine. Neurology 1980:30:867–871.
12. Jackson DV, Wells HB, Zehan PJ, White DR, et al. Amelioration of vincristine neuropathy by glutamic acid. JAMA 1988:84:1016–1022.
13. van Kooten B, van Diemen HAM, Groenhout KM, et al. A pilot study on the influence of a corticotropin (4–9) analogue on vinca alkaloid–induced neuropathy. Arch Neurol 1992:49:1027–1031.
14. Binet S, Chaineau E, Fellous A, et al. Immunofluorescence study of the action of Navelbine, vincristine and vinblastine on mitotic and axonal microtubules. Int J Cancer 1990:46:262–266.
15. Toso C, Lindley C. Vinorelbine: A novel alkaloid. Am J Health-Syst Pharm 1995:52:1287–1304.
16. Parimoo D, Jeffers S, Muggia FM. Severe neurotoxicity from vinorelbine–paclitaxel combinations. J Natl Cancer Inst 1996:88:1079–1080.
17. Sweeny DJ, Diasio RB. Toxicity of antimetabolites. In: G Powis, MP Hacker, eds. The Toxicity of Anticancer Drugs. New York: Pergamon Press, 1991, pp 63–81.
18. Quinn CT, Griener JC, Bottiglieri T, et al. Elevation of homocysteine and excitatory amino acid neurotransmitters in the CSF of children who receive methotrexate for the treatment of cancer. J Clin Oncol 1997:15:2800–2806.
19. Lipton SA, Rosenberg PA. Mechanism of disease: Excitatory amino acids as a final common pathway for neurologic disorders. N Engl J Med 1994:330:613–622.
20. Allen JC, Rosen G, Metha B, Horten B. Leukoencephalopathy following high-dose i.v. methotrexate chemotherapy with Leucovorin rescue. Cancer Treatment Rep 1980:64:1261–1273.
21. Bleyer WA, Drake JC, Chabner BA. Neurotoxicity and elevated cerebrospinal fluid methotrexate concentrations in meningeal leukemia. N Engl J Med 1973:289:770–773.
22. Nelson RW, Frank JT. Intrathecal methotrexate-induced neurotoxicities. Am J Hosp Pharm 1981:38:65–68.
23. Blaney SM, Balis FM, Poplack DG. Current pharmacological treatment approaches to central nervous system leukemia. Drugs 1991:41(5):702–716.
24. Borsi JD, Sagen E, Romslo I, et al. 7-Hydroxymethotrexate concentrations in serum and cerebrospinal fluid of children with acute lymphoblastic leukemia. Cancer Chemother Pharmacol 1990:27:164–167.

25. Bleyer WA, Coccia PF, Sather HN, et al. Reduction in central nervous system leukemia with a pharmacokinetically derived intrathecal methotrexate dosage regimen. J Clin Oncol 1983:1:317–325.
26. O'Marcaigh AS, Johnson CM, Smithson WA, et al. Successful treatment of intrathecal methotrexate overdose by using ventricolumbar perfusion and intrathecal instillation of carboxypeptidase G2. Mayo Clin Proc 1996:71:161–165.
27. Watterson J, Toogood I, Nieder M, Morse M, et al. Excessive spinal cord toxicity from intensive central nervous system–directed therapies. Cancer 1994:74:3034–3041.
28. Herzig RH, Hines JD, Herzig GP, Wolff SN. Cerebellar toxicity with high-dose cytosine arabinoside. J Clin Oncol 1987:5:927–932.
29. Baker WJ, Royer GJ, Weiss RB. Cytarabine and neurologic toxicity. J Clin Oncol 1991:9:679–693.
30. Burns LJ. Ocular toxicities of chemotherapy. Semin Oncol 1992:19:492–500.
31. Kintzel PE, Dorr RT. Anticancer drug renal toxicity and elimination: Dosing guidelines for altered renal function. Cancer Treatment Rev 1995:21:33–64.
32. DeAngelis LM, Kreis W, Chan K, et al. Pharmacokinetics of Ara-C and Ara-U in plasma and CSF after high-dose administration of cytosine arabinoside. Cancer Chemother Pharmacol 1992:29:173–177.
33. Rubin EH, Andersen JW, Berg DT, et al. Risk factors for high-dose cytarabine neurotoxicity: An analysis of a cancer and leukemia group B trial in patients with acute myeloid leukemia. J Clin Oncol 1992:10:948–953.
34. Smith GA, Damon LE, Rugo HS, et al. High-dose cytarabine dose modification reduces the incidence of neurotoxicity in patients with renal insufficiency. J Clin Oncol 1997:15:833–839.
35. Capizzi RL, White JC, Powell BL, Perrino F. Effect of dose on the pharmacokinetic and pharmacodynamic effects of cytarabine. Semin Hematol 1991: 28(suppl 4):54–69.
36. Resar LM, Phillips PC, Kastan MB, et al. Acute neurotoxicity after intrathecal cytosine arabinoside in two adolescents with acute lymphoblastic leukemia of B-cell type. Cancer 1993:71:117–123.
37. Crawford M, Rustin GJ, Bagshawe KD. Acute neurologic toxicity of intrathecal cytosine arabinoside. Cancer Chemother Pharmacol 1986:16:306–307.
38. Moertel CG, Reitemeier RJ, Bolton CF, Schorter RG. Cerebellar ataxia associated with fluorinated pyrimidine therapy. Cancer Chemother Rep 1964: 41:15–18.
39. Koenig H, Patel A. Biochemical basis for fluorouracil neurotoxicity: The role of Krebs cycle inhibition by fluoroacetate. Arch Neurol 1970:23:155–160.
40. Diasio RB, Zu L. Dihydropyrimidine dehydrogenase activity and fluorouracil chemotherapy. J Clin Oncol 1994:12:2239–2242.
41. Barberi-Heyob M, Weber B, Merlin JL, et al. Evaluation of plasma 5-fluorouracil nucleoside levels in patients with metastatic breast cancer: Relationships with toxicities. Cancer Chemother Pharmacol 1995:37:110–116.
42. Lemaire L, Malet-Martino MC, Longo S, et al. Fluoroacetalydehyde as cardiotoxic impurity in fluorouracil (Roche). Lancet 1991:337:560.

43. Lemaire L, Arellano M, Malet-Martino MC, Martino R, De Forni M. Cardiotoxicité du 5-fluorouracile: Une question de formulation. Bull Cancer 1994: 81:1057–1059.
44. Miller LJ, Eaton VE. Ifosfamide-induced neurotoxicity: A case report and review of the literature. Ann Pharmacother 1992:26:183–187.
45. Kamen BA, Frenkel E, Colvin OM. Ifosfamide: Should the honeymoon be over? J Clin Oncol 1995:13:307–309.
46. Watkin SW, Husband DJ, Green JA, Warenius HM. Ifosfamide encephalopathy: A reappraisal. Eur J Cancer Clin Oncol 1989:25:303–310.
47. Cerny T, Küpfer A. The enigma of ifosfamide encephalopathy. Ann Oncol 1992:3:679–681.
48. Bhardwaj A, Badesha PS. Ifosfamide-induced nonconvulsive status epilepticus. Ann Pharmacother 1995:29:1237–1239.
49. Cerny T, Castiglione M, Brunner K, et al. Ifosfamide by continuous infusion to prevent encephalopathy. Lancet 1990:335:175.
50. Patel SR, Forman AD, Benjamin RS. High-dose ifosfamide-induced exacerbation of peripheral neuropathy. J Natl Cancer Inst 1994:86:305–306.
51. Goren MP, Wright RK, Pratt C, Bell FE. Dechloroethylation of ifosfamide and neurotoxicity [letter]. Lancet 1986:II:1219–1230.
52. Walker D, Flinois J-P, Monkman SC, et al. Identification of the major human hepatic cytochrome P450 involved in activation and N-dechloroethylation of ifosfamide. Biochem Pharmacol 1994:47:1157–1163.
53. Wainer IW, Ducharme J, Granvil CP, et al. Ifosfamide stereoselective dechloroethylation and neurotoxicity. Lancet 1994:343:982–983.
54. Lewis LD, Meanwell CA. Ifosfamide pharmacokinetics and neurotoxicity. Lancet 1990:335:175–176.
55. Bohnenstengel F, Hofmann U, Eichelbaum M, Kroemer HK. Characterization of the cytochronme P450 involved in side-chain oxidation of cyclophosphamide in humans. Eur J Clin Pharmacol 1996:51:297–301.
56. Boddy AV, Yule SM, Wyllie R, et al. Intrasubject variation in children of ifosfamide pharmacokinetics and metabolism during repeated administration. Cancer Chemother Pharmacol 1996:38:147–154.
57. Transon C, Lecoeur S, Leemann T, et al. Interindividual variability in catalytic activity and immunoreactivity of three major human liver cytochrome P450 isoenzymes. Eur J Clin Pharmacol 1996:51:79–85.
58. Spatzenegger M, Jaeger W. Clinical importance of hepatic cytochrome P450 in drug metabolism. Drug Metab Rev 1995:27(3):397–417.
59. Zulian GB, Tullen E, Maton B. Methylene blue for ifosfamide-associated encephalopathy. N Engl J Med 1995:332:1239–1240.
60. Highley MS, Momerency G, van Cauwenberghe K, et al. Formation of chloroethylaminc and 1,3-oxazolidine-2-one following ifosfamide administration in humans. Drug Metab Dispos 1995; 195:23:433–437.
61. Aeschlimann C, Cerny T, Küpfer A. Inhibition of (mono)amine oxidase activity and prevention of ifosfamide encephalopathy by methylene blue. Drug Metab Dispos 1996:24:1336–1339.

62. Hofmann U, Eichelbaum M, Seefried S, Meese CO. Identification of thiodiglycolic acid sulfoxide, and (3-carboxymethylthio)lactic acid as major human biotransformation products of *S*-carboxymethyl-L-cysteine. Drug Metab Dispos 1991:19:222–226.
63. Lauterburg BH, Nguyen T, Hartmann B, Junker E, Küpfer A, Cerny T. Depletion of total cysteine, glutathione, and homocysteine in plasma by ifosfamide/mesna therapy. Cancer Chemother Pharmacol 1994:35:132–136.
64. Pecci L, Montefoschi G, Fontana M, Cavallini D. Aminoethylcysteine ketimine decarboxylated dimer inhibits mitochondrial respiration by impairing electron transport at complex I level. Biochem Biophys Res Commun 1994:199: 755–760.
65. Cavallini D, Ricci G, Dupré S, et al. Sulfur-containing cyclic ketimines and imino acids. Eur J Biochem 1991:202:217–223.
66. Küpfer A, Aeschlimann C, Wermuth B, Cerny T. Prophylaxis and reversal of ifosfamide encephalopathy with methylene blue. Lancet 1994:343:763–764.
67. Küpfer A, Aeschlimann C, Cerny T. Methylene blue and the neurotoxic mechanisms of ifosfamide encephalopathy. Eur J Clin Pharmacol 1996:50:249–252.
68. van der Wall E, Beijnen JH, Rodenhuis S. High-dose chemotherapy regimens for solid tumors. Cancer Treatment Rev 1995:21:105–132.
69. Gregg RW, Molepo JM, Monpetit VJA, et al. Cisplatin neurotoxicity: The relationship between dosage, time and platinum concentration in neurologic tissues, and morphological evidence of toxicity. J Clin Oncol 1992:10:795–803.
70. Hacker MP. Toxicity of platinum-based anticancer drugs. In: G Powis, MP Hacker, eds. The Toxicity of Anticancer Drugs. New York: Pergamon Press, 1991, pp 82–105.
71. Chu G, Mantin R, Shen Y-M, et al. Massive cisplatin overdose by accidental substitution for carboplatin. Cancer 1993:72:3707–3714.
72. Laurell G, Beskow C, Frankendal B, Borg E. Cisplatin administration to gynecologic cancer patients—long-term effects on hearing. Cancer 1996:78: 1798–1804.
73. Laurell G, Jungnelius U. High-dose cisplatin treatment. Hearing loss and plasma concentrations. Laryngoscope 1990:100:724–734.
74. Cattaneo MT, Filipazzi V, Piazza E, et al. Transient blindness and seizure associated with cisplatin therapy. J Cancer Res Clin Oncol 1988:14:528–530.
75. Ongerboer de Visser BW, Tiesseus G. Polyneuropathy induced by cisplatin. Proc Exp Tumor Res 1985:29:190–196.
76. Higa GM, Wise TC, Crowell EB. Severe, disabling neurologic toxicity following cisplatin treatment. Ann Pharmacother 1995:29:134–137.
77. Christian MC. The current status of new platinum analogs. Semin Oncol 1992: 19:720–733.
78. Donehower RC, Rowinsky EK. An overview of experience with Taxol (paclitaxel) in the USA. Cancer Treatment Rev 1993:19(suppl C):63–78.
79. Rowinsky EK, Chaudhry V, Cornblath DR, Donehower RC. Neurotoxicity of Taxol. Monogr Natl Cancer Inst 1993:15:107–115.

80. Hainsworth JD, Thompson DS, Greco FA. Paclitaxel by 1-hour infusion: An active drug in metastatic non-small-cell-lung cancer. J Clin Oncol 1995:13: 1609–1614.
81. Tsavaris N, Polzos A, Kosmas C, et al. A feasibility study of 1-h paclitaxel infusion in patients with solid tumors. Cancer Chemother Pharmacol 1997: 40:353–357.
82. Hidalgo M, Benito J, Colomer R, Paz-Ares L. Recall reaction of a severe local peripheral neuropathy after paclitaxel extravasation. J Natl Cancer Inst 1996:88:1320.
83. Cavaletti G, Boglium G, Marzorati L, Zincone A, et al. Peripheral neurotoxicity of Taxol in patients previously treated with cisplatin. Cancer 1995:75: 1141–1150.
84. Glantz MJ, Choy H, Kearns CM, Mills PC, et al. Paclitaxel disposition in plasma and central nervous systems of humans and rats with brain tumors. J Natl Cancer Inst 1995:87:1077–1081.
85. Rowinsky EK, Donehower RC, Jones RJ, et al. Microtubule changes and cytotoxicity in leukemic cells treated with Taxol. Cancer Res 1988:48:4093–4100.
86. Cheson BD, Vena DA, Foss FM, Sorensen JM. Neurotoxicity of purine analogs: A review. J Clin Oncol 1994:12:2216–2228.
87. Kane BJ, Kuhn JG, Roush MK. Pentostatin: An adenosine deaminase inhibitor for the treatment of hairy cell leukemia. Ann Pharmacother 1992:26:939–947.
88. Brogden RN, Sorkin EM. Pentostatin: A review of its pharmacodynamic and pharmacokinetic properties, and therapeutic potential in lymphoproliferative disorders. Drugs 1993:46(4):652–677.
89. Spriggs DR, Stopa E, Mayer RJ, Schoene W, Kufe DW. Fludarabine phosphate (NSC 312878) infusions for the treatment of acute leukemia: Phase I and neuropathological study. Cancer Res 1986:46:5953–5958.
90. Bryson HM, Sorkin EM. Cladribine: A review of its pharmacodynamic and pharmacokinetic properties, and therapeutic potential in haematological malignancies. Drugs 1993:46(5):872–894.
91. Phyllis JW, Kostopoulos JK, Edstrom JP, et al. Role of adenosine and adenine nucleotides in central nervous system function. In: HP Bauer, GI Drummond, eds. Physical and Regulatory Functions of Adenosine and Adenine Nucleotides. New York: Raven Press, 1979, pp 343–360.
92. Buggia I, Locatelli F, Regazzi MB, Zecca M. Busulfan. Ann Pharmacother 1994:28:1055–1062.
93. Murphy CP, Harden EA, Thompson JM. Generalized seizures secondary to high-dose busulfan therapy. Ann Pharmacother 1992:26:30–31.
94. Vassal G, Deroussent A, Hartmann O, Challine D, et al. Dose-dependent neurotoxicity of high-dose busulfan in children: A clinical and pharmacological study. Cancer Res 1990:50:6203–6207.
95. Fitzsimmons WE, Ghalie R, Kaizer H. The effect of hepatic enzyme inducers on busulfan neurotoxicity and myelotoxicity. Cancer Chemother Pharmacol 1990:27:226–228.

96. Ames MM. Hexamethylmelamine: Pharmacology and mechanism of action. Cancer Treatment Rev 1991:18(suppl A):3–14.
97. Ames MM, Sanders ME, Tiede WS. Role of *N*-methylolpentamethylmelamine in the metabolic activation of hexamethylmelamine. Cancer Res 1983:43:500–504.
98. Wyllie ARJ, Bayliff CD, Kovacs MJ. Myoclonus due to chlorambucil in two adults with lymphoma. Ann Pharmacother 1997:31:171–174.
99. Wolfson S, Onley MB. Accidental ingestion of a toxic dose of chlorambucil: Report of a case in a child. JAMA 1957:165:239–240.
100. Newell DR, Gore ME. Toxicity of alkylating agents: Clinical characteristics and pharmacokinetic determinations. In: G Powis, MP Hacker, eds. The Toxicity of Anticancer Drugs. New York: Pergamon Press, 1991, pp 44–62.
101. Prough RA, Tweedie DJ. Procarbazine. In: G Powis, RA Prough, eds. Metabolism and Action of Anticancer Drugs. Oxford: Taylor & Francis, 1987, pp 29–47.
102. Henry MC, Marlow M. Preclinical toxicologic study of procarbazine. Cancer Chemother Rep 1973:4:97–102.
103. Goria-Gatti L, Iannone A, Tomasi A, Poli G, Albano E. In vitro and in vivo evidence for the formation of methyl radical from procarbazine: A spin-trapping study. Carcinogenesis 1992:13(5):799–805.
104. Chabner BA, DeVita VT, Considine N, et al. Plasma pyridoxal phosphate depletion by the carcinostatic procarbazine. Proc Soc Exp Biol Med 1969:132:1119–1122.
105. Cairo MS, Lazarus K, Gilmore RL, Baehner RL. Intracranial hemorrhage and focal seizures secondary to use of L-asparaginase during induction therapy of acute lymphocytic leukemia. J Pediatr 1980:97:829–833.

10

Pulmonary Toxicity of Chemotherapeutic Agents

JOST NIEDERMEYER
Medizinische Hochschule Hannover, Hannover, Germany

H. FABEL
Medizinische Hochschule Hannover, Hannover, Germany

CARSTEN BOKEMEYER
University of Tübingen Medical Center, Tübingen, Germany

HANS-PETER LIPP
University of Tübingen, Tübingen, Germany

10.1 INTRODUCTION

When patients who receive antineoplastic agents or have been exposed to such treatment develop clinical or radiological evidence of pulmonary disease, a broad range of diagnoses must be considered. Infections, tumor recurrences, or extension to the lungs and radiation injury, particularly chemotherapy-related lung disease, have to be differentiated from each other. Since there is no specific marker or laboratory test to prove the diagnosis of drug-induced injury to the lungs this is a diagnosis of exclusion.

Serial pulmonary function tests and especially determination of the diffusion capacity for carbon monoxide (DLCO) are the most widely used methods of detecting treatment-associated toxicity to the lung. When patients are weakened by underlying disease, chemotherapy, recent surgery, or pain, however, these tests are often difficult to perform and interpret. Most patients undergoing intensive chemotherapy will show some deterioration in lung function.

Chest radiographs neither reliably predict the onset of clinical toxicity nor allow a differentiation between infection and drug-related disease. High-resolution CT scanning (HRCT) is of proven value in the detection of subtle inflammatory and fibrotic changes in the lung [1], but again no specific pattern has been described for drug-related lung disease. Therefore fiber-optic bronchoscopy supplemented by bronchoalveolar lavage (BAL) and if possible by transbronchial biopsy (TBB) is still the central procedure in the investigation of these patients. The search for a possible cause for respiratory deterioration, however, may well prove fruitless even after one has proceeded further and performed open lung biopsy. At autopsy a definite diagnosis is still not made in up to 15% of patients who die of respiratory complications while receiving chemotherapy [2].

The pathological findings attributed to the pulmonary toxicity of antineoplastic agents is highly variable and often unspecific (Table 1). According to the location of such effects, alveolar, interstitial, and vascular changes can be differentiated. *Desquamative interstitial pneumonitis* refers to a histological pattern in which the alveoli are packed with dense collections of alveolar macrophages and generally mild interstitial infiltrates of lymphocytes and plasma cells with minimal interstitial fibrosis. In *usual interstitial pneumonitis* the number of interstitial inflammatory cells is decreased and the alveolar interstitium is broadened by fibroblastic proliferation, the deposition of collagen, and in some instances smooth muscle proliferation. *Eosinophilic pneumonitis* refers to an accumulation of eosinophils

Table 1 Spectrum of Clinical and Histologic Changes in the Lung Attributed to Anticancer Therapy

Desquamative interstitial pneumonitis (DIP)
Usual interstitial pneumonitis (UIP)
Diffuse alveolar damage (DAD)
Pulmonary fibrosis
Eosinophilic pneumonitis
Bronchiolitis obliterans with organizing pneumonia (BOOP)
Alveolar proteinosis
Pulmonary veno-occlusive disease
Spontaneous pneumothorax
Pleural effusion
Noncardiogenic pulmonary edema

in the interstitium and alveolar spaces. *Bronchiolitis obliterans with organizing pneumonia* (BOOP) is characterized by polyploid proliferation of connective tissue in the lumen of small airways with chronic inflammatory changes in the surrounding alveoli. Immunologic injury to blood vessels may present as *veno-occlusive disease, vasculitis, or diffuse alveolar hemorrhage.* Often lesions occur simultaneously in all three anatomical compartments. Desquamation, proliferation, and metaplasia of the alveolar epithelium are common features of desquamative interstitial pneumonitis and usual interstitial pneumonitis (UIP).

Pulmonary toxicity due to the use of antineoplastic agents is primarily based on one of three mechanisms: direct cytotoxicity, hypersensitivity reactions, or idiosyncrasy.

A drug that is directly *cytotoxic* will severely impair the permeability of endothelial membranes, causing diffuse alveolar damage that may proceed to progressive fibrosis. Despite extensive animal studies, the underlying mechanisms are not yet fully understood. It is postulated that the generation of reactive superoxide and hydroxyl radicals released from the drug itself by electron transfer reactions or by inflammatory cells may play an important role in pathogenesis. Additionally, fibroblast growth factor (FGF) production appears to be involved. *Hypersensitivity reactions* are cosegregated, with the formation of immune complexes or the reaction of the drug with sensitized lymphocytes. Typically, but not always, peripheral or tissue eosinophilia may be present. Symptoms can develop within hours or weeks after drug administration; sometimes they occur after corticosteroids implemented in a multidrug regimen are withdrawn. *Idiosyncratic reactions*, which have acute onset and are acute self-limiting, are characterized by a nonpermeable pulmonary edema without diffuse alveolar damage.

The number of reports concerning pulmonary toxicity of anticancer drugs is growing at a fast rate [3–5]. Most of the publications, however, convey anecdotal information or report small, uncontrolled casuistic studies. Therefore morbidity and mortality rates attributed to pulmonary toxicity of chemotherapy are not precisely known. The presence of certain risk factors seem to reduce pulmonary tolerance to various antineoplastic agents. For several drugs a dose–response relationship for pulmonary toxicity has been postulated (Table 2). Other risk factors include the presence of previous lung disease, old or very young age, concurrent or sequential radiation therapy, high-dose, multiple-drug regimens, surgery, and oxygen therapy.

10.2 BLEOMYCIN

Bleomycin is a mixture of antibiotics isolated from *Streptomyces verticillus*, which is used in the treatment of lymphomas, cancer of the head and neck,

Table 2 Pulmonary Toxicity of Different Cytotoxic Agents

Drug	Pulmonary manifestation	Risk factors[a]	Notes
Cytotoxic antibiotics			
Actinomycin D	ARDS-like syndrome; noncardiogenic pulmonary edema	Potentiation of radiotherapy	
Bleomycin	Pneumonitis–fibrosis; ARDS; BOOP; spontaneous pneumothorax; acute substernal pain syndrome; hypersensitivity reaction; pulmonary veno-occlusive disease	Age > 70 years, cumulative dose > 400–500 mg; high F_{IO_2}; non-Hodgkin lymphoma; radiotherapy to chest; emphysema; smoking history; bolus application	Dose-dependent toxicity; if toxicity is suspected, discontinue therapy and administer corticosteroids. Overall 1% fatal pulmonary fibrosis.
Doxorubicin	ARDS-like syndrome; noncardiogenic pulmonary edema; pneumonitis–fibrosis	Potentiation of radiotherapy	Following radiotherapy, ARDS may occur in 15% of patients treated with doxorubicin.
Mitomycin	Pneumonitis–fibrosis; noncardiogenic pulmonary edema associated with hemolytic uremic syndrome; pleural effusion, bronchospasm; hypersensitivity reaction; pulmonary veno-occlusive disease	Radiotherapy; $F_{IO_2} > 0.3$; combination with vinca alkaloids	Variable incidence of pulmonary toxicity 3–36%; therapy prophylaxis with corticosteroids may be beneficial.

Alkylating agents and nitrosoureas			
BCNU (carmustine)	Pneumonitis–fibrosis; pulmonary veno-occlusive disease	Cumulative dose > 1500 mg/m^2; preexisting lung disease; smoking history	Incidence of 30–50% with dose > 1500 mg/m^2; 20% incidence with 900–1200 mg/m^2; combination with high-dose etoposide or cyclophosphamide may increase risk. Steroids probably inefficient; concomitant therapy with ambroxol may decrease the risk.
Chlorambucil	Acute or "late"-onset pneumonitis; progressive fibrosis; hypersensitivity pneumonitis (very rare)	Cumulative dose > 2.5 g	Rare incidence; toxicity occurs after 5–56 months. Despite corticosteroids, prognosis may be poor in "late"-onset pneumonitis.
Cyclophosphamide	Early-onset pneumonitis–fibrosis; pleural thickening; pulmonary veno-occlusive disease	High-dose intermittent cyclophosphamide; interactions with radiotherapy/BCNU	Reactive metabolites may be involved in lung toxicity; rare incidence.
Ifosfamide	Pulmonary edema; interstitial pneumonitis	Previous therapy with cyclophosphamide	
Melphalan	Pneumonitis–fibrosis		Very rare incidence.
Procarbazine	Hypersensitivity pneumonitis		Incidence is very rare.

Table continued on following page

Table 2 Continued

Drug	Pulmonary manifestation	Risk factors[a]	Notes
Busulfan	Pneumonitis–fibrosis; alveolar proteinosis	Radiation therapy; smoking history	"Busulfan lung" occurs after 6 weeks–10 years. Estimated incidence 6%; prognosis is poor.
Antimetabolites			
Methotrexate	Hypersensitivity pneumonitis; endothelial injury; capillary-leak pulmonary edema; pneumonitis–fibrosis; pleural effusion; bronchospasm	Daily or weekly drug therapy; underlying pulmonary disease or renal failure; adrenalectomy	Incidence is about 5–8%; anecdotal reports of uneventful rechallenge.
Cytarabine (Ara-C)	Capillary-leak pulmonary edema; pleural effusion	High-dose regimens (esp. as continuous infusion); severe diarrhea	Incidence is about 22% (mortality rate 6–10%); treatment with high-dose methylprednisolone.
Gemcitabine	Tachypnea, marked hypoxemia; pulmonary edema; interstitial pneumonitis; ARDS	Unknown	Incidence is about 3–4%. Withdrawal of drug and administration of corticosteroids and diuretics may help to avert a fatal outcome.

Fludarabine monophosphate	Interstitial pneumonitis; pleural effusions	Unknown	Treatment with corticosteroids.
Mitotic inhibitors			
Vinca alkaloids	Pulmonary edema; pleural effusion; bronchospasm; pneumonitis–fibrosis	Coadministration of other cytotoxic agents particularly mitomycin C	Incidence with combination chemotherapy is 5%; treatment with corticosteroids is recommended.
All-*trans*-retinoic acid (ATRA)	Noncardiogenic pulmonary edema sometimes proceeding to ARDS; interstitial lung disease	Early increase in leukocytes during treatment with ATRA	Prophylaxis with corticosteroids significantly reduces pulmonary toxicity; pulmonary toxicity as part of "ATRA syndrome."
Paclitaxel, docetaxel	Hypersensitivity reaction causing bronchospasm		Premedication with H_1 and H_2 blockers and corticosteroids is obligatory.

[a]F_{IO_2}, fraction of inspired oxygen.

and germ cell tumors. Almost every pattern of lung injury has been observed after administration of the drug, and several modes of its toxicity have been demonstrated in animal models.

To exert cytotoxicity, bleomycin intercalates between DNA base pairs with its bithiazole moiety and binds molecular oxygen as a sixth ligand to the central atom Fe(II) (Fig. 1). Upon the transfer of one electron from Fe(II), oxygen is reduced to the corresponding superoxide radical anion, which is released and converted to highly toxic hydroxyl radicals in the presence of Fe(III) ions. The bleomycin hydrolyase catalyzes the hydrolysis of the β-aminoalanine side chain, resulting in deamidobleomycin. The latter does not exert any cytotoxic effects because it is unable to bind oxygen as a ligand. This is explained by noting that the carboxylic acid released by the hydrolysis reaction occupies the fifth coordination site, which results in a conformation change of the complex and reduces the binding affinity of molecular oxygen. If tumor cells have a very high constitutive expression of bleomycin hydrolase, they will be resistant to the glycopeptide. The comparatively high sensitivity of the lung tissue toward bleomycin can be explained by its very low constitutive expression of the detoxifying enzyme, bleomycin hydrolase. In contrast to other tissues like the heart or the bone marrow, which do not seem to be adversely affected by this glycopeptide, the low constitutive level in the lung cannot overcome bleomycin-induced radical formation. This release of superoxide or hydroxyl anion radicals that are generated in the presence of oxygen seems to be the most common mechanisms in bleomycin-induced pulmonary toxicity. In addition, hyper-

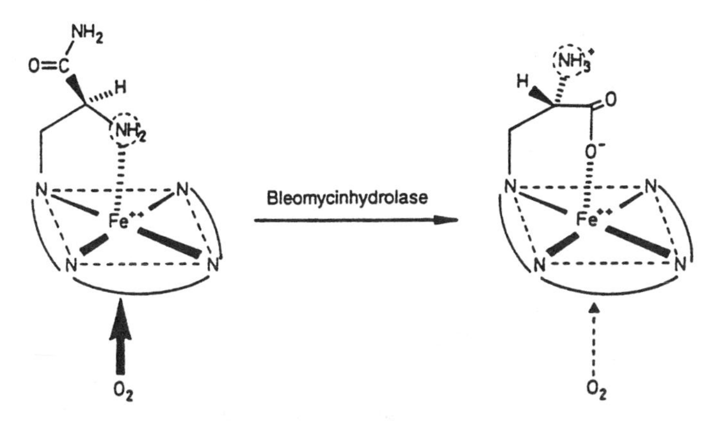

Fig. 1 Bleomycin hydrolase plays an essential role in the detoxification of the anticancer drug. The hydrolysis of the aminoalanine amide side chain results in a complex that can no longer bind oxygen with high affinity.

sensitivity reactions as well as immune-complex-related reactions may also occur.

Rapidly progressing pulmonary bleomycin–oxygen toxicity leading to adult respiratory distress syndrome (ARDS) has been observed within 24 hours after administration of hyperbaric oxygen in patients who had received bleomycin during the preceding 6–12 months [6,7]. Therefore, no elective surgery with anesthesia should be performed during this period.

A more common form of bleomycin-related lung disease, however, is a slowly progressive pulmonary fibrosis syndrome that occurs in 2–40% of patients who received the drug [8]. There appears to be a critical cumulative dose of 400–450 mg above which the risk for interstitial fibrosis rises sharply and a dose–response relationship becomes evident. Fatal cases have, however, also been published at a total dose of as little as 50 mg [4]. Since bleomycin is predominantly excreted in the urine, the dose must be adjusted to renal function. To detect the fibrosis syndrome early, monitoring of total lung capacity has been proposed as a more specific marker than the carbon monoxide diffusing capacity [7]. Upon diagnosis, discontinuation of the drug and the administration of glucocorticosteroid have been recommended. The prophylactic use of 100 mg of hydrocortisone has not been systematically evaluated. As a complication of interstitial fibrosis due to bleomycin treatment, spontaneous pneumothorax must be considered when patients present with acute severe dyspnea or chest pain [9].

Other rarer forms of bleomycin-related lung disease include BOOP, the appearance of nodular lesions mimicking metastasis, acute substernal or pleuritic chest pain during infusion of the drug, and hypersensitivity reactions [3].

10.3 CARMUSTINE (BCNU)

Carmustine (BCNU) and other nitrosurea drugs (lomustine, semustine), easily cross the blood–brain barrier owing to their high lipophilicity. Therefore these drugs are used primarily in the treatment of central nervous system malignancies. Recently carmustine has also been incorporated into several combination high-dose chemotherapy regimens for breast cancer and lymphoma. The mechanism of nitrosourea-induced pulmonary toxicity is not fully understood. During the rapid decomposition of nitrosoureas, very reactive isocyanates are released which are able to bind covalently to several macromolecules. This reaction can irreversibly change the structure and function of the macromolecules. Thus, it has been hypothesized that particularly the pulmonary enzyme glutathione reductase, which is important for lung protection against a variety of oxidative agents, may be inactivated by these isocynates.

Pulmonary toxicity was noticed soon after the introduction of carmustine in the 1970s and was first described as an acute pulmonary fibrotic reaction occurring days or months after treatment, with an incidence of up to 40% and a mortality of 12% during the first 3 years posttreatment [10]. A dose-related toxicity has been proposed with rising pulmonary complication rates if total doses above 1500 mg/m^2 carmustine and 1100 mg/m^2 lomustine are used. If carmustine was given as part of combination high-dose chemotherapy in female patients with Hodgkin disease, doses above 475 m/m^2 were associated with a higher rate of fatal pulmonary toxicity [11]. In addition, some investigators have suggested that age, previous chest radiotherapy, or smoking habit might be additional risk factors for the development of pulmonary toxic reactions when BCNU is used as part of high-dose chemotherapy regimen [12,13]. Other studies, however, have failed to confirm such factors predictive of BCNU lung injury [14–16].

Recently a delayed onset of fatal pulmonary fibrosis occurring 8–20 years posttreatment was reported in children who survived carmustine therapy for brain tumors. Mortality was 35% for the "late pulmonary fibrosis," which seemed more likely to occur in children treated at ages younger than 6 years [17].

In patients who manifest symptoms or signs of BCNU lung injury, or have asymptomatic decreases in DLCO, empirical treatment with prednisone is recommended [18]. In addition, ambroxol has been proposed as a useful protectant against subclinical BCNU injury.

10.4 MITOMYCIN C (MMC)

Mitomycin C (MMC) is a naturally occurring antibiotic that has been isolated from *Streptomyces caesipotus*. It is used in the treatment of lung, gastrointestinal, prostate, and breast cancer, sometimes alone but often also in combination with other drugs.

MMC is a prodrug that must be reduced to its corresponding hydroquinone system. There are two distinct pathways resulting in the corresponding hydroquinone (Fig. 2). A two-electron pathway catalyzed by the enzyme DT diaphorase is unimpeded by molecular oxygen and seems to be the critical pathway for antitumor activity. Through a one-electron pathway, which is catalyzed by the NADPH-dependent cytochrome P450 reductase and is impeded by molecular oxygen, semiquinone free radical intermediates are formed which release superoxide radicals during redox cycle.

The combination of free radical formation and lipid peroxidation has been suggested as the underlying mechanism of MMC, which may be responsible for the induction of pulmonary complications. However, under-

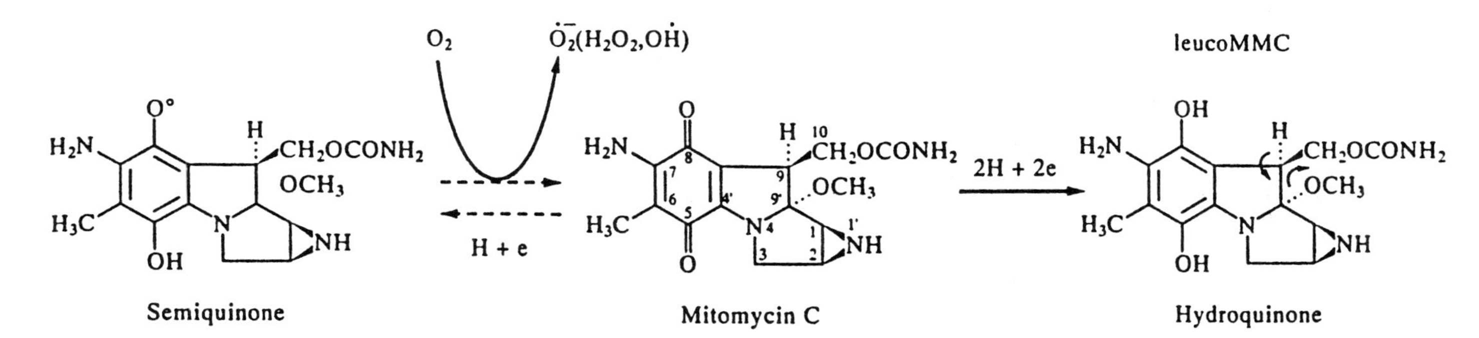

Fig. 2 It has been postulated that the redox cycling of mitomycin C (MMC) results in the release of reactive oxygen radicals that may be partially responsible for MMC-induced pulmonary toxicity.

lying hypersensitivity reactions as well as immune-complex-related reactions may also occur. The incidence of pulmonary toxicity has been reported to range from 3 to 12% [19–21]. It is uncertain whether there is a correlation between cumulative total dose and increased risk for developing pulmonary fibrosis.

The most common form of MMC-induced lung disease is pneumonitis–fibrosis, which usually develops 2–4 months after therapy. The first clinical symptoms are dyspnea, dry, unproductive cough, and fatigue [20,21]. Unusual clinical presentations are noncardiogenic pulmonary edema in association with hemolytic uremic syndrome and acute bronchospasm in patients who have received both MMC and vinca alkaloids [21]. A recent prospective study reported a significant decline in DLCO in 28% of MMC-treated patients after only three cycles of chemotherapy. This result, however, was not associated with adverse prognosis or the development of other pulmonary complications.

Discontinuation of MMC and treatment with corticosteroids has been recommended as soon as the first symptoms become obvious.

10.5 BUSULFAN

Busulfan, which has been used in the treatment of chronic myelogenous leukemia, was the first cytotoxic agent known to induce pulmonary toxicity [22]. The recognition of this association resulted in the coining of the term "busulfan lung"; however, other alkylating agents (e.g., chlorambucil, the oxazaphosphorines, and melphalan) may also cause an identical pneumonitis–fibrosis syndrome. The incidence of clinically evident pneumonitis caused by busulfan has been estimated to be about 6% [23]. So far a close dose–response relationship has not been observed, but some authors advise the use of threshold doses above 500 mg or cumulative dose above 2.9 g/m^2 [24]. Symptoms can occur as early as 6 weeks after initiation of treatment, but a much later manifestation, averaging about 41 months after therapy, is more common [23]. The precise mechanisms by which alkylating agents cause lung toxicity have not been fully elucidated. The histologic pattern seen in the pneumonitis–fibrosis syndrome is similar to ultrastructural changes induced by bleomycin and includes hyperplasia and dysplasia of type II pneumocytes. Prognosis of busulfan-induced pulmonary fibrosis is grave, with mortality rate between 60 and 84%. The discontinuation of therapy and immediate onset of steroid application has been recommended as soon as the first symptoms are noted.

Apart from pulmonary fibrosis, busulfan may also cause an acute hypersensitivity reaction or pulmonary ossification after long-term therapy

[25]. Another very rare manifestation of busulfan pulmonary toxicity is the development of alveolar proteinosis.

10.6 ANTIMETABOLITES

10.6.1 Methotrexate

Methotrexate (MTX) is used alone or in combination with several other antineoplastic drugs in different cancer treatment programs as well as in the management of nonmalignant diseases. It can cause a special form of desquamative interstitial and eosinophilic pneumonitis that is only rarely fatal. Because of frequently observed blood and tissue eosinophilia, pathogenesis has been interpreted as a hypersensitivity-type reaction. However, there have been several reports of uneventful readministration of the drug in the same patient. Other pathogenic hypotheses include endothelial injury causing noncardiogenic pulmonary edema and interstitial pneumonitis with diffuse alveolar damage. Respiratory symptoms may occur after oral, intravenous, or intrathecal administration of the drug. The incidence of pulmonary toxicity caused by MTX ranges from 1 to 8% [26]. A clear dose–response relationship has not been established. Little is known about risk factors for methotrexate-induced lung injury. It has been suggested that there may be a greater likelihood of pulmonary toxicity in patients receiving the drug daily or weekly. Rheumatoid arthritis, previous lung disease, old age, diabetes, rheumatoid lung disease, and hypoalbuminemia have been identified as important risk factors [27,28].

Recovery seems to be common within 10–45 days after discontinuation of therapy, and the development of irreversible pulmonary fibrosis is unusual. Leucovorin rescue does not seem to prevent pulmonary complications.

10.6.2 Cytarabine

The antimetabolite cytarabine is used in the treatment of adult acute leukemia. It may cause capillary-leak syndrome involving primary the lung and occurring 2–21 days after the first dose—especially after high-dose therapy. In addition capillary leakage can involve pleural, pericardial, and peritoneal surfaces. The disorder is frequently misdiagnosed as ARDS due to other causes and may not be recognized as a drug-induced problem [3]. Establishing the correct diagnosis, however, is important, since discontinuation of therapy and initiation of high-dose methylprednisolone leads to a mortality below 10% [29].

10.6.3 Gemcitabine

Recently, a fatal pulmonary toxicity following treatment with gemcitabine was reported after several cycles of about 1200 mg/m^2. The incidence of severe dyspnea with gemcitabine was 2–3% in one study. For patients who develop unexplained noncardiogenic pulmonary edema after repeated administration of the drug, treatment with diuretics and corticosteroids is recommended, although the underlying mechanism is not known [30].

10.7 CYCLOPHOSPHAMIDE

Cyclophosphamide is an immunosuppressive alkylating agent used in the treatment of a wide variety of malignant and nonmalignant conditions. The spectrum of pulmonary toxicity that can be specifically attributed to this drug has recently been reviewed meticulously [31]. Over the last 20 years the authors collected fewer than 20 cases, including reports from literature, in which cyclophosphamide could be identified as the only etiologic agent for lung toxicity. From this study two distinct patterns of cyclophosphamide-associated injury emerged: an early-onset pneumonitis syndrome developing 1–6 months after administration of the drug and a "late-onset" pneumonitis presenting months to years after treatment and even after discontinuation of the drug. The latter form of toxicity was observed after prolonged treatment with low daily cyclophosphamide doses and differed clinically from idiopathic pulmonary fibrosis in that digital clubbing or "Velcro" rales were not detectable. In contrast to early-onset pneumonitis, the "late" manifestation frequently took a fatal course despite discontinuation of cyclophosphamide and treatment with corticosteroid. When high-dose cyclophosphamide is administered together with other antineoplastic agents or in association with radiotherapy, several types of pulmonary toxicity have been observed. These include acute alveolar hemorrhage, bronchiolitis obliterans, and noncardiogenic pulmonary edema [4,31,32]. In the setting of allogenic bone marrow transplantation, about 30% of patients develop an "idiopathic pneumonitis" after receiving busulfan and cyclophosphamide [33].

10.8 CYTOTOXIC DRUGS ONLY RARELY CAUSING PULMONARY TOXICITY

Mainly based on case reports, causal relationships between cytotoxic agents and lung injury have been suggested for vinca alkaloids, procarbazine, podophyllotoxin derivatives, fludarabine monophosphate, azathioprin, or 6-mercaptopurin, and melphalan (Table 2). However, in most cases drug combinations or concomitant radiotherapy were administered, which makes any interpretation of such data difficult.

REFERENCES

1. Wells AU, Rubens MB, du Bois RM, Hansell DM. Serial CT in fibrosing alveolitis: Prognostic significance of the initial pattern. Am J Roentgenol 1993; 161:1159–1165.
2. Rosenow EC. Diffuse pulmonary infiltrates in the immunocompromised patient. Clin Chest Med 1990;11:55–64.
3. Rosenow EC, Myers JL, Swensen SJ, Pisani RJ. Drug induced pulmonary disease. Chest 1992;102:239–250.
4. Cooper JAD, White DA, Matthay RA. Drug-induced pulmonary disease. 1: Cytotoxic drugs. Am Rev Respir Dis 1986;133:321–340.
5. Foucher P, Biour M, Blayac JP, Godard P, Sgro C, Kuhn M, Vergnon JM, Vervloet D, Pfitzenmeyer P, Ollagnier M, Mayaud C, Camus P. Drugs that may injure the respiratory system. Eur Respir J 1997;10:265–279.
6. Van Barneveld PWC, Sleijfer DT, van der Mark TW, Mulder NH, Scharffordt KH, Sluiter HJ, et al. Natural course of bleomycin-induced pneumonitis. Am Rev Respir Dis 1987;135:48–51.
7. Wolkowicz J, Sturgeon J, Rawji M, Chan CK. Bleomycin-induced pulmonary function abnormalities. Chest 1992;101:97–101.
8. Jules-Elysee K, White DA. Bleomycin-induced pulmonary toxicity. Clin Chest Med 1990;11:1–20.
9. Hsu JR, Chang SC, Perng RP. Pneumothorax following cytotoxic chemotherapy in malignant lymphoma. Chest 1990;98:1512–1513.
10. O'Driscoll BR, Hastleton S, Taylor PM, et at. Active lung fibrosis up to 17 years after chemotherapy with carmustine (BCNU) in childhood. N Engl J Med 1990;323:378–382.
11. Rubio C, Hill ME, Milan S, O'Brien ME, Cunningham D. Idiopathic pneumonia syndrome after high-dose chemotherapy for relapsed Hodgkin's disease. Br J Cancer 1997;75:1044–1048.
12. Pecego R, Hill R, Applebaum F, et al. Interstitial pneumonitis following autologous bone marrow transplantation. Transplantation 1986;42:515–517.
13. Aronin PA, Mahaley MS, Rudnick SA. Prediction of BCNU pulmonary toxicity in patients with malignant gliomas. N Engl J Med 1980;303:183–188.
14. Jochelson M, Tarbell NJ, Freedman AS, et al. Acute and chronic pulmonary complications following autologous bone marrow transplantation in non-Hodgkin's lymphoma. Bone Marrow Transplant 1990;6:329–331.
15. Valteau D, Hartmann O, Benhamou E, et al. Nonbacterial nonfungal pneumonitis following autologous bone marrow transplantation in children treated with high-dose chemotherapy without total-body-irradiation. Transplantation 1988;45:737–740.
16. Ghalie R, Szidon J, Thompson L, et al. Evaluation of pulmonary complications after bone marrow transplantation: The role of pretransplant pulmonary function tests. Bone Marrow Transplant 1992;10:359–365.

17. O'Driscoll BR, Kalra S, Gattamaneni HR, Woodcock AA. Late carmustine lung fibrosis. Age at treatment may influence severity and survival. Chest 1995;107: 1355–1357.
18. Kalaycioglu M, Kavuru M, Tuason L, Bolwell B. Empiric prednisone therapy for pulmonary toxic reaction after high-dose chemotherapy containing carmustine (BCNU). Chest 1995;107:482–487.
19. Verweij J, van Zanten T, Sourem T, et al. Prospective study on the dose relationship of mitomycin C–induced interstitial pneumonitis. Cancer 1987;60: 756–761.
20. Orwoll ES, Kiessling PJ, Patterson JR. Interstitial pneumonia from mitomycin. Ann Intern Med 1978;89.
21. Castro M, Veeder MH, Mailliard JA, Tazelaar HD, Jett JR. A prospective study of pulmonary function in patients receiving mitomycin. Chest 1996;109:939–944.
22. Oliner H, Schwartz R, Rubio F, Dameshek W. Interstitial pulmonary fibrosis following busulfan therapy. Am J Med 1961;31:134–139.
23. Massin F, Fur A, Reybet-Degat O, Camus P, Jeannin L. Busulfan-induced pneumopathy. Rev Mal Respir 1987;4:3–10.
24. Ginsberg SJ, Comis RL. The pulmonary toxicity of antineoplastic agents. Semin Oncol 1982;9:34–51.
25. Kuplic JB, Higley CS, Niewoehner DE. Pulmonary ossification associated with long-term busulfan therapy in chronic myeloid leukemia. Am Rev Respir Dis 1972;106:759–762.
26. Sostman HD, Matthay RA, Putman CE, Smith GJW. Methotrexate-induced pneumonitis. Medicine 1976;55:371–388.
27. Golden MR, Katz RS, Balk RA, Golden HE. The relationship of preexisting lung disease to the development of methotrexate pneumonitis in patients with rheumatoid arthritis. J Rheumatol 1995;22:1043–1047.
28. Alarcon GS, Kremer JM, Macaluso M, Weinblatt ME, et al. Risk factors for methotrexate-induced lung injury in patients with rheumatoid arthritis. Ann Intern Med 1997;127:356–364.
29. Tham RT, Peters WG, DeBruine FT, Willemze R. Pulmonary complications of cytosine–arabinoside therapy: Radiographic findings. Am J Roentgenol 1987; 49:23–27.
30. Pavlakis N, Bell DR, Millward MJ, Levi JA. Fatal pulmonary toxicity resulting from treatment with gemcitabine. Cancer 1997;80:286–291.
31. Malik SW, Myers JL, DeRemee RA, Specks U. Lung toxicity associated with cyclophosphamide use. Two distinct patterns. Am J Respir Crit Care Med 1996; 154:1851–1856.
32. Spector JI, Zimbler H, Ross JS. Early-onset cyclophosphamide-induced interstitial pneumonitis. JAMA 1979;242:2852–2854.
33. Bandini G, Belcardinelli A, et al. Toxicity of high-dose busulphan and cyclophosphamide as conditioning therapy for allogeneic bone marrow transplantation in adults with haematological malignancies. Bone Marrow Transplant 1994;13:577–581.

11

Cardiotoxicity of Cytotoxic Drugs

HANS-PETER LIPP
University of Tübingen, Tübingen, Germany

11.1 INTRODUCTION

Several cytostatics are able to impair heart function to an extent that may result in arrhythmia, congestive cardiomyopathy, or even myocardial infarction (Table 1) [1–3]. The pathogenesis is often rather complex and partially involves an extensive superoxide radical formation, particularly in the case of the anthracycline glycosides and related compounds (Fig. 1) [4,5]. There appears to be a good correlation between the risk of anthracycline-induced cardiotoxicity and the corresponding cumulative dosages. However, because of the underlying high variability of the individual pharmacokinetics, as well as sensitivity and risk factors, described limits of cumulative dosages must be interpreted with caution [1,6,7]. As a consequence, one patient may develop severe symptoms even at half the defined cumulative dosage, whereas another will tolerate much more.

The mechanism of cardiotoxicity induced by paclitaxel, 5-fluorouracil, or high-dose cyclophosphamide is not fully understood [8–10]. Cardiotoxic events associated with the use of bleomycin or vincristine are very rare [11,12].

11.2 ANTHRACYCLINE GLYCOSIDES

11.2.1 Side Effects

Three distinct types of anthracycline-induced cardiotoxic side effects must be kept in mind when the anthracycline glycosides are used [13–19].

Table 1 Cardiotoxicity Induced by Cytostatics: A brief Overview

Cytostatics	Comment
Anthracyclines	Acute cardiotoxic side effects (mostly reversible)
	Cumulative dose-related cardiomyopathy: several risk factors exist; dexrazoxane (ICRF-187) appears to be a promising agent for cardioprotection.
	Late cardiotoxic side effects
Mitoxantrone, amsacrine	See Anthracyclines
5-Fluorouracil	Most common symptoms: angina, ECG changes
	Incidence of cardiac ischemia or arrhythmia appears to be higher in patients with a history of coronary artery diseases
	Response to nitroglycerin
High-dose cyclophosphamide	Acute hemorrhagic myocarditis, ECG changes
	An inverse relationship between cyclophosphamide AUC and cardiotoxicity cannot be excluded
Paclitaxel	Asymptomatic and reversible arrhythmias, particularly bradycardia
	Paclitaxel-induced cardiotoxicity does not seem to be associated with cumulative dose
Others	
Bleomycin	Rare events of acute chest pain syndrome and severe pericarditis
Cisplatin	Rare events of transient ECG changes and transient coronary ischemia
Vincristine	Rare events of acute myocardial infarction (by affecting the cardiac parasympathetic system?)

Source: Refs. 1–3.

11.2.1.1 Transient Effects

Immediately after administration of drugs in this class of cytotoxics, transient cardiac dysfunction (e.g., nonspecific ST-T changes in the ECG or supraventricular tachycardia) may occur. However, a pericarditis–myocarditis syndrome and even life-threatening ventricular arrhythmias rep-

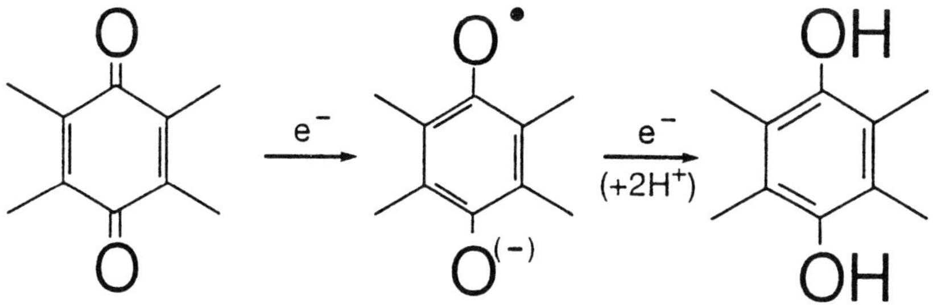

Fig. 1 Reactive superoxide radicals appear to play an important role in cytostatic-induced cardiotoxicity. In particular, quinone-containing structures are able to release such reactive oxygen species via redox cycling.

resent very rare events due to acute cardiotoxic side effects of anthracyclines. It has been estimated that up to 40% of the patients treated with doxorubicin may suffer from temporary abnormalities [14].

11.2.1.2 Chronic Effects

In contrast to the acute or subacute side effects, whose incidence is not dependent on the cumulative anthracycline dosage, chronic cardiotoxicity is primarily characterized by congestive hear failure (CHF). The clinical symptoms of this cardiac insufficiency include tachycardia, arrhythmia, difficult breathing, unproductive cough, edemas, and cardiomegaly. Its incidence can be strongly correlated with the cumulative total dosage of the respective anthracycline. If the total doxorubicin dosage is less than 550 mg/m^2, the incidence of congestive cardiomyopathy in adult patients is supposed to be less than 1% (e.g., about 0.14% at total dosages <400 mg/m^2, whereas dosages of 550 and 700 mg/m^2 are associated with a cumulative probability of developing doxorubicin-induced heart failure of 7 and 18%, respectively (Fig. 2) [20]. There is some evidence that therapeutic intervention based on the use of digoxin, angiotensin-converting enzyme inhibitors, or diuretics may help to improve the prognosis if congestive cardiomyopathy is already manifest [1,17].

However, there is strong evidence that in some patients severe chronic cardiotoxic symptoms may occur after cumulative dosages of less than 200 mg/m^2 (Table 2), whereas others tolerate dosages up to even more than 5000 mg/m^2 [1]. The underlying reasons may have primarily to do with highly different clinical pharmacokinetics between individuals as well as the role of individual predisposition (Table 3) [6,7]. It has been suggested that previous mediastinal radiation, advanced or younger age, female sex, preexisting heart disease or hypertension, as well as bolus injections rather than a

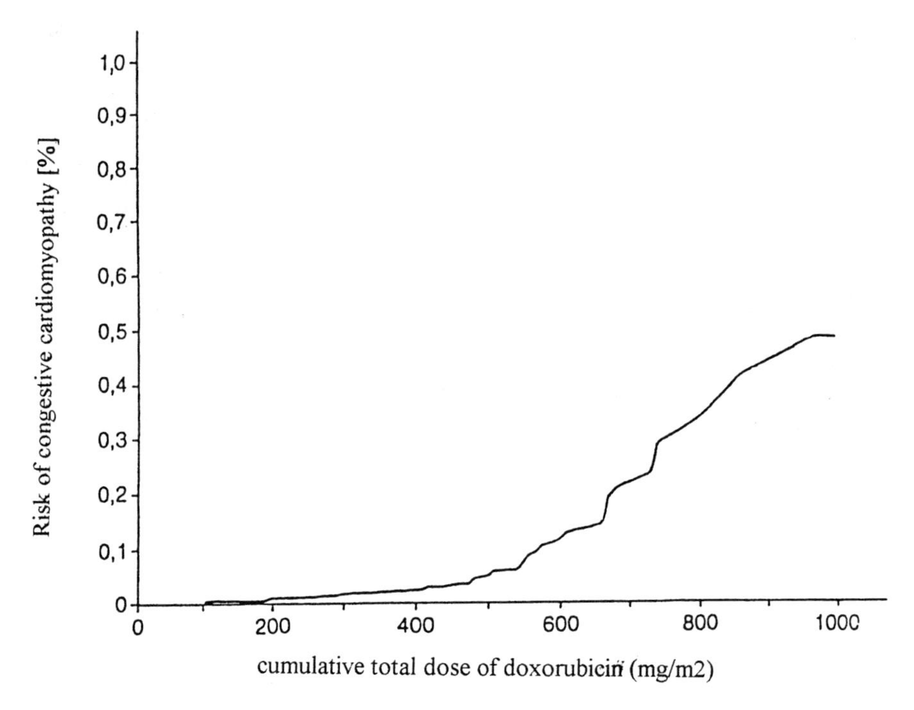

Fig. 2 There is a strong correlation between the increased risk of congestive cardiomyopathy and the total cumulative anthracycline dose. (From Ref. 20.)

Table 2 Cumulative Anthracycline Dosages That Should Not Be Exceeded in the Interest of Minimizing the Risk of Congestive Cardiomyopathy[a]

Anthracycline	Cumulative total dosage (mg/m^2)	Usual dosage (mg/m^2)
Daunorubicin i.v.	500–600	20–80 q21d
Doxorubicin i.v.	550	60–75 q21d
Epirubicin i.v.	850–1000	50–90 q21d
Idarubicin i.v.	120–(290)	8–12 d1–3 q21d
Idarubicin orally	600–720	15–30 d1–3 q21d
DaunoXome i.v.	>1000	40 q14d
Doxil (Caelyx) i.v.	>860	20 q21d
Mitoxantrone	160–(200)	10–12 d1(–5) q21d
Amsacrine	580–(800)	90–150 d1–5 q7–21d

Notice: It is not recommended to substitute one anthracycline for another when the cumulative dose threshold of one of the drugs has been reached.

[a]There is a strong correlation between the increased risk for congestive cardiomyopathy and the total cumulative dosage of anthracyclines given as bolus applications.

Table 3 Factors that Increase the Risk for Congestive Cardiomyopathy by Anthracyclines

Cumulative total dosage
Age (infants and older patients)
Radiation of the mediastinum
Preexisting cardiac diseases
Flow rate: There may be correlation between the risk of cardiomyopathy and peak concentrations of anthracyclines in plasma. Continuous infusions and application of lower doses in shorter intervals may be preferable in this respect.
Malnutrition (especially vitamin E deficiency) It has even been proposed that 2 g tocopherol per day beginning one week before anthracycline therapy may allow the total cumulative dosage to be exceeded.
Simultaneous therapy with drugs that may impair the elimination and inactivation of anthracyclines

prolonged infusion time are important risk factors for the development of chronic heart failure after anthracycline administration [6,7,19–22].

11.2.1.3 Late-Onset Effects

More than one year or even later after treatment, severe late-onset cardiotoxicity has been reported. Patients may develop ventricular dysfunction, heart failure, and arrhythmias. Steinherz and colleagues calculated an 18% incidence of reduced fractional shortening on resting echocardiograms in patients followed for 4–10 years after the end of anthracycline therapy. These abnormalities may develop at lower cumulative dosages than congestive cardiomyopathy. The pathogenesis as well as the underlying risk factors have not yet been fully understood [18].

11.2.2 Calculation of Total Dosages

As indicated in Table 2, the different anthracyclines vary greatly in the cumulative dosages that seem to represent thresholds of incurring the risk of cardiomyopathy. Particularly in the case of doxorubicin and epirubicin, which are similar in efficacy, it is of clinical importance that their corresponding cumulative dosages, which should not be exceeded in clinical practice, have been defined to average 550 and 800 mg/m^2, respectively. As a consequence, treatment cycles containing epirubicin rather than doxorubicin can be repeated much more often [23–26]. Indeed, recently Dranitsaris and Tran demonstrated that the fluorouracil, epirubicin, and cyclophosphamide (FEC) protocol was associated with significantly fewer cardiac abnormalities than the corresponding fluorouracil, Adriamycin, and cyclophosphamide (FAC) protocol containing doxorubicin [27].

However, one has to be careful if the anthracycline therapy is switched from doxorubicin, daunorubicin, or epirubicin to idarubicin or mitoxantrone (Table 2) because the cumulative dosages must first be mathematically converted. For example, if a patient is switched from daunorubicin to idarubicin, a cumulative dose of 360 mg/m^2 daunorubicin (divided by 4) resembles about 90 mg/m^2 cumulative idarubicin IV. As a consequence, a further total dose of 30 mg/m^2 idarubicin can be administered without exceeding the recommended total intravenous idarubicin dose of 120 mg/m^2 (Table 2) [28–30].

Whereas a total dosage of 120 mg/m^2 idarubicin IV should not be exceeded over one year for patients with newly diagnosed acute myeloblastic leukemia (AML), a total dosage of 230 mg/m^2 appears to be applicable over 2 years for patients with newly diagnosed acute promyelocytic leukemia. Recently it has been estimated that the probability of idarubicin-related cardiomyopathy may average 5% at a cumulative dose of 150 to 290 mg/m^2 IV [31]. Oral idarubicin (about 45–50 mg/m^2 PO is nearly bioequivalent to 15 mg/m^2 IV) appears to be tolerable in regard to a change of left ventricular ejection fraction up to cumulative dosages of 600–720 mg/m^2 [32–34].

11.2.3 Mechanism of Anthracycline-Induced Congestive Heart Failure

There is strong evidence that the development of anthracycline-induced chronic CHF is mainly due to the progressive formation of cardiotoxic free oxygen radicals, particularly superoxide anion and hydroxyl radicals (Fig. 3) [4,35].

The NADPH-dependent cytochrome P 450 reductase serves to transfer an electron to the quinone system of the anthracycline aglycones. The resulting semiquinone that is formed during this process can be reversed to the quinone by releasing this electron. If oxygen accepts this electron, the reactive superoxide anion radical will be formed, and then further converted into a highly toxic hydroxyl radical in the presence of ferric ions (Fe^{3+}). Very probably these hydroxyl radicals are primarily responsible for severe DNA damage and lipid peroxidation within cardiac tissue [4,35].

The high sensitivity of the heart tissue to such oxygen radicals can be explained by its constitutive low amount of radical scavenging enzymes and coenzymes, particularly superoxide dismutase and catalase [36]. The hypothesis that highly reactive radicals are formed particularly in the presence of ferric ions is strengthened by the ability of dexrazoxane (ICRF-187), which represents a lipid-soluble analogue of ethylenediamine tetraacetate

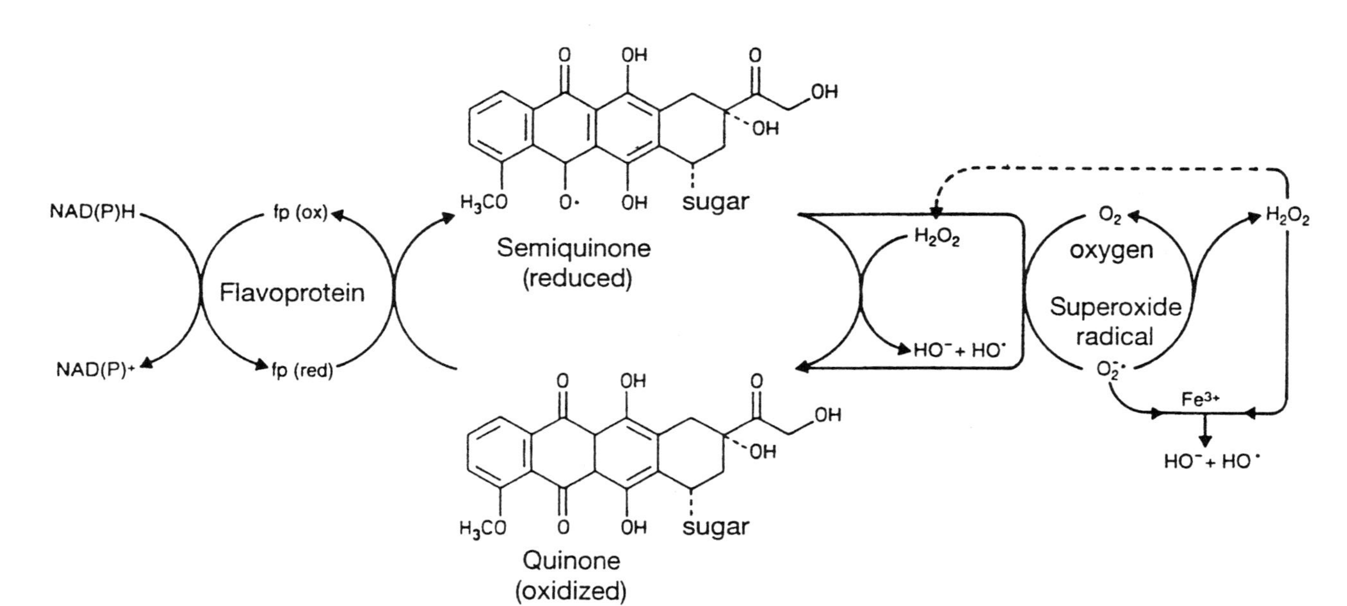

Fig. 3 There is strong evidence that the formation of superoxide and hydroxyl radicals, particularly in the presence of ferric ions, is an important mechanism of anthracycline-induced cardiotoxicity.

(EDTA), to decrease the risk of chronic anthracycline-induced cardiotoxicity at the defined cumulative doses [37].

There is some evidence that anthracycline-induced CHF also results from the interaction between the cytotoxic drug and certain phospholipids, particularly cardiolipin. Since the highest level of cardiolipin is detectable in the mitochondrial membranes of cardiac cells, this interaction permeability of membranes is severely impaired [36,38,39].

11.2.4 The Cardioprotective Role of Dexrazoxane

Within the last few years, several strategies have been tried to overcome the anthracycline-induced risk of congestive cardiomyopathy. The possible benefits of radical scavengers like ubiquinone as well as tocopherol are still somewhat controversial, whereas more promising data exist that favor the use of dexrazoxane as a first-line cardioprotective agent [1,3,37,40].

Dexrazoxane, which is structurally related to EDTA, is rapidly hydrolyzed to the corresponding carboxylamine, ICRF-198, within the cell (Fig. 4). The latter is able to form a stable chelated complex with ferric ions, which results in a decrease in the bioavailability of free Fe^{3+}. As a consequence, the formation of reactive hydroxyl radicals is impaired. Indeed, several clinical studies indicate that the concomitant use of dexrazoxane allows higher cumulative anthracycline doses without an increased risk of CHF [3,37,40].

However, three aspects regarding the use of ICRF-187 have not yet been evaluated precisely. First, more data are necessary to prove that this supportive agent does not impair antineoplastic efficacy; second, the optimal dosage of ICRF-187 has not yet been defined with precision (e.g., 500 or 1000 mg/m^2 ICRF-187 in combination with 50 mg/m^2 doxorubicin); third, it remains to be determined whether ICRF-187 influences the duration or severity of anthracycline-induced neutropenia [3].

In the meantime, dexrazoxane has been approved by the U.S. Food and Drug Administration for the prophylaxis of Adriamycin-induced CHF if cumulative doses exceed 300 mg/m^2. The drug is generally administered in a dose ratio of 10:1 in combination with doxorubicin. It has been recommended that the interval between ICRF-187 short-time infusion and the start of anthracycline administration not exceed 30 minutes [3].

→

Fig. 4 Dexrazoxane is a promising cardioprotective agent to be used to counteract the risk of anthracycline-induced congestive cardiomyopathy. The chelation of ferric ions strongly diminishes the formation of very toxic hydroxyl radicals. (Modified from Ref. 37.)

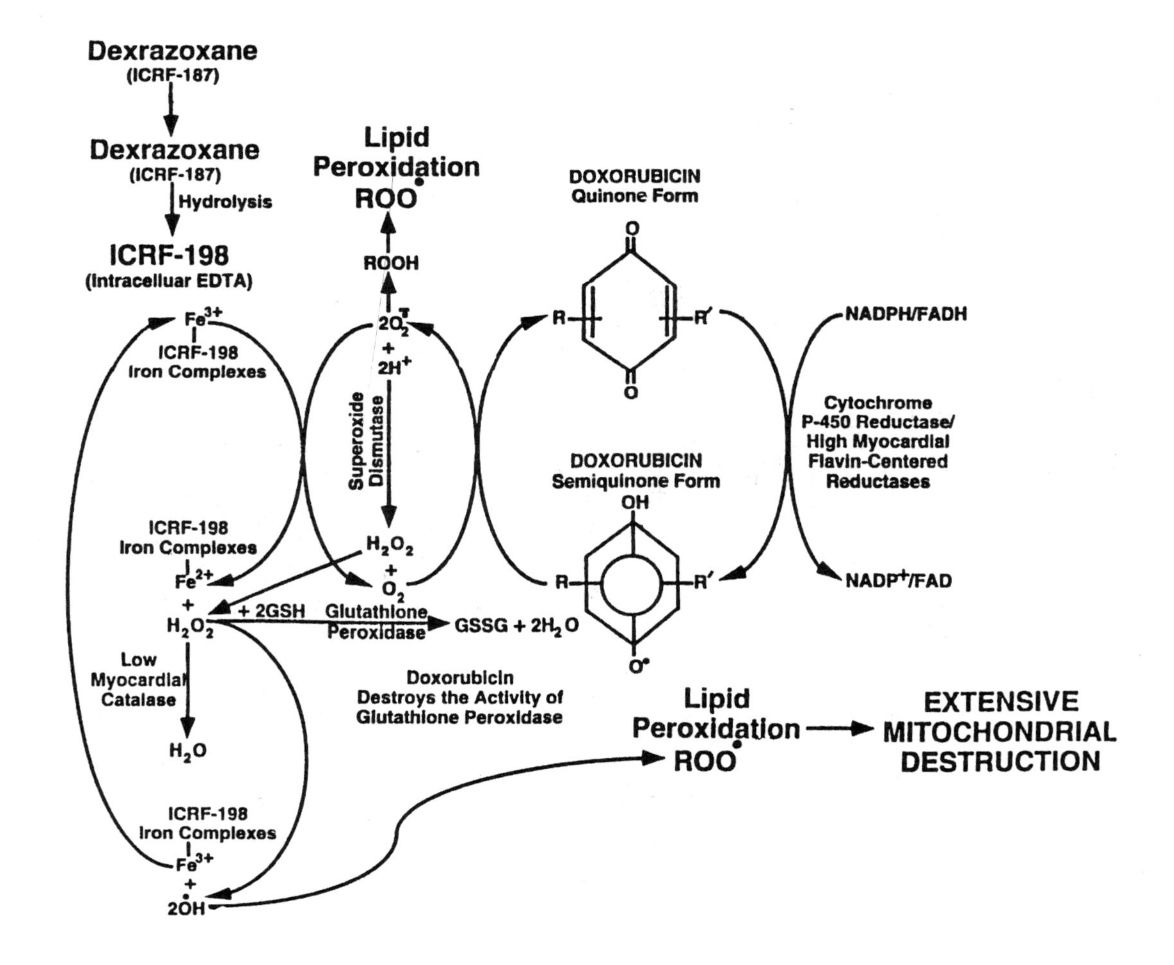
Dexrazoxane
(ICRF-187)
Dexrazoxane
(ICRF-187)
Hydrolysis
ICRF-198
(Intracellular EDTA)
Lipid
Peroxidation
ROO•
ROOH
DOXORUBICIN
Quinone Form
O
O
R
R′
NADPH/FADH
Fe^{3+}
ICRF-198
Iron Complexes
$2O_2^{\cdot-}$
+
$2H^+$
Superoxide
Dismutase
Cytochrome
P-450 Reductase/
High Myocardial
Flavin-Centered
Reductases
DOXORUBICIN
Semiquinone Form
OH
ICRF-198
Iron Complexes
Fe^{2+}
+
H_2O_2
H_2O_2
+
O_2
R
R′
O•
$NADP^+$/FAD
+ 2GSH
Glutathione
Peroxidase
GSSG + $2H_2O$
Low
Myocardial
Catalase
H_2O
Doxorubicin
Destroys the Activity of
Glutathione Peroxidase
Lipid
Peroxidation
ROO•
EXTENSIVE
MITOCHONDRIAL
DESTRUCTION
ICRF-198
Iron Complexes
Fe^{3+}
+
2OH•

11.2.5 Anthracycline Dose Adaptation in Patients with Hepatic Dysfunction

To avoid an increased risk of CHF, it has been recommended to adapt the anthracycline dose to the individual's underlying hepatic function, for otherwise severe drug cumulation cannot be excluded [41,42]. Dosage recommendations for anthracyclines in patients with hepatic dysfunction were listed in Chapter 2 (Table 13).

11.2.6 Accidental Overdosage of Anthracyclines and Related Compounds

Only a few case reports exist that deal with therapeutic intervention in cases of accidental anthracycline overdosage. One may speculate that cardiotoxicity will be fatal if doxorubicin or mitoxantrone is accidentally overdosed tenfold. However, acute cardiac complications appear to be transient and reversible after overdosage, whereas mucositis gets a predominant clinical problem. If hemoperfusion with a charcoal filter is started after several hours, the plasma concentration of doxorubicin and doxorubicinol probably will not be changed significantly by this therapeutic intervention because of the high and rapid affinity of anthracyclines (and related compounds) for plasma constituents [43,44].

11.2.7 Liposomal Drug Delivery

In the meantime, three liposomally encapsulated anthracycline formulations have been emerged for recent clinical trials: Doxil (Caelyx), DaunoXome, and TLC D-99 [45–48].

In contrast to conventional doxorubicin, which is associated with an increased risk of irreversible cardiomyopathy when cumulative doses exceed 550 mg/m^2, no comparable signs of cardiotoxicity were observed in cancer patients treated with cumulative polyethylene glycol–liposomal doxorubicin doses ranging from 760 to 860 mg/m^2.

The same appears to be true for liposomal daunorubicin (DaunoXome). Even after cumulative doses exceeding 1000 mg/m^2, no significant declines in cardiac function were observed after treatment with liposomal daunorubicin [49].

Future randomized clinical trials will show whether the significantly improved tolerability (particularly in regard to chronic cardiotoxicity) of liposomal anthracyclines is cosegregated with an improved therapeutic efficacy [45–49].

11.3 OTHER CARDIOTOXIC DRUGS STRUCTURALLY RELATED TO THE ANTHRACYCLINES

The bis(substituted aminoalkylamino) anthraquinone mitoxantrone differs from the common chemical structure of the anthracyclines. Its antineoplastic efficacy may be primarily based on an interaction with the topoisomerase II that results in single- and double-strand breaks of DNA. It cannot be excluded that reactive intermediates released during metabolism may be responsible for the antiproliferative mechanism. However, superoxide anions and hydroxyl radicals appear to be released to a lower extent than the anthracyclines [50–56].

There is some evidence that such anthrapyrazole derivatives as DUP 937, losoxantrone [biantrazole], and piroxantrone [oxantrazole], which represent a new class of anticancer drugs, may induce less cumulative cardiotoxicity than the established anthracyclines, even though they appear to exert comparable antiproliferative activity in comparison to the anthracyclines on an equimolar basis. For example, the use of piroxantrone was not associated with an increased risk of CHF even at dosages up to 1200 mg/m^2. As a consequence, these novel antineoplastic agents may represent promising candidates for dose escalation studies [57].

The use of amsacrine, which is primarily provided for the treatment of acute lymphatic and acute myelogenous leukemia in adults, has also been associated with the development of CHF [58–60]. Particularly if amsacrine is given when more than 500 mg/m^2 of doxorubicin has already been administered, if the amsacrine dose exceeds 200 mg/m^2 within 48 hours, or if the cumulative dose of amsacrine and doxorubicin exceeds 900 mg/m^2, the risk of CHF is severely increased [61,62]. It has been suggested that the release of superoxide radicals during metabolism may be responsible for the development of amsacrine-induced CHF [63].

11.4 5-FLUOROURACIL

There is some evidence that in a few patients the use of 5-fluorouracil (5-FU) is associated with such cardiotoxic side effects as angina pectoris or even myocardial infarction [8,64]. The overall incidence of cardiac ischemia or arrhythmias has been estimated to approximate 4.5% in predisposed patients, whereas the incidence in cancer patients with no history of coronary artery diseases may average 1.1% [65]. Possibly continuous infusion as well as the concomitant use of cisplatin may increase the risk of 5-FU-induced cardiotoxicity [8,66].

If chest pain is evident during 5-FU continuous infusion, it would seem to be mandatory to stop the infusion immediately as well as to administer spasmolytic drugs (e.g., nitroglycerin).

The underlying mechanism by which 5-FU exerts cardiotoxic effects is yet fully understood [67]. As in the case of 5-FU-induced neurotoxicity, it has not been speculated that the highly cardiotoxic 5-FU catabolites fluoroacetate and fluorocitrate may be released during metabolism. However, this hypothesis has not been confirmed thus far by pharmacokinetic studies. It is more probable that impurities rather than 5-FU metabolites are responsible for the formation of fluorocitrate. Indeed, fluoroacetate was isolated from the urine of cancer patients treated with 5-FU preparations containing small amounts of fluoroacetaldehyde [68–70].

Other proposed mechanisms of 5-FU-induced coronary spasms and ischemic manifestations include an autoimmune response, interindividually different drug accumulation in the myocardium, or a change in blood viscosity [71–73]. Interindividually, different expression of the dihydropyrimidine dehydrogenase (DPDH), which is the responsible enzyme for 5-FU catabolism, does not appear to be a predisposing factor because cancer patients with DPDH deficiency do not generally suffer from extended cardiotoxic side effects [74].

11.5 HIGH-DOSE CYCLOPHOSPHAMIDE

High-dose cyclophosphamide (HD cyclophosphamide), which is often used in transplant regimens, is reported to cause transient cardiac decompensation as well as fatal cardiomyopathy [3,75,76].

The incidence of severe cardiotoxic side effects has been estimated to range from 2 to 10%. Patients show progressive hypotension associated with a marked decrease in systemic and pulmonary vascular resistance [77,78].

The pathogenesis of HD-cyclophosphamide-induced cardiotoxicity is not fully understood. An increase of free oxygen radicals mediated by elevated intracellular phosphoramide mustard levels may be causative [79,80]. As a consequence, one would expect that the supportive use of such radical scavengers as ascorbic acid might counteract the development of cardiac toxicity. However, clinical data regarding the prophylactic use of antioxidants during HD cyclophosphamide are still lacking.

The hypothesis that phosphoramide mustard (or other reactive intermediates) rather than the parent compound may be responsible for the onset of cardiotoxic side effects is strengthened by the clinical data of Ayash and colleagues. These researchers observed a significantly lower AUC of unchanged cyclophosphamide in cancer patients who developed cardiotoxicity

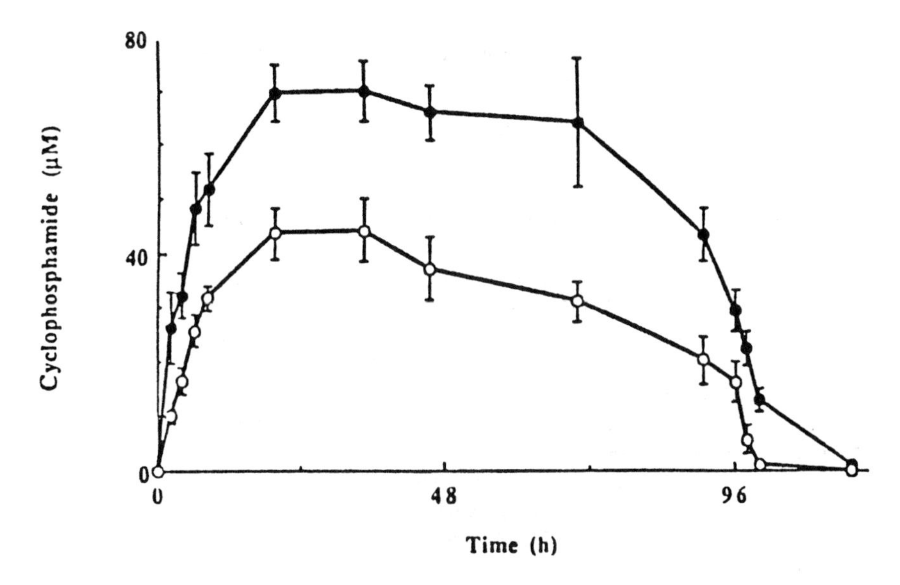

Fig. 5 AUC of total cyclophosphamide performed in six patients who developed reversible cardiotoxicity (open circles: mean, 3.189; median, 2.888 µmol/L/h) is significantly lower than in 13 patients who did not develop cardiotoxicity (solid circles: mean, 6.052; median, 6.121 µmol/L/h; $p < 0.002$) (SE bars included). Tumor response durability was significantly longer ($p = 0.008$) in the lower AUCs. (From Ref. 9.)

and concluded that an increased rate of metabolic conversion may increase antineoplastic activity but also end-organ toxicity (Fig. 5) [9].

11.6 PACLITAXEL

The taxoid paclitaxel has been reported to cause arrhythmias (e.g., sinus bradycardia and atrial fibrillation) as well as ischemia in cancer patients. However, cardiotoxicity is generally mild and reversible, whereas severe forms of cardiac complications (e.g., ventricular tachycardia and myocardial infarction) appear to be primarily restricted to patients with preexisting heart disease [81–83].

Ultrastructural abnormalities in the myocardium have been described in patients with palitaxel-induced cardiotoxicity [82]. The exact pathogenetic mechanism of this side effect remains still unknown and does not appear to be due directly to the mitotic inhibitory drug action, since the structurally related docetaxel has not been associated with the same incidence of cardiotoxicity thus far [84–86].

REFERENCES

1. Allen A. The cardiotoxicity of chemotherapeutic drugs. Semin Oncol 1992:19: 529–542.
2. Brestescher C, Pautier P, Farge D. Chemotherapy and cardiotoxicity. Ann Cardiol Angiol Paris 1995:44:443–447.
3. Hochster H, Wasserheit C, Speyer J. Cardiotoxicity and cardioprotection during chemotherapy. Curr Opin Oncol 1995:7:304–309.
4. Powis G. Toxicity of free radical forming anticancer agents. In: G Powis, MP Hacker, eds. The Toxicity of Anticancer Drugs. New York: Pergamon Press, 1991, pp 106–132.
5. Riggs CE, Bachur NR. Clinical pharmacokinetics of anthracycline antibiotics. In: MM Ames, G Powis, JS Kovach, eds. Pharmacokinetics of Anticancer Agents in Humans. Amsterdam: Elsevier Science Publishers, 1983, pp 229–277.
6. Minow RA, Benjamin RS, Lee ET, Gottlieb JA. Adriamycin cardiomyopathy: Risk factors. Cancer 1977:39:1397–1402.
7. von Hoff DD, Layard MW, Basa P, et al. Risk factors of doxorubicin-induced congestive heart failure. Ann Intern Med 1979:91:710–717.
8. Anand AJ. Fluorouracil cardiotoxicity. Ann Pharmacother 1994:28:374–378.
9. Ayash LJ, Wright JE, Tretyakov O, et al. Cyclophosphamide pharmacokinetics: Correlation with cardiac toxicity and tumor response. J Clin Oncol 1992:10: 995–1000.
10. Goldberg MA, Antin JH, Guinan EC, Rappeport JM. Cyclophosphamide cardiotoxicity: An analysis of dosing as a risk factor. Blood 1986:68:1114–1118.
11. White DA, Schwartzberg LS, Kris MG, et al. Acute chest pain during bleomycin infusions. Cancer 1987:59:1582–1585.
12. Mandel EM, Lewinsky U, Djaldetti M. Vincristine-induced myocardial infarction. Cancer 1975:36:1561–1562.
13. Giantris A, Abdurrahman L, Hinkle A, et al. Anthracycline-induced cardiotoxicity in children and young adults. Critical Reviews in Oncology/Hematology 1998:27:53–68.
14. Brenner DE, Wiernik PH, Wesley M, Bachur NR. Acute doxorubicin toxicity. Cancer 1984:53:1042–1048.
15. Krischer JP, Epstein S, Cuthbertson DD, et al. Clinical cardiotoxicity following anthracycline treatment for childhood cancer: The Pediatric Oncology Group experience. J Clin Oncol 1997:15:1544–1552.
16. Massidda B, Fenu MA, Ionta MT, et al. Early detection of the anthracycline-induced cardiotoxicity. A non-invasive haemodynamic study. Anticancer Res 1997:17:663–668.
17. Shan K, Lincoff M, Young JB. Anthracycline-induced cardiotoxicity. Ann Intern Med 1996:125:47–58.

18. Steinherz LJ, Steinherz PG, Tan CTC, Heller G, Murphy ML. Cardiac toxicity 4 to 20 years after completing anthracycline therapy. JAMA 1991:266:1672–1677.
19. Shapira J, Gotfried M, Lishner M, Ravid M. Reduced cardiotoxicirty of doxorubicin by a 6-hour infusion regimen. Cancer 1990:65:870–873.
20. von Hoff DD, Layard MW, Basa P, et al. Risk factors for doxorubicin-induced heart failure. Ann Intern Med 1979:91:710–717.
21. Bielack SS, Erttman R, Winkler K, Landbeck G. Doxorubicin: Effect of different schedules on toxicity and antitumor efficacy. Eur J Cancer Clin Oncol 1989:25:873–882.
22. Basser RL, Green MD. Strategies for prevention of anthracycline cardiotoxicity. Cancer Treatment Rev 1993:19:57–77.
23. Bonnadonna G, Gianni L, Santoro A, et al. Drugs ten years later: Epirubicin. Ann Oncol 1993:4:359–369.
24. Coukell A, Faulds D. Epirubicin—A review of its pharmacodynamic and pharmacokinetic properties, and therapeutic efficacy in the management of breast cancer. Drugs 1997:53(3):453–482.
25. Launchbury AP, Habboubi N. Epirubicin and doxorubicin: A comparison of their characteristics, therapeutic activity and toxicity. Cancer Treatment Rev 1993:19:197–228.
26. Weiss RB. The anthracyclines: Will we ever find a better doxorubicin? Semin Oncol 1992:19:670–686.
27. Dranitsaris G, Tran TM. Economic analysis of toxicity secondary to anthracycline-based breast cancer chemotherapy. Eur J Cancer 1995:31A: 2174–2180.
28. Lopez M, Contegiacomo A, Vici P, et al. A prospective randomized trial of doxorubicin versus idarubicin in the treatment of advanced breast cancer. Cancer 1989:64:2431–2436.
29. von Hoff DD, Rozencweig M, Layard M, et al. Daunomycin-induced cardiotoxicity in children and adults. A review of 110 cases. Am J Med 1977:62: 200–208.
30. Martoni A, Piana E, Guaraldi M, et al. Comparative phase II study of idarubicin versus doxorubicin in advanced breast cancer. Oncology 1990:47:427–432.
31. Anderlini P, Benjamin RS, Wong FC, et al. Idarubicin cardiotoxicity: A retrospective study in acute myeloid leukemia and myelodysplasia. J Clin Oncol 1995:13:2827–2834.
32. Berger DP, Winterhalter BR, Schick U, Höffken K. Idarubicin—intravenös und oral. Onkologe 1995:1:154–166.
33. Bertelli G, Amoroso D, Pronzato P, Rosso R. Idarubicin: An evaluation of cardiac toxicity in 77 patients with solid tumors. Anticancer Res 1988:8:645–646.
34. Villani F, Galimberti M, Comazzi R. Evaluation of cardiac toxicity of idarubicin (4-demethoxydaunorubicin). Eur J Cancer Clin Oncol 1989:25:13–18.
35. Lown JW, Chen H, Plambeck JA. Further studies on the generation of reactive oxygen species from activated anthracyclines and the relationship to cyctotoxic action and cardiotoxic effects. Biochem Pharmacol 1982:31:575–581.

36. Ehrke MJ, Mihich E, Berd D, Mastrangelo MJ. Effects of anticancer drugs on the immune system in humans. Semin Oncol 1989:16:230–253.
37. Seifert CF, Nesser ME, Thompson DF. Dexroxazone in the prevention of doxorubicin-induced cardiotoxicity. Ann Pharmacother 1994:28:1063–1072.
38. Goormaghtigh E, Chatelain P, Caspers J, et al. Evidence of a complex between Adriamycin derivatives and cardiolipin: Possible role in cardiotoxicity. Biochem Pharmacol 1980:29:3003–3010.
39. Myers CE, McGuire WP, Liss RH, et al. Adriamycin: The role of lipid peroxidation in cardiac toxicity and tumor response. Science 1977:197:165–167.
40. Bates M, Lieu D, Zagari M, Spiers A, Williamson T. A pharmacoeconomic evaluation of the use of dexrazoxane in preventing anthracycline-induced cardiotoxicity in patients with stage IIIB or IV metastatic breast cancer. Clin Ther 1997:19(1):167–184.
41. Benjamin RS, Riggs CE, Bachur NR. Plasma pharmacokinetics of Adriamycin and its metabolites in humans with normal hepatic and renal function. Cancer Res 1977:37:1416–1420.
42. Twelves CJ, Dobbs NA, Michael Y, et al. Clinical pharmacokinetics of epirubicin: The importance of liver biochemical tests. Br J Cancer 1992:66:765–769.
43. Hachimi-Idrissi S, Schots R, Dewolf D, et al. Reversible cardiopathy after accidental overdose of mitoxantrone. Pediatr Hematol Oncol 1993:10:35–40.
44. Bäck H, Gustavsson A, Eksborg S, Rödjer S. Accidental doxorubicin overdosage. Acta Oncol 1995:34:533–536.
45. Coukell AJ, Spencer CM. Polyethylene glycol–liposomal doxorubicin: A review of its pharmacodynamic and pharmacokinetic properties, and therapeutic efficacy in the management of AIDS-related Kaposi's sarcoma. Drugs 1997: 53(3):520–538.
46. Kim S. Liposomes as carriers of cancer chemotherapy. Drugs 1993:46(4):618–638.
47. Ranson M, Howell A, Cheeseman S, Margison J. Liposomal drug delivery. Cancer Treatment Rev 1996:22:365–379.
48. Gabizon A, Isacson R, Libson E, et al. Clinical studies of liposome-encapsulated doxorubicin. Acta Oncol 1994:33:779–786.
49. Gill PS, Espina BM, Muggia F, et al. Phase I/II clinical and pharmacokinetic evaluation of liposomal daunorubicin. J Clin Oncol 1995:35(4):996–1003.
50. Crossley RJ. Clinical safety and tolerance of mitoxantrone. Semin Oncol 1984: 11(suppl 1):54–58.
51. Ehninger G, Schuler U, Proksch B, Zeller KP, Blanz J. Pharmacokinetics and metabolism of mitoxantrone, a review. Clin Pharmacokinet 1990:18(5):365–380.
52. Henderson IC, Allegra JC, Woodcock T, et al. Randomized clinical trial comparing mitoxantrone with doxorubicin in previously treated patients with breast cancer. J Clin Oncol 1989:7:560–571.
53. Feldman EJ, Alberts DS, Arlin Z, et al. Phase I clinical and pharmacokinetic evaluation of high-dose mitoxantrone in combination with cytarabine in patients with acute leukemia. J Clin Oncol 1993:11:2002–2009.

54. Mewes K, Blanz J, Ehninger G, Gebhardt R, Zeller KP. Cytochrome P450-induced cytotoxicity of mitoxantrone by formation of electrophilic intermediates. Cancer Res 1993:53:5135–5142.
55. Posner LE, Dukart G, Goldberg J, Bernstein T, Cartwright K. Mitoxantrone: An overview of safety and toxicity. Invest New Drugs 1985:3:123–132.
56. Poirier TI. Mitoxantrone. Drug Intell Clin Pharm 1986:20:97.
57. Judson IR. The anthrapyrazoles: A new class of compounds with clinical activity in breast cancer. Semin Oncol 1992:19:687–694.
58. De Lena M, Rossi A, Bonnadonna G. Phase II trial of AMSA in patients with refractory breast cancer. Cancer Treatment Rep 1979:63:1961–1964.
59. Rivera G, Evans W, Dahl G, Yee GC, Pratt CB. Phase I clinical and pharmacokinetic study of 4′-(9-acridinylamino)methanesulfan *m*-anisidine (AMSA) in children with cancer. Cancer Res 1980:40:4250–4253.
60. van Mouwerik TJ, Caines P, Ballentine R. Amsacrine evaluation. Drug Intell Clin Pharm 1987:21:330–334.
61. Vorobiof DA, Iturralde M, Falkson G. Amsacrine cardiotoxicity: Assessment of ventricular function by radionuclide angiography. Cancer Treatment Rep 1983:67:1115–1117.
62. Weiss RB, Grillo-López AJ, Marsoni S, et al. Amsacrine associated cardiotoxicity: An analysis of 82 cases. J Clin Oncol 1986:4:918–928.
63. Lee HH, Palmer D, Denny W. Reactivity of quinone imine and quinone diimine metabolites and the antitumor drug amsacrine and related compounds to nucleophiles. J Org Chem 1988:53:6042–6047.
64. Burger AJ, Mannino S. 5-Fluorouracil-induced vasospasm. Am Heart J 1987: 114:433–436.
65. Labianca R, Beretta G, Clerici M, et al. Cardiac toxicity of 5-fluorouracil: A study on 1083 patients. Tumori 1982:68:505–510.
66. Forni MD, Malet-Martino M, Jaillais P, et al. Cardiotoxicity of high-dose continuous infusion fluorouracil: A prospective clinical trial. J Clin Oncol 1992: 10:1795–1801.
67. Lieutaud T, Brain E, Golgran-Toledano D, et al. 5-Fluorouracil cardiotoxicity: A unique mechanism for ischaemic cardiopathy and cardiac failure? Eur J Cancer 1996:32A:369–370.
68. Lemaire L, Arellano M, et al. Cardiotoxicité du 5-fluorouracile: Une question de formulation. Bull Cancer 1994:81:1057–1059.
69. Lemaire L, Malet-Martino MC, de Forni M, et al. Cardiotoxicity of commercial 5-fluorouracil vials stems from the alkaline hydrolysis of the drug. Br J Cancer 1992:66:119–127.
70. Lemaire L, Malet-Martino MC, Longo S, et al. Fluoroacetaldehyde as cardiotoxic impurity in fluorouracil (Roche) [letter]. Lancet 1991:337:560.
71. Cwikiel M, Persson SU, Larsson H, et al. Changes of blood viscosity in patients treated with 5-fluorouracil—A link to cardiotoxicity? Acta Oncol 1995:34: 83–85.
72. McLachlan SA, Millward MJ, Toner GC, Guiney MJ, Bishop F. The spectrum of 5-fluorouracil cardiotoxicity. Med J Aust 1994:161:207–209.

73. Robben NC, Pippas AW, Moore JO. The syndrome of 5-fluorouracil cardiotoxicity. Cancer 1993:71:493–499.
74. Beuzeboc P, Pierga J-Y, Stoppa-Lyonnet D, et al. Severe 5-fluorouracil toxicity possibly secondary to dihydropyrimidine dehydrogenase deficiency in a breast cancer patient with osteogenesis imperfecta. Eur J Cancer 1996:32A:370–371.
75. Demirer T, Buckner CD, Appelbaum FR, et al. Busulfan, cyclophosphamide and fractionated total body irradiation for autologous or syngenic marrow transplantation for acute and chronic myelogenous leukemia: Phase I dose escalation of busulfan based on targeted plasma levels. Bone Marrow Transplant 1996: 17:491–495.
76. van der Wall E, Beijnen JH, Rodenhuis S. High-dose chemotherapy regimens for solid tumors. Cancer Treatment Rev 1995:21:105–132.
77. Braverman AC, Antin JH, Plappert MT, et al. Cyclophosphamide cardiotoxicity in bone marrow transplantation: A prospective evaluation of new dosing regimens. J Clin Oncol 1991:9:1215–1223.
78. Lee CK, Harman GS, Hohl RJ, Gingrich RD. Fatal cyclophosphamide cardiomyopathy: Its clinical course and treatment. Bone Marrow Transplant 1996: 18:573–577.
79. Burton KP, Morris AC, Massey KD, et al. Free radicals after ionic calcium levels and membrane phospholipids in cultured rat ventricular myocytes. J Mol Cell Cardiol 1990:22:1035–1047.
80. Levine ES, Friedman HS, Griffith OW, et al. Cardiac cell toxicity induced by 4-hydroxycyclophosphamide is modulated by glutathione. Cardiovasc Res 1993:27:1248–1253.
81. Finley RS, Rowinsky EK. Patient-care issues: The management of paclitaxel-related toxicities. Ann Pharamacother 1994:28:S27–S34.
82. Shek TWH, Luk ISC, Ma L, Cheung KL. Paclitaxel-induced cardiotoxicity. Arch Pathol Lab Med 1996:120:89–91.
83. Rowinsky EK, McGuire WP, Guarnieri T, et al. Cardiac disturbances during the administration of Taxol. J Clin Oncol 1991:9:1704–1712.
84. Verweij J. Docetaxel (Taxotere): A new anti-cancer drug with promising potential? Br J Cancer 1994:70:183–184.
85. Mross K, Unger C. Docetaxel—ein Taxoid mit breiter Antitumorwirksamkeit. Arzneimitteltherapie 1996:14:195–199.
86. Burris H, Irvin R, Kuhn J, et al. Phase I clinical trial of Taxotere administered as either a 2-hour or 6-hour intravenous infusion. J Clin Oncol 1993:11:950–958.

V

LATE SIDE EFFECTS OF CANCER CHEMOTHERAPY

12

Gonadal Toxicity and Teratogenicity After Cytotoxic Chemotherapy

ELIZABETH B. LAMONT
University of Chicago Pritzker School of Medicine, Chicago, Illinois

ROBERT L. SCHILSKY
Cancer Research Center, University of Chicago Pritzker School of Medicine, Chicago, Illinois

12.1 INTRODUCTION

With the advent of curative combination chemotherapy regimens for the malignancies that commonly affect young people, oncologists now have both the luxury and the burden of documenting the late side effects of therapy. Chief among these are secondary malignancies, long-term immunosuppression, and infertility. Treatment-related infertility in patients with curable cancers is a complex topic, made more confusing by the association of several of the most curable tumors in young patients with infertility prior to the initiation of therapy. Posttreatment infertility in patients has become predictable now that mouse models and human epidemiologic data have identified the agents most toxic to the germinal epithelium. Because of concerns that chemotherapy might irreparably damage gametes, many investigators have sought to determine the effects of chemotherapy on the progeny of cancer survivors. Finally, efforts to prevent infertility by hormone manipulation in patients undergoing chemotherapy have not shown success, but new methods of manipulating gametes prior to and after cytotoxic chemotherapy offer patients hope of retaining fertility posttreatment.

12.2 PRETREATMENT INFERTILITY

12.2.1 Introduction

Hodgkin's disease, testicular cancer, and perhaps breast cancer are associated with varying degrees of pretreatment infertility. In males with testis cancer or Hodgkin's disease, who are often quite young and have not yet planned to have children, the infertility may not be clinically apparent at the time of cancer diagnosis. Infertility is often noted incidentally when such fertility surrogates as sperm count and gonadotropin levels are evaluated prior to treatment. The important breast cancer risk factors of parity and lactation, the known trophic effects of sex hormones on breast cancer, and the case reports describing newly diagnosed breast cancer in women undergoing infertility evaluation have led many investigators to examine the relationship between infertility and subsequent breast cancer.

12.2.2 Testis Cancer

Consistently 50–80% of patients with testicular tumors present with oligospermia* [1–4]. Reasons for the pretreatment infertility are both speculative and far-ranging. Some investigators postulate that an increase in scrotal temperature from the contralateral tumor is enough to decrease spermatogenesis in the unaffected testicle. Others hypothesize that a fundamental defect in testicular morphogenesis predisposes to both infertility and cancer. In favor of the latter theory are results from contralateral testis biopsies of 200 consecutive patients with unilateral testis cancer sampled after orchiectomy but before chemotherapy and/or radiation therapy. Twenty-four percent of patients had abnormalities in the contralateral testis, including 12% with the Sertoli cell only syndrome (a condition in which the germinal epithelium is ablated, leaving only the supportive Sertoli cells), 11% with hyalinized seminiferous tubules, 10% with complete arrest of spermatogenesis, and 5% with carcinoma in situ [5]. In a study by Skakkebaek, testicular biopsy samples from 555 infertile, but otherwise healthy men presenting to a fertility clinic revealed a 1.1% incidence of carcinoma in situ. Sixty-seven percent of those men went on to develop invasive germ cell tumors within 5 years [6]. Like the observation that cryptorchism is associated with an increased risk of testis cancer in both the descended and undescended testes, these findings

*In this chapter, *oligospermia* refers to sperm counts of below 20×10^6 or 40×10^6 sperm/mL semen as both definitions are used in the literature. *Azoospermia* refers to sperm counts of 0×10^6 sperm/mL semen.

suggest that a diffuse testicular abnormality is the etiology for cancer, rather than a discrete single somatic cell mutation [7].

Other theories offered to explain the observed pretreatment infertility of patients with testis cancer include endocrine dysfunction from the circulating human chorionic gonadotropin (βhCG) produced by 20% of testis cancers. Morrish et al. have shown that elevated serum βhCG levels in testis cancer patients is associated with hypersecretion of 17-β estradiol (E2) from normal testicular tissue that reciprocally suppresses follicle-stimulating hormone (FSH) [8]. Others have not reported FSH suppression, but rather elevation, as would be expected with a testicular origin of infertility [5]. Finally, autoimmunity has also been suggested as a mechanism of pretreatment infertility, since 21% of testis cancer patients prior to orchiectomy have detectable antisperm antibodies [9]. Malignant disruption of the blood–testis barrier is presumed to be the cause of antigen exposure.

12.2.3 Hodgkin's Disease

Studies of pretreatment sperm counts in patients with Hodgkin's disease have found that 20% of such patients are oligospermic, and as many as 30–60% have abnormal semen analyses as assessed by indices of sperm count, sperm motility, and sperm density [10–15]. Results of testicular biopsies of newly diagnosed patients, obtained prior to treatment, reveal a number of abnormalities. Chapman and colleagues reported the results of biopsies of nine patients, only one of whom had normal histology. The remaining eight patients had abnormalities ranging from complete loss of germinal epithelium, hyalinization of tubules, and loss of Sertoli cells to early tubular hyalinization and occasional loss of germinal epithelium [10].

Several hypotheses to explain Hodgkin's-related infertility have been suggested, but few have been substantiated. Previously, constitutional illness was assumed to be the mechanism of the observed infertility. Although it has been shown that a small percentage of patients with Hodgkin's disease (10%) are either impotent or too weak to provide semen samples, several authors have excluded both B symptoms and stage as causal factors of infertility [10,14–16]. A central rather than testicular origin of the infertility has been proposed by two groups of investigators who have described low baseline FSH and testosterone levels in newly diagnosed Hodgkin's disease patients compared with controls [10,11]. However, these observations have not been confirmed by other investigators [15]. An additional hypothesis proposes that the infertility is related to imbalances in cellular immunity. Since suppressor T lymphocytes are normally found in both seminal fluid and testicular tissue, some investigators postulate that the fluctuations in T4:

T8 cell ratios seen in Hodgkin's disease patients may result in immune-mediated damage to the testes [17]. This interesting theory deserves further investigation. Though a definitive explanation for the pretreatment infertility of patients with Hodgkin's disease has not been discovered, the independence of the phenomenon of stage and testicular involvement suggests a paraneoplastic etiology.

12.2.4 Breast Cancer

The inverse relationship of parity to risk of developing breast cancer was described in the 1960s by MacMahon's group, who reported an increased risk of breast cancer in women with first births occurring after the age of 30 [18]. Given estrogen's known trophic effect on malignant mammary tissue, Korenman reasoned in his "estrogen window" hypothesis that tonic estrogen exposure, unopposed by the progesterone provided by pregnancy, resulted in an increased risk of malignant transformation of breast tissue [19]. A natural test of the hypothesis was to determine the relationship of anovulatory infertility, a condition with diminished or absent normal luteal progesterone elevations, to breast cancer.

Several groups have examined this question by calculating the relative risk of infertility in breast cancer cohorts compared to controls or by calculating the relative risk of breast cancer in infertile cohorts compared to controls [20–26]. After the early paper by Cowan's group [20] that described a 5.4-fold increased relative risk of breast cancer in women suffering from progesterone deficiency infertility, subsequent groups have reported no increased risk of breast cancer in infertile women in general nor in the subset of progesterone-deficient infertile women [21,23–26]. Three groups have also examined the effect of ovulatory stimulating drugs like clomiphene on risk of breast cancer, and all three have determined that the drugs conferred no added risk [22,26,27].

12.2.5 Summary

While both testis cancer and Hodgkin's disease are associated with high rates of pretreatment infertility in men, breast cancer is not associated with preexisting infertility. The etiology of the observed infertility remains unknown. In testis cancer, a generalized testicular abnormality is believed to be the source of infertility, inasmuch as histologic abnormalities are observed in contralateral, "noncancerous" testicles. In Hodgkin's disease, the testicular failure is felt to be paraneoplastic in origin. Several large epidemiologic studies have refuted the concern that breast cancer is associated with infertility.

12.3 CHEMOTHERAPY-RELATED INFERTILITY

12.3.1 Males

12.3.1.1 Pathophysiology

Human male infertility secondary to treatment with cytotoxic chemotherapy is almost entirely a function of damage to the seminiferous tubule germinal epithelium that results in decreased sperm counts. A review of the physiology of human spermatogenesis, the available clinical data from men treated with chemotherapy, and the experimental data from mice treated with chemotherapy suggests that there are two phases to chemotherapy-related infertility, an acute and a chronic phase.

The duration of development from stem cell to mature spermatozoa is 12 weeks in humans. This period is divided into a slowly cycling stem cell phase and a rapidly cycling spermatogonia stage. The rapid cell divisions of the spermatogonia stage give rise to spermatocytes that undergo two meiotic divisions to become spermatids and then morphologic changes to become spermatozoa.

The acute infertility from cytotoxic chemotherapy is a result of inhibition of the rapid division of spermatogonia. Since the time from the spermatocyte to the mature spermatozoa is approximately 6 weeks, it is not surprising that the acute infertility from cytotoxic chemotherapy is not noted until approximately 6 weeks after treatment. As the full cycle length would suggest, sperm counts often return to normal in men with selective suppression of the spermatogonial stage of spermatogenesis about 12 weeks after the discontinuation of therapy.

Unfortunately, the chronic phase of posttreatment infertility is clinically more significant and is often irreversible. Chemotherapeutic damage to germinal epithelial stem cells can result in prolonged or even permanent infertility. Although the cells cycle far less frequently than those in the spermatogonia phase, their repopulation after damage is at best slow and the control of their repopulation is not well understood. Table 1 summarizes the literature regarding the precise location of chemotherapy effects on the mouse spermatic cycle [28].

Although scientists believe that there is a degree of homology between mouse and human spermatogenesis, mouse models arc not always predictive of chemotherapy effects in humans. For example, single-agent doxorubicin is very toxic to mice but has little reproductive toxicity in humans. Table 2 classifies chemotherapeutic agents by observed human reproductive toxicity and mouse stem cell toxicity [29]. Since it would be unethical to study the

Table 1 Site of Toxicity of Antineoplastic Drugs in the Germinal Epithelium

Drug	Cell type affected	Literature reference
Actinomycin D	Stem cells; early spermatogonia	a
BCNU	Stem cells; intermediate spermatogonia	a
Bleomycin	Intermediate spermatogonia	b
Busulfan	Type A spermatogonia	c,d
CCNU	Intermediate spermatogonia; spermatocytes	a
Cisplatin	Spermatogonia; spermatocytes	a
Cytosine arabinoside	Late spermatogonia; spermatocytes	b
Cyclophosphamide	Late spermatogonia; spermatocytes	b
Doxorubicin	Stem cells	b
Methotrexate	Early spermatogonia	a
Mitomycin C	Stem cells; spermatogonia	a
Nitrogen mustard	Intermediate and late spermatogonia	a
Procarbazine	Stem cells; early spermatogonia	a

[a]Meistrich ML, Finch M, da Cunha MF, Hacker U, Au WW. Damaging effects of fourteen chemotherapeutic drugs on mouse testis cells. Cancer Res 1982:42:122–131.
[b]Lu CC, Meistrich ML. Cytotoxic effects of chemotherapeutic drugs on mouse testis cells. Cancer Res 1979:39:3575.
[c]Jackson H. The effects of alkylating agents on fertility. Br Med Bull 1964:20:107–113.
[d]Jackson H, Fox BW, Craig AW. Antifertility substances and their assessment in the male rodent. J Reprod Fertil 1961:2:447–465.
Reprinted from Crit Rev Oncol Hematol, 8(2), Gradishar WE, Schilsky RL. Effects of cancer treatment on the reproductive system, 1988, with permission from Elsevier Science Ireland, Ltd., Bay 15K, Shannon Industrial Estate, County Clare, Ireland.

effects of chemotherapy agents in humans the way they have been studied in mice, our understanding of the effects of chemotherapy on human male fertility comes from studying men treated with chemotherapy for neoplastic and nonneoplastic medical conditions. Because few data regarding actual posttreatment paternity are available, fertility surrogates such as sperm counts, gonadotropin levels, and, occasionally, the results of testicular biopsies are used to infer infertility. With germinal epithelial damage, sperm counts fall, FSH increases, and biopsy samples reveal arrest of spermatogenesis and variable numbers of stem cells.

12.3.1.2 Clinical History

After the mucocutaneous and aerodigestive toxicities of mustard gas vapors were observed in soldiers during World War I, scientists in the postwar period studied the effects of systemic injection of nitrogen mustard in animals. Autopsies revealed destruction of rapidly dividing cell types in these

Table 2 Comparison of the Relative Gonadal Toxicity of Antineoplastic Agents in Mouse and in Humans

	Potency for stem cell killing in mice[a]		
Effects in humans	High	Moderate	Negligible
Cause long-term azoospermia in man			
Single agents	Radiation Busulfan Chlorambucil		
Combination agents		Procarbazine	Cisplatin Cyclophosphamide
Have additive effects with agents above in causing long-term azoospermia	Adriamycin		Cytosine arabinoside
Unknown effects because always given with highly sterilizing agents			Nitrogen mustard
Permanent recovery of sperm count in a majority of patients with no demonstrated additive effects at doses used in conventional regimens	Thiotepa	Actinomycin D Daunorubicin 5-Fluorouracil	AMSA Bleomycin Dacarbazine 6-Mercaptopurine Methotrexate Mitoxantrone Prednisone Vinblastine Vincristine

[a]When given in single doses up to maximally tolerated doses.
Source: Meistrich, ML. Effect of chemotherapy and radiotherapy on spermatogenesis. Eur Urol 1993:23:136–142. Reproduced with permission of S. Karger AG, Basel, Switzerland.

animals, including lymphoid tissue, hematopoietic tissue, mucous membranes, and testicular tissue [30,31]. In the 1940s when nitrogen mustards were first given to patients with neoplasms, human autopsy studies revealed numerous testicular changes in most male patients, including arrest of spermatogenesis with an absence of spermatocytes and spermatids, decreased seminiferous tubule size, thickened basement membranes, and Sertoli cell only syndrome [32].

The use of cyclophosphamide in the 1960s for the treatment of nephrotic renal disease revealed that the drug could cause predictable, long-lasting azoospermia in a dose-dependent fashion. Fairley et al. compared results of semen analyses to duration of daily oral cyclophosphamide therapy in men with nephrotic syndrome and found that all men treated for 6 months or more developed azoospermia. He also found that with discontinuation of the drug, only 20% of patients had even minimal recovery in sperm counts after 3–9 months [33]. Similar results were reported by physicians treating lymphoma patients with busulfan [34]. Several years after the development of curative combination chemotherapy regimens for Hodgkin's disease and testis cancer, oncologists in the 1980s began to report infertility in young men cured of these previously incurable malignancies.

12.3.1.3 Testis Cancer

Cisplatin-based combination chemotherapy is the standard of care for stage II and III testis cancer and is associated with an 80% survival rate. Four cycles of bleomycin, etoposide, and cisplatin (BEP) or cisplatin, vinblastine, and bleomycin (PVB) are the two most commonly used regimens and are associated with similar fertility outcomes. While 50–80% of patients will be oligospermic prior to cytotoxic chemotherapy, all patients will be oligospermic one year after treatment (with 50–75% of those azoospermic), and 75% will be oligospermic 2 years after treatment (with one-third of those persistently azoospermic) [2,4,35]. Five years after therapy, more patients will have improved sperm counts, but a full 50% of patients remain oligospermic [36]. Hansen et al. studied posttreatment paternity in 158 patients with unilateral germ cell tumors and found that 41 patients had wished to have children after the completion of chemotherapy. Of these 41 patients, 16 men (39%) had become fathers at a median of 5 years after treatment, had median sperm counts of 50×10^6, and had no gross anomalies in their offspring. Another 25 patients (61%) had unsuccessfully attempted to induce conception at a median of 4 years after treatment and had median sperm counts below 20×10^6 [37]. In summary, 4–5 years after therapy with four cycles of BEP or PVB combination chemotherapy for testis cancer, roughly half of all men will have persistent oligospermia and will be clinically infertile.

12.2.1.4 Hodgkin's Disease

Like testis cancer, Hodgkin's disease is curable with combination chemotherapies that carry substantial risks of posttreatment male infertility. In 1964 the MOPP (nitrogen mustard, vincristine, procarbazine, and prednisone) regimen was developed at the National Cancer Institute for the treatment of

Hodgkin's disease and was associated with complete remission rates of 70–80%, with 80% of those patients still in remission at 20 years. During the 1970s several combination chemotherapy regimens as efficacious as MOPP were developed, among them ABVD (Adriamycin, bleomycin, vinblastine, and dacarbazine). In 1979 in his Karnofsky Memorial Lecture, Devita summarized the successful history of the MOPP regimen and was the first to comment on its substantial sterilizing effects [38]. A review of the MOPP literature reveals that six cycles of MOPP are associated with azoospermia rates of 100% immediately following treatment, 100% after 1 year, 90% after 2 years, and 86% after 3–7 years [10,12,39–41]. Six cycles of ABVD have a far better infertility profile, with azoospermia rates of only 33% immediately following treatment, and recovery of sperm counts in 70–100% of patients at 18 months [40,41]. The hybrid regimen of six to nine cycles of MOPP alternating with ABVD has azoospermia rates that reflect the component regimens, with immediate posttreatment azoospermia in 75–85% patients and recovery of sperm counts in 40–60% of patients at 2 years [15,41]. These results are consistent with the established threshold for permanent infertility of greater than or equal to five cycles of MOPP described by da Cunha et al. [16]. In summary, the posttreatment infertility of ABVD is far less than that of MOPP or MOPP/ABVD.

12.3.1.5 Bone Marrow Transplantation

Despite 15–20 years of experience with bone marrow transplantation, data regarding its effects on human fertility remain limited. The technique of treating patients with conditioning myeloablative chemotherapy with or without radiation therapy followed by infusion of either autologous or allogeneic blood progenitor cells has been applied to hematologic malignancies, solid tumors, and nonmalignant blood disorders. Two groups have examined the end points of fertility in such patients. Sanders' group analyzed data from small numbers of patients with aplastic anemia who were conditioned with high-dose cyclophosphamide (200 mg/kg) alone and from small numbers of acute leukemia patients who were conditioned with both high-dose cyclophosphamide (120 mg/kg) and total body irradiation (TBI). Of male aplastic anemia patients who received cyclophosphamide (200 mg/kg) only, 33% were azoospermic from 1 to 7 years after transplant. Thirteen percent of patients fathered children after therapy. Of the male acute leukemia patients who received both cyclophosphamide (120 mg/kg) and TBI, 94% were azoospermic at an unspecified follow-up period. Only 2% of patients fathered children after therapy [42]. Keilholz and colleagues examined FSH as a fertility surrogate in 19 men with lymphoma or leukemia conditioned with high-dose cyclophosphamide and TBI or cyclophosphamide, carmustine, and etoposide (CBV) prior to stem cell reinfusion. At a median follow-up period of 15.8 months, 89% of all men had elevated FSH consistent with damage to the germinal epithelium. Five patients with elevated FSH underwent semen analysis and all were azoospermic. At 5-year follow-up, 68% of men had persistently elevated FSH levels suggestive of persistent germinal aplasia [43,44]. A subset analysis determining the contribution of TBI to this observed infertility was not performed. In summary, high-dose cyclophosphamide used as conditioning therapy preceding stem cell reinfusion has sterilizing effects in men, and regimens using TBI in combination with cyclophosphamide appear to be far more sterilizing than cyclophosphamide alone.

12.3.1.6 Summary

Chemotherapy-induced infertility in men can be predicted by agent and schedule. Alkylating agents appear to be the most toxic to the germinal epithelium. Alkylating agents given as daily single agents above a threshold dose or combined in multidrug regimens like MOPP are by far the most toxic to the germinal epithelium. Although there appears to be slow repopulation of germinal epithelial stem cells over time, little improvement in sperm counts is observed 5 years after therapy. The addition of total body irradiation to alkylating agent conditioning regimens for bone marrow transplant results in dramatic increases in posttransplant infertility compared with regimens utilizing alkylator therapy alone.

12.3.2 Females

12.3.2.1 Pathophysiology

Cytotoxic chemotherapy causes female infertility through primary ovarian failure. Patients with primary ovarian failure develop amenorrhea, menopausal symptoms related to estrogen deficiency, and elevated FSH levels; in addition, there are ovarian findings of arrested follicular maturation with diminished or absent primordial follicles. The details of the pathophysiology of postchemotherapy infertility in females are less well understood than those relating to postchemotherapy infertility in males. The location of the female gonad and gamete kinetics preclude safe, simple, and rapid gamete analysis. Therefore what is known about chemotherapy toxicity to the ovaries is largely inferred from the menstrual histories, serum gonadotropin levels, and ovarian biopsy results of women treated with cytotoxic drugs.

12.3.2.2 Clinical History

Concerns about the effects of alkylating agents on female reproductive function were raised in the 1950s by physicians treating premenopausal women with daily busulfan (Myleran) for chronic granulocytic leukemia. In three small series, investigators reported cessation of menses in all patients after the initiation of busulfan therapy, two of the groups noting the onset of amenorrhea within 6 months of therapy [45–47]. By comparing the time to onset of amenorrhea with the dose of busulfan, Belohorsky's group determined that amenorrhea occurred in a dose-dependent manner [47]. These investigators also reported results of two postmortem examinations of women who had had "Myleran amenorrhea" at the time of death: ovarian "atrophy" was found in one patient, and fibrosis and single follicles in the second.

These results were reinforced in the 1960s and 1970s by the observations of rheumatologists and nephrologists who reported larger series of women treated with daily cyclophosphamide for glomerular disease or rheumatoid arthritis [48–51]. Not only was amenorrhea noted in most patients, but it was found to persist at one year in 90% [49]. Warne et al. localized the etiology of the amenorrhea to the ovary and termed the condition "ovarian failure" after endocrinologic evaluations revealed elevated urinary gonadotropins. From a cohort of amenorrheic patients, Warne obtained five ovarian biopsy samples that confirmed a lack of follicular maturation with a complete absence of primordial follicles in all cases [50]. Similar pathologic findings have been reported by other groups [51].

12.3.2.3 Breast Cancer

In the last 20 years, studies from the National Surgical Adjuvant Breast and Bowel Project (NSABP) and other large cooperative groups have proven that adjuvant chemotherapy confers a substantial survival advantage for women with node positive and high-risk node negative breast cancer. A review of adjuvant breast cancer treatment data that includes the end point of fertility reveals that in addition to agent and dose, age is an important determinant of postchemotherapy infertility.

Koyama's group reported that postoperative daily oral cyclophosphamide led to permanent amenorrhea from ovarian failure in 83% of patients, but only after a cumulative dose of 9.3 grams in women in their thirties compared with 5.2 grams in women aged 40 years or older [52]. Fisher et al. reinforced this point in reports from NSABP B-05 and B-07. After 17 cycles of L-phenylalanine mustard (PAM) or PAM with fluorouracil, 65–77% of women aged 40 years or older experienced permanent amenorrhea compared with only 12–30% of women aged 39 years or less [53]. Dnistrian et al. published similar results for women treated with 24 cycles of adjuvant cyclophosphamide, methotrexate, and 5-fluorouracil (CMF), reporting amenorrhea in 100% of women over 35 years old and in 0% of women younger than 30 [54].

Boccardo et al. evaluated the sterilizing effect of tamoxifen in a study comparing the antitumor effects of CMF versus tamoxifen versus CMF plus tamoxifen and found that 66% of women had persistent amenorrhea in the tamoxifen-only arm, compared with 74% in the CMF arm and 76% in the CMF-and-tamoxifen arm [55]. The relative contribution of doxorubicin to posttreatment infertility was questioned in a study by Hortobagyi et al. in which the investigators recorded amenorrhea in patients receiving several doxorubicin-containing regimens. Because each regimen also included the known ovarian toxin cyclophosphamide, isolation of a doxorubicin effect was difficult. The results were similar to those reported previously, with amenorrhea in 96% of women 40 years of age and older, in 33% of those ages 30–39, and in 0% of those under 30 [56].

In summary, adjuvant chemotherapy for breast cancer is associated with predictable agent-, dose-, and age-related posttreatment infertility in the course of multiple cycles of treatment with alkylating agents the most sterilizing for women 40 years old and older were most likely to become sterile. What is not known yet is the timing of the onset of menopause in the younger cohort (age < 30 years), who had no acute change in menses during the studies. It is likely that longer follow-up will reveal a shortened period of fertility, with early-onset menopause in these patients.

12.3.2.4 Hodgkin's Disease

Unlike men with Hodgkin's disease, women with newly diagnosed Hodgkin's disease have no significant pretreatment infertility. Chapman et al. evaluated ovarian tissue in three women with newly diagnosed Hodgkin's disease and found a normal number of primordial follicles, normal corpora lutea, and normally developing secondary follicles [57]. Indeed, there are many reports of women who became pregnant during the course of their illness [58–60]. Most remarkable was a series from Walter Reed Army Hospital reported by Smith et al., in which over 30% of patients became pregnant during the course of their illness [59].

Like men with Hodgkin's disease, women with Hodgkin's disease are at a substantial risk of developing posttreatment infertility. Several groups examined the long-term effects of MOPP, MVPP (nitrogen mustard, vinblastine, procarbazine, and prednisone), and ChVPP (chlorambucil, vinblastine, procarbazine, and prednisone) on female fertility and found significant ovarian toxicity [39,57,61,62]. In Chapman's cohort of 41 patients (40 MVPP, 1 ChVPP), followed for a median of 36 months after chemotherapy, overall 62% experienced ovarian failure, with 84% of women 30 years of age and older experiencing ovarian failure, and only 31% of women under 30 experiencing ovarian failure [57]. Others have reported persistent amenorrhea in 45–57% of women treated with six or more cycles of MOPP or MVPP [62–64]. Horning et al. performed a multivariate analysis that identified treatment with concomitant total lymphoid irradiation and chemotherapy as a predictor of posttreatment infertility [61]. Several investigators have identified age less than 30 at the time of treatment as a predictor of preservation of fertility after treatment with MOPP [61,65].

As is the case in male patients, the ABVD regimen appears to be far less sterilizing than the MOPP regimen in female patients. A small study by Santoro et al. reports that 25% of women treated with three cycles of MOPP followed by irradiation developed persistent amenorrhea, compared with none of the women treated with three cycles of ABVD followed by irradiation [65].

12.3.2.5 Bone Marrow Transplantation

As noted earlier, few studies report the effects of bone marrow transplantation on human fertility. Sanders reported results on 24 women with aplastic anemia who were conditioned with high-dose cyclophosphamide (200 mg/kg) and 38 women with acute leukemia who were conditioned with high-dose cyclophosphamide (120 mg/kg) and TBI. In the chemotherapy only group, 33% of women over 26 years of age were amenorrheic at a median follow-up of 6 months posttransplant, while none of the women younger than 26 were amenorrheic at that time. Twenty-one percent of the women subsequently became pregnant. These results contrast sharply with those of the acute leukemia patients who received both high-dose cyclophosphamide and TBI, 92% of whom experienced primary ovarian failure with amenorrhea and elevated serum FSH levels. Only 5% of the women became pregnant [42]. Keilholz and colleagues describe similar results in women with hematologic malignancies conditioned primarily with cyclophosphamide and TBI, reporting primary ovarian failure in 100% of women at 15.8 months of follow-up [43]. At 5-year follow-up, 100% of women conditioned with the TBI-containing regimen remained amenorrheic, while the single patient conditioned with CBV experienced a return of menses and had given birth to two children [43,44]. As with the male patients, women who are treated with conditioning regimens that include TBI have a higher likelihood of posttransplant infertility than women conditioned with cyclophosphamide alone.

A problem with interpreting thc results of transplantation studies is that most patients who are treated on protocols with high-dose chemotherapy followed by stem cell reinfusion have been heavily pretreated with standard therapies that were unsuccessful. The relative contribution of the prior treatment regimens to posttransplantation infertility in these studies is impossible to determine. Fertility results in the small number of chemotherapy-naive patients undergoing transplant (e.g., inflammatory breast cancer patients, Ph + acute lymphoblastic leukemia (ALL) patients) need to be examined before the sterilizing effects of "transplantation" regimens can be evaluated fairly.

12.3.2.6 Summary

Postchemotherapy infertility in women can be predicted by agent, dose, schedule, and age. Exposure to alkylating drugs like busulfan and cyclophosphamide causes infertility in women in a dose-dependent manner. When alkylating agents are combined in multidrug regimens like MOPP or MVPP, infertility is more frequent. Single-agent tamoxifen appears to have a sterilizing effect in women, and doxorubicin combined with cyclophosphamide may increase the risk of subsequent sterility. Patient age at exposure appears to be a critical determinant of posttreatment infertility, with women 30 or more years of age at a much higher risk of subsequent infertility than women under 30.

12.3.3 Children

12.3.3.1 Introduction

Much of our understanding of the effects of cytotoxic chemotherapy on developing gonads comes from reports of children treated with combination chemotherapy for leukemia and Hodgkin's disease and with cyclophosphamide for nephrotic syndrome. The literature is difficult to interpret because of the heterogeneity introduced by the patients' wide spectrum of pubertal development, by the wide range of cytotoxic agents utilized, and by the varied schedules of administration. Perhaps most important, follow-up time sufficient to evaluate full pubertal development is often lacking in these studies. The fertility indices most frequently used in these studies are degree of pubertal development defined by Tanner stage and onset of menarche, sex hormone and gonadotropin levels, sperm counts, and histology of gonadal biopsy samples. Results are often stratified by patients' pubertal stage at the initiation of treatment, with the most common subdivisions being prepubertal, pubertal, and postpubertal.

12.3.3.2 Boys

Acute Leukemia

Several groups have examined the fertility indices of testicular biopsy results and pubertal development in boys undergoing therapy for acute lymphoblastic leukemia (ALL), and the results reveal that treatment with regimens that include cyclophosphamide and/or cytarabine are associated with significantly greater histologic changes in the gonad than regimens that do not include these agents. Examining a cohort of 35 primarily prepubertal boys in complete remission 30–48 months after cessation of chemotherapy, Uderzo et al. found that 100% of patients treated with a regimen that included cyclophosphamide and cytarabine had abnormal testicular biopsy results, compared with only 26% of patients treated with regimens that did not include those agents. The abnormalities included thickened basement membranes, reduced or absent spermatogenesis, germinal aplasia, and reduced tubular fertility indices.[†] All the patients treated with cyclophosphamide and cytarabine had TFIs of 30% or less, while none of the patients treated with other regimens had abnormal TFIs. Interestingly, clinical indices of pubertal development [testosterone, FSH, luteinizing hormone (LH), bone age, pubertal stage] were normal in all but one patient. Data analysis revealed the testicular changes to be independent of age at the start of treatment and to be unaccompanied by developmental delays [66]. Similar results have been reported by other investigators [67–69].

Hodgkin's Disease

The timing of MOPP chemotherapy relative to puberty appears to be critical to subsequent fertility. Both Sherins and Whitehead reported high infertility indices in pubertal or late pubertal boys treated with MOPP compared with their prepubertal counterparts. Sherins et al., described gynecomastia, depressed serum testosterone, elevated LH and FSH levels, and testicular biopsy samples with germinal cell aplasia in 69% of pubertal Ugandan boys treated with MOPP [70]. None of the prepubertal boys had gynecomastia nor significant abnormalities in hormone or gonadotropin levels. Whitehead et al. have reported similar endocrinologic profiles [71]. Some disagree with the importance of timing of treatment relative to puberty, citing papers that show equal degrees of posttreatment infertility in prepubertal and pubertal patients [72,73]. However, most patients in these studies were also treated with radiation therapy, often to the inguinal region, which makes determination of an isolated chemotherapy effect on gonadal development impossible.

Nephrotic Syndrome

Review of the available data regarding the long-term effects of cyclophosphamide administration during childhood on the testes of patients treated for nephrotic syndrome suggests both a dose-related and age-related risk of subsequent infertility. In a study of 29 boys treated with daily cyclophosphamide

---

[†]Tubular fertility index (TFI) is an estimate of fertility defined as the number of seminiferous tubules out of 100 containing spermatogonia. A normal value is ≥80%.

for nephrotic syndrome, Lentz et al. determined that a cumulative dose exceeding 365 mg/kg was associated with a 75% risk of azoospermia at a median follow-up of 3.5 years. None of the patients treated with cumulative doses of less than 365 mg/kg developed azoospermia [74]. Age at treatment was not an indicator of subsequent infertility in this study. Parra and colleagues reported the hormone profiles of 13 nephrotic boys treated with cumulative doses lower than 365 mg/kg, from 1 to 5 years after cessation of treatment. They found that 50% of boys pubertal (Tanner 2–3) at the time of treatment had elevated FSH levels compared to 0% of prepubertal boys. Additionally, half the patients with elevated FSH levels underwent semen analyses and all were azoospermic [75].

12.3.3.3 Girls

Leukemia

There are few studies documenting the effects of leukemia treatment on the developing ovary. Siris et al. reported fertility indices from 35 girls with leukemia, 34 of whom had ALL and were treated with steroid, vincristine, methotrexate, and 6-mercaptopurine, and one of whom had CML and was treated with busulfan. The patients were stratified into three groups by level of pubertal development: prepubertal, pubertal, and postmenarchal. The results revealed only 3 cases of primary ovarian failure: one pubertal patient and two postmenarchal patients. In both postmenarchal patients, the primary ovarian failure was characterized by amenorrhea, depressed serum estrogen, and elevated serum FSH and was transient. In the single case in the pubertal group, the primary ovarian failure was characterized by depressed serum estrogen and elevated serum FSH and occurred in the one patient treated with busulfan [76]. Wallace et al. reported a 15-year follow-up of 40 girls with childhood ALL who were treated with vincristine, prednisolone, 6-mercaptopurine, and methotrexate with or without asparaginase, cytosine arabinoside, doxorubicin, and cyclophosphamide and with or without cranial and spinal radiation therapy. Ninety-three percent of patients had regular menses, and only 10% suffered "ovarian damage," as defined by low serum estradiol and elevated gonadotropin levels. Almost all patients with "ovarian damage" had received cranial and spinal irradiation, suggesting that radiation to the spine may be a major risk factor for subsequent ovarian dysfunction in girls treated for ALL [77].

Nephrotic Syndrome

In the papers described above, neither Lentz nor Parra found evidence that daily cyclophosphamide leads to primary ovarian failure in small numbers of girls treated for nephrotic syndrome [74,75]. At a median follow-up period of 5 years, Lentz found that basal body temperature patterns and serum gonadotropin levels were normal in all patients, suggesting normal ovulation.

12.3.3.4 Summary

Data from studies of children who received chemotherapy for medical illnesses reveal that the developing male gonad is more sensitive to chemotherapy than the female gonad. Alkylating agents used singly or in combination are highly toxic to developing male germinal epithelium. Further, the cumulative dose of alkylator and the timing of administration are critical predictors of subsequent male infertility. In boys, the highest risks of infertility are associated with cumulative cyclophosphamide doses exceeding 365 mg/kg regimens containing two alkylators, or treatment during puberty. Data from a small number of studies of girls receiving single-agent or combination chemotherapy for childhood illnesses suggest that while alkylating agents may be toxic to the developing ovary, the incidence of infertility is far lower than in boys and does not appear to be dose dependent at the doses employed. These results are corroborated by Byrne et al., who undertook a retrospective study of 2283 long-term survivors of childhood cancers, comparing patient fertility outcome to sibling controls. These researchers reported fertility deficits in 60% of men treated with alkylating agents with or without subdiaphragmatic radiation therapy. They found no fertility deficits in women treated with alkylating agents and only modest fertility deficits in women treated with both alkylating agents and subdiaphragmatic radiation therapy [78]. However, longer follow-up studies that report the onset of menopause in similar patients are needed before definitive statements can be made about the effects of chemotherapy during childhood on reproductive life expectancy in women.

12.4 EFFECT ON PROGENY

12.4.1 Introduction

Logical concerns regarding a potential increase in birth defects in the progeny of people who had previously received chemotherapy have led several investigators to examine the pregnancy outcomes of cancer survivors.

12.4.2 Patients Treated in Childhood

Pregnancy outcomes in survivors of childhood cancer have been evaluated in general and by specific tumor type. Two groups evaluating patients treated with chemotherapy for "childhood cancer" reported no increase in the frequency of congenital malformations in offspring compared to controls [79,80]. Green's subset analysis, however, revealed excess structural congenital cardiac defects in the children of women treated with dactinomycin in childhood [81]. Investigators examining the effects of therapy for Hodgkin's disease or ALL on subsequent progeny reported no excess in fetal malformations [81–84]. A study of the children of Wilms tumor survivors reported no excess in fetal malformations when analysis was limited to those who had received chemotherapy, excluding subjects who had received abdominal radiation [85]. Excluding hereditary retinoblastoma and bilateral Wilms tumors, no excess in malignancies was reported in offspring described in these papers.

12.4.3 Patients Treated in Adulthood

Pregnancy outcomes in patients treated with cytotoxic chemotherapy in adulthood are similar to those of patients treated with cytotoxic chemotherapy in childhood. No excess of fetal malformations was reported by several authors who examined adults with "cancer" previously treated with chemotherapy [86,87]. Several groups evaluated children of Hodgkin's disease survivors and noted no excess in fetal malformations compared with controls [61,63,64,88,89]. Although there is surprisingly scant literature on the pregnancy outcomes of breast cancer survivors treated with adjuvant chemotherapy, one study of 227 consecutive breast cancer patients reported no increase in fetal malformations among progeny [90]. Similarly, one report revealed no increase in congenital malformations among offspring of male patients treated with cisplatin-based chemotherapy for unilateral germ cell tumors [37].

12.4.4 Summary

With the exception of a possible association of dactinomycin treatment in childhood with congenital cardiac defects in offspring, treatment with cytotoxic chemotherapy in either childhood or adulthood does not appear to be associated with an increase risk of congenital malformations in patients' subsequent offspring.

12.5 TERATOGENICITY OF CHEMOTHERAPY

What is known of the teratogenicity of chemotherapy in humans is largely inferred from the results of animal studies and clinical case reports. Both the chemotherapeutic agent employed and the gestational timing of the exposure appear to be important determinants of chemotherapy-induced teratogenicity in humans.

Nearly all chemotherapeutic agents have been associated with adverse fetal outcomes in mice or humans. Several authors have culled case reports from either the literature or single institutions to compile case series identifying agents teratogenic to humans [91–96]. Among the agents described, the antimetabolites (aminopterin, cytarabine, 5-fluorouracil, 6-mercaptopurine, methotrexate) and alkylating agents (chlorambucil, busulfan, cyclophosphamide) appear to be the most frequently teratogenic, particularly when administered during the period of organogenesis.

Defined as ranging from the second through the eighth week of gestation, organogenesis is a period of intense fetal cellular division and differentiation leading to organ development. Disruption of this orderly process by cytotoxic chemotherapy can result in deformities in any organ system. The congenital abnormalities caused by chemotherapy drugs in humans are not predictable, likely because of the wide spectrum of organ development during this interval. For example, in the series of Sieber and Adamson, methotrexate given to three women at the same early stage of pregnancy resulted in three different outcomes: a normal pregnancy, a premature delivery, and a baby with multiple cranial and digital anomalies [92]. Reports like these, as well as results from animal experiments, have led the U.S. Food and Drug Administration (FDA) to develop pregnancy risk categories that may be applied to all drugs. Table 3 lists chemotherapy drugs by risk category.

In summary, case reports and experimental animal data have identified nearly all chemotherapeutic agents as potentially teratogenic when administered to pregnant women. From the human literature, the alkylating agents and antimetabolites appear to be the most consistently teratogenic, particularly when administered to during the first trimester of pregnancy. A thorough and frank discussion between physician and patient regarding the risk/benefit ratio of first-trimester chemotherapy must occur before a decision to treat is made.

12.6 PREVENTION AND TREATMENT OF CHEMOTHERAPY-INDUCED INFERTILITY

12.6.1 Males

12.6.1.1 Introduction

Chemotherapy-related infertility in men is due to irreversible germ cell damage. Some investigators have attempted to prevent chemotherapy-induced

Table 3 Chemotherapy Drugs Classified by FDA Pregnancy Risk

Drug	FDA classification[a]	Common clinical use
Alkylating agents		
Busulfan	D	Chronic leukemias
Carboplatin	D	Lung cancer
		Ovarian cancer
Carmustine	D	CNS malignancies
		Lymphomas
Cisplatin	D	Lung cancer
		Ovarian cancer
		Sarcomas
Cyclophosphamide	D	Breast cancer
		Lymphomas
Melphalan	D	Chronic leukemias
		Multiple myeloma
Thiotepa	D	Breast cancer
		Ovarian cancer
Antiestrogen		
Tamoxifen	D	Breast cancer
		Uterine cancer
Antimetabolites		
Cytarabine	C	Acute leukemias
		Lymphomas
Fludarabine	D	Chronic lymphocytic leukemia
		Lymphomas
5-Fluorouracil	D	Breast cancer
		Gastrointestinal tumors
6-Mercaptopurine	D	Acute leukemias
Methotrexate	D	Breast cancer
		Leukemias
		Lymphomas
Antitumor antibiotics		
Bleomycin	D	Lymphomas
Dactinomycin	C	Sarcomas
		Uterine cancer
Daunorubicin	D	Acute leukemias
Doxorubicin	D	Acute leukemias
		Breast cancer
		Sarcomas
Mitoxantrone	D	Acute leukemias
		Lymphomas

Table 3 Continued

Drug	FDA classification[a]	Common clinical use
Steroid		
Prednisone	B	Leukemias Lymphomas
Vinca alkaloids		
Vincristine	D	Acute leukemias Lymphomas Multiple myeloma
Vinblastine	D	Lymphomas
Others		
Etoposide	D	Leukemias Lung cancer Lymphomas
Taxol	D	Breast cancer Ovarian cancer

[a]A, Adequate studies in pregnant women have failed to show a risk to the fetus in the first trimester, and there is no evidence of risk in later trimesters. B, Animal studies have not shown an adverse effect on the fetus, but there are no adequate clinical studies in pregnant women. C, Animal studies have shown an adverse effect on the fetus, but there are no adequate studies in human. The drug may be useful in pregnant women despite its potential risks. D, There is evidence of risk to the human fetus, but the potential benefits of use in pregnant women may be acceptable despite potential risks.
Used with permission from Physician's Drug Handbook, 8th ed., Springhouse Corp., 1999, p. vi.

germ cell damage with use of gonadotropin-releasing hormone (GnRH) agonists and antagonists. Others have attempted to overcome the sterility associated with germ cell damage by micromanipulation of gametes. Both approaches are reviewed.

12.6.1.2 GnRH Agonists and Antagonists

The pulsatile release of GnRH is a feature of the normal male hypothalamic–pituitary–gonadal axis. GnRH leads to the release of LH, which stimulates testicular Leydig cells to release testosterone. In the presence of testosterone, FSH stimulates Sertoli cells to support the development of the germinal epithelium. Although the exact endocrinology of spermatogenesis and the control of stem cell division is not well understood, it is likely that testosterone, LH, and FSH are critical components of its regulation. Tonic treatment of both men and mice with GnRH agonists, GnRH antagonists, or sex hormones like testosterone, produces suppression of the pituitary–gonadal axis, eventually resulting in low levels of FSH, LH, and testosterone. Such treatment is associated acutely with azoospermia and eventually with structural changes like testicular atrophy, as demonstrated by Giberti et al., who examined testicular biopsy samples from seven patients with prostate cancer who had been treated for 24–36 months with LHRH agonists. These investigators reported decreased numbers of Leydig cells, tubular derangement, and fibrosis [97].

It has been postulated that limited treatment with these agents might result in germ cell cycle arrest that could be exploited to protect stem cells from the damage of cytotoxic chemotherapy. In several preclinical studies, investigators have shown improved stem cell survival and full stem cell recovery after cytotoxic chemotherapy in animals pretreated with these agents [98–104].

Unfortunately, the success has not carried over to human experiments, where not a single study has shown benefit of treatment with GnRH agonists, GnRH antagonists, or sex hormones prior to cytotoxic chemotherapy [105–108]. The problem may be one of biology, with murine stem cells responding differently to hormonal manipulations, or it may simply be related to duration of therapy. In the successful mouse experiments, mice were pretreated for 6 weeks with GnRH agonists prior to receiving chemotherapy. In the human studies, treatment either preceded chemotherapy by 7 days or was coincident with chemotherapy. From what we know of the kinetics of spermatogenesis in humans and mice (murine cycles last 6 weeks and human cycles last 12 weeks), it would stand to reason that humans require twice the pretreatment period of mice. However, given the urgency of treatment initiation in potentially curable malignancies like Hodgkin's disease and testis cancer, it may not be appropriate to delay potentially curative therapy for 3 months to allow suppression of spermatogenesis to occur.

12.6.1.3 Gamete Manipulation

In the past, paternity prospects for azoospermic and oligospermic cancer survivors were limited to adoption, or artificial insemination of their partners by donor sperm. However over the last 20 years, fertility specialists in the fields of reproductive endocrinology, obstetrics and gynecology, and urology have developed multidisciplinary approaches to couples with male factor infertility that seem ideally suited for oligospermic and azoospermic cancer survivors. These include artificial insemination with banked sperm and in vitro fertilization with or without micromanipulation of gametes.

Sperm Banking

The American Fertility Society's guidelines for banking (vizi, sperm counts of $\geq 50 \times 10^6$ sperm/mL semen, $\geq 60\%$ motility, normal morphology) preclude most testis cancer patients and many Hodgkin's disease patients from banking sperm prior to receiving chemotherapy [109]. Although this set of figures has been a deterrent for many patients and physicians, a number of investigators have challenged these guidelines and have shown that pregnancies can be achieved by means of artificial insemination techniques with substandard sperm samples from Hodgkin's disease patients [3,14,110–112]. Through artificial insemination techniques, successful pregnancies are reported with sperm counts as low as $10–50 \times 10^6$ in such patients [110–112]. Although the success rates of artificial insemination in cancer survivors with low sperm counts are not commonly published, one small series had a successful pregnancy rate of 45% [112].

In Vitro Fertilization

Standard in vitro fertilization (IVF) is the technique of oocyte fertilization by sperm outside the body. In the application of IVF to male factor infertility, women are required to take follicle-stimulating drugs, undergo ovarian aspiration of stimulated oocytes, and then receive uterine implantation of the fertilized egg. Men are required to have minimum sperm counts of 100,000 sperm/mL semen, a number substantially lower than that required for artificial insemination. The sperm are manipulated in the laboratory and incubated with the oocytes, and the zygote is transferred to the uterus after the eight-cell stage. Although IVF is a seemingly promising technique for cancer survivors, success rates with testicular cancer patients have been reported to be much lower than those for other IVF patients who have not received chemotherapy, with pregnancy rates per cycle of only 8%, compared with 50% in the other group [113]. This discrepancy is likely explained by the lower median sperm counts and motility observed in the testicular cancer survivors compared with other IVF patients.

Gamete Micromanipulation

"Gamete micromanipulation" is a broad term used to describe several techniques that can be used in the setting of IVF to increase pregnancy rates in couples with extreme male factor infertility who fail or do not qualify for standard IVF. The subject has recently been reviewed in detail [114]. Intracytoplasmic sperm injection (ICSI) is a type of gamete micromanipulation that holds particular promise for azoospermic and oligospermic cancer survivors. ICSI is the direct injection of a single sperm into the cytoplasm of an oocyte in the context of in vitro fertilization. Patients with semen samples devoid of sperm are still candidates for the procedure, since sperm may be obtained through epididymal aspiration or testicular sperm extraction (TESE). Through TESE, testicular biopsy tissue is macerated, centrifuged, and examined for the presence of sperm. TESE is a critical avenue of sperm recovery for patients who have undergone cytotoxic chemotherapy and suffer from apparent germinal aplasia. One group showed that 76% of patients with either complete germinal aplasia or maturation arrest on biopsy had recoverable sperm after TESE, presumably because of adjacent areas of intact spermatogenesis [115]. The reported pregnancy rates per cycle range from 30 to 40% and do not appear to be significantly altered by the source of sperm or the testicular histology [115–118].

12.6.1.4 Summary

While hormone manipulation with GnRH agonists and antagonists has not proved protective against the sterilizing effects of chemotherapy in men, micromanipulation of gametes with ICSI in the context of IVF currently offers great hope for paternity in cancer survivors who are azoospermic or oligospermic before or after cytotoxic chemotherapy. Patients should not be dissuaded from pretreatment sperm banking, since successful pregnancies have been reported from single immotile sperm through ICSI.

12.6.2 Females

12.6.2.1 Introduction

Maternity prospects for women with failing gonads after cytotoxic chemotherapy remain poor. Efforts to pharmacologically prevent ovarian damage with hormone manipulation prior to chemotherapy have not been consistently successful. Traditional IVF has limitations in women anticipating chemotherapy and in women postchemotherapy. New techniques of cryopreserving ovarian tissue prior to chemotherapy hold great promise for fertile women anticipating potentially sterilizing treatments.

12.6.2.2 Hormone Manipulation

As is the case in men, efforts to use hormone manipulation to prevent the gonadal damage caused by chemotherapy have generally been unsuccessful. Interest was initially raised by Chapman's group, who reported follicle preservation in women treated with oral contraceptives during MVPP treatment for Hodgkin disease compared with a control group who did not receive hormone therapy [119]. However, other investigators have not been able to reproduce those results. [64,90].

12.6.2.3 Gamete Manipulation

In Vitro Fertilization

As described previously, in vitro fertilization is a technique of egg fertilization by sperm that is performed outside of the body. Women are treated with clomiphene to induce ovulation, and stimulated oocytes are harvested for fertilization by sperm in the laboratory. The fertilized zygote can then be frozen for implantation in a human uterus at a later date. For women with new cancer diagnoses, this series of events can be problematic. First, there may be such urgency to start treatment with chemotherapy that a delay of 1–2 months for adequate oocyte harvest may be inadvisable. Second, the patient may not have a sperm donor. Third, the trophic effects of clomiphene and other stimulators of ovulation on tumors have not been well explored, and these drugs may therefore pose a risk to the patient's health. This last concern has been addressed by Brown and colleagues, who are experimenting with "natural cycle" IVF, where eggs are harvested during the patient's natural ovulatory cycle rather than a pharmacologically induced egg-rich cycle [120]. Historically, women who attempt IVF after cytotoxic chemotherapy have pregnancy rates of less than 10%, substantially lower than the average reported success rate of 30–45% [121,122].

Ovarian Autografting

A new technique that holds great promise for women anticipating treatment with potentially sterilizing chemotherapy is ovarian autografting. Already in clinical trials in England, the technique relies on the removal of oocyte-rich ovarian cortical tissue that is then slowly cooled and stored in a cryopreservative. At a later date, the tissue may be thawed and reimplanted near the fallopian tubes for potentially natural ovulation and fertilization. Gosden's group, which pioneered this technique, reported successful pregnancies in sheep and are now applying the technique to humans [123–125].

12.6.2.4 Summary

Although attempts at hormone manipulation during chemotherapy have not been successful at preventing posttreatment infertility, and although IVF may be an imperfect solution to the problem of chemotherapy-related sterility, new techniques of ovarian autografting currently provide the greatest hope for women anticipating potentially sterilizing chemotherapy who also wish to later become pregnant. Until recently, technology has not provided women with a way to store unfertilized gametes outside the body in the way that is possible for men through sperm banking. With ovarian autografting, cryopreservation of pretreatment oocytes may become possible and may return fertility to women sterilized by chemotherapy.

REFERENCES

1. Thachil JV, Jewett MAS, Rider WD. The effects of cancer and cancer therapy on male fertility. J Urol 1981:126:141–145.

2. Drasga RE, Einhorn LH, Williams SD, Patel DN, Stevens EE. Fertility after chemotherapy for testicular cancer. J Clin Oncol 1983:1:179–183.
3. Hendry WF, Stedronska J, Jones CR, Blackmore CA, Barrett A, Peckham MJ. Semen analysis in testicular cancer and Hodgkin's disease: Pre- and posttreatment findings and implications for cryopreservation. Br J Urol 1983:55: 769–773.
4. Nijman JM, Koops HS, Kremer J, Sleijfer D. Gonadal function after surgery and chemotherapy in men with stage II and III nonseminomatous testicular tumors. J Clin Oncol 1987:5:651–656.
5. Berthelsen JG, Skakkebaek NE. Gonadal function in men with testis cancer. Fertil Steril 1983:39:68–75.
6. Skakkebaek NE. Carcinoma in situ of the testis: Frequency and relationship to invasive germ cell tumours in infertile men. Histopathology 1978:2:157–170.
7. Batata MA, Whitmore WF Jr, Hilaris BS, Tokita N, Grabstald H. Cancer of the undescended testis. Am J Roetgenol 1976:126:302.
8. Morrish DW, Venner PM, Siy O, Barron G, Bhardwaj D, Outhet D. Mechanisms of endocrine dysfunction in patients with testicular cancer. J Natl Cancer Inst 1990:82:412–418.
9. Foster RS, Rubin LR, McNulty A, Bihrle R, Donohue JP. Detection of antisperm-antibodies in patients with primary testicular cancer. Int J Androl 1991:14:179–185.
10. Chapman RM, Sutcliffe SB, Malpas JS. Male gonadal dysfunction in Hodgkin's disease. JAMA 1981:245:1323–1328.
11. Vigersky RA, Chapman RM, Berenberg J, Glass AR. Testicular dysfunction in untreated Hodgkin's disease. Am J Med 1982:73:482–486.
12. Whitehead E, Shalet SM, Blackledge G, Todd I, Crownther D, Beardwell CG. The effects of Hodgkin's disease and combination chemotherapy on gonadal function in the adult male. Cancer 1982:49:418–422.
13. Marmor D, Elefant E, Dauchez C, Roux C. Semen analysis in Hodgkin's disease before the onset of treatment. Cancer 1986:57:1686–1687.
14. Redman JR, Bajorunas DR, Goldstein MC, Evenson DP, Gralla RJ, Lacher MJ, Koziner B, Lee BJ, Straus DJ, Clarkson BD, Feldschuh R, Feldschuh J. Semen cryopreservation and artificial insemination for Hodgkin's disease. J Clin Oncol 1987:5:233–238.
15. Viviani S, Ragni G, Santoro A, Perotti L, Caccamo E, Negretti E, Valagussa P, Bonadonna G. Testicular dysfunction in Hodgkin's disease before and after treatment. Eur J Cancer 1991:27:1389–1392.
16. da Cunha MF, Meistrich ML, Fuller LM, Cundiff JH, Hagemeister FB, Velasquez WS, McLaughlin P, Riggs SA, Cabanilas FF, Salvador PG. Recovery of spermatogenesis after treatment for Hodgkin's disease: Limiting dose of MOPP chemotherapy. J Clin Oncol 1984:2:571–577.
17. Barr RD, Booth C, Booth JD. Dyspermia in men with localized Hodgkin's disease. A potentially reversible, immune-mediated disorder. Med Hypotheses 1993:40:165–168.

18. MacMahon B, Cole P, Lin TM, Mirra AP, Ravnihar B, Salber EJ, Valaoras VG, Yuasa S. Age at first birth and breast cancer risk. Bull World Health Organ 1970:43(2):209–221.
19. Korenman SG. Oestrogen window hypothesis of the aetiology of breast cancer. Lancet 1980:1:700–701
20. Cowan LD, Gordis L, Tonascia JM, Jones GS. Breast cancer incidence in women with a history of progesterone deficiency. Am J Epidemiol 1981:114: 209–217.
21. Vessey MP, McPherson K, Roberts MM, Neil A, Jones L. Fertility in relation to the risk of breast cancer. Br J Cancer 1985:52:625–628.
22. Ron E, Lunefeld B, Menczer J, Blumstein T, Katz L, Oelsner G, Serr D. Cancer incidence in a cohort of infertile women. Am J Epidemiol 1987:125: 780–790.
23. Morabia A, Szklo M. Nulliparity, infertility and risk of breast cancer among premenopausal women. Abstract presented at the 22nd Annual Meeting of the Society for Epidemiologic Research, Birmingham, AL, June 14–16, 1989. Am J Epidemiol 1989:130:811–812.
24. Brinton LA, Melton LJ III, Malkasian GD Jr, Bond A, Hoover R. Cancer riak after evaluation for infertility. Am J Epidemiol 1989:129:712–722.
25. Gammon MD, Thompson WD. Infertility and breast cancer: A population-based case–control study. Am J Epidemiol 1990:132:708–716.
26. Rossing MA, Daling JR, Weiss NS, Moore DE, Self SG. Risk of breast cancer in a cohort of infertile women. Gynecol Oncol 1996:60:3–7.
27. Venn A, Watson L, Lumley J, Giles G, King C, Healy D. Breast and ovarian cancer incidence after infertility and in vitro fertilization. Lancel 1995:346: 995–1000.
28. Schilsky RL, Gradishar WJ. Effects of cancer treatment on the reproductive system. Crit Rev Oncol Hematol 1988:8(2):153–171.
29. Meistrich ML. Effect of chemotherapy and radiotherapy on spermatogenesis. Eur Urol 1993:23:136–142.
30. Warthin AS, Weller CV. The Medical Aspects of Mustard Gas Poisoning. St. Louis: Mosby, 1919.
31. Pappenheimer AM, Vance M. The effects of intravenous injections of dichloroethylsulfide in rabbits, with special reference to its leucotoxic action. J Exp Med 1920:31:71–95.
32. Spitz S. The histological effects of nitrogen mustards on human tumors and tissues. Cancer 1948:1(3):383–398.
33. Fairley KF, Barrie JU, Johnson W. Sterility and testicular atrophy related to cyclophosphamide therapy. Lancet 1972:1:568–569.
34. Richter P, Calamera JC, Morgenfeld MC, Kierszenbaum AL, Lavieri JC, Mancini RE. Effect of chlorambucil on spermatogenesis in the human with malignant lymphoma. Cancer 1970:25:1026–1030.
35. Stephenson WT, Poirier SM, Rubin L, Einhorn LH. Evaluation of reproductive capacity in germ cell tumor patients following treatment with cisplatin, etoposide and bleomycin. J Clin Oncol 1995:13:2278–2280.

36. Petersen PM, Hansen SW, Giwercman A, Rorth M, Skakkebaek NE. Dose-dependent impairment of testicular function in patients treated with cisplatin-based chemotherapy for germ cell cancer. Ann Oncol 1994:5:355–358.
37. Hansen PV, Glavind K, Panduro J, Pedersen M. Paternity in patients with testicular germ cell cancer: Pretreatment and post-treatment findings. Eur J Cancer 1991:27:1385–1389.
38. DeVita VT. The consequences of the chemotherapy of Hodgkin's disease: The 10th David A. Karnofsky Memorial Lecture 1979, published 1981. Cancer 1981:47:1–13.
39. Cunningham J, Mauch P, Rosenthal DS, Canellos GP. Long-term complications of MOPP chemotherapy in patients with Hodgkin's disease. Cancer Treatment Rep 1982:66:1015–1022.
40. Viviani S, Santoro A, Ragni G, Vonfante V, Bestetti O, Bonadonna G. Gonadal toxicity after combination chemotherapy for Hodgkin's disease. Comparative results of MOPP vs ABVD. Eur Cancer Clin Oncol 1985:21(5):601–605.
41. Anselmo AP, Carton C, Bellantuono P, Maurizi-Enrici R, Aboulkair N, Ermini M. Risk of infertility in patients with Hodgkin's disease treated with ABVD vs MOPP vs ABVD/MOPP. Haematologica 1990:75:155–158.
42. Sanders JE, Buckner CD, Leonard JM, Sullivan KM, Witherspoon RP, Deeg HJ, Storb R, Thomas ED. Late effects on gonadal function of cyclophosphamide, total-body irradiation, and marrow transplantation. Transplantation 1983:36:252–255.
43. Keilholz U, Korbling M, Fehrentz D, Bauer H, Hunstein W. Long-term endocrine toxicity of myeloablative treatment followed by autologous bone marrow/blood derived stem cell transplantation in patients with malignant lymphohematopoietic disorders. Cancer 1989:64:641–645.
44. Keilholz U, Max R, Scheibenbogen C, Wuster C, Korbling M, Haas R. Endocrine function and bone metabolism 5 years after autologous bone marrow/blood-derived progenitor cell transplantation. Cancer 1997:79:1617–1622.
45. Louis J, Limarizi LR, Best WR. Treatment of chronic granulocytic leukemia with Myleran. Arch Intern Med 1956:97:299–308.
46. Galton DAG, Till M, Wiltshaw E. Busulfan (1,4-dimethanesulfonyloxybutane, Myleran): Summary of clinical results. Ann NY Acad Sci 1958:68:967–973.
47. Belohorsky B, Siracky J, Sandor L, Klauber E. Comments on the development of amenorrhea caused by Myleran in cases of chronic myelosis. Neoplasma 1960:7:397–402.
48. Fosdick WM, Parsons JL, Hill DF. Long-term cyclophosphamide therapy in rheumatoid arthritis. Arthritis Rheum 1968:11:151–161.
49. Uldall PR, Kerr DNS, Tacchi D. Sterility and cyclophosphamide [letter]. Lancet 1972:1:693–694.
50. Warne GL, Fairley KF, Hobbs JB, Martin FIR. Cyclophosphamide-induced ovarian failure. N Engl J Med 1973:289:1159–1162.
51. Miller JJ, Williams GF, Leissring JC. Multiple late complications of therapy with cyclophosphamide, including ovarian destruction. Am J Med 1971:50:530–535.

52. Koyama H, Wada T, Nishizawa Y, Iwanaga T, Aoki Y, Terasawa T, Kosaki G, Yamamoto T, Wada A. Cyclophosphamide-induced ovarian failure and its therapeutic significance in patients with breast cancer. Cancer 1977:39:1403–1409.
53. Fisher B, Sherman B, Rockette H, Redmond C, Margolese R, Fisher ER. L-Phenylalanine mustard (L-PAM) in the management of premenopausal patients with primary breast cancer. Cancer 1979:44:847–857.
54. Dnistrian AM, Schwartz MK, Fracchia AA, Kaufman RJ, Hakes TB, Currie VE. Endocrine consequences of CMF adjuvant therapy in premenopausal and postmenopausal breast cancer patients. Cancer 1983:51:803–807.
55. Boccardo F, Rubagotti A, Bruzzi P, Cappellini M, Isola G, Nenci I, Piffanelli A, Scanni A, Sismondi P, Santi L, Genta F, Saccani F, Sassi M, Malacarne P, Donati D, Farris A, Castagnetta L, De Carlo A, Traina A, Galletto L, Smerieri F, Buzzi F. Chemotherapy versus tamoxifen versus chemotherapy plus tamoxifen in node-positive, estrogen receptor-positive breast cancer patients: Results of a multicentric Italian study. J Clin Oncol 1990:8:1310–1320.
56. Hortobagyi GN, Buzdar AU, Marcus CE, Smith TL. Immediate and long-term toxicity of adjuvant chemotherapy regimens containing doxorubicin in trials at M. D. Anderson Hospital and Tumor Institute. Natl Cancer Inst Monogr 1986:1:105–109.
57. Chapman RM, Sutcliffe SB, Malpas JS. Cytotoxic-induced ovarian failure in women with Hodgkin's disease. JAMA 1979:242:1877–1881.
58. Myles TJM. Hodgkin's disease and pregnancy. J Obstet Gynaecol Bri Emp 1955:62:884–891.
59. Smith RBW, Sheehy TW, Rothberg H. Hodgkin's disease and pregnancy. Arch Intern Med 1958:102:777–789.
60. Carcassonne Y, Dodemant P, Favre R. Hodgkin's disease and pregnancy. Acta Haematol 1981:66:67–68.
61. Horning SJ, Hoppe RT, Kaplan HS, Rosenberg SA. Female reproductive potential after treatment for Hodgkin's disease. N Engl J Med 1981:304:1377–1382.
62. Sherins R, Winokur S, DeVita VT Jr, Vaitukaitis J. Surprisingly high risk of functional castration in women receiving chemotherapy for lymphoma. Clin Res 1975:23:343A (Abstr).
63. Schilsky RL, Sherins RJ, Hubbard SM, Wesley MN, Young RC, DeVita VT. Long-term follow up of ovarian function in women treated wtih MOPP chemotherapy for Hodgkin's disease. Am J Med 1981:714):552–556.
64. Whitehead E, Shalet SM, Blackledge G, Todd I, Crowther D, Beardwell CG. The effect of combination chemotherapy on ovarian function in women treated for Hodgkin's disease. Cancer 1983:52:988–993.
65. Santoro A, Bonadonna G, Valagussa P, Zucali R, Viviani S, Villani F, Pagnoni AM, Bonfante V, Musumeci R, Crippa F, Tess JDT, Banfi A. Long-term results of combined chemotherapy-radiotherapy approach in Hodgkin's disease: Superiority of ABVD plus radiotherapy versus MOPP plus radiotherapy. J Clin Oncol 1987:5(1):27–37.

66. Uderzo C, Locasciulli A, Marzorati R, Adamoli L, Di Natale B, Nizzoli G, Cazzaniga M, Masera G. Correlation of gonadal function with histology of testicular biopsies at treatment discontinuation in childhood acute leukemia. Med Pediatr Oncol 1984:12:97–100.
67. Lendon M, Palmer MK, Hann IM, Shalet SM, Jones PHM. Testicular histology after combination chemotherapy in childhood for acute lymphoblastic leukemia. Lancet 1978:2:439–441.
68. Blatt J, Poplack DG, Sherins RJ. Testicular function in boys after chemotherapy for acute lymphoblastic leukemia. N Engl J Med 1981:304:1121–1124.
69. Hensle TW, Burbige KA, Shepard BR, Marboe CC, Blanc WA, Wigger JH. Chemotherapy and its effects on testicular morphology in children. J Urol 1984:131:1142–1144.
70. Sherins RJ, Olweny CLM, Ziegler JL. Gynecomastia and gonadal dysfunction in adolescent boys treated with combination chemotherapy for Hodgkin's disease. N Engl J Med 1978:299:12–16.
71. Whitehead E, Shalet SM, Jones PHM, Beardwell CG, Deakin DP. Gonadal function after combination chemotherapy for Hodgkin's disease in childhood. Arch Dis Child 1982:47:287–291.
72. Jaffe N, Sullivan MP, Ried H, Boren H, Marshal R, Meistrich M, Maor M, da Cunha M. Male reproductive function in long-term survivors of childhood cancer. Med Pediatr Oncol 1988:16:241–247.
73. Shafford EA, Kingston JE, Malpas JS, Plowman PN, Pritchard J, Savage MO, Eden OB.Testicular function following the treatment of Hodgkin's disease in childhood. Br J Cancer 1993:68:1199–1204.
74. Lentz RD, Bergstein J, Steffes MW, Brown DR, Prem K, Michael AF, Vernier RL. Postpubertal evaluation of gonadal function following cyclophosphamide therapy before and during puberty. J Pediatr 1977:91:385–394.
75. Parra A, Santos D, Cervantes C, Sojo I, Carranco A, Cortes-Gallegos V. Plasma gonadotropins and gonadal steroids in children treated with cyclophosphamide. J Pediatr 1978:92:117–124.
76. Siris ES, Leventhal BG, Vaitukaitis JL. Effects of childhood leukemia and chemothrapy on puberty and reproductive function in girls. N Engl J Med 1976:294:1143–1146.
77. Wallace WHB, Shalet SM, Tetlow LJ, Morris-Jones PH. Ovarian function following the treatment of childhood acute lymphoblastic leukemia. Med Pediatric Oncol 1993:21:333–339.
78. Byrne J, Mulvihill JJ, Myers MH, Connelly RR, Naughton MD, Krauss MR, Steinhorn SC, Hassinger DD, Austin DF, Bragg K, Holmes GF, Holmes FF, Latourette HB, Weyer PJ, Meigs JW, Teta MJ, Cok JW, Strong LC. Effects of treatment on fertility in long-term survivors of childhood or adolescent cancer. N Engl J Med 1987:317:1315–1321.
79. Li FP, Fine W, Jaffe N, Holmes GE, Holmes FF. Offspring of patients treated for cancer in childhood. J Natl Cancer Inst 1979:62:1193–1197.
80. Green DM, Zevon MA, Lowrie G, Seigelstein N, Hall B. Congenital anomalies in children of patients who received chemotherapy for cancer in childhood and adolescence. N Engl J Med 1991:325:141–146.

81. Green DM, Hall B. Pregnancy outcome following treatment during childhood or adolescence for Hodgkin's disease. Pediatr Hematol Oncol 1988:5:269–277.
82. Green DM, Hall B, Zevon MA. Pregnancy outcome after treatment for acute lymphoblastic leukemia during childhood or adolescence. Cancer 1989:64:2335–2339.
83. Ortin TT, Shostak CA, Donaldson SS. Gonadal status and reproductive function following treatment for Hodgkin's disease in childhood: The Stanford experience. Int J Radiat Oncol Biol Phys 1990:19:873–880.
84. Nygaard R, Clausen N, Siimes MA, Marky I, Skjeldestad FE, Kristinsson JR, Vuoristo A, Wegelius R, Moe PJ. Reproduction following treatment for childhood leukemia: A population-based prospective cohort study of fertility and offspring. Med Pediatr Oncol 1991:19:459–466.
85. Li FP, Gimrere K, Gelber RD, et al. Outcome of pregnancy in survivors of Wilms' tumor. JAMA 1987:257:216–219.
86. Blatt J, Mulvihill JJ, Ziegler JL, Young RC, Poplack DG. Pregnancy outcome following cancer chemotherapy. Am J Med 1980:69:828–832.
87. Mulvihill JJ, McKeen A, Rosner F, Zarrabi MH. Pregnancy outcome in cancer patients. Cancer 1987:60:1143–1150.
88. Holmes GE, Holmes FF. Pregnancy outcomes of patients treated for Hodgkin's disease: A controlled study. Cancer 1978:41:1317–1322.
89. Specht L, Hansen MM, Geisler C. Ovarian function in young women in long-term remission after treatment for Hodgkin's disease stage I or II. Scand J Haematol 1984:32:265–270.
90. Sutton R, Buzdar AU, Hortobagyi GN. Pregnancy and offspring after adjuvant chemotherapy in breast cancer patients. Cancer 1990:65:847–850.
91. Nicholson HO. Cytotoxic drugs in pregnancy. J Obstet Gynaecol Br Commonw 1968:75:307–312.
92. Sieber SM, Adamson RH. Toxicity of antineoplastic agents in man: Chromosomal aberrations, antifertility effects, congenital malformations, and carcinogenic potential. Adv Cancer Res 1975:22:57–155.
93. Sweet DL, Kinzie J. Consequences of radiotherapy and antineoplastic therapy for the fetus. J Reprod Med 1976:17(4):241–246.
94. Doll DC, Ringenberg S, Yarbro JW. Management of cancer during pregnancy. Arch Intern Med 1988:148:2058–2064.
95. Aviles A, Diaz-Maqueo JC, Talavera A, Guzman R, Garcia EL. Growth and development of children of mothers treated with chemotherapy during pregnancy: Current status of 43 children. Am J Hematol 1991:36:243–248.
96. Wiebe VJ, Sipila PEH. Pharmacology of antineoplastic agents in pregnancy. Crit Rev Oncol Hematol 1994:16:75–112.
97. Giberti C, Barreca T, Martorana G, Truini M, Franceschini R, Roland E, Guiliani L. Hormonal pattern and testicular histology in patients with prostatic cancer after long-term treatment with a gonadotropin-releasing hormone agonist analogue. Eur Urol 1988:15:125–127.
98. Glode LM, Robinson J, Gould SF. Protection from cyclophosphamide-in-

duced testicular damage with an analogue of gonadotropin-releasing hormone. Lancet 1981:1:1132–1134.

99. Nseyo UO, Huben RP, Klioze SS, Pontes JE. Portection of germinal epithelium with luteinizing hormone-releasing hormone analogue. J Urol 1985:34: 187–190.
100. Delic JI, Bush C, Peckham MJ. Protection from procarbazine-induced damage of spermatogenesis in the rat by androgen. Cancer Res 1986:46:1909–1914.
101. Karashima T, Zalatnai A, Schally AV. Protective effects of analogs of luteinizing hormone-releasing hormone against chemotherapy-induced testicular damage in rats. Proc Natl Acad Sci USA 1988:85:2329–2333.
102. Cepedes RD, Peretsman SJ, Thompson IM, Jackson C. Protection of the germinal epithelium in the rat from the cytotoxic effects of chemotherapy by a luteinizing hormone–releasing hormone agonist and antiandrogen therapy. Urology 1995:46:688–691.
103. Meistrich ML, Wilson G, Ye WS, Thrash C, Huhtaniemi I. Relationship among hormonal treatments, suppression of spermatogenesis, and testicular protection from chemotherapy-induced damage. Endocrinology 1996:137: 3823–3831.
104. Manabe F, Takeshima H, Akaza H. Protecting spermatogenesis from damage induced by doxorubicin using the luteinizing hormone-releasing hormone agonist leuprorelin. Cancer 1997:79:1014–1021.
105. Johnson DH, Linde R, Hainsworth JD, Vale W, Rivier J, Stein R, Flexner J, Van Welch R, Greco FA. Effect of a luteinizing hormone releasing hormone agonist given during combination chemotherapy on posttherapy fertility in male patients with lymphoma: Preliminary observations. Blood 1985:65: 832–836.
106. Waxman JH, Ahmed R, Smith D, Wrigley PFM, Gregory W, Shalet S, Crowther D, Rees LH, Besser GM, Malpas JS, Lister TA. Failure to preserve fertility in patients with Hodgkin's disease. Cancer Chemother Pharmacol 1987:19:159–162.
107. Fossa SD, Klepp O, Norman N. Lack of gonadal protection by medroxyprogesterone acetate-induced transient medical castration during chemotherapy for testicular cancer. Br J Urol 1988:449–453.
108. Kreuser ED, Hetzel WD, Hautmann R, Pfeiffer E. Reproductive toxicity with and without $LHRH_A$ administration during adjuvant chemotherapy in patients with germ cell tumors. Horm Metab Res 1990:22:494–498.
109. American Fertility Society. Guidelines for therapeutic donor insemination: Sperm. Fertil Steril 1993:59(2 suppl 1):1–9.
110. Milligan DW, Hughes R, Linday KS. Semen cryopreservation in men undergoing cancer chemotherapy—A UK survey. Br J Cancer 1989:60:966–967.
111. Rhodes EA, Hoffman DJ, Kaempfer SH. Ten years of experience with semen cryopreservation by cancer patients: Follow-up and clinical considerations. Fertil Steril 1985:44:512–516.
112. Scammell GE, White N, Stedronska J, Hendry WF, Edmonds DK, Jeffcoate SL. Cryopreservation of semen in men with testicular tumour or Hodgkin's

disease: Results of artificial insemination of their partners. Lancet 1985:2: 31–32.
113. Hakim LS, Lobel SM, Oates RD. The achievement of pregnancies using assisted reproductive technologies for male factor infertility after retroperitoneal lymph node dissection for testicular carcinoma. Fertil Steril 1995:64(6):1141–1146.
114. Schlegel PN. Micromanipulation of gametes for male factor infertility. Urol Clin North Am 1994:21:477–486.
115. Tournaye H, Liu J, Nagy PZ, Camus M, Goosens A, Silber S, Van Steiteghem AC, Devroey P. Correlation between testicular histology and outcome after intracytoplasmic sperm injection using testicular spermatozoa. Hum Reprod 1996:11:127–132.
116. Palmero GD, Cohen J, Alikani M, Adler A, Rosenwaks Z. Intracytoplasmic sperm injection: A novel treatment for all forms of male factor infertility. Fertil Steril 1995:63:1231–1240.
117. Oehninger S, Veeck L, Lanzendorf S, Maloney M, Toner J, Muasher S. Intracytoplasmic sperm injection achievement of high pregnancy rates in couples with severe male factor infertility is dependent primarily upon female not male factors. Fertil Steril 1995:64:977–981.
118. Harari O, Bourne H, McDonald M, et al. Intracytoplasmic sperm injection: A major advances in the management of severe male subfertility. Fertil Steril 1995:64:3690–368.
119. Chapman RM, Sutcliffe SB. Protection of ovarian function by oral contraceptives in women receiving chemotherapy for Hodgkin's disease. Blood 1981:58:849–851.
120. Brown JR, Modell E, Obasaju M, Ying YK. Natural cycle in-vitro fertilization with embryo cryopreservation prior to chemotherapy for carcinoma of the breast. Hum Reprod 1996:11:197–199.
121. Pados G, Camus M, Van Waesberghe L, Liebaers I, Van Steirteghem A, Devroey P. Oocyte and embryo donation: Evaluation of 412 consecutive trials. Hum Reprod 1992:7:1111–1117.
122. Tan SL, Royston P, Campbell S, Jacobs HS, Betts J, Mason B, Edwards RG. Cumulative conception and live birth rates after in-vitro fertilization. Lancet 1992:339:1390–1394.
123. Gosden RG, Baird DT, Wade JC, Webb R. Restoration of fertility to oophorectomized sheep by ovarian autografts stored at −196°C. Hum Reprod 1994: 9:597–603.
124. Newton H, Aubard Y, Rutherford A, Sharma V, Gosden R. Low temperature storage and grafting of human ovarian tissue. Hum Reprod 1996:11:1487–1491.
125. Law C. Freezing ovary tissue may help cancer patients preserve fertility. J Natl Cancer Inst 1996:88:1184–1185.

13

Secondary Malignancies

CARSTEN BOKEMEYER and CHRISTIAN KOLLMANNSBERGER
University of Tübingen Medical Center, Tübingen, Germany

13.1 INTRODUCTION

With the increase in survival and overall cure rate of tumor patients, the potential risk of therapy-associated secondary malignancies has become of growing interest. This problem is even more significant in that today, large groups of patients with breast or colorectal cancer receive adjuvant chemotherapy following complete surgical resection. Initially, secondary malignancies following prior tumor therapy were presented as case reports; subsequently, the first more complete risk assessments were performed in patients with Hodgkin's disease. Additionally, increasingly larger studies including patients with other potentially curative treatable tumors are also being presented.

Whereas initially most reports concentrated on the risk for therapy-related secondary acute myeloid leukemia (AML), at present, more and more studies examining the risk of solid secondary tumors are being conducted. In principle, both radiation and chemotherapy are able to induce malignant tumors. In most studies, radiation is predominantly associated with solid secondary tumors, which usually occur following a period of more than 5–10 years. Most secondary solid tumors arise within the previously radiated area.

A threshold radiation dose for the induction of cancerous effects has not been defined. Moreover, cases of secondary leukemias are also reported following radiation therapy alone. Relatively low doses of radiation applied to large bone marrow volumes seem to be much more leukemogenic than high doses applied to small bone marrow volumes.

resulting from treatment with topoisomerase II inhibitors (e.g., etoposide). The characteristics of each form are summarized in Table 2 [2–4].

Secondary nonlymphocytic leukemias following therapy with alkylating agents are often preceded by a preleukemic period of myelodysplasia and usually occur after an average interval of 5–7 years, whereas secondary leukemias associated with epipodophyllotoxins seem to have a significantly shorter latency period and are characterized by a sudden onset, without a myelodysplastic prephase. Alkylating agent induced secondary leukemias often represent an M1 or M2 phenotype (French-American-British co-operative (FAB) classification). In contrast, epipodophyllotoxin-related secondary leukemias most commonly exhibit an M4 or M5 morphological type.

Secondary lymphoblastic leukemias have been reported following alkylating agent therapy, as well as following epipodophyllotoxin treatment, although together these represent less than 5% of all secondary leukemias. Unlike primary leukemias, secondary alkylating agent induced leukemias often exhibit alterations of chromosomes 5 and 7 (60–90%), whereas in topoisomerase II associated leukemias translocations affecting the long arm of chromosome 11 (11q23) are frequently present [5].

The prognosis for alkylating agent induced secondary leukemia is worse than that for spontaneously occurring leukemias. More favorable results are reported for the treatment of epipodophyllotoxin-associated leukemias. However, these data require further confirmation. Epipodophyllotoxin-associated secondary leukemias were described most commonly following treatment of lung cancer, of AML in children, and of testicular cancer. In epipodophyllotoxin-induced secondary leukemia, both treatment schedule and epipodophyllotoxin dosage seem to be important for the development of secondary leukemias. Children receiving weekly or twice weekly epipodophyllotoxin maintenance therapy were at an increased risk for secondary leukemia compared to children receiving less intensive epipodophyllotoxin schedules or maintenance therapy without these drugs [6]. Several studies

Table 2 Characteristics of Secondary Leukemias Following Chemotherapy with Alkylating Agents or Epipodophyllotoxins

	Treatment	
Characteristic	Alkylating agent	Epipodophyllotoxin
Interval following therapy, years	5–7	2–3
Morphology (FAB classification)	M1/M2	M4/M5
Preceding myelodysplasia	Frequent	Rare
Chromosomes bearing aberrations	5; 7	(11q23)

[2,7,8] have investigated the correlation between epipodophyllotoxin dose and risk for secondary AML, following Pedersen-Bjergaard's report of an extremely high risk (336-fold) for patients treated with chemotherapy containing a cumulative dose of more than 2 g/m^2 of etoposide [9] (see also Testicular Cancer, Section 13.2.2.3).

13.2.2 Incidence of Secondary Leukemias

13.2.2.1 Hodgkin's Disease

The cumulative 10-year incidence of secondary nonlymphocytic leukemias is substantially increased following curative treatment for Hodgkin's disease, with various studies reporting incidence rates of between 1.5 and 10% [10–12]. The relative risk in larger studies is about 20–40 times that of the general population 5–10 years following therapy. Yearly incidence rates peak 4–8 years following therapy and equal those of the general population 10 years after treatment. Although the use of radiation therapy is definitely associated with a risk for developing leukemia, to date the largest published study, with nearly 30,000 patients [13], does not show a further increase in risk of chemotherapy-induced leukemias for patients receiving additional radiotherapy. However, this issue remains to be addressed conclusively. The highest leukemia risk is associated with the MOPP regimen and increases considerably with the cumulative dose of mechlorethamine used (relative risk doubles after more than six cycles). The regimen of Adriamycin, bleomycin, vinblastine and dacarbazine (ABVD) appears to be associated with a substantially lower secondary leukemia rate [14]. Splenectomy or radiation of the spleen seems to approximately double the risk for developing leukemia [13,14]. Equally, the risk among patients over 40–45 years of age at the time of treatment seems to be twice as high as for younger patients [15,16].

A recent study has indicated that the AML risk may be associated with treatment-related acute bone marrow toxicity. Study results showed a significantly increased risk of leukemia among patients with low platelet counts, both in response to initial therapy and during follow-up (approximately fivefold higher in patients with $\geq$70% decrease in platelet count) [17]. It is possible that severe thrombocytopenia indicates a greater bioavailability of cytotoxic agents, which might be a causal factor in the development of leukemia. Alternatively, it is also possible that severe thrombocytopenia is an indicator of a specific type of preexisting bone marrow damage. It remains to be seen whether this observation can be used as a predictive factor for the development of secondary leukemias. Overall, the long-term survival of patients cured from Hodgkin's disease is reduced by approximately 2–3% after 15 years by the occurrence of secondary myelogenous leukemias

Table 3 Risk of Secondary Leukemia Following Therapy for Hodgkin's Disease[a]

Number of patients	Number of secondary leukemias	Relative risk at different time intervals since Hodgkin's disease (years)[b]				Cumulative incidence at 10 years (%)[b]
		1–4	5–10	>10	Total	
744	16	32	76	36	46	5.1
1,507	28	77	63	0	72	3.3
1,579	17	—	—	—	37	1.7
1,681	18	—	—	—	89	2.3
12,411	158	31	32	11	26	1.8
29,552	163	7	11	3	NR	NR
1,939	31	36	60	21	35	NR
10,472	122	22	15	6	24	NR
794	8	96	85	38	66	NR

[a]Results of larger studies.
[b]NR, not reported.
Source: Modified from Henry-Amar and Dietrich [18], Kaldor et al. [13,19], and others [14,16,20].

and myelodysplastic syndromes. Data concerning the risk assessment of secondary leukemias in patients with Hodgkin's disease are summarized in Table 3 [13,14,16,18–20].

13.2.2.2 Ovarian Cancer

A substantial risk for developing secondary leukemias is associated with the cumulative dose of the alkylating agents administered. Cyclophosphamide, chlorambucil, melphalan, thiotepa, and treosulfan appear, independently of one another, to increase the risk of secondary leukemia, with chlorambucil and melphalan resulting in the highest risk. The largest study, which included nearly 100,000 surviving ovarian cancer patients, showed a relative risk of 12 (4–32) following chemotherapy [19,21]. Further prospective data are needed for the risk assessment of standard regimens and high dose chemotherapy regimens.

13.2.2.3 Testicular Cancer

Approximately half of all larger studies examining secondary leukemia risk show a significantly elevated risk following treatment for testicular cancer, this risk being three to eight times higher than that found in the general population. Since older regimens not containing epipodophyllotoxins appear

Table 4 Secondary Leukemias Following Chemotherapy of Testicular Cancer Containing Cumulative Etoposide Doses <2 g/m^2

Number of patients	Number of secondary leukemias		Median follow-up (years)	Ref.
	Total	Etoposide-related		
636	4	3	5.7	22
538	2	2	4.9	2
343	2	1	≥5	8
221	1	1	5.5	23
130	0	0	5.4	9
1868	9 (0.5%)	7 (0.4%)	≈5	

to have a very small risk, epipodophyllotoxins may be an important cause for secondary leukemia. As mentioned previously, several studies have addressed the possibility of a correlation between the risk for secondary AML and the administered cumulative dose of etoposide. As shown in Tables 4 and 5, etoposide doses of more than 2 g/m^2 appear to be associated with a substantially increased risk for developing secondary leukemias [2,8,9,22,22a,23]. However, studies investigating etoposide doses of more than 2 g/m^2 included far fewer patients than those investigating etoposide doses of less than 2 g/m^2. Additionally factors such as concomitant radiotherapy or high cisplatin doses may influence the reported etoposide-related secondary leukemia risk. Thus more data are necessary for a final risk assessment, particularly regarding the correlation between secondary leukemia risk and the cumulative dose of etoposide [2,4,7].

Table 5 Secondary Leukemias Following Chemotherapy for Testicular Cancer Containing Cumulative Etoposide Doses ≥ 2 g/m^2

Number of patients	Number of secondary leukemias		Median follow-up (years)	Ref.
	Total	Etoposide-related		
82	5	4	5.4	9
25	2	2	5.7	22
128	1	1	4.5	7
302	6	4	~5	22a
537	14 (2.6%)	11 (2.0%)	~5	

13.2.2.4 Breast Cancer

The cumulative 10-year incidence of secondary leukemias occurring in patients treated with chemotherapy, including melphalan, reached 1.5%. However, this is significantly higher than for the surgery-only group. For both melphalan and cyclophosphamide, the risk of AML increases significantly with increasing cumulative drug doses. Cumulative cyclophosphamide doses of 20 g or less resulted in an approximately two-fold increase in risk, whereas doses of 20 g or more were associated with a 5.7-fold increase in risk for developing secondary AML [24]. Based on a large survey that included 83,000 women treated for breast cancer, five therapy-related secondary leukemias can be expected per 10,000 patients within a 10-year interval following 6 months of adjuvant therapy with CMF: cyclophosphamide, methotrexate, and 5-fluorouracil (5-FU) [25].

The low risk of secondary AML following CMF-based adjuvant chemotherapy was recently confirmed by the Milan Cancer Institute [26]. Among 2241 patients treated with CMF-based adjuvant chemotherapy and a median follow-up of 12 years, 3 cases of AML were observed. This results in a 15-year cumulative AML risk of 0.23% and a nonsignificant 2.3-fold increase in risk as compared to the general population.

5-FU, Adriamycin, and cyclophosphamide (FAC)-based adjuvant chemotherapy also seems to have an approximately two-fold increase in risk compared to the general population [27]. Since this increase in risk is most probably attributable to cyclophosphamide, the possible leukemogenic potential of the anthracyclines remains unclear.

However, there is concern over the recent occurrence of six cases of M4 or M5 AML, with three patients exhibiting 11q23 abnormalities, in the high-dose cyclophosphamide/high-dose doxorubicine treatment arm of the National Surgical Adjuvant Breast and Bowel Project (NSABP) B25 trial of adjuvant chemotherapy with Adriamycin and cyclophosphamide for breast cancer [28]. This indicates that anthracyclines may induce the topoisomerase II related type of secondary leukemias. Recently, three cases of secondary AML were observed following therapy with mitomycin C, methotrexate, and mitoxantrone, all of which were attributed to the anthrancycline-like agent mitoxantrone [29].

13.2.2.5 Non-Hodgkin's Lymphoma [Including Chronic Lymphocytic Leukemia (CLL), Immunocytoma, Multiple Myeloma]

Several individual leukemia cases in patients with CLL, immunocytoma, and multiple myeloma have been observed following treatment with alkylating agents. Patients treated for multiple myeloma were found to have the highest incidence, with 9.2% of secondary leukemias 10 years after treatment. This extremely high incidence is mostly attributed to prolonged treatment with melphalan. The average interval until onset of secondary leukemia was 60 months [30]. For patients who received prednimustine or mechlorethamine, the risk for developing secondary leukemia seems to increase up to 12- to 14-fold [31].

A significantly increased risk of AML (50- to 100-fold excess risk) has been found to be associated with long-term maintenance chemotherapy, total body irradiation (TBI), total nodal irradiation (TNI), and hemibody irradiation (HBI) [32–34]. The contribution of radiotherapy is still controversially discussed, with two other studies not showing an increased risk following combined-modality treatment. However, the latter reports had included only a few patients receiving TBI, TNI, or HBI [31,35].

Recently, etoposide has also been incorporated in treatment regimens for non-Hodgkin's lymphoma (NHL). In the only study published so far, no etoposide-induced secondary AML was observed in patients receiving a median etoposide dose of 1600 mg/m^2, which is consistent with the observation made in patients treated for testicular cancer [36].

Purine analogues, such as fludarabine (FLU), 2-deoxycoformycin (DCF), and 2-chlorodeoxyadenosine (CdA), are increasingly used in the treatment of indolent lymphoid malignancies. The data available to date demonstrate only an identifiable increase in risk in CLL patients treated with CdA [37]. A follow-up of more than 5 years is needed to more accurately assess the risk of secondary malignancies in these patients.

13.2.2.6 Secondary Leukemias/Myelodysplastic Syndrome (MDS) Following High-Dose Chemotherapy Plus Autologous Stem Cell Support (PBSCT or ABMT)

Dose-intensified strategies are being increasingly investigated in chemotherapy-sensitive malignancies, especially breast cancer, NHL, and testicular and ovarian cancers. High-dose chemotherapy approaches are used not only for patients with metastatic disease, but also as adjuvant treatment in patients with a high risk for relapse (e.g., patients with breast cancer with more than 10 involved lymph nodes). In view of the intended aim of an increased life expectancy of those treated, it becomes exceedingly important to evaluate the carcinogenic potential of high-dose chemotherapy treatment, particularly in the adjuvant setting. There is emerging evidence that the combination of dose-intensified anthracyclines and alkylating agents is leukemogenic and carcinogenic, with a strongly increased risk for developing secondary AML or MDS, resulting in a cumulative incidence of approximately 9% at 5 years [38,39]. Some studies suggest a significantly elevated risk for developing secondary myelodysplasic syndromes with subsequent AML following autologous bone marrow transplantation (ABMT) or peripheral blood stem cell transplantation (PBSCT) as treatment for Hodgkin's or non-Hodgkin's lymphoma (Table 6) [39,41–44].

It remains unclear whether the increased risk for secondary MDS is due to the myeloablative high-dose chemotherapy itself or whether it is related to the previous chemotherapy. There is evidence to support the possibility that this complication may be related to pretransplant bone marrow damage caused by chemotherapy prior to transplantation. First, all patients received intensive induction chemotherapy and, for the most part, additional chemotherapy and/or radiotherapy for the treatment of one or more relapses. Second, as shown in Table 6, the time interval between initial therapy and MDS development is approximately 4–7 years, which corresponds closely to the known incubation period for MDS induced by an alkylating agent. Apart from this, MDS rarely occurs after allogenic bone marrow transplantation, indicating that the reinfused stem cells rather than residual damaged host cells will develop MDS.

Larger studies will need to quantify the risk for developing secondary leukemia following high-dose chemotherapy, as well as to further investigate the cause for secondary MDS. Patients treated with high-dose chemotherapy and autologous stem cell or bone marrow transplantation should therefore be followed to assess the long-term side effects of these intensive chemotherapy strategies.

13.2.2.7 Secondary Leukemia in Allogenic Bone Marrow Transplant (BMT) Patients

As shown in Table 7, patients receiving allogenic BMT as treatment for leukemia, lymphoma, or aplastic anemia are at higher risk for developing secondary leukemia or myelodysplastic syndrome than the general population [45–48]. The highest incidence is seen within the first 8 years after allogenic BMT, plateauing at 8–10 years posttransplant [45]. It is not known which possible risk factors contribute to the development of secondary leukemias or myelodysplastic syndrome in patients treated with allogenic bone marrow transplantation.

13.2.2.8 Incidence of Secondary Leukemias in Patients with Nonmalignant Diseases

Antineoplastic agents are also used for the treatment of nonmalignant diseases, such as psoriasis and rheumatoid arthritis.

Table 6 MDS Following Autologous Bone Marrow Transplantation for Lymphoid Malignancies:

Number of patients	Number of MDS/AML cases (crude incidence)	Cumulative incidence	Time to MDS/AML from Dx to Tx (months)[a]	Ref.
117	4 (3%)	6.8% (at 5 years)	NR/8–70	39
275	10 (4%)	6.4% (at 2 years)	47/17	41
262	20 (7%)	18% (at 6 years)	69/31	42
206	9 (4%)	14.5% (at 5 years)	65/34	43
511	12 (2%)	4% (at 5 years)	4–249/44	47
1371	55 (4%)	≈9% (at 5 years)	—	

[a]Dx, diagnosis; Tx, transplantation; NR, not reported.

Secondary AMLs have been repeatedly described following therapy for psoriasis with alkylating agents such as chlorambucil and cyclophosphamide. In 61 patients with nonmalignant primary diseases and secondary leukemia, more than two-thirds had received alkylating agents. Ten patients were treated with antimetabolites only (azathioprin, 6-mercaptopurine) [49].

Thus far, no secondary leukemias have been reported for methotrexate [50]. High cumulative doses of alkylating agents correlate with an increased leukemia risk in patients with rheumatic diseases (>1 g of chlorambucil or >50 g of cyclophosphamide).

In organ transplant patients receiving immunosuppressive therapy, the incidence of leukemias appears not to be elevated. Other secondary malignancies are dominant (e.g., skin tumors, lymphomas).

Table 7 Secondary AML/MDS Following Allogeneic Bone Marrow Transplantation for Hematologic Malignancies and Aplastic Anemia: Four Reports, 1989–1996

Number of patients	Number of cases of AML/MDS	Relative risk	Median follow-up (years)	Ref.
2145	6	40	NR	46
557	1	NR	NR (1–24)	47
1400	1	25	3.1	45
748	2	28.6	3.9	48
5600	10	~25 to 40-fold	—	

13.3 SOLID TUMORS FOLLOWING ANTICANCER TREATMENT

Following antineoplastic therapy, solid tumors occur chronologically later than acute secondary leukemias. As in secondary leukemias, the largest data pools exist for patients with Hodgkin's disease and for survivors of childhood cancer.

13.3.1 Characteristics of Nonleukemic Secondary Neoplasias

Solid secondary neoplasias are primarily reported following radiation therapy, and for the most part they develop within the radiated area. Additional chemotherapy, however, appears to significantly increase the risk for some specific tumors.

Thus far, cytogenetic investigation of nonleukemic secondary tumors has been performed only sporadically; molecular testing also has not revealed any systematic pattern or specific aberrations. Yet distinct genetic syndromes, such as the Li–Fraumeni syndrome (which has a germ cell line defect of the p53 tumor suppressor gene and an increased incidence of secondary neoplasia following first tumor treatment), show that in some patients, the risk for developing a secondary cancer is influenced by molecular changes [51].

Secondary NHLs following therapy of malignant disease are heterogeneous in morphology, but a higher incidence of central nervous system involvement is found in immunosuppressed patients. In these patients, NHLs most commonly originate from the B-cell lineage and are often associated with Epstein–Barr virus (EBV) infection.

It remains unclear whether the prognosis of solid secondary neoplasias differs from the prognosis of primary neoplasias having the same location and histology.

13.3.2 Incidence of Solid Tumors

13.3.2.1 Hodgkin's Disease

As the interval following treatment lengthens, the risk for solid secondary tumors and non-Hodgkin's lymphomas constantly increases. After a 15-year interval, the cumulative incidence of solid secondary tumors is 13–14% and for non-Hodgkin's lymphomas 1–2%. A plateau or a decline in the incidence of secondary solid tumors following therapy has not been observed. The most common secondary solid tumors are lung cancer, gastric cancer, and soft tissue and bone sarcomas, now being considered as typical radiation-induced secondary neoplasias [23,52,53]. Approximately 15 years after treatment, the risk for secondary non-Hodgkin's lymphomas equals the risk for secondary AML in patients with Hodgkin's disease. A direct relationship between the administered therapy and secondary NHLs does not exist, and therefore it is possible that this form of secondary neoplasia is related to the reduced immunstatus of Hodgkin's disease patients. However, in contrast to immunosuppressed organ transplant recipients, fewer intracerebral lymphomas are found following treatment for Hodgkin's disease, and the percentage of EBV-associated lymphomas is also substantially lower. It appears therefore also possible that diagnostic misclassification contributes to the relatively high risk for secondary NHL. That is, misdiagnosis of the primary tumor as Hodgkin's disease while it was NHL. Therefore, a secondary NHL would, in actuality, be a relapse of the primary NHL. It is also possible that transformation into the non-Hodgkin's form is part of the natural course of some subtypes of Hodgkin's disease (e.g., the lymphocyte-predominant type).

The risk for secondary lung cancer is approximately two to eight times higher in patients with Hodgkin's disease than is found in the general population [16,54]. While this increase has, in the past, been largely attributed to radiation therapy, more recent studies indicate that an added chemotherapy may further increase this risk [55]. Furthermore, the risk for smokers is considerably higher than that for nonsmokers [56].

An increased risk for developing breast cancer also exists following therapy for Hodgkin's disease [16,57]. As with lung cancer, adding chemotherapy seems to elevate the risk of secondary breast cancer associated with radiation therapy alone. In particular, the risk in women receiving radiotherapy under the age of 30 is increased 12-fold and further increases up to 30-fold in patients younger than 20 years of age at the time of treatment [57,58].

The risk for developing secondary gastric cancer appears to correlate with radiation therapy, with a continuous increase being observed as the interval following treatment lengthens. The risk for melanoma appears to be at least twice as high in Hodgkin's patients than in the general population. Since this risk is not dependent on the form of administered therapy, an underlying immunologic component appears to play an important role [59].

A 16-fold increase in risk for thyroid cancer is found following mantle field radiation in Hodgkin's patients [60]. Studies conducted in children and adolescents describe a much higher risk, which appears to be increased 25- to 75-fold [61].

The risk for osteosarcoma seems to be particularly dependent on previous radiation therapy. A 5- to 10-fold elevated risk is described in adult patients [54].

Table 8 Relative Risk for Developing Solid Secondary Cancers After Therapy for Hodgkin's's Disease: Relative Risks Significantly Elevated Compared to Control Group

Tumor type	Number of patients	Number of secondary malignancies	Relative risk
Non-Hodgkin's lymphoma	60,591	224 (0.4%)	16 (1.5–32)
Lung cancer	59,769	380 (0.6%)	5.3 (1.9–7.7)
Thyroid cancer	56,540	44 (0.08%)	17 (2.4–68)
Osteosarcoma	43,416	17 (0.04%)	37 (4.5–106)
Melanoma	56,315	54 (0.1%)	6 (1.6–16)
Breast cancer	34,416	180 (0.5%)	2.2 (1.3–6.5)

Source: Modified from Tucker [3] and others [16,20,21].

In general, the risk for developing secondary solid tumors following therapy for Hodgkin's disease appears to be primarily dependent on radiation therapy, although there is an additional risk with added chemotherapy in certain secondary carcinomas such as breast cancer or lung cancer. This risk also has a pronounced dependency on the age of the patient at the time of treatment, with more unfavorable results being reported in younger patients. Further large studies are needed to appropriately address unclear aspects, such as length of follow-up or age-specific risks, and to be able to define preventive measures [62]. The relative risk found in large studies for various tumors following therapy for Hodgkin's disease is shown in Table 8.

13.3.3.2 Malignant Germ Cell Tumors

Since 80–85% of all patients with metastatic testicular cancer can be cured with adequate chemotherapy or radiation therapy, the rate of secondary tumors is of great importance in these patients.

A summary of the available data generally shows a two- to threefold increase in risk for developing secondary solid malignancies following therapy for testicular cancer. Investigations of the various treatment forms suggest that radiation therapy may increase the risk for developing secondary tumors by a factor of 2–3 in comparison to the general population. Radiation-induced cancers particularly affect the gastrointestinal tract (e.g., gastric or colon cancer) and the genitourinary tract (e.g., bladder or kidney cancer), and they may also occur as sarcomas. The relative risk for these subtypes following radiation therapy is somewhat elevated, and is estimated as being three to seven times that of the general population. It appears that the risk of solid secondary cancer following radiation increases significantly over time. Chemotherapy alone does not seem to be associated with a significant increase in secondary solid tumors [23,63].

Regardless of the form of therapy, testicular cancer does not appear to be inherently accompanied by an increased secondary cancer risk, as shown in several observation-only studies. However, 3–5% of all patients develop contralateral secondary testicular cancer, resulting from a contralateral carcinoma in situ at the time of the first tumor's diagnosis and not being treatment related [64].

13.3.3.3 Breast Cancer

Incidence rates significantly higher than those found in the general population have been observed for cancers of the ovary, uterus, lung, thyroid, colon–rectum, and the contralateral breast, as well as for soft tissue sarcoma and melanoma. For some of these secondary cancers, such as those of the contralateral breast, ovary, uterus, and melanoma, the increased risk may be fully or partly explained by a common etiology (e.g., genetic predisposition, such as being a *BRCA* gene carrier for ovarian or breast cancer; hormonal risk factors). Contralateral breast cancer accounts for 40–50% of all secondary tumors in women with breast cancer, with a cumulative risk of 10–13% at 15 years [65,66]. Radiation therapy appears to significantly increase the risk for contralateral disease in women who are less than 45 years old at the time of radiation treatment (radiation-associated risk 1.9), whereas radiation does not appear to influence the risk for contralateral disease when administered to women older than 45 years of age [67]. Excess lung cancer risk following treatment for breast cancer has been attributed to radiotherapy. Larger studies show that lung cancer risk increases with increasing radiation doses to the affected lung, resulting in an approximately threefold excess risk for patients who receive a lung dose of 5–10 Gy [68].

13.3.3.4 Solid Secondary Tumors Following Treatment of Other Malignant Diseases

The development of secondary bladder cancer following treatment with the oxazaphosphorines cyclophosphamide and ifosfamide is well known and experimentally documented. Transitorial cell carcinomas of the urinary tract are most common histologic type. Prophylactic application of mesna appears to remove this risk or, at least, to greatly reduce it [69]. No interference with the antitumor activity of cyclophosphamide or ifosfamide was observed.

An increased risk for the development of osteosarcoma is described following skeletal radiation therapy, particularly when the dosage reaches 40–50 Gy. This risk is also dependent on the type of underlying disease and is highest for patients with retinoblastoma. However, the observed 1000-fold higher risk is most likely due to a genetic characteristic of both diseases [70].

An increased risk for developing breast cancer, lung cancer, and thyroid cancer has been described for various primary tumors treated with radiation therapy.

13.3.3.5 Secondary Solid Neoplasias Following Allogenic BMT

Patients who undergo allogenic BMT are at risk for developing solid secondary tumors following transplantation. According to studies with long-term follow-up, this risk increases steadily over time. A strong correlation appears to exist between the age at the time of transplantation and the risk for developing secondary solid tumors, with children transplanted under the age of 10 being at the highest risk [71]. Total body irradiation (TBI), as part of the conditioning regimen, appears to be an independent risk factor for developing secondary solid tumors [45,47,71]. It remains controversial whether immune dysfunctions (e.g., HLA-mismatched marrow transplants, T-cell depletion, graft-versus-host disease, or the application of antithymocyte globulin) are linked to an elevated risk of solid secondary cancer [45,46,71]. Table 9 shows the relative risk for developing secondary solid tumors as described in several larger studies.

13.3.3.6 Secondary Solid Neoplasia Following Treatment for Nonmalignant Diseases and Following Organ Transplantation

Subsequent to immunosuppressive therapy with alkylating agents, azathioprin, or steroids, an increase in non-Hodgkin's lymphomas and skin malignancies has been found in organ transplant recipients. In particular, NHL occurring during or immediately after treatment are usually associated with EBV found in the lymphoma cells. Individual cases of remission following the reduction of immunosuppressive treatment have been reported [72].

Osteosarcomas and thyroid cancer have been occasionally observed following radiation therapy for Bechterew's disease or thymus enlargement, respectively. Similarly, individual cases of breast cancer have been documented following fluoroscopy for tuberculosis.

The use of cytostatic drugs for the treatment of rheumatic disease appears to at least double the risk for developing non-Hodgkin's lymphomas.

Recently, an increased melanoma incidence 15 years following PUVA treatment (psoralens and ultraviolet A) for psoriasis has been reported, with patients who received more than 250 treatments being at highest risk [73].

Table 9 Relative Risk for Developing Secondary Solid Tumors Following Allogeneic Bone Marrow Transplantation: Five Reports, 1989–1997

Number of patients	Number of secondary tumors	Relative risk	Median follow-up (years)	Ref.
2,145	12	3.8	NR	46
748	7	5.74	3.9	48
557	8	NR	1–24	47
1,400	8	2.2	3.1	45
19,229	80	2.7	3.5	71
24,829	115	≈2.2 to 5.8-fold	—	

13.4 SUMMARY AND CLINICAL IMPLICATIONS

Because of their rather long latency period, secondary neoplasias particularly endanger patients who enjoy long-term survival after successful primary tumor treatment. Tragically, these are the patients who profited most from primary therapy and thus were able to reach the treatment's objective. On the other hand, the discussion regarding the incidence of secondary neoplasias has been made possible only by the dramatic successes of new therapy strategies for various malignant diseases. Additionally, it must be remembered that not all second cancers are due to treatment, since other factors may be involved, as stated above.

The majority of patients developing secondary leukemia following chemotherapy were treated with alkylating agents. As observed from the large number of patients treated for Hodgkin's disease, the following risk factors constitute a particularly high risk for developing secondary leukemia: a high cumulative dose of alkylating agents, long-term and maintenance therapy, added radiation therapy, and old age at the time of primary tumor treatment. With the increasing number of reports regarding subgroup analysis of patients with secondary neoplasias, a future objective should be the ability to estimate the individual patient's risk of developing secondary malignancies already at the time of primary tumor treatment. It will also be necessary to monitor the late effects of new treatment modalities such as new antineoplastic agents, combination regimens, and high-dose chemotherapy regimens. Since large data pools are lacking and the number of patients treated with high-dose chemotherapy followed by ABMT or PBSCT is constantly increasing—not only in advanced disease patients, but especially in the adjuvant situation—these patients must be closely observed for the development of secondary malignancies. At the same time it must be remembered that it takes 15–20 years before the extent of therapy's harmful late effects can be somewhat accurately determined. Only these data will allow researchers to perform a risk–benefit analysis for new treatment strategies in oncology. Thus, the research for less toxic therapy regimens with equal therapeutic efficacy should continue. Early diagnosis is necessary if secondary neoplasias are to be cured. Thus, patients who may be cured of malignant disease should, in particular, be followed with emphasis on therapy-associated late effects. Additional risk factors for the induction of secondary neoplasias should be avoided, such as smoking by patients who receive mantle field radiation for Hodgkin's disease and therefore have a substantially increased risk for developing lung cancer. Women under the age of 30 who receive radiation therapy should be informed about the increased risk of secondary breast cancer and should be instructed in the technique of breast self-examination. Screening tests for dysplastic nevi may additionally result in a decrease in incidence of malignant melanoma in previously treated tumor patients.

An exact documentation of the type of malignant disease, the administered therapy, the application schedules and dosages, as well as long-term follow-up are necessary to answer the numerous remaining questions concerning the development of secondary malignancies [74]. International cooperation is required to obtain adequate patient numbers to permit statistically relevant subgroup analyses to be performed, with the goal of detecting specific risk constellations and the accumulation of rare secondary cancers.

REFERENCES

1. Boivin J-F. Second cancers and other late side effects of cancer treatment—A review. Cancer 1990:65:770–775.
2. Nichols C, Breeden E, Loehrer P, Williams S, Einhorn LH. Secondary leukemia associated with a conventional dose of etoposide: Review of serial germ cell tumor protocols. J Natl Cancer Inst 1993:85:36–40.
3. Whitlock JA, Greer JP, Lukas JN. Epipodophyllotoxin-related leukemia. Cancer 1991:68:600–604.
4. Bokemeyer C, Schmoll HJ, Poliwoda H. Sekundäre Leukämien nach Etoposid-hältiger Chemotherapie. Dtsch Med Wochenschr 1994:119:707–713.
5. Pedersen-Bjergaard J, Philip P, Larson SO, Jensen G, Bryting K. Chromosome aberrations and prognostic factors in therapy-related myelodysplasia and acute nonlymphocytic leukemia. Blood 1990:6:1083–1091.
6. Pui CH, Ribeiro C, Hancock ML, Rivera GK, Evans WE, Raumondi SC, Head DR, Behr FG, Mahmond MH, Sandlund JT. Acute myeloid leukemia in children treated with epipodopyllotoxins for acute lymphoblastic leukemia. N Engl J Med 1991:325:1682–1687.

7. Bokemeyer C, Kuczk M, Beyer J, Siegert W. Risk of secondary leukemia following high cumulative doses of etoposide during chemotherapy for testicular cancer. J Natl Cancer Inst 1995:87:58–59.
8. Bajorin D, Motzer R, Rodriguez E, Murphy B, Bosl G. Acute nonlymphocytic leukemia in germ-cell tumor patients treated with etoposide-containing chemotherapy. J Natl Cancer Inst 1993:85:60–62.
9. Pedersen-Bjergaard J, Daugaard G, Werner-Hansen S, Philip P, Larsen OS, Rorth M. Increased risk of myelodysplasia and leukemia after etoposide, cisplatin and bleomycin for germ-cell tumours. Lancet 1991:338:159–363.
10. Kaldor JM, Day NE, Band P, Choi NW, Clarke EA, Coleman MP, Hakama M, Koch M, Langmark F, Neal FE. Second malignancies following testicular cancer, ovarian cancer and Hodgkin's disease: An international collaborative study among cancer registries. Int J Cancer 1987:39:571–585.
11. Nelson DF, Cooper S, Weston M, Rubin P. Second malignant neoplasms in patients treated for Hodgkin's disease with radiotherapy or radiotherapy and chemotherapy. Cancer 1981:48:2286–2393.
12. Coltman CA, Dixon DO. Second malignancies complicating Hodgkin's disease: A southwest oncology group 10-year follow-up. Cancer Treatment Rep 1982:676:1023–1033.
13. Kaldor JM, Day NE, Clarke A, van Leeuwen FE, Henry-Amar M, Fiorentino MV, Bell J, Pedersen D, Band P, Avonline D. Leukemia following Hodgkin's disease. N Engl J Med 1990:322:7–13.
14. Boivin JF, Hutchinson GB, Zauber AG, Bernstein L, David FG, Michel RP, Zanke B, Tan CT, Fuller LM, Mauch P, Ultman LE. Incidence of second cancers in patients treated for Hodgkin's disease. J Natl Cancer Inst 1995:87:732–741.
15. Henry-Amar M. Second cancer after the treatment for Hodgkin's disease: A report from the international database on Hodgkin's disease. Ann Oncol 1992:3(suppl 4):117–121.
16. van Leeuwen FE, Klohman WJ, Hagenbeeck A, Noyon R, van den Belt-Dusebout AW, van Kerkhoff EH, van Heerde P, Somers R. Second cancer risk following Hodgkin's disease: A 20 year follow-up-study. J Clin Oncol 1994:12:312–325.
17. van Leeuwen FE, Chorus AM, van den Belt-Dusebout A, Hagenbeeck A, Noyon R, van Kerkhoff E, Pinedo H, Somers R. Leukemia risk following Hodgkin's disease: Relation of cumulative dose of alkylating agents, treatment with teniposide combinations, number of episodes of chemotherapy, and bone marrow damage. J Clin Oncol 1994:12:1063–1073.
18. Henry-Amar M, Dietrich PY. Acute leukemia after treatment of Hodgkin's disease. Hematol Oncol Clin North Am 1993:7(2):368–387.
19. Kaldor JM, Day NE, Petterson F, Pedersen D, Mehnert W, Bell J, Host H, Prior P, Karjalainen J. Leukemia following chemotherapy for ovarian cancer. N Engl J Med 1990:322:1–6.
20. Mauch PM, Kalish LA, Marcus KC, Coleman CN, Shulman LN, Krill E, Come S, Silver B, Canellos GP, Torbell NJ. Second malignancies after treatment for laparotomy staged IA–IIIB Hodgkin's disease: Long-term analysis of risk factors and outcome. Blood 1996:87:3625–3632.

21. Greene MH, Boice JD, Greer BE, Blessing JA, Dembo AJ. Acute nonlymphocytic leukemia after therapy with alkylating agents for ovarian cancer. N Engl J Med 1982:307:1416–1421.
22. Boshoff C, Begent RH, Oliver RT, Rustin GJ, Newlands ES, Andrews R, Shelton M, Holden L, Ong J. Secondary tumours following etoposide containing therapy for germ cell cancer. Ann Oncol 1995:6:35–40.
22a. Kollmannsberger C, Beyer J, Droz J-P, Harstick A, Hartman JT, Biron P, Fléchon A, Schoffski P, Kuczyk M, Schmoll H-J, Kanz L, Bokemeyer C. Secondary leukemia following high cumulative doses of etoposide in patients treated for advanced germ cell tumors. J Clin Oncol 1998 (In press).
23. Bokemeyer C, Schmoll HJ. Secondary neoplasms following treatment of malignant germ cell tumors. J Clin Oncol 1993:11:1703–1709.
24. Curtis RE, Boice JD, Stovall M, Bernstein L, Greenberg RS, Flannery JT, Schwartz AG, Weyer P, Moloney WC, Hoover RN. Risk of leukemia after chemotherapy and radiation treatment for breast cancer. N Engl J Med 1992: 326:1745–1751.
25. Portugal MA, Falkson HC, Stevens K, Falkson G. Acute leukemia as a complication of long-term treatment of advanced breast cancer. Cancer Treatment Rep 1979:63:177–181.
26. Valagussa P, Moliterni A, Terenziani M, Zambetti M, Bonadonna G. Second malignancies following CMF-based adjuvant chemotherapy in resectable breast cancer. Ann Oncol 1994:5:803–808.
27. Diamandidou E, Buzdar A, Smith T, Frye D, Witjahsono M, Hortobogyi G. Treatment-related leukemia in breast cancer patients treated with fluorouracil-doxorubicin-cyclophosphamide combination adjuvant chemotherapy. The University of Texas MD Anderson Cancer Center experience. J Clin Oncol 1996:14:2722–2730.
28. DeCillis A, Anderson S, Wickerham D, Brown A, Fisher B. Acute myeloid leukemia (AML) in NSABP B25. Proc Am Soc Clin Oncol 1995:98(Abstr 92).
29. Sajeva M, Musto P, Melillo L, Cascaville N, Perla G, DÀrena G, Carotenuto M. Secondary acute myeloid leukemia (s-AML) after 3M (mitoxantrone, methotrexate, mitomycin) chemotherapy for metastastic breast cancer: Report of three cases. Proc Am Soc Clin Oncol 1997:189a(Abstr 664).
30. Greene MH, Hoover RN, Fraumeni JF Jr. Subsequent cancer in patients with chronic lymphocytic leukemia—A possible immunologic mechanism. J Natl Cancer Inst 1978:61:337–340.
31. Travis LB, Curtis RE, Stovall M, Holowaty EJ, van Leeuwen FE, Glimelius B, Lynch CF, Hagenbeeck A, Li C-Y, Banks PM, Gospodarowicz MK, Adami J, Wacholder S, Inskip PD, Tucker MA, Boice JD Jr. Risk of leukemia following treatment for non-Hodgkin's lymphoma. J Natl Cancer Inst 1994:86: 1450–1457.
32. Greene MH, Young RC, Merrill LM, DeVita VT. Evidence of a treatment dose response in acute nonlymphocytic leukemias which occur after therapy for non-Hodgkin's lymphoma. Cancer Res 1983:43:1891–1898.

33. Gomez GA, Aggarwall KK, Han T. Post-therapeutic acute malignant myeloproliferative syndrome and acute nonlymphocytic leukemia in non-Hodgkin's lymphoma. Cancer 1982:50:2285–2288.
34. Travis LB, Weeks J, Curtis RE, Chaffey JT, Stovall M, Banks PM, Boice JB, Jr. Leukemia following low-dose irradiation and chemotherapy for non-Hodgkin's lymphoma. J Clin Oncol 1996:14:565–571.
35. Pedersen-Bjergaard J, Ersboll J, Sorensen HM, Keiding N, Larson SO, Philip P, Larsen MS, Schultz H, Nissen NJ. Risk of acute nonlymphocytic leukemia and preleukemia in patients treated with cyclophosphamide for non-Hodgkin's lymphomas. Ann Intern Med 1985:103:195–200.
36. Karakas T, Rummel M, Bergmann L, Hoelzer D, Mitrou P. Secondary malignancies following treatment of malignant lymphomas with etoposide-containing chemotherapy. Proc Am Soc Clin Oncol 1997:24a(Abstr 82).
37. Cheson B, Vena D, Freidlin B, Barrett J, Sorensen J. The risk of secondary malignancies following purine analog therapy of chronic lymphocytic leukemia (CLL) and hairy cell leukemia (HCL). Proc Am Soc Clin Oncol 1997: 15a(Abstr 52).
38. Guyotat D, Coiffier B, Campos L, Archimband E, Treille D, Ehrsam A, Fiere D. Acute leukemia following high-dose chemotherapy with bone marrow rescue for ovarian teratoma. Acta Hematol 1988:80:52–53.
39. Armitage J, Vose J, Anderson J, Bierman P, Bishop M, Kessinger A. Complete remission (CR) following high-dose chemotherapy (HDC) and autologous hematopoietic rescue for non-Hodgkin's lymphoma: A valuation of CR-durability and incidence of secondary myelodysplastic syndrome. Proc Am Soc Clin Oncol 1993:12:363(Abstr 1225).
40. Stone R. Myelodysplastic syndrome after autologous transplantation for lymphoma: The price of progress? Blood 1994:83:3437–3440.
41. Traweek S, Slovak M, Nademanee A, Brynes R, Niland J, Forman S. Myelodysplasia occurring after autologous bone marrow transplantation (ABMT) for Hodgkin's disease (HD) and non-Hodgkin's lymphoma (NHL). Blood 1993:82:455a(Abstr 1805).
42. Stone R, Neuberg D, Soiffer R, Takvorian T, Whelan M, Rabinowe S, Aster J, Learitt P, Mauch P, Freedman A, Nadler L. Myelodysplastic syndrome as a complication after autologous bone marrow transplantation for non-Hodgkin's lymphoma. J Clin Oncol 1994:12:2535–2542.
43. Miller J, Arthur D, Litz C, Neglia J, Miller W, Weisdorf D. Myelodysplastic syndrome after autologous bone marrow transplantation: An additional late complication of curative cancer therapy. Blood 1994:12:3780–3786.
44. Darrington D, Vose J, Andersen J, Bierman P, Bishop M, Chan W, Morris M, Reed E, Sanger W, Tarantolo S, Weisenburger D, Kessinger A, Armitage J. Incidence and characterisation of secondary myelodysplastic syndrome and acute myelogenous leukemia following high-dose chemotherapy and autologous stem-cell transplantation for lymphoid malignancies. J Clin Oncol 1994: 12:2527–2534.

45. Bhatia S, Ramsay N, Steinbuch M, Dusenberg K, Shapiro R, Weisdorf D, Robison L, Miller J, Neglia J. Malignant neoplasms following bone marrow transplantation. Blood 1996:87:3633–3639.
46. Witherspoon R, Fisher L, Schoch G, Martin P, Sullivan K, Sanders J, Deeg J, Doney K, Thomas D, Storb R, Thomas E. Secondary cancers after bone marrow transplantation for leukemia or aplastic anemia. N Engl J Med 1989: 321:784–789.
47. Lowsky R, Lipton J, Fyles G, Minden M, Meharchand J, Tegpar J, Atkins H, Sutcliffe S, Messner H. Secondary malignancies after bone marrow transplantation in adults. J Clin Oncol 1994:12:2187–2192.
48. Socie G, Henry-Amar M, Bagigalupa A, Hows J, Tichelli A, Ljungman P, McCann S, Friekhofen N, Van't Veer-Korthof E, Gluckman E. Malignant tumors occurring after treatment of aplastic anemia. N Engl J Med 1993:329: 1152–1157.
49. Grünwald HW, Rosner F. Acute leukemias and immunosuppressive drug use: A review of patients undergoing immunosuppressive therapy for non-neoplastic disease. Arch Intern Med 1979:139:461–466.
50. Penn I. The occurrence of cancer in immune deficiencies. Curr Probl Cancer 1982:6:1–64.
51. Malkin D, Jolly KW, Barbier N, Look At, Friend SH, Gebhardt MC, Andersen TI, Borresen AL, Li FP, Garber J. Germline mutations of the p53 tumor-suppressor gene in children and young adults with second malignant neoplasms. N Engl J Med 1992:326:1309–1315.
52. Tester WJ, Kinsella TJ, Waller B, Makuch RW, Kelley PA, Glastein E, DeVita VT. Second malignant neoplasms complicating Hodgkin's disease. The National Cancer Institute experience. J Clin Oncol 1984:2:762–769.
53. Tucker MA. Solid second cancers following Hodgkin's disease. Hematol Oncol Clin North Am 1993:7(2):389–415.
54. Tucker MA. Risk of second cancers after treatment for Hodgkin's disease. N Engl J Med 1988:318:76–81.
55. Kaldor JM, Day NE, Bell J. Lung cancer following Hodgkin's disease: A case-control study. Int J Cancer 1992:52:677.
56. van Leeuwen FE, Klokman WJ, Stovall M. Roles of radiotherapy and smoking in lung cancer following Hodgkin's disease. J Natl Cancer Inst 1995:87: 153.
57. Hancock SL, Tucker MA, Hoppe RT. Breast cancer after treatment of Hodgkin's disease. J Natl Cancer Insti 1993:85:25.
58. Bathia S, Robinson L, Oberlin O, Greenberg M, Bunin C, Fossati-Bellani F, Meadows A. Breast cancer and other second neoplasms after childhood Hodgkin's disease. N Engl J Med 1996:334:745–751.
59. Tucker MA, Mifeldt D, Coleman CN, Clark WH Jr, Rosenberg SA. Cutaneous malignant malanoma after Hodgkin's disease. Ann Intern Med 1985:102:37–42.
60. Hancock SL, Cox RS, McDougall IR. Thyroid diseases after treatment for Hodgkin's disease. N Engl J Med 1991:325:599–608.

61. Tucker MA, Jones PH, Boice JD Jr. Therapeutic radiation at young age is linked to secondary thyroid cancer. The late effect study group. Cancer Res 1991:51:2885–2891.
62. Valagussa P, Santoro A, Fossati-Bellani F, Franchi F, Banfi A, Bonadonna G. Absence of treatment-induced second neoplasms after ABVD in Hodgkin's disease. Blood 1982:59:488–494.
63. van Leeuwen FE, Stiggelbout AM, van den Belt-Dusenbaut AW, Noyon R, Eliel MR, van Kerkhoff EH, Delemarre JF, Somers R. Second cancer risk following testicular cancer. J Clin Oncol 1993:11:415–424.
64. Bokemeyer C, Schmoll H-J. Bilateral testicular tumors: Prevalence and clinical implications. Eur J Cancer 1993:29:874–876.
65. Chaudary MA, Millis RR, Hoskins EO, Halder M, Bulbrook RD, Cuzich J, Hayward JL. Bilateral primary breast cancer: A prospective study of disease incidence. Br J Surg 1984:71:711–714.
66. Kurtz JM, Amdrice R, Brandone H, Ayme Y, Spitalier JM. Contralateral breast cancer and other second malignancies in patients treated by breast conserving therapy with radiation. Int J Radiat Oncol Biol Phys 1988:15:277–284.
67. Storm HH, Andersson M, Boice JD, Blettner M, Stovall M, Mouridsen HT, Dombernowsky P, Rose C, Jacobson A, Pedersen M. Adjuvant radiotherapy and risk of contralateral breast cancer. J Natl Cancer Inst 1992:84:1245–1250.
68. Inskip PD, Stovall M, Flannery JT. Lung cancer risk and radiation dose among women treated for breast cancer. J Natl Cancer Inst 1994:86:983–988.
69. Fairchild WV, Spence CR, Solomon HD, Gangai MP. The incidence of bladder cancer after cyclophosphamide therapy. J Urol 1979:122:163–164.
70. Hansen FM. Osteosarcoma and retinoblastoma: A shared chromosomal mechanism revealing recessive predisposition. Proc Natl Acad Sci USA 1985:82: 6216–6220.
71. Curtis R, Rowlings P, Deeg J, Shriner D, Socie G, Travis L, Horowitz M, Witherspoon R, Hoover R, Sobocinski A, Fraumeni J, Boice J Jr. Solid cancers after bone marrow transplantation. N Engl J Med 1997:226:897–904.
72. Penn I. Tumors after renal and cardiac transplantation. Hematol Oncol Clin North Am 1993:7:431–445.
73. Stern R, Nichols K, Vaheva L. Malignant melanoma in patients treated for psoriasis with methoxsalen (psoralen) and ultraviolet A radiation (PUVA). N Engl J Med 1997:336:1041–1045.
74. Smith MA, Rubinstein L, Cazenave L, Ungerleider RS, Maurer HM, Heyn R, Khan FM, Gehan E. Report of the cancer therapy evaluation program monitoring plan for secondary acute myeloid leukemia following treatment with epipodopyllotoxins. J Natl Cancer Inst 1993:85:554–558.

Index

Aclarubicin, 81, 82, 96
  class II anthracycline, 81
  metabolic pathways, 96, 98
  pharmacokinetic characteristics, 88
  therapeutic use, 96
ACNU (*see* Nimustine)
Acrolein, 27, 28
Actinomycin D, 107, 108
  alopecia, 264
  elimination, 108
  emetogenic potency, 240
  hepatotoxicity, 355
  extravasation, 280, 292
  gonadal toxicity, 496–497
  mucositis and oral complications, 247
  therapeutic use, 107
Adenosine Deaminase Inhibitors, 143–148
  chemical structures, 144
  CNS toxicity, 146
  cytotoxic mechanism, 145
  mechanism of action, 143
  neurotoxicity, 445–446
  therapeutic use, 146
  toxicity profile, 146
Adjuvants, 263, 265
Adriamycin (*see* Doxorubicin)
Alkane sulphonate, 19–24
Alkylating agents, 11–60
  carcinogenicity, 527
  extravasation, 292–296
  infertility, 507
  pregnancy risk, 510
All-trans-retinoic acid, 461
Alopecia, 263–264
Altretamine, 14, 40
  emetogenic potency, 240
  metabolic pathways, 40, 41, 44
  neurotoxicity, 446–447
  therapeutic use, 40
  toxicity pattern, 40
Amifostine, 74, 75
  pharmacokinetics, 74
  prodrug, 75
Amsacrine, 84, 104–106
  alopecia, 264
  biotransformation pathways, 105
  cardiotoxicity, 472
  extravasation, 291
  gonadal toxicity, 497
  reduction of dose, 106
  therapeutic use, 104
  toxicity profile, 104
Anthracyclines, 81–100
  accidental overdosage, 480
  cardiotoxic side effects, 472
  chemical structures, 82

[Anthracyclines]
cumulative cardiotoxicity, 83, 84
emetogenic potency, 240
extravasation, 84, 280
intercalation, 83
liposomal drug delivery, 81, 480
mechanism of action, 81
nephrotoxicity, 322
pregnancy risk, 510
toxicity pattern, 81
Anthrapyrazole derivatives, 102, 104, 481
Antiemetic agents, 238, 239, 241–246
Antifolates, 114–125
Antimetabolites, 114–156
neurotoxicity, 432
pregnancy risk, 510
Asparaginase, 194–197, 360–391
analytical problems, 361–362
bleeding and thrombosis, 370–381
dose dependency of liver damage, 368–369
hepatotoxicity, 349, 360–391
hypersensitivity, 266, 270
liver, pancreas and coagulation disorders, 194, 360–391
neurotoxicity, 432, 448
pancreatitis, 370–373
preparations, 194–197, 360–361
time-dependence of liver damage, 369
toxicity profile, 362–363
Azacytidine, 322
Azathioprine, 128–130, 349, 354
Aziridines, 24–26

BCNU (*see* Carmustine)
Bendamustine, 19
Bleomycin, 106–107
alopecia, 264
bleomycin hydrolase, 106
cardiotoxicity, 472
dosage adjustment, 107
emetogenic potency, 241
[Bleomycin]
gonadal toxicity, 496, 497
mucositis and oral complications, 247
pregnancy risk, 510
pulmonary toxicity, 106, 457, 458, 462, 463
Busulfan, 14, 19–23
carcinogenicity, 527
dosage, 19–20
emetogenic potency, 241
gonadal toxicity, 496, 497
GST induction, 20
hepatic veno-occlusive disease (HVOD), 20, 23, 349, 352–353
high-dose therapy, 21–23
interindividual variations in AUC, 22
major metabolites, 20, 21
neurotoxicity, 432, 446
ocular toxicity, 433
oral administration, 19–21
pulmonary fibrosis, 460, 466–467
simplified busulfan TDM, 23
therapeutic use, 19–20
toxicity profile, 20

Calcium folinate (*see* Leucovorin)
Camptothecin, 168–169
Capecitabine, 142–143
Carboplatin, 61, 66–73
AUC values, 66, 67
clinical pharmacokinetics regarding efficacy and toxicity, 67–73
distribution, 66
emetogenic potency, 240
excretion, 66
interindividual variability of pharmacokinetics, 68
mathematical calculations
Calvert formula, 67, 69–72
Chatelut formula, 69–72
Chatelut formula (pediatric formula), 72, 73
Cockcroft-Gault formula, 69, 71

[Carboplatin]
Jeliffe formula (modified form), 69
Newell formula (pediatric formula), 72, 73
nephrotoxicity, 322, 332–333
protein-bound platinum, 67
target carboplatin AUC, 70
Carcinogenicity (*see* secondary malignancies)
Cardiotoxicity, 471–488
anthracycline glycosides, 471–480
dexrazoxane, 478–479
fluorouracil, 472, 481–482
high-dose cyclophosphamide, 31, 471, 482–483
paclitaxel, 472, 483–484
Carmustine, 14, 41, 45–50
alopecia, 264
AUC determination, 46
elimination, 45
emetogenic potency, 240
gonadal toxicity, 496
hepatotoxicity, 349
metabolic inactivation, 46
neurotoxicity, 432
pulmonary toxicity, 46, 459, 463–464
therapeutic use, 41
CCNU (*see* Lomustine)
Chlorambucil, 13–16
carcinogenicity, 527, 530
dosage, adjustment, 13, 16
emetogenic potency, 241
gonadal toxicity, 497
metabolism, 13, 16
neurotoxic symptoms, 447
pulmonary toxicity, 459
pharmacokinetics, 13
therapeutic use, 13
toxicity profile, 13
Chloroacetaldehyde, 327, 441–443
Chloroethylamine, 443
Cisplatin, 61–66
cardiotoxicity, 472
[Cisplatin]
clinical pharmacokinetics regarding efficacy and toxicity, 65, 66
cytochrome P450, 64
dialyzability, 64
dosage adjustment, 64
elimination, 62
emetogenic potency, 240
gonadal toxicity, 496–497
interaction with other drugs, 64
intraperitoneal administration, 64
ligand exchange, 62, 63
nephrotoxicity, 65, 322, 328–332
neurotoxicity, 65, 443–445
ocular toxicity, 433
platinum-protein complexes, 64
therapeutic use, 61, 62
toxicity pattern, 61, 62
tumoral platinum concentrations, 65
Cladribine, 143, 144, 147
Cold caps, 265
Constipation, 254
CPT-11 (*see* Irinotecan)
Cremophor EL, 263, 267
Cyclophosphamide, 14, 27–31
acrolein, 27, 28
alopecia, 264
autoinduction, 30
carcinogenicity, 527, 532, 539
cardiotoxicity, 31, 472, 482–483
clinical pharmacokinetics regarding efficacy and toxicity, 31
cytochrome P450, 27, 28, 30
dosage reduction, 30
emetogenic potency, 240
genetic polymorphism, 29
gonadal toxicity, 496, 497
hemorrhagic cystitis, 336–337
high-dose cyclophosphamide, 31
4-hydroxycyclophosphamide, 28
mesna, 27, 336
metabolism, 27–29
ocular toxicity, 433
oral application, 27
phosphoramide mustard, 28–30
prodrug, 27

[Cyclophosphamide]
pulmonary toxicity, 459, 468
therapeutic use, 27, 31
toxicity pattern, 27
urotoxicity, 27, 336–337
Cytarabine, 132–135
alopecia, 264
clinical pharmacokinetics, 132, 134–135
dosage recommendations, 134
emetogenic potency, 240
gonadal toxicity, 496, 497
high-dose chemotherapy, 132
intrathecal administration, 132
neurotoxicity, 438–439
ocular toxicity, 433
pharmacological aspects, 115
pulmonary toxicity, 460, 467
therapeutic use, 132
toxicity profile, 132
Cytostasane (*see* Bendamustine)

Dacarbazine, 14, 37–39
emetogenic potency, 240
extravasation, 298
gonadal toxicity, 497
hepatotoxicity, 353
light exposure, 37
metabolism, 37, 38
therapeutic use, 37
toxicity pattern, 37
Dactinomycin (*see* Actinomycin D)
Daunorubicin, 82, 84, 92–93
alopecia, 264
cardiotoxicity, 474
dose reduction, 88, 93
excretion, 93
extravasation, 280
gonadal toxicity, 497
liposomal drug delivery, 84, 99
metabolic pathways, 92
pharmacokinetic characteristics, 88
DaunoXome, 84, 99 (*see also* liposomal daunorubicin)
Dermatological toxicity, 263–272
Dexarzoxane, 478–479
Diarrhea, 252–254
Docetaxel, 188–190
alopecia, 264
dose modification, 190
emetogenic potency, 240
extravasation, 303–306
hypersensitivity reactions, 268
metabolic pathways, 189
neurotoxicity, 445
Dolasetron, 244
Doxorubicin, 81, 82, 84–89
alopecia, 264
cardiotoxicity, 473, 474
clinical pharmacokinetics, 88, 89
dose reduction, 85, 88
elimination, 85
emetogenic potency, 240
extravasation, 280
gonadal toxicity, 496, 497
liposomal drug delivery, 84, 97, 99, 100
metabolic pathways, 85–87
mucositis and oral complications, 247
pharmacokinetic characteristics, 88
pulmonary toxicity, 458
therapeutic use, 84
DTIC (*see* Dacarbazine)

Edatrexate, 123, 124
Emesis, 236–246
anticipatory emesis, 236
antiemetic agents, 238, 239, 241–246
delayed nausea and vomiting, 236, 237, 238
emetogenic potency of cytostatic drugs, 239–241
5-HT3-antagonists, 238
pathophysiology of nausea and vomiting, 236–237
Eniluracil, 137
Epirubicin, 82–84
cardiotoxicity, 84, 89, 474
clinical pharmacokinetics, 88–92
dose reduction, 88, 90

[Epirubicin]
emetogenic potency, 240
extravasation, 280
therapeutic use, 89
Erwinase, 194–197 (*see also* Asparaginase)
Etoposide, 156, 161, 163–166
alopecia, 264
carcinogenicity, 528, 531
clinical pharmacokinetics, 161, 163–166
cytotoxic action, 158
dosage adjustment, 163
emetogenic potency, 240
excretion, 159
extravasation, 307
hepatic biotransformation, 159
high-dose etoposide, 157–158, 165–166
hypersensitivity reactions, 267
limited sampling method, 165
metabolic pathways, 162
oral administration, 158
pharmacokinetic parameters, 159
potential interactions, 163, 165, 166
pregnancy risk, 511
therapeutic drug monitoring, 164
therapeutic use, 156–157
toxicity profile, 158
Etoposide phosphate, 156–161
Extravasation, 279–318
antidotes, 308
exited catheters, 281–282
implanted VADs, 282–284
treatment
alkylating agents, 292–296
amsacrine, 291
anthracyclines, 285–290
dacarbazine, 298
dactinomycin, 292
epipodophyllotoxins, 307
liposomal anthracyclines, 290–292
mechlorethamine, 293–294
mitomycin C, 294–296
[Extravasation]
mitoxantrone, 291
platinum-containing agents, 296–297
taxanes, 303–306
vinca alkaloids, 298–303

Fludarabine Monophosphate, 143, 144, 148, 241, 433
Fluorouracil, 136–143
cardiotoxicity, 472, 481–482
chronomodulation, 140
clinical pharmacokinetics, 139–141
cytotoxic mechanism, 116
diarrhea, 253
dihydropyrimidine dehydrogenase, 137, 139
dosage adjustment, 137
emetogenic potency, 240
first-pass effect, 137
gonadal toxicity, 497
hand-foot syndrome, 137, 139, 272
hepatotoxicity, 354–355
intratumoral concentrations, 140–141
metabolites, 137–139
mucositis and oral complications, 247
neurotoxicity, 439–441
ocular toxicity, 433
pharmacogenetics, 139
pharmacological aspects, 115, 136
therapeutic use, 137
Fotemustine, 14, 48–50

Gemcitabine, 132, 135–136
emetogenic potency, 240
pharmacological aspects, 115
pulmonary toxicity, 460, 468
therapeutic use, 135
toxicity profile, 135
GFR determination, 67
Gonadal Toxicity, 491–508
Granisetron, 244

Granulocyte colony-stimulating factor (G-CSF) (*see* Hematopoietic growth factors)
Granulocyte-macrophage colony-stimulating factor (GM-CSF) (*see* Hematopoietic growth factors)
Granulocytopenia (*see* Neutropenia)

Hematopoietic growth factors, 206–221
  acute agranulocytosis, 213
  aplastic anemia, 212–213
  high-dose myeloablative therapy, 216–219
  HIV-infected patients, 214–215
  indications, 206–211
  myeloid malignancies, 213–214
  reasons for using G-CSF and GM-CSF, 206
  recommended dosage, 220
  treatment duration, 221
  treatment of febrile neutropenia, 212
Hemorrhagic cystitis, 336–337
Hepatotoxicity induced by cytostatic drugs, 347–391
  assessment, 348–450
  interpretation of abnormal liver function tests, 350–352
  MGEX liver function test, 351
Hexamethylmelamine (*see* Altretamine)
5-HT3-Antagonists, 238, 242, 244
  dolasetron, 244
  granisetron, 244
  ondansetron, 244
  tropisetron, 244
Hyaluronidase, 179
Hydroxyurea, 198, 199, 241, 264
Hypersensitivity reactions, 266–271

Idarubicin, 82–84, 93–96
  cardiotoxicity, 84, 474
  dosage reduction, 96
  emetogenic potency, 240
[Idarubicin]
  idarubicinol, 95, 96
  oral administration, 93, 95
  pharmacokinetic characteristics, 88, 94
  therapeutic use, 93
Ifosfamide, 14, 31
  acrolein, 33, 337
  alopecia, 264
  autoinduction, 34
  carcinogenicity, 539
  chloroacetaldehyde, 33, 34
  chloroethylamine, 34
  clinical pharmacokinetics regarding efficacy and toxicity, 34–35
  conventional dosage, 31
  cytochrome P450, 32, 33, 35
  dechloroethylation, 33–35
  dosage modification, 34
  emetogenic potency, 240
  Fanconi syndrome, 325
  hemorrhagic cystitis, 336–337
  high-dose ifosfamide, 31, 32
  isophosphoramide mustard, 33
  mesna, 32, 336
  metabolism, 32, 33
  nephrotoxicity, 35, 322, 324–328
    clinical consequences, 326
    pathogenesis, 327
    risk factors, 325, 326
  neurotoxiciy, 432, 441–443
  pulmonary toxicity, 459
  therapeutic use, 31
  toxicity pattern, 31, 34
  urotoxicity, 32, 336–337
Individualization of anticancer drug therapy, 3–6
Infertility, 491–508, 509–523
  chemotherapy-related infertility, 495–508
    antineoplastic drugs, 496
    clinical history, 496–507
    effect on progeny, 507–508
    gamete manipulation, 512–525
  pretreatment infertility, 492–494
  prevention and treatment, 509–515

Irinotecan, 167–173
  biliary index, 171–172
  clinical pharmacokinetics, 171–172
  diarrhea, 171, 253–254
  elimination, 171
  emetogenic potency, 240
  metabolic pathways, 169, 170
  therapeutic use, 169

Ketimine structures, 443

Leucovorin, 114
  antidote, 114
  rescue, 118
Liposomal Anthracyclines, 97–100
  extravasation, 290–291
  formulations, 290–291
Liver disorders (*see* Hepatotoxicity)
Lometrexol, 124, 125
Lomustine, 14, 46–47
  degradation, 46
  gonadal toxicity, 496
  isocyanates, 46
  metabolites, 47
  therapeutic use, 46
Losoxantrone, 102
Lung toxicity (*see* Pulmonary Toxicity)

Malignancies (*see* Secondary Malignancies)
Mechlorethamine, 13
  alopecia, 264
  carcinogenicity, 527
  emetogenic potency, 240
  extravasation, 280, 293–294
  gonadal toxicity, 496
  hydrolysis, 13
  mechanism of action, 13
Melphalan, 16–19
  carcinogenicity, 530, 532
  clinical pharmacokinetics regarding efficacy and toxicity, 18–19
  dosage, adjustment, 16, 17
  emetogenic potency, 241
  high-dose melphalan, 17–19
[Melphalan]
  hydrolysis, 17
  hypersensitivity, 268, 271
  intravenous administration, 17
  nonenzymatic deactivation, 17, 18
  oral administration, 17
  therapeutic use, 16
  toxicity, 17
6-Mercaptopurine (and related compounds), 125–128, 392–429 (*see also* Thiopurines)
  bioavailability, 125
  clinical pharmacokinetics, 126–128, 392–429
  gonadal toxicity, 497
  hepatotoxicity, 349, 354
  metabolic pathways, 127
  pharmacogenetic aspects, 392–429
  therapeutic use, 125
Mesna, 27
Methotrexate (MTX), 114–123
  albumin binding-sites, 118
  alopecia, 264
  antidote, 114
  clinical pharmacokinetics, 120–123
  cytotoxic mechanism, 114, 116
  DAMPA, 117, 199
  dosage adjustment, 119
  emetogenic potency, 240, 241
  gonadal toxicity, 496, 497
  hepatotoxicity, 349
  Leucocorin-Rescue, 121, 122
  metabolism, 117
  monitoring of MTX blood levels, 122
  mucositis and oral complications, 247
  nephrotoxicity, 322, 333–334
  neurotoxicity, 435–438
  ocular toxicity, 433
  pharmacokinetic-pharmacodynamic relationships, 122–123
  pharmacological aspects, 115
  polyglutamate, 117
  pulmonary toxicity, 460, 467
  synergism with fluorouracil, 136

[Methotrexate]
therapeutic use, 114
toxicity profile, 118
treatment regimens, 118
Methylene blue, 441–443
Mitomycin C, 14, 39
emetogenic potency, 240
extravasation, 40, 280, 294–296
gonadal toxicity, 496
metabolic pathways, 43, 43
nephrotoxicity, 40, 322, 335
ocular toxicity, 433
prodrug, 40
pulmonary toxicity, 458, 464–466
redox cycling, 465
therapeutic use, 39
toxicity pattern, 40
Mitotane, 198–200
Mitotic Inhibitors, 178–194, 461
vinca alkaloids, 178–183
taxanes, 183–190
Mitoxantrone, 84, 100–103
cardiotoxicity, 84, 101, 472, 474
chemical structure, 102, 103
clinical pharmacokinetics, 101, 102
dosage adjustment, 101
emetogenic potency, 240
extravasation, 291
gonadal toxicity, 497
therapeutic use, 100, 101
toxicity profile, 101
MOPP-combination therapy, 502–505, 527, 529
MTA, 125
Mucositis, 246–252
prevention and treatment, 246–252
oral decontamination regimens
allopurinol, 251
amifostine, 250
chlorhexidine, 249
G-CSF, 251
oral cryotherapy, 250
plant extracts, 252
propantheline, 250
prostaglandins, 252
PTA lozenges, 249
[Mucositis]
sucralfate, 251
vitamins, 252
Myelosuppression (*see* neutropenia)

N-Lost-derivatives, 11–19
Nausea (*see* Emesis)
Nephrotoxicity, 321–335
assessment, 322–324
carboplatin, 332–333
chemotherapeutic agents, 322
cisplatin, 328–332
clinical consequences, 330
clinical features, 329
nephroprotection, 331–332
doxorubicin, 334
ifosfamide, 324–328
clinical consequences, 326
clinical features, 325
risk factors, 325, 326
melphalan, 334
methotrexate, 333–334
mitomycins, 335
nitrosourea compounds, 334–335
protocol for investigation, 323
Neurotoxicity, 431–454
Neutropenia, 205–221
congenital, cyclic or chronic idiopathic neutropenia, 219
Felty syndrome, 219
risk factors, 208
Nimustine, 47, 48
hydrolysis, 47
metabolic pathways, 47
therapeutic use, 47
Nitrogen mustard, 11
Nitrosoureas, 12, 41
clinical pharmacokinetics, 45
hepatotoxicity, 353–354
nephrotoxicity, 322, 334–335

Ocular toxicity, 433
Oligospermia (*see* Infertility)
Ondansetron, 244
Oral and Gastrointestinal Toxicity, 235–261

Oxaliplatin, 61, 62, 73, 74
chronomodulated infusion, 74
neurotoxicity, 74
therapeutic use, 73
toxicity pattern, 73, 74
Oxazaphosphorines, 12, 26–36, 336–337

Paclitaxel, 186–188
alopecia, 264
cardiotoxicity, 472, 483–484
clinical pharmacokinetics, 186–188
emetogenic potency, 240
extravasation, 303–306
hepatotoxicity, 349, 355
high-dose paclitaxel, 186
hypersensitivity reactions, 185, 267–270, 461
metabolic pathways, 184, 187
neuropathy, 445
pregnancy risk, 511
therapeutic use, 186
Paravasation (*see* Extravasation)
Pegaspargase, 194–197
Pentostatin, 143–147
Piritrexim, 123, 124
Piroxantrone, 102
Platinum compounds, 61–81, 240–241
extravasation, 296–297
hypersensitivity, 270–271
nephrotoxicity, 331–332
neurotoxicity, 432
Podophyllotoxin derivatives, 157
Prednimustine, 527
Procarbazine, 14, 36–39
dosage reduction, 37
emetogenic potency, 240
gonadal toxicity, 496
neurotoxicity, 432, 448
pharmacokinetics, 37
therapeutic use, 36, 37
toxicity pattern, 37
Pulmonary Toxicity of Chemotherapeutic Agents, 455–470
alkylating agents, 459
[Pulmonary Toxicity of Chemotherapeutic Agents]
busulfan, 460, 466–467
carmustine (BCNU), 459, 463–464
chlorambucil, 459
cyclophosphamide, 459
ifosfamide, 459
mitomycin C, 458, 464–466
antimetabolites
cytarabine, 460
gemcitabine, 460
methotrexate, 460
bleomycin, 457, 458, 462, 463
doxorubicin, 458
underlying mechanisms, 457
Purine Antimetabolites, 125–132
Pyrimidine- and pyrimidine nucleoside antimetabolites, 132–143

Ralitrexed, 123–125

Secondary Malignancies, 525–542
Carcinogenicity of Antineoplastic Agents, 527
Secondary Leukemias, 526–535
Solid Tumors, 536–541
Streptozocin, 14, 48
dosage adjustment, 50
emetogenic potency, 240
hepatotoxicity, 349
metabolites, 49
nephrotoxicity, 48
Sulfir mustard gas, 11

Taxanes, 183–190
chemical structures, 184, 189
cytotoxic effect, 178
emetogenic potency, 240
extravasation, 303–306
hypersensitivity, 185
interaction with other drugs, 185
schedule-dependent administration, 185
toxicity profile, 183

Taxol (*see* Paclitaxel)
Tegafur, 141–142
Teniposide, 157, 162, 167, 307
TEPA (triethylene phosphoramide), 24
Teratogenicity, 508–509
Therapeutic drug monitoring (TDM), 3–6
6-Thioguanine, 130–132, 393–403 (*see also* Thiopurines)
  emetogenic potency, 241
  metabolic pathways, 130, 131
  oral administration, 130
  pharmacological aspects, 115
  therapeutic use, 130
Thiopurines, 393–403
  cytotoxic effect of mercaptopurine and thioguanine, 393–403
  metabolism and mechanism of action, 393–403
  thiopurine-S-methyltransferase (TPMT), 403–421
    biochemistry, 403–405
    detection of the TPMT deficiency, 416–420
    genetic polymorphism, 126, 408–411
    molecular genetics, 405–407
    mutant proteins, 411–416
    variability of TPMT activity, 407–408
Thiotepa, 14, 24–26
  alopecia, 264
  carcinogenicity, 527
  clinical pharmacokinetics regarding efficacy and toxicity, 26
  conventional doses, 24, 26
  dosage adjustment, 26
  gonadal toxicity, 497
  high-dose thiotepa, 24, 26
  metabolism, 24–25
  neurotoxicity, 26, 432
  nonenzymatic transformation, 25
  toxicity pattern, 24
Tomudex (*see* Ralitrexed)
Topoisomerase-I-Inhibitors, 156, 167–173
Topoisomerase-II-Inhibitors, 156–167
Topotecan, 167, 168, 172–173, 240
Treosulfan, 14, 24, 527
Trimetrexate, 123, 124
Trofosfamide, 14, 35–36
Tropisetron, 244

UFT (Uracil/Tegafur), 141–142
Urotoxicity, 336–337
  characteristics, 336–337

Vinblastine, 178, 180–182, 254
  alopecia, 264
  emetogenic potency, 241
  extravasation, 280
  gonadal toxicity, 497
  metabolism, 181
  mucositis and oral complications, 247
  preganany risk, 511
Vinca alkaloids, 178–183
  constipation, 254
  extravasation, 179, 280, 298–303
  extravasation antidotes, 301
  neurotoxicity, 431–435
  ocular toxicity, 433
  pharmacokinetic characteristics, 180
  pulmonary toxicity, 461
  toxicity profile, 179
Vincristine, 178–180
  alopecia, 264
  cardiotoxicity, 472
  constipation, 254
  dosage modification, 180
  emetogenic potency, 241
  extravasation, 280
  metabolism, 179
  neurotoxicity, 431–435
  pharmacokinetic characteristics, 180
  therapeutic use, 179
Vindesine, 178, 180, 182, 264
Vinorelbine, 178, 182–183, 241
  emetogenic potency, 241
  extravasation, 280, 302
  pharmacokinetic characteristics, 180
Vomiting, 236–246 (*see also* Emesis)